Immunopotentiators in Modern Vaccines

Immunopotentiators in Modern Vaccines

Virgil E.J.C. Schijns (Professor, Dr, PhD)
Head of Vaccine Technology & Immunology R&D
Intervet International B.V. and Principal Immunologist
Nobilon Akzonobel, The Netherlands and
part-time Professor in Immunology and Virology
Department of Population Health and Pathobiology
NC State University, Raleigh, USA

Derek T. O'Hagan (B.Pharm., MRPharmS., PhD)
Senior Director and Head of Vaccine Delivery Research
Chiron Vaccines, Emeryville, USA

ELSEVIER

AMSTERDAM • BOSTON • HEIDELBERG • LONDON
NEW YORK • OXFORD • PARIS • SAN DIEGO
SAN FRANCISCO • SINGAPORE • SYDNEY • TOKYO
Academic Press is an imprint of Elsevier

ACADEMIC
PRESS

Elsevier Academic Press
30 Corporate Drive, Suite 400, Burlington, MA 01803, USA
525 B Street, Suite 1900, San Diego, California 92101-4495, USA
84 Theobald's Road, London WC1X 8RR, UK

This book is printed on acid-free paper. ⊚

Library of Congress Cataloging-in-Publication Data
Immunopotentiators in modern vaccines / [edited] by Virgil Schijns and
  Derek O'Hagan. – 1st ed.
     p. ; cm
  Includes bibliographical references and index.
  ISBN-13: 978-0-12-088403-2 (casebound : alk. paper)
  ISBN-10: 0-12-088403-8 (casebound : alk. paper)
  1. Immunological adjuvants. 2. Immune response–Regulation.
  3. Vaccines. I. Schijns, Virgil E. J. C.   II. O'Hagan, Derek T.
  [DNLM: 1. Vaccines–immunology. 2. Adjuvants, Immunologic.
  3. Drug Delivery Systems. 4. Immunotherapy.   QW 805 1337 2005]
  QR187.3.I56 2005
  615′.372–dc22   2005016429

British Library Cataloguing in Publication Data
A catalogue record for this book is available from the British Library

ISBN 13: 978-0-12-088403-2
ISBN 10: 0-12-088403-8

For information on all Elsevier Academic Press publications
visit our Web site at www.books.elsevier.com

Printed in the United States of America
05 06 07 08 09 10   9 8 7 6 5 4 3 2 1

Contents

Preface

Vaccine adjuvants are becoming increasingly necessary to enable successful vaccine development, since new-generation antigens, including those identified through genomic screening of microorganisms, are predominantly recombinant purified proteins, which are often poorly immunogenic. New-generation adjuvants may also be sufficiently potent to allow vaccination strategies to be applied to novel areas, including "therapeutic" vaccines designed to control allergies, auto-immune diseases, malignancies, drug dependencies, neural diseases, or fertility.

As novel adjuvants advance to clinical testing, there is a greater need to better understand the mechanisms controlling their effects on the immune response. This is helped by the recent dramatic expansion in our knowledge about molecular details of antigen presentation and T cell activation. There is a growing awareness of how some adjuvants activate innate immune cells, while others influence the delivery and residence of antigen in lymphoid organs. Increasingly, these effects are being used in synergy to design optimal adjuvant formulations. Adjuvants can now be classified functionally, according to current immunological concepts, which allows a more in-depth understanding of how they achieve their effects *in vivo*.

This book includes chapters on all the vaccine adjuvant approaches that are currently available, incorporating those that are included in licensed vaccines, those that are working their way through the regulatory approval process, and those that are still in early stages of preclinical research. However, in contrast to existing books on the subject, this book provides recent data on the critical mechanisms governing the activity of vaccine adjuvants and delivery systems. This book aims to better define the biological effect(s) of adjuvants and to categorize these effects by function. Current knowledge of immunological pathways and the impact of adjuvants on cellular and molecular interactions of immune cells are described and depicted in comprehensive illustrations. Such information will provide a helpful reference for the reader to assess different types of adjuvants. The adjuvants described in this book include those that mainly function via a "delivery" mechanism and by immunopotentiators, which are effective through activating components of the innate immune response. Moreover, the attractiveness of combined delivery system/immunopotentiator formulations are discussed in detail, with examples of how this approach may be applied to enhance potency and reduce potential toxicities. The book extends from examples of preclinical research all the way through to clinical evaluation, with chapters covering clinical assessment of novel adjuvants, including competitive evaluations of different approaches. In addition, the book provides a regulatory perspective from the US Food and Drug Administration to highlight which data will be required to allow the approval of adjuvants within new-generation vaccines.

Virgil E.J.C. Schijns and Derek T. O'Hagan

List of contributors

Martin Bachmann
Cytos Biotechnology AG
Zurich-Schlieren
Switzerland

Jory Baldridge
Corixa Corporation
Hamilton
USA

Tom Barr
University of Edinburgh
Edinburgh
UK

Filippo Belardelli
Instituto Superiore di Sanità
Rome
Italy

Imerio Capone
Instituto Superiore di Sanità
Rome
Italy

Jennifer Carlring
University of Sheffield
Sheffield
UK

Christopher Cluff
Corixa Corporation
Hamilton
USA

Cecil Czerkinsky
INSERM
Nice
France

Giuseppe Del Guidice
Chiron Vaccines
Siena
Italy

Debbie Drane
CSL Ltd
Parkville
Australia

Robert Edelman
University of Maryland School of Medicine
Baltimore
USA

Jay Evans
Corixa Corporation
Hamilton
USA

Nathalie Garçon
GlaxoSmithKline Biologicals
Rixensart
Belgium

Gregory Glenn
Iomai Corporation
Gaithersburg
USA

Reinhard Glück
Berna Biotech Ltd
Bern
Switzerland

Marion Gruber
CBER/FDA
Rockville
USA

Ali Harandi
Göteborg University
Göteborg
Sweden

Andrew Heath
University of Sheffield
Sheffield
UK

Jan Holmgren
Göteborg University
Göteborg
Sweden

David Johnson
Corixa Corporation
Hamilton
USA

Richard Kenney
Iomai Corporation
Gaithersburg
USA

Charlotte Kensil
Antigenics Inc.
Lexington
USA

Michael Lebens
Göteborg University
Göteborg
Sweden

Erik Lindblad
Brenntag Biosector
Frederikssund
Denmark

Stephen Martin
Cytos Biotechnology AG
Zurich-Schlieren
Switzerland

Michael McCluskie
Coley Pharmaceutical Group
Kanata
Canada

Patrick McGowan
Corixa Corporation
Hamilton
USA

Ian Metcalfe
Berna Biotech Ltd
Bern
Switzerland

Philippe Moingeon
Stallergenes
Antony
France

Sally Mossman
Corixa Corporation
Seattle
USA

Derek O'Hagan
Chiron Vaccines
Emeryille
USA

Achal Pashine
Chiron Corporation
Emeryville
USA

Martin Pearse
CSL Ltd
Parkville
Australia

David Persing
Corixa Corporation
Seattle
USA

Audino Podda
Chiron Vaccines
Siena
Italy

Paola Rizza
Instituto Superiore di Sanità
Rome
Italy

Virgil Schijns
Intervet International BV
Boxmeer
The Netherlands

Jakub Simon
University of Maryland School of Medicine
Baltimore
USA

Jia-Bin Sun
Göteborg University
Göteborg
Sweden

Elizabeth Sutkowski
CBER/FDA
Rockville
USA

Jeffrey Ulmer
Chiron Corporation
Emeryville
USA

Nicholas Valiante
Chiron Corporation
Emeryville
USA

Marcelle Van Mechelen
GlaxoSmithKline Biologicals
Rixensart
Belgium

Laurence Van Overvelt
Stallergenes
Antony
France

Risini Weeratna
Coley Pharmaceutical Group
Kanata
Canada

Martine Wettendorff
GlaxoSmithKline Biologicals
Rixensart
Belgium

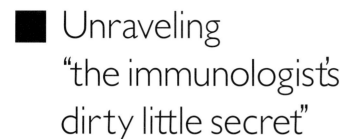

Unraveling "the immunologist's dirty little secret"

Virgil E. J. C. Schijns

Intervet International BV, Boxmeer, The Netherlands

■ Introduction

The immune system has evolved to free the host from potentially noxious pathogens. Upon first exposure to a pathogen, the immune system reacts with innate and primary adaptive immune responses. Primary adaptive immune responses need at least a few days to develop before they become effective immune effector responses. This delay is the reason for the variable success of the naive host to attack the invading microorganism in the case of a rapidly replicating invader. Vaccination against microorganisms ideally facilitates the formation of long-lived T and B memory cells to conserved antigens and may also generate readily available immune effector elements, such as circulating antibodies with various functional capacities.

Classic vaccines come in various forms, either as attenuated, less virulent, replicating microorganisms, which carry the risk of reversion to virulence, or as nonreplicating inactivated microbes or their components. The latter category is most safe and therefore preferred. But immunization with purified antigen alone is usually insufficient for proper immune induction. Initiation, amplification and guidance of an appropriate adaptive immune response of sufficient magnitude and duration requires coadministration of immunostimulatory components called adjuvants (adjuvare (Latin) = to help). Many different types of adjuvants have been described, which are not unified by a common structure. However, the choice of adjuvant for the vaccine formulation is difficult. This is due to the fact that little is known about the mechanisms underlying adjuvant activity in general. In addition, depending on the antigen–adjuvant combination, the local and systemic reactions may vary. Therefore, it is difficult to predict what type of immune reaction will be elicited by the chosen adjuvant. Moreover, the side effects often cannot be foreseen. Therefore, adjuvants have been called "the immunologist's dirty little secret" (Janeway, 1989). Although vaccines are the most successful medical invention of the last century, it is obvious that future vaccines require adjuvants with predictable activity.

Today we know that adaptive immune responses in a normal individual initially involve the activation of antigen-specific T helper cells which amplify and regulate – via either soluble cytokines or membrane-bound costimulatory molecules – the activities of antimicrobial effector cells, microbiocidal macrophages, cytolytic T cells, and/or B cells. Activation of naive antigen-specific T helper cells occurs in lymphoid organs by dendritic cells (DC), so-called professional antigen presenting cells (APC). Upon delivery or expression of antigen in peripheral tissues, DC take up the antigen via pinocytosis, phagocytosis, or following infection by the microorganism. During virulent infection, DC receive stimuli from (structures of) the pathogen, leading to maturation and activation. In the absence of these stimuli, DC are presumed to tolerarize antigen-specific T helper cells; hence, there is insufficient priming for an effective T helper cell-dependent immune response.

Currently, a number of immunological theories may explain the critical mechanisms underlying adjuvanticity, each of them championing either distinct pathways or different key steps in immunological pathways. Here, the most important concepts are discussed in relation to the most recent advances in vaccine adjuvant research.

Adjuvants provide start signals for immune reactivity and guide the response to an acceptable magnitude

As mentioned earlier, vaccination aims to generate memory immune effector responses of adaptive T and/or B cells specific for a preferentially conserved epitope of the pathogen, tumor, or allergen of interest. T helper cells are critical amplifiers and guiders of antigen-specific immune reactions, such as those of B cells and cytolytic T cells. In addition, they amplify microbiocidal activity of macrophages. Hence, the priming and clonal expansion of antigen-specific T helper cells is initially critical for adequate adaptive immunity. According to the two-signal model of immune reactivity, activation of T helper cells is, apart from the delivery of antigen signals to T cell receptors (signal 1), critically dependent on costimulatory signals (signal 2) in the form of soluble cytokines or membrane-bound surface molecules. According to the classic two-signal model, antigen presentation in the absence of costimulation results in T cell anergy, tolerance, or deletion (Bretscher and Cohn, 1970; Lafferty and Woodnough, 1977; Cohn and Langman, 1990).

Following on from these thoughts, efficient vaccines should be able to amplify and direct adaptive immune responses, most of which are under regulatory control of antigen-specific MHC class II restricted T helper cells. Although the two-signal theory is well accepted and sustained by numerous publications, it does not explain all immunological events and is at variance with other experimental data.

Regulation of immune responses by antigen deliverance (signal I)

Naive antigen-specific T cells continuously survey and recirculate between lymph nodes and spleen. They are unable to access non-lymphoid areas of the body. Only memory and effector cells can do this. In order to be recognized by antigen-specific T and B cells of the adaptive immune system, antigen administered to peripheral tissues must first reach peripheral lymphoid organs. Mice lacking secondary lymph nodes, due to a genetic mutation or surgical ablation, are strongly compromised in cellular and humoral responses (Karrer et al., 1997). Also, interruption of afferent lymphatic vessels prevents immune responses (Frey and Wenk, 1957; Barker and Billingham, 1967). Antigen within peripheral tissues drains to regional lymph nodes, either in free form or after uptake by local immature DC. Only DC can prime naive T cells and are, therefore, called "nature's adjuvant" (Steinman et al., 1998; Banchereau et al., 2000). Upon arrival in the lymph node, DC have processed the antigen in peptide fragments, which are then exposed in MHC molecules on the cell surface (signal 1).

According to the geographical concept of immune induction (Zinkernagel et al., 1997) and the classic depot theory (Freund, 1937, 1956; Herbert, 1966), this facilitation of signal 1 expression in secondary lymphoid organs is most critical for immune reactivity and a durable immune response, respectively (see Figures 1.1 (upper panel) and 1.2).

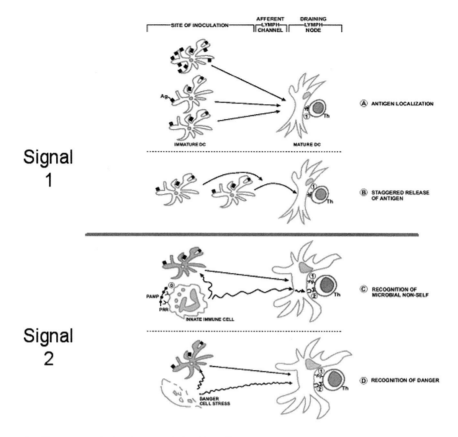

Signal 1

Signal 2

Figure I.I **Schematic of key events during immune induction.** (A) Antigen localization in the lymph node determines immune induction. (B) Staggered release of antigen from the inoculation site facilitates immune induction. (C) Nonself-discrimination by innate immune cells starts an immune response by upregulation of costimulatory signals. (D) Necrotic or stressed cells evoke increased costimulation of antigen-presenting cells. Each step may explain the mechanism underlying a particular type of adjuvant: (0) signal 0, (I) signal I, (2) signal 2. (After Schijns, V.E.J.C. (2001). *Crit. Rev. Immunol.* 21, 75–85. With permission.) (See Color Plate Section.)

A number of observations are in accordance with this view. Kündig et al. (1996) noted that repeated immunization with peptide leads to a functional T cell response even in CD28-deficient mice, while one immunization resulted in T cell anergy.

Immunization of syngenic mice with fibroblasts transfected with glycoprotein G of lymphocytic choriomeningitis virus (LCMV) evoked CTL-mediated immunity against lethal LCMV challenge and resistance to challenge infection with recombinant vaccinia virus expressing LCMV-G protein. Intraperitoneal injection of the transfected cells required only 1% of the cells if injected subcutaneously to induce CTL, whereas as few as 500 cells were sufficient following direct injection into the spleen (Kündig et al., 1995).

The fibrosarcoma cell line (MC57), capable of CTL induction, was in fact a prototypic nonprofessional antigen-presenting cell (APC), expressing only MHC–peptide complexes without any other known costimulatory molecule (Kündig et al., 1995). This study shows that immune responsiveness can occur in the absence of signal 2 if the antigen is able to reach the secondary lymphoid organs in sufficient amounts.

Also, direct injection of vesicular stomatitis virus (VSV) particles into the mesenteric lymph nodes of splenectomized and anti-CD4 treated mice, primed for IgM responses largely without T cell help (Ochsenbein et al., 2000), while injection of comparable amounts of antigen subcutaneously does not reach the spleen or lymph nodes in sufficient amounts and fails to activate B cells without T cell help.

From these studies, it was concluded that the presence of a sufficient amount of antigen in secondary lymphoid tissues over a given time period (i.e., 'immunoavailability') is critical for immune reactivity. Hence, localization, dose, and time of antigen within secondary lymphoid organs determine immune reactivity (Ochsenbein et al., 2000; Zinkernagel, 2000).

◼ Facilitation of signal I

We observed that, upon intramuscular injection of antigen in a saline solution stained with the colorant methylene blue, the majority of the inoculum is detected in the liver and urine within minutes (Schijns et al., unpublished observations). Arguably, higher doses of injected antigen are less rapidly cleared by phagocytes or degraded by enzymatic reactions, and have an increased chance to be sampled by resident immature DC or B cells. The half-life of labelled gD2 antigen after intramuscular injection is only 2.5 hours. Only trace amounts of antigen reach the lymph nodes (Dupuis et al., 2000).

Cytokines, such as GM-CSF and Flt3-ligand, influence the level of influx and type of DC migrating towards the antigen injection site and their migration capacity towards the draining lymph node. Thereby, they regulate the amount of antigen (signal 1) presented as processed peptide–MHC complexes on the APC surface that can be recognized (Pulundran et al., 1998; Mwangi et al., 2002).

As early as 1966 Herbert demonstrated that repeated, daily immunizations of minute amounts of antigen (1 μg/dose) in saline solution for a period of 50 days evoked antibody formation with kinetics similar to responses evoked by one single immunization of a high dose of antigen (2000 μg) formulated in a water-in-oil depot (Herbert, 1966). From this experiment, Herbert concluded that a slow release of antigen could fully explain the great effectiveness of depot-forming adjuvant (Herbert, 1966). Remarkably, the minute amounts of antigen are apparently able to increase antibody titers in the face of circulating antigen-specific antibodies. It is also remarkable that, under *in vitro* conditions, antigen included in a water-in-oil emulsion adjuvant is not released from this depot for a period of more than 3 weeks while, given *in vivo*, such a formulation evokes significant antibody responses within the same 3-week period after inoculation (Aucouturier et al., 2001; Jansen et al., 2005). By contrast, antigen dissolved in saline or antigen formulated with an oil-in-water adjuvant emulsion is released quickly *in vitro*, but evokes generally less antibody responses despite immediate availability of antigen.

According to the geographical concept of immune induction and the depot theory, the facilitation of signal 1 expression is most critical and sufficient for immune reactivity. Hence, immune induction critically depends on facilitation of antigen delivery and presentation in the lymph node. This site is visited by circulating, potentially reactive, resting T or B cells and, importantly, contains sufficient amounts of signal 2 molecules which do not necessarily need to be upregulated (Zinkernagel, 2000). Indeed, antigen unable to reach the lymph node does not elicit a response (Karrer et al., 1997).

Apart from antigen localization, dose, and timing, the antigenic structure also influences immune reactivity. In particular, highly ordered, repetitive structures mimic pathogen signatures and, therefore, are able to induce immune responses without adjuvants, when given at high concentrations (Ochsenbein et al., 2000). This may explain why purified virus-like particles (VLP), or even virosomes devoid of genetic material, lacking presumed danger signals such as RNA or DNA, are able to evoke an immune response in the apparent absence of any danger signal (Moser et al., 2003). Instead, they possess a surface structure in a highly repetitive configuration, ordered such that they may crosslink B cell receptors and thereby provide a direct activation signal for proliferation and antibody synthesis (Fehr et al., 1998; Bachmann, et al., 1997). In addition, they can target surface receptors on antigen-presenting cells (Zurbriggen, 2003). This may explain why viral antigens, when decorated in a highly ordered pattern on a particulate carrier, are more immunogenic than solubilized antigens (Katayama et al., 1999; Jegerlehner et al., 2002). In 1968 Dresser noted that repeated immunization with aggregate-free soluble bovine γ globulin (BGG) caused immunological tolerance, unless particle aggregates of BGG were removed (Dresser, 1968). This observation is in apparent conflict with the data described by Herbert (1966). Indeed, empty microparticles *per se*, with no antigen incorporated or adsorbed, may exert adjuvant activity for antigen that is just admixed (Aucouturier et al., 2001; Schijns et al., unpublished data).

While is it nowadays accepted that a minimal amount of antigen (concentration) has to reach the secondary lymphoid organs, the optimal kinetics of antigen delivery are unknown. Studies using osmotic pumps, or solid implants continuously delivering antigen over a prolonged time period of weeks or months, readily evoked adequate immune reactions (Walduck and OpdeBeeck, 1997; Kemp et al., 2002; for a review, see Lofthouse, 2002). These recent observations contrast with older reports suggesting that continuous antigen delivery leads to tolerance or so-called "immunological paralysis" (Dixon and Maurer, 1955; Dresser, 1962; Mitchison, 1968). However, in those studies, exceptionally high or low antigen doses were used.

Although an immune response can be evoked by soluble antigen when it is able to reach the lymph nodes, in general, the strengths and the duration of the reaction strongly benefits from co-delivery of an adjuvant, i.e., an immunopotentiator or a delivery system. This is particularly true for the subcutaneous or intramuscular immunization routes, with reduced chances of antigen uptake by the lymphoid organs before antigen degradation (Ochsenbeim et al., 2000).

The activity of a number of well-known facilitating adjuvants fits precisely within this concept. All adjuvants that prolong the presence of antigen after inoculation, not necessarily leading to upregulation of signal 2 molecules on DC, can be categorized accordingly. In this respect, an interesting study of Sun et al. (2003) showed that alum, nonionic surfactant vesicles (NISV), and, to limited levels, also poly(lactide-co-glycolide) (PLGA) failed to upregulate the important classic signal 2 molecules (such as CD80, CD86, and CD40) on DC, in contrast to lipopolysaccharide (LPS), but proved to stimulate antigen-specific T cells *in vitro* (Sun et al., 2003).

Although not formally proven, signal 1-facilitating adjuvants likely include the above-mentioned depot type water-in-oil adjuvants (Herbert, 1966) and, for a limited time and amount of antigen, also oil-in-water microemulsions, as well as double-oil emulsions (Aucouturier et al., 2001), aluminum or calcium salts (Iyver et al., 2003; He et al., 2000), liposome-based delivery systems (Kersten and Crommelin, 2003), and the diverse group of antigen delivery systems based on polymers. They may briefly prolong antigen retention and/or half-life after administration. In addition, all adjuvants that facilitate recruitment of increased numbers of APC, or which facilitate the targeting, loading, processing, and presentation of antigen on APC, fit within this concept. Such adjuvants include certain recombinant host-derived chemokines as well as fetal liver tyrosine kinase 3 (Flt3) ligand and GM-CSF, as well as interferon (IFN)-γ or inducers of such molecules (Pulendran et al., 1998; Mwangi et al., 2002; Westerman et al., 2002; Sang et al., 2003). Due to their ability to stimulate proliferation of hematopoietic progenitor cells of both lymphoid and myeloid origin, they all lead to increased numbers of antigen sampling DC at the inoculation site.

In addition, host opsonins, such as complement or (natural) antibodies, naturally targeting receptors on APC, can be engaged to improve receptor-mediated delivery of antigen to APC. Dempsey et al. (1996) showed that fusion of 2–3 copies of complement Cd3 to a recombinant model antigen, hen egg lysozyme (HEL), made the antigen 100- to 1000-fold more immunogenic, as evidenced by facilitated antibody formation, when compared with HEL alone. Similarly, targeting of poorly immunogenic antigen to DC for example, through selective engagement of receptors for Fc portions of immunoglobulin (Fc γ R), has been shown to overcome nonresponsiveness and induce immunity to model and tumor antigens (Regnault et al., 1999; Kalergis and Ravetch, 2002; Akiyama et al., 2003). The recognition and concentration of pathogen-derived proteins by natural antibodies can act as a trigger for complement-dependent pathways, leading to improved immune responses, including interleukin (IL)-4 production and CD8+ T cell priming (Stäger et al., 2003).

■ Regulation of signal 2

■ Signal 0 (recognition of stranger) concept

The immune system evolved to protect the host from potentially noxious pathogens. In particular, innate immune cells, including immature DC in peripheral tissues, are able to recognize molecular patterns on the surface of microorganisms that provide a microorganism-specific signal and an initiation stimulus for the immune system. These patterns represent a conserved signature of certain classes of pathogens and are not found on host cells. The recognition of these so-called pathogen-associated patterns (PAMP) occurs by pathogen recognition receptors (PRR), such as the recently described toll-like receptors (TLR), mannose receptors, and complement receptors (Janeway, 1989, 1992;

Yamamoto et al., 1997; Barrington et al., 2001). These receptors are germ-line encoded, evolutionary conserved and found in evolutionary distinct species, from drosophila to mammals. Activation of PRR, defined as signal 0, leads to transcriptional activation of proinflammatory cytokine ad chemokine genes. In addition, PRR engagement leads to upregulation of costimulatory molecules, such as members of the B7 family of molecules expressed on the surface of APC, like DC and accessory innate immune cells, e.g., macrophages. The upregulated soluble and membrane-bound costimulatory signals on DC are designated signal 2 and considered essential for activation of resting T cells and the productive prolongation of the immune response. Indeed, MyD88-deficient mice, which cannot signal through most known TLR, showed reduced inflammatory responses and selectively impaired immune responses following exposure to microbial stimuli, such as *Mycobacterium tuberculosis* in complete Freund's adjuvant (CFA) (Schnare et al., 2001) (see Figures 1.1 (lower panel) and 1.3).

Signaling via different PRRS, expressed by different subsets of innate immune cells, may evoke qualitatively different types of immune reactions that are necessary for proper elimination of the pathogens (Kadowaki et al., 2001). Also, expression of TLR is regulated by infection-associated signals. Hence, IFN-α/β and IFN-γ activate a number of different TLR on macrophages (Miettinen et al., 2001). Also, TLR expression is inducible by LPS (Alexopoulou et al., 2001). Analysis of gene expression profiles of human DC exposed to different pathogens or their components revealed both common and pathogen-specific gene activation programs. Interestingly, microbial components of these pathogens (like LPS from the *E. coli* cell wall, yeast cell wall-derived mannan and double-stranded RNA evoked by influenza infection, which act as ligands for known PRR) induced only a subset of genes of those induced by the complete infectious pathogen. Moreover, the levels of gene expression upon recognition

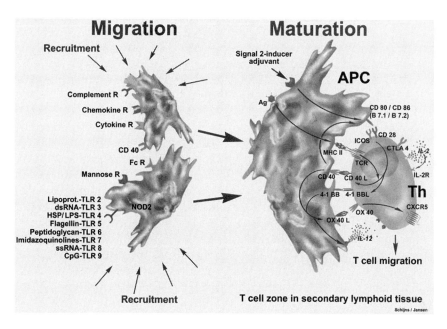

Figure I.2 **Adjuvants recruit, target, or activate antigen-presenting dendritic cells (DC).** Hence, DC/antigen-presenting cell (APC) migration (signal I facilitation) or maturation (signal 2 facilitation) by microbial or nonmicrobial immunopotentiators is key to primary immune induction. (See Color Plate Section.)

of the microbial ligand were reduced when compared with the infection of the DC by the live pathogen (Huang et al., 2001). Both in humans and mice, specialized DC have been identified which sense the presence of viruses, even without the need to become infected, and respond with rapid production of type IFN (Siegal et al., 1999; Asselin-Paturel et al., 2001).

In accordance with the two-signal model, agonistic engagement of pathogen structures with PRR leads to upregulation of signal 2 molecules on APC, as a result of direct maturation of DC; indirectly, this may be supported by cytokines produced by bystander macrophages or other accessory cells (Figures 1.1 and 1.2).

■ Danger concept

A related though distinct concept is the proposed "danger" theory championed by Matzinger (1994) and co-workers. The danger theory is largely in accordance with the two-signal model, but stresses that phenotypic and functional maturation of APC results especially from the presence of so-called danger signals. This model emphasizes that, rather than distinguishing between microbial nonself (stranger) and nonmicrobial self, the immune system only discriminates between harmless, healthy signals and signals resulting from tissue destruction (danger). The stress signals may be released endogenously and are not necessarily provided by conserved structures of microbial origin. They can be generated from organelles of cells undergoing pathological necrotic death from stressed, damaged tissue, but are not clearly defined at the molecular level. However, it was proved that mitochondrial and nuclear fractions of necrotic cells (Li et al., 2001), as well as heat shock proteins (HSP), are responsible for DC maturation and subsequent immune activation. Interestingly, TLR4-deficient C3H/HeJ mice failed to respond to HSP60-induced macrophage activation (Ohashi et al., 2000), suggesting that HSP60 is a putative endogenous ligand for the TLR-4 complex. By contrast, apoptotic cells, which maintain intact cell membranes and do not release cell content, before being cleared by phagocytosis, are unable to phenotypically and functionally mature DC (Li et al., 2001). Besides TLR4, HSP are also claimed to activate TLR2, although there has been speculation about the possibility of endotoxin contamination (Wallin et al., 2002). Recently, steroidal ginseng saponins, known to cause substantial muscle necrosis at the injection site, proved to mature DC *in vitro* and to drive Th-1 polarization (Takei et al., 2004).

Transplantation of skin grafts evokes immune-activating danger signals, leading to transplant rejection, even a month after adoptive transfer of repopulating fetal liver stem cells (Anderson, 2001). Also, mammalian double-stranded DNA proved to activate APC (Ishii et al., 2001). At conflict with this hypothesis is the observation that both necrotic and apoptotic cells failed to induce maturation of human monocyte-derived immature DC, except in cases when the cells were contaminated by mycoplasma, an exogenous microbial stimulus. When mycoplasma was eliminated by cyprorin treatment, the maturation-inducing effect was lost (Salio et al., 2000). Recently, Shi et al. (2003) identified a molecule purified by chromatography in fractionated cytoplasm of necrotic cells that acts as an alarming endogenous danger signal. They identified uric acid as an activator of DC and adjuvant for particulate HIVgp120 antigen.

■ Facilitation of signal 2

A number of well-known experimental adjuvants are likely to act via microbe recognition receptors. This is the case for various bacterial lipoproteins that have been shown to engage TLR2. Examples include *Mycobacterium tuberculosis* in complete Freund adjuvants, or mycobacterial derivatives, such as PPD, muramyl dipeptide (MDP), and threonyl MDP, coadministered in free form or included as a component in well-known commercially available adjuvants. Also, synthetic poly I:C, mimicking double-stranded DNA (dsDNA),

provides a conserved pattern characteristic of a natural viral infection. This pattern is recognized by TLR-3 leading to IFN-α/β production (Alexopoulou et al., 2001). IFN-α/β upregulates expression of TLR 1, 2, 3, and 7 (Miettinen et al., 2001), activates DC (Cella et al., 1999), and is required for Th1-dependent responses following vaccination with naked DNA plasmids in mice (Tudor et al., 2001). In addition, LPS and monophosphoryl lipid A (MPL) is recognized by TLR-4, while a highly conserved structure of bacterial flagellin is seen by TLR-5 (Akira et al., 2001; McSorley et al., 2002). Both nonmethylated CpG motifs, found abundantly on bacterial DNA, including naked DNA of vaccine plasmids (but to limited amounts in self, eukaryotic DNA), and synthetic CpG-rich oligodeoxynucleotides (ODN) are recognized as a molecular pattern by TLR 9 (Hemmi et al., 2000). Terminal α-D-mannopyranosyl residues are common glycoprotein structures of parasites, bacteria, yeasts, and enveloped virus. Mannose receptors (MR) found on macrophages and immature DC have been described to recognize such carbohydrate patterns on microorganisms (Sallusto et al., 1995; Stahl and Ezekowitz, 1998). These receptors also recognize chitin structures in chitosan or mannans in yeast cell walls, both common vaccine adjuvants (Shibata, 1997, 2001). MR may act as signal-transducing receptors and have been shown to trigger cytokine secretion and DC activation (Sallusto et al., 1995; Shibata et al., 1997; Yamamoto et al., 1997). In the last few years the list of identified receptors on innate immune cells has expanded dramatically. For a number of microbial structures, the innate immune cell pattern recognition receptors have yet to be determined. Among viruses, the viral surface G protein of respiratory syncytial virus (RSV) has been identified as a potential ligand for TLR 4 (Kurt-Jones, 2000; Haynes et al., 2001). However, purified inactivated, nonreplicating viral particles of distinct virus families are able to evoke immune responses in the absence of adjuvants. Repetitive highly organized surface antigens on various virus types, such as the prototypic rhabdoviruses, are likely to crosslink B cell receptors in the presumed absence of signal 2 (Jegerlehner et al., 2002). However, even randomly or poorly organized antigens on other virus families, e.g., herpes or corona viridae, are able to evoke T helper and IgG responses without the help of adjuvant (De Wit et al., 2004). These viruses contain ds-DNA or RNA sequences, which, upon cell entry, possibly activate MHC gene expression and genes involved in antigen presentation (Suzuki et al., 1999). Indeed, TLR 8 recognizes single-stranded RNA (Diebold et al., 2004; Heil et al., 2004), while TLR 2 and TLR9 recognize herpesviral elements (Compton et al., 2003; Hochrein et al., 2004). Also, the non-microbial, low molecular weight adenine or guanosine analogs, such as imidazoquinoline compounds and loxoribine, are able to activate inflammatory responses of immune cells via TLR 7 (Hemmi et al., 2002).

Terminal α-D-mannopyranosyl residues are glycoprotein PAMP, common on bacteria, yeasts, parasites, and viruses, and less abundantly expressed on eukaryotic cells. They are recognized with relatively high specificity by mannose receptors, C-type lectins, on macrophages and DC (Sallusto et al., 1995; Agnes et al., 1997; Engering et al., 1997). Antigens naturally exposing mannosylated glycoproteins or engineered to express mannose residues are efficiently internalized by DC and concentrated in the endocytotic pathway. This leads to more efficient presentation to specific T cells when compared with internalization by fluid phase antigens (Engering et al., 1997; Copland et al., 2003). In addition, IFN-α is induced following recognition of enveloped viruses (Milone et al., 1998). Similarly, artificial synthetic particles of nonmicrobial origin, decorated with terminal sugar residues, including mannose, fucose, or N-acetyl-D-glucosamine, are recognized by mannose or β-glucan receptors on macrophages, resulting in IL-12, tumor necrosis factor (TNF), and IFN-γ production (Shibata et al., 1997, 2001). The increased immunogenicity of the latter

particulate structures is probably explained by the activation of innate immune cells upon recognition of mimics of microbes in phago-cytosable form (<10 μm). Larger particles of 50–100 μm fail to activate such events. Therefore, mannosylation of antigens is assumed to facilitate immunogenicity.

When using such microbe component-based adjuvants, it is important to realize that receptors for microbial patterns can be differentially expressed among species, and on innate immune cells or their subtypes residing in different tissues, including vaccine inoculation sites. The qualitative and quantitative variation in microbial recognition receptor expression may explain differences in the quality of immunological responses.

Interestingly, in mice studies, it has been shown that endogenous type I IFN proved essential for Th-1 type humoral immune responses induced by typical adjuvants, including LPS, Poly I:C (Hoebe et al., 2003), IFA, CFA, and CpG motifs (Proietti et al., 2002).

Endogenous IL-12, but not IL-6, proved essential for ISCOM adjuvanticity (Smith et al., 1999), while IL-4 and IL-13 function (Brewer et al., 1999) and MyD88 (Schnare et al., 2001) proved redundant for adjuvant activity of aluminum hydroxide.

Signal 2 molecules themselves have been demonstrated to act as molecular adjuvants. Prototypic molecules include soluble cytokines, facilitating either APC subtype recruitment and activation, or acting more downstream at the level of T helper–CTL or T helper–B cell interaction. Examples include various cytokines such as the earlier mentioned hematopoietic growth factors, GM-CSF, and Flt-3 ligand, which may selectively recruit response modulating APC, as well as the proinflammatory IFN, IL-1, IL-6, IL-12, IL-18, or T cell-derived IL-2, IL-4, etc. (Pulendran et al., 1999; Hanlon et al., 2001; Proietti et al., 2002).

Many recombinant cytokines have proven successful in murine model systems (Schijns et al., 1994, 2000, 2002; Proietti et al., 2002) or in veterinary species (Hanlon et al., 2001);

some are in clinical trials whereas others are already components of registered products (IFN, IL-2, GM-CSF). However, the degree and duration of efficacy boosting may depend on the nature and dose of antigen and may vary between distinct cytokines and the species of interest (Schijns, unpublished data).

In addition to secreted cytokines, membrane-bound costimulatory molecules exert adjuvant activity, e.g., TNF ligand super family members, such as CD40 ligand (Mendoza et al., 1997; Ninomiya et al., 2002; Manoj et al., 2003), OX40-ligand (Linton et al., 2003), B cell activating factor (BAFF) (Mackay and Browning, 2002), etc., or the lymphocyte activation gene-3 (LAG-3) (Andreae et al., 2002). Under physiological conditions, these molecules act as natural amplifiers of Ag presentation by APC, as products of activated T cells. Activation by these ligands of their natural receptors on APC induces further expression of immune costimulatory molecules, thereby further enhancing APC activity.

When administered as recombinant molecules, expressed *in vivo* either by plasmids or recombinant vectors, or delivered as recombinant (Ag-fusion) proteins, immunopotentiation may result (Heath, 1995; Gurunathan et al., 1998; El Mir and Triebel, 2000; Weinberg, 2002).

■ Adjuvants provide signal 3, regulating the quality of immunity

As outlined before, T helper cells amplify Ag-specific adaptive immune response pathways. Under extreme conditions, they can polarize these responses into either Th1- or Th2-type responses by the pattern of cytokines they produce. The instructive signals for this Th1/Th2 polarization may originate most upstream in the activation cascades during APC activation (Figure 1.3). According to the geographical concept, immune induction and potentiation benefits from delivery of antigen in secondary lymphoid tissues. For this concept, the antigen regulates the extent

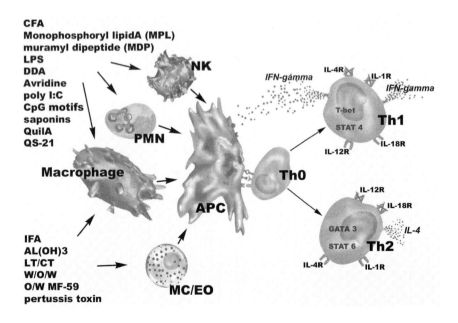

Figure I.3 **Immunopotentiators influence the quality of immune reactions.** Recognition of adjuvants by innate immune cells generates soluble, secreted, or membrane-bound signals, which shape the direction of downstream Th phenotypes upon priming by activated and conditioned antigen-presenting dendritic cells. (See Color Plate Section.)

of immune responses. Consequently, the quality of immune response may be an intrinsic feature of the antigen or its structure. Depending on the route of inoculation or the type of adjuvant, functionally different APC will sample the antigen, which may potentially influence the nature of the immune response. For example, recruitment of DC precursors by pretreatment with GM-CSF favors polarization towards Th2-type immunity, while pretreatment with Flt3 ligand facilitates Th1-associated IgG2a formation for the same ovalbumin antigen (Pulendran et al., 1999).

Apart from antigen (signal 1), the quality of immune responses is under the influence of signal 2 molecules (Figures 1.1, 1.2, and 1.3). This may occur by endogenous danger signals or by PRR activation by exogenous microbial structures, leading to predominant Th1 differentiation as a result of IL-12 and IL-18 production, or IFN-γ production by NK. Conversely, commitment for the Th2 pathway is proposed to develop in the absence of such microbial stimuli, resulting in the alternative default Th2 pathway (Jankovic et al., 2001). This pathway is more dependent on the constellation of membrane-bound costimulatory molecules like CD28 or CTLA-4 (Jankovic et al., 2001). However, signal 0 activation may not always be associated with Th1 responses. For example, LPS from *Porphyromas gingivalis*, which activates via a TLR-4-independent pathway, stimulates IL-4 production, while hyphae from *Candida albicans* and a filarial nematode product stimulate IL-4 production by DC and subsequent Th2 responses (d'Ostiani et al., 2000; Hirschfeld et al., 2001). Also, cholera toxin polarizes the maturation of DC into Th2 priming APC (Gagliardi et al., 2000). In addition, protein extracts from the helminth, *Schistosoma mansoni*, were able to induce DC-promoting Th2 cell (designated DC2 cells) development *in vitro* (De Jong et al., 2002). Notably, typical PRR conditioning for a Th2-type response has not been identified yet.

MyD88 is an adaptor protein mediating signal transduction by TLR. Interestingly, MyD88 knockout mice, which have an impaired ability to signal through many TLR, show no defects in immune responses against ovalbumin when coadministered with alum (Schnare et al., 2001), while they lacked an inflammatory response to bacterial components (Kawai et al., 1999). This indicates that certain adjuvants, especially those of a nonmicrobial nature, do not necessarily trigger the recently delineated TLR/NF-kB pathway in DC, but possibly other PRR or PRR-independent pathways.

Dendritic cells come in various forms related to their localization, phenotype, and function (Liu et al., 2001). They may express different sets of PRR or danger receptors depending on their origin and their surrounding tissue signals (Kadowaki et al., 2001). Professional APC judge the conditions during antigen uptake and, depending on the cytokine or endogenous danger, molecule constellation may be stably conditioned to differentiate into so-called DC1-, DC2-, or DC3-type APC (Liu et al., 2001, de Jong et al., 2002; Lavelle et al., 2003), associated with imprinting of Th1-, Th2-, and Th3-type immune reactions, respectively (d'Ostiani et al., 2000; Hirschfeld et al., 2001). A cell type lacking classic DC phenotype markers with plasmacytoid morphology has been identified as the major type I IFN-producing cell, sensing the presence of viruses (Asselin-Paturel et al., 2001; Giliet et al., 2002). However, when addressing the capacity and response skewing ability of distinct DC subsets following interaction with viral structures, we recently came to the conclusion that the nature of the antigen dictates the type of immune response rather than the DC subset (De Wit et al., 2005).

■ Outlook

The majority of new-generation vaccines will consist of purified recombinant, synthetic, or natural antigens. Unfortunately, purified antigens are rather passive elements unable to prime proper immune responses. They require the co-localization of adjuvants to induce, amplify, and guide an innate and subsequent adaptive immune response of sufficient magnitude and quality. Without a proper adjuvant, even the most suitable antigen will not result in an efficacious vaccine. Adjuvants for new-generation vaccines will be designed as precision instruments able to trigger appropriate immunological target molecules with minimal local or systemic side reactions. These modern immunopotentiators can nowadays be searched for in a rational approach by addressing one or more of the above described concepts. Combinations of differentially acting molecules may further enhance vaccine efficacy.

The following chapters detail characteristics of modern immunopotentiators and their presumed or confirmed mode(s) of action.

■ Acknowledgments

The technical expertise of John Jansen, Monique Teeuwen, and Dick Coppus in the preparation of the illustrations is gratefully acknowledged. The author is grateful to Dr. William Enright for the critical reading of the manuscript and many colleagues from Intervet for helpful discussions.

■ References

Akira, S., Takeda, K., and Kaisho, T. (2001). Toll-like receptors: critical proteins linking innate and acquired immunity. *Nature Immunol.* 2, 675–680.

Akiyama, K., Ebihara, S., Yada, A., Matsumura, K., Aiba, S., Nukiwa, T., and Takai, T. (2003). Targeting apoptotic tumor cells to Fc gamma R provides efficient and versatile vaccination against tumors by dendritic cells. *J. Immunol.* 170, 1641–1648.

Alexopoulou, L., Czopik Holt, A., Medzhitov, R., and Flavell, R. (2001). Recognition of double-stranded RNA and activation of NF-kappaB by Toll-like receptor 3. *Nature* 413, 732–738.

Anderson, C.C., Carroll, J.M., Gallucci, S., Ridge, J.P., Cheever, A.W., and Matzinger, P. (2001). Testing, time-, ignorance-, and danger-based models of tolerance. *J. Immunol.* 166, 3663–3671.

Andreae, S., Piras, F., Burdin, N., and Triebel, F. (2002). Maturation and activation of dendritic cells induced by lymphocyte activation gene-3 (CD223). *J. Immunol.* 168, 3874–3880.

Asselin-Paturel, C., Boonstra, A., Dalod, M., Durand, I., Yessaad, N., Dezutter-Dambyuant, C.,Vicari, A., O'Garra, A., Biron,C., Briere, F., and Trinchieri, G. (2001). Mouse type I IFN-producing cells are immature APCs with plasmacytoid morphology. *Nature Immunol.* 2, 1144–1150.

Aucouturier, J., Dupuis, L., and Ganne, V. (2001). Adjuvants designed for veterinary and human vaccines. *Vaccine* 19, 2666–2672.

Bachmann, M.F. and Kopf, M. (1999). The role of B cells in acute and chronic infections. *Curr. Opin. Immunol.* 11, 332–339.

Bachmann, M.F. and Zinkernagel, R.M. (1997). Neutralizing antiviral B cell responses. *Ann. Rev. Immunol.* 15, 235–270.

Bancherau, J., Briere, F., Caux, C., Davoust, J., Lebecque, S., Liu, Y.J., Pulendran, B., and Palucka, K. (2000). Immunobiology of dendritic cells. *Ann. Rev. Immunol.* 18, 767–811.

Barker, C.F. and Billingham, R.E. (1967). The role of regional lymphatics in the skin homograft response. *Transplantation* 5, 962–966.

Barrington, R., Zhang, M., Fisher, M., and Carroll, M.C. (2001). The role of complement in inflammation and adaptive immunity. *Immunol. Rev.* 180, 5–15.

Bretscher, P. and Cohn, M. (1970). A theory of self-nonself discrimination. *Science* 169, 1042–1049.

Brewer, J.M., Conacher, M., Hunter, C.A., Mohrs, M., Brombacher, F., and Alexander, J. (1999). Aluminium hydroxide adjuvant initiates strong antigen-specific Th2 responses in the absence of IL-4- or IL-13-mediated signaling. *J. Immunol.* 163, 6448–6454.

Cella, M., Salio, M., Sakakibara, Y., Langen, H., Julkunen, I., and Lanzavecchia, A. (1999). Maturation, activation and protection of dendritic cells by double-stranded RNA. *J. Exp. Med.* 189, 821–829.

Cohn, M. and Langman, R.E. (1990). The protection: the unit of humoral immunity selected by evolution. *Immunol. Rev.* 115, 11–147.

Compton, T., Kurt-Jones, E., Boehme, K.W., Belko, J., Latz, E., Golenbock, and Finberg R.W. (2003). Human cytomegalovirus activates inflammatory cytokine responses via CD14 and toll-like receptor 2. *J. Virol.* 77, 4588–4596.

Copland, M.J., Baird, M.A., Rades, T., McKenzie, J.L., Becker, B., Reck, F., Tyler, P.C., and Davies, N.M. (2003). Liposomal delivery of antigen to human dendritic cells. *Vaccine* 21, 883–890.

De Jong, E.C., Vieira, P.L., Kalinski, P., Schuitemanker, J.H., Tanaka, Y., Wierenga, E.A., Yazdanbakhsh, M., and Kapsenberg, M.L. (2002). Microbial compounds selectively induce Th1 cell-promoting or Th2 cell-promoting dendritic cells in vitro with diverse Th cell-polarizing signals. *J. Immunol.* 168, 1704–1709.

De Wit, M., Horzinek, M.C., Haagmans, B.L., and Schijns, V.E.J.C. (2004). Host-dependent type-1 cytokine response driven by inactivated viruses may fail to default in the absence of IL-12 and IFN-α/β. *J. Gen. Virol.* 85, 795–803.

De Wit, M., Horzinek, M.C., Haagmans, B.L., and Schijns, V.E.J.C. (2005). Immunisation with virion-loaded plasmacytoid or myeloid dendritic cells induces primary Th-1 immune responses. *Vaccine* 23, 1343–1350.

Dempsey, P.W., Allison M.E., Akkaraju, S., Goodnow, C.C., and Fearon, D.T. (1996). C3d of complement as molecular adjuvant: bridging innate and acquired immunity. *Science* 271, 348–350.

Diebold, S.S., Kaisho, T., Hemmi, H., Akira, S., and Reis e Sousa, C. (2004). Innate antiviral responses by means of TLR7-mediated recognition of single-stranded RNA. *Science* 303, 1529–1531.

Dixon, F.J. and Maurer, P.H. (1955). Immunologic unresponsiveness induced by protein antigens. *J. Exp. Med.* 101, 237–245.

D'Ostiani C., Del Sero, G. Bacci, A., Montagnoli, C., Spreca, A., Mencacci, A.P., Ricciardi-Castagnoli, P., and Romani, L. (2000) Dendritic cells discriminate between yeasts and hyphae of the fungus *Candida albicans*: implications for initiation of T helper cell immunity in vitro and in vivo. *J. Exp. Med.* 191, 1661–1674.

Dresser, D.W. (1968). Adjuvanticity of vitamin A. *Nature* 217, 527–529.

Dresser, D.W. and Gowland, G. (1964). Immunological paralysis induced in adult rabbits by small amounts of protein antigen. *Nature* 203, 275–292.

Dupuis, M., McDonald, D.M., and Ott, G. (2000). Distribution of adjuvant MF59 and antigen gD2 after intramuscular injection in mice. *Vaccine* 18, 434–439.

El Mir, S. and Triebel, F. (2000). A soluble lymphocyte activation gen-3 molecule used as vaccine adjuvant elicits greater humoral and cellular immune responses to both particulate and soluble antigens. *J. Immunol.* 164, 5583–5589.

Engering, A.J., Cella, M., Fluitsma, D., Brockhaus, M., Hoefsmit, E.C.M., Lanzavecchia, A., and Pieters, J. (1997). The mannose receptor functions as a high capacity and broad specificity antigen receptor in human dendritic cells. *Eur. J. Immunol.* 27, 2417–2425.

Fehr, T., Bachmannn, M.F., Bluethmann, Kikutani, H., Hengartner, H., and Zinkernagel, R.M. (1996). T-independent activation of B cells by vesicular stomatitis virus: no evidence for the need for a second signal. *Cell. Immunol.* 15, 184–192.

Fehr, T., Skrastina, D., Pumpens, P., and Zinkernagel, R. (1998). T cell-independent type I antibody response against B cell epitopes expressed repetitively on recombinant viral particles. *Proc. Natl. Acad. Sci. USA* 95, 9477–9481.

Freund, J. (1956). The mode of action of immunological adjuvants. *Adv. Tuberc. Res.* 7, 130–147.

Freund, J., Casals, J., and Page Hosmer, E. (1937). Sensitization and antibody formation after injection of tubercle bacilli and paraffin oil. *Proc. Soc. Exp. Biol. Med.*37, 509–513.

Frey, J.R. and Wenk, P. (1957). Experimental studies on the pathogenesis of contact eczema in the guinea pig. *Int. Arch. Allergy Appl. Immunol.* 11, 81–100.

Gagliardi, M.C., Sallusto, F., Marinaro, M., Langenkamp, A., Lanzavecchia, A., and De Magistris, M.T., (2000). Cholera toxin induces maturation of human dendritic cells and licenses them for Th2 priming. *Eur. J. Immunol.* 30, 2394–2403.

Gallucci, S., Lolkema, M., and Matzinger, P. (1999). Natural adjuvants: endogenous activators of dendritic cells. *Nature Med.* 5, 1249–1225.

Giliet, M., Boonstra, A., Paturel, C., Antonenko, S., Xu, X.L., Trinchieri, G., O'Garra, A., and Liu, Y.J. (2002). The development of murine plasmacytoid dendritic cell precursors is differentially regulated by Flt3-ligand and granulocyte/macrophage colony stimulating factor. *J. Exp. Med.* 195, 953–958.

Glenny, A.T., Buttle, G.A.H., and Stevens, M.F. (1931). Rate of disappearance of diphtheria toxoid injected into rabbits and guinea pigs: toxoid precipitated with alum. *J. Pathol. Bacteriol.* 34, 267–275.

Gurunathan, S., Irvine, K.R., Wu, C.Y., Cohen, J.I., Thomas, E., Prussin, C., Restifo, N.P., and Seder, R.A. (1998). CD40 ligand/trimer DNA enhances both humoral and cellular immune responses and induces protective immunity to infectious and tumour challenge. *J. Immunol.* 161, 4563–4571.

Hanlon, L., Argyle, D., Bain, D., Nicolson, L., Dunham, S., Golder, M.C., McDonald, M., McGillivray, C., Jarrett, O., Neil, J.C., and Onions, D.E. (2001). Feline leukemia virus DNA vaccine efficacy is enhanced by coadministration with interleukin-12 (IL-12) and IL-18 expression vectors. *J. Virol.* 75, 8424–8433.

Haynes, L.M., Moore, D.D., Kurt-Jones, E.A., Finberg, R.W., Anderson, L.J., and Tripp, R.A. (2001). Involvement of toll-like receptor 4 in innate immunity to respiratory syncytial virus. *J. Virol.* 75, 10730–10737.

He, Q., Mitchell, A.R., Johnson, S.L., Wagner-Bartak C., Morcol, T., and Bell, S. (2000). Calcium phosphate nanoparticle adjuvant. *Clin. Diagn. Lab. Immunol.* 7, 899–903.

Heath, A.W. (1995). Cytokines as immunological adjuvants. *Pharm. Biotechnol.* 6, 645–658.

Hemmi, H., Takeuchi, O., Kawai, T., Kaisho, T., Sato, S., Sanjo, H., Matsumoto, M., Hoshino, K., Wagner, H., Takeda, K., and Akira, S. (2000). A Toll-receptor recognizes bacterial DNA. *Nature* 408, 740–745.

Hemmi, H., Kaisho, T., Takeuchi, O., Sato, S., Sanjo, H., Hoshino, K., Horiuchi, T., Tomizawa, H., Takeda, K., and Akira, S. (2002). Small anti-viral compounds activate immune cells via TLR7 MyD88-dependent signalling pathway. *Nature Immunol.* 3, 196–200.

Heil, F., Hemmi, H., Hochrein, H., Ampenberger, F., Kirschning C., Akira, S., Lipford, G., Wagner, H., and Bauer, S. (2004). Species-specific recognition of single-stranded RNA via toll-like receptor 7 and 8. *Science* 303, 1526–1529.

Herbert, W.J. (1966). Antigenicity of soluble protein in the presence of high levels of antibody: a possible mode of action of the antigen adjuvants. *Nature* 210, 747–748.

Hirschfeld, M., Weis, J.J., Toshchakov, V., Salkowski, C.A., Cody, M.J., Ward, D.C., Qureshi, N., Michalek, S.M., and Vogel, S.N. (2001). Signalling by Toll-like receptor 2 and 4 agonists results in differential gene expression in murine macrophages. *Infect. Immun.* 69, 1477–1482.

Hochrein, H., Schlatter, B., O'Keeffe, M., Wagner, C., Schmitz, F., Schiemann, M., Bauer, S., Suter, M., and Wagner, H. (2004). Herpes simplex virus type-1 induces IFN-α production via toll-like receptor 9-dependent and independent pathways. *Proc. Natl. Acad. Sci. USA* 101, 11416–11421.

Hoebe, K., Janssen, E.M., Kim, S.O., Alexopoulou, L., Flavell, R.A., Han, J., and Beutler, B. (2003). Upregulation of costimulatory molecules induced by lipopolysaccharide and double stranded RNA occurs by Trif-dependent and Trif-independent pathways. *Nature Immunol.* 4, 1223–1229.

Huang, Q., Liu, D., Majewski, P., Schulte, L.C., Korn, J., Young, R.A., Lander,E.S., and Hacohen, N. (2001). The plasticity of denditic cells to pathogens and their components. *Science* 294, 870–875.

Ishii, K.J., Suzuli, K., Coban, C., Takeshita, F., Itoh, Y., Matoba, H., Kohn, L.D., and Klinman, D.M. (2001). Genomic DNA released by dying cells induces the maturation of of APCs. *J. Immunol.* 167, 2602–2607.

Iyver, S., Hogenesch, H., and Hem, S.L. (2003). Relationship between the degree of antigen adsorption to aluminium hydroxide adjuvant in interstitial fluid and antibody production. *Vaccine* 21, 1219–1223.

Janeway, Ch.A. Jr. (1989). Approaching the asymptote? Evolution and revolution in immunology. *Cold Spring Harbor Symp. Quant. Biol.* 54, 1–13.

Janeway, Ch.A. Jr. (1992). The immune system evolved to discriminate infectious nonself from noninfectious self. *Immunol. Today* 13, 11–16.

Jankovic, D., Liu, Z., and Gause, W.C. (2001). Th1 and Th2-cell commitment during infectious disease: asymmetry in divergent pathways. *Trends Immunol.* 22, 450–457.

Jansen, Th., Hofmans, M.P., Theelen, M.J.G., and Schijns, V.E.J.C. (2004). Structure–activity relations of water-in-oil vaccine formulations and induced antigen-specific antibody responses. *Vaccine* 23, 1053–1060.

Jegerlehner, A., Storni, T., Lipowski, G., Schmid, M., Pumpens, P., and Bachmann M.F. (2002). Regulation of IgG antibody responses by epitope density and CD21-mediated costimulation. *Eur. J. Immunol.* 32, 2205–3314.

Kadowaki, N., Ho, S., Antonenko, S., De WaalMalefyt, R., Kastelein, R.A., Bazan, F., and Liu, Y.-J. (2001). Subsets of human dendritic cells precursors express different Toll-like receptors and respond to different microbial antigens. *J. Exp. Med.* 194, 863–869.

Karrer, U., Althage, A., Odermatt, B., Roberts, C.W.M., Korsmeyer, S.J., Miyawaki, S., Hengartner, H., and Zinkernagel, R.M. (1997). On the key role of secondary lymphoid organs in antiviral immune responses studied in alymphoplastic (aly/aly) and spleenless (Hox11–/–) mutant mice. *J. Exp. Med.* 185, 2157–2170.

Katayama, S., Oda, K., Ohgitani, T., Hirahara, T., and Shimizu, Y. (1999). Influence of antigenic forms and adjuvants on the Ig subclass antibody response to Aujeszky's disease virus. *Vaccine* 17, 2733–2739.

Kawai, T., Adachi, O., Ogawa, T., Takeda, K., and Akira, S. (1999). Unresponsiveness of MyD88-deficient mice to endotoxin. *Immunity* 11, 115–122.

Kemp, J.M., Kajihara, M., Nagahara, S., Sano, A., Brandon, M., and Lofthouse, S. (2002). Continuous antigen delivery from controlled release implants induces significant and anamnestic immune responses. *Vaccine* 20, 1089–1098.

Kersten, G.F.A. and Crommelin, D.J.A. (2003). Liposomes and ISCOMS. *Vaccine* 21, 915–920.

Kündig, T.M., Bachmann, M.F., DiPaolo, C., Simard, J.J.L., Battegay, M., Lother, H., Gessner, A., Kuhlcke, K., Ohashi, P., Hengarten, H., and Zinkernagel, R.M. (1995). Fibroblasts as efficient antigen-presenting cells in lymphoid organs. *Science* 268, 1343–1347.

Kündig, T.M., Shahinian, A., Kawai, K., Mittrucker, H.W., Sebzda, E., Bachmann, M., Mak, T.W., and Ohashi, P. (1996). Duration of TCR stimulation determines costimulatory requirements of cells. *Immunity* 5, 41–52.

Kurt-Jones, E.A., Popova, L., Kwinn, L., Haynes, L.M., Jones, L.P., Tripp, R.A., Walsh, E.E., Freeman, M.W., Golenbock, D.T., Anderson, L.J., and Finberg, R.W. (2000). Pattern recognition receptors TLR4 and CD19 mediate response to respiratory syncytial virus. *Nature Immunol.* 1, 398–401.

Lafferty, K.J. and Woodnough, J. (1977). The origin and mechanism of allograft reaction. *Immunol. Rev.* 35, 231–262.

Lavelle, E.C., McNeela, E., Armstrong, M.E., Leavy, O., Higgins, S.C., and Mils, K.H. (2003). Cholera toxin promotes the induction of regulatory T cells specific for bystander antigens by modulating dendritic cell activation. *J. Immunol.* 171, 2384–2392.

Li, M., Carpio, D.F., Zheng, Y., Bruzzo, P., Singh, V., Ouaaz, F., Medzhitov, R.M., and Beg, A.A. (2001). An essential role of the NF-KB/toll-like receptor (TLR) pathway in induction of inflammatory and tissue-repair gene expression by necrotic cells. *J. Immunol.* 166, 7128–7135.

Linton, P.J., Bautista, B., Biederman, E., Bradley, E.S., Harbertson, J., Kondrack, R.M., Padrick, R.C., and Bradley, L.M. (2003). Costimulation via OX40L expressed by B cells is sufficient to determine the extent of primary CD4 cell expansion and Th2 cytokine secretion in vivo. *J. Exp. Med.* 197, 875–883.

Liu, Y.-J., Kanzler, H., Soumelis, V., and Gillet, M. (2001) Dendritic cell lineage, plasticity and cross-regulation. *Nature Immunol.* 2, 585–589.

Lofthouse, S. (2002). Immunological aspects of controlled antigen delivery. *Adv. Drug Delivery Rev.* 54, 863–870.

Mackay, F. and Browning, J.L. (2002). BAFF: a fundamental survival factor or B cells. *Nature Rev. Immunol.* 2, 465–475.

Manoj, S., Griebel, P.J., Babiuk, L.A., Van Drunen Littel van den Hurk, S. (2003). Targeting with bovine CD154 enhances humoral immune responses induced by a DNA vaccine in sheep. *J. Immunol.* 170, 989–996.

Matzinger P. (1994). Tolerance, danger and the extended family. *Ann. Rev. Immunol.* 12, 991–1045.

McSorely S.J., Ehst B.D., Yu, Y., and Gerwitz, A.T. (2002). Bacterial flagellin is an effective adjuvant for CD4+ T cells in vivo. *J. Immunol.* 169, 3914–3929.

Mendoza, R.B., Cantwell, M.J., and Kipps, T.J. (1997). Immunostimulatory effects of a plasmid expressing CD40 ligand (CD154) on gene immunization. *J. Immunol.* 159, 5777–5781.

Miettinen, M., Savereva, T., Julkunen, I., Matikainen, S. (2001) IFNs activate toll-like receptor gene expression in viral infections. *Genes Immunity* 2, 349–355.

Milone, M.C. and Fitzgerald-Bocarsly, P. (1998). The mannose receptor mediates induction of IFN-alpha in peripheral blood dendritic cells by enveloped RNA and DNA viruses. *J. Immunol.* 161, 2391–2399.

Mitchison, N.A. (1968). The dose requirements for immunological paralysis by soluble proteins. *Immunology* 15, 509–530.

Moser, C., Metcalfe I.C., and Viret, J.-F. (2003). Virosomal adjuvanted antigen delivery systems. *Expert Rev. Vaccines* 2, 189–196.

Mwangi, W., Brown, W.C., Lewin, H.A., Howard, C.J., Hope, J.C., Baszler, T.V., Caplazi, P., Abbott, J., and Palmer, G.H. (2002). DNA-encoded fetal liver tyrosine kinase 3 ligand and granulocyte macrophage-colony-stimulating factor increase dendritic cell recruitment to the inoculation site and enhance antigen-specific CD4+ T cell responses induced by DNA vaccination of outbred animals. *J. Immunol.* 169, 3837–3846.

Ninomiya, A., Ogasawara, K., Kajino, K., Takada, A., and Kida, H. (2002). Intranasal administration of a synthetic peptide vaccine encapsulated in liposome together with anti-CD40 antibody induces protective immunity against influenza A virus in mice. *Vaccine* 20, 3123–3029.

Ochsenbein, A.F., Pinschewer, D.D., Odermatt, B., Ciurea, A., Hengartner, H., and Zinkernagel, R.M.(2000). Correlation of T cell independence of antibody responses with antigen dose reaching secondary lymphoid organs: implications for splenectomized patients and vaccine design. *J. Immunol.*164, 6296–6302.

Ohashi, K., Burkart, V., Flohe, S., and Kolb, (2000). Heat shock protein 60 is a putative endogenous ligand of toll-like receptor-4 complex. *J. Immunol.* 164, 558–561.

Proietti, E., Bracci, L., Puzelli, S., Di Pucchio, T., Sestili, P., De Vincenzi, E., Venditti, M., Capone, I., Seif, I., De Maeyer, E., Tough, D., Donatelli, I., and Belardelli, F. (2002). Type I IFN as a natural adjuvant for a protective immune response: lessons from the influenza model. *J. Immunol.* 169, 375–383.

Pulendran, B., Smith, J.L., Jenkins, M., Schoenborn, M., Maraskovsky E., and Maliszewski, C.R. (1998). Prevention of peripheral tolerance by a dendritic cell growth factor: flt3 ligand as an adjuvant. *J. Exp. Med.* 188, 2075–2082.

Pulendran, B., Smith, J.L., Caspary, G., Brasel, K., Pettit, D., Maraskovsky, E., and Maliszewski, C.R. (1999). Distinct dendritic cell subsets differentially regulate the class of immune response in vivo. *Proc. Natl. Acad. Sci. USA* 96, 1036–1041.

Regnault A., Lankar, D., Lacabanne, V., Rodriguez, A., Thery, C., Rescigno, M., Saito, T., Verbeek, S., Bonnerot, C., Ricciardi-Castagnoli, P., and Amigorena, S. (1999). Fc gamma receptor-mediated induction of dendritic cell maturation and major histocompatibility complex class I-restricted antigen presentation after immune complex internalization. *J. Exp. Med.* 189, 371–380.

Salio, M., Cerundolo, V., and Lanzavechia, A. (2000). Dendritic cell maturation is induced by mycoplasma infection but not by necrotic cells. *Eur. J. Immunol.* 30, 705–708.

Sallusto, F., Cella, M., Danieli, C., and Lanzavecchia, A. (1995). Dendritic cells use macropinocytosis and the mannose receptor to concentrate macromolecules in the major histocompatibility complex class II compartment: down-regulation by cytokines and bacterial products. *J. Exp. Med.* 182, 389–400.

Sang, H., Pisarev, V.M., Munger, C., Robinson, S., Chavez, J., Hatcher, L., Parajuli, P., Guo, Y., and Talmadge, J.E. (2003). Regional, but not systemic recruitment/expansion of dendritic cells by a pluronic-formulated Flt3-ligand plasmid with vaccine adjuvant activity. *Vaccine* 21, 3019–3029.

Schijns, V.E.J.C. (2000). Immunological concepts of vaccine adjuvant activity. *Curr. Opin. Immunol.* 12, 456–463.

Schijns, V.E.J.C. (2001). Activation and programming of adaptive immune responses by vaccine adjuvants. Veterinary Science Tomorrow 3 (http://www.vetscite.org).

Schijns, V.E.J.C. (2001). Induction and direction of immune responses by vaccine adjuvants. *Crit. Rev. Immunol.* 21, 75–85.

Schijns, V.E.J.C., Claassen, I.J., Vermeulen, A.A., Horzinek, M.C., and Osterhaus, A.D. (1994). Modulation of antiviral immune responses by exogenous cytokines: effects of tumour necrosis factor-alpha, interleukin-1 alpha, interleukin-2 and interferon-gamma on the immunogenicity of an inactivated rabies virus vaccine. *J. Gen. Virol.* 75, 55–63.

Schijns, V.E.J.C., Weining, K.C., Nuijten, P., Rijke, E.O., and Staeheli, P. (2000). Immunoadjuvant activities of E. coli- and plasmid expressed recombinant chicken IFN-α/β, IFN-γ and IL-1β in day- and 3-week-old chickens. *Vaccine* 18, 2147–2154.

Schijns, V.E.J.C., Scholtes, N.C., van Zuilekom, H.I., Sanders, L.H.H., Nicolson, L. and Argyle, D. (2002). Facilitation of antibody forming responses to viral antigens in young cats by recombinant baculovirus-expressed feline IFN-γ. *Vaccine* 20, 1718–1724.

Schnare, M., Barton, G.M., Holt, A.C., Takeda, K., Akira, S., and Medzhitov, R. (2001). Toll-like receptors control activation of adaptive immune responses. *Nature Immunol.* 2, 947–950.

Shi, Y., Evans, J.E., and Rock, K.L. (2003). Molecular identification of a danger signal that alerts the immune system to dying cells. *Nature* 425, 516–521.

Shibata, Y., Metzger, W.J., and Myrvik, Q.N. (1997). Chitin particle-induced cell-mediated immunity is inhibited by soluble mannan. Mannose receptor-mediated phagocytosis initiates Il-12 production. *J. Immunol.* 159, 2462–2467.

Shibata, Y., Honda, I., Justice, P., van Scott, M., Nakamura, R.M., and Myrvik, Q.N. (2001). Th1 adjuvant N-acetyl-D-glucosamine polymer up-regulates Th1 immunity but down-regulates Th2 immunity against a mycobacterial protein (MPB-59) in interleukin-10-knockout and wild-type mice. *Infect. Immun.* 69, 6123–6130.

Siegal, F.P., Kadowaki, N., Shodell, M., Fitzgerald-Bocarsky, P.A., Shah, K., Ho, S., Antonenko, S., and Liu, Y.S. (1999). The nature off the principle type I IFN-producing cells in human blood. *Science* 284, 1835–1837.

Smith, R.E., Donachie, A.M., Grdic, D., Lycke, N., and Mowat, A.McI. (1999). Immune-stimulating complexes induce an IL-12-dependent cascade of innate immune responses. *J. Immunol.* 162, 5536–5546.

Stäger, S., Alexander J., Kirby, A.C., Botto, M., Van Rooijen, N., Smith, D.F., Brombacher, F., and Kaye, P.M. (2003). Natural antibodies and complement are endogenous adjuvants for vaccine-induced CD8+ T-cell responses. *Nature Med.* 9, 1287–1292.

Stahl, P.D. and Ezekowitz, R.A. (1998). The mannose receptor is a pattern recognition receptor involved in host defense. *Curr. Opin. Immunol.* 10, 50–55.

Steinman, R.M., Metlay, J., Bhardwaj, N., Freudenthal, P., Langhoff, E., Crowly, M., Lau, L., Witmer-Pack, M., Young, J.W., Pure, E., Romani, N., and Inaba, K. (1998). Dendritic cells: nature's adjuvant. In Janeway, Jr. C.A., Sercarz, E.E., and Sprent, J. (Eds) *Immunogenicity*, Alan R. Liss/John Wiley, New York, pp. 155–165.

Sun, H., Pollock, K.G.J., and Brewer, J.M. (2003). Analysis of the role of vaccine adjuvants in modulating dendritic cell activation and antigen presentation in vitro. *Vaccine* 21, 849–855.

Suzuki, K., Mori, A., Ishii, K.J., Saito, Singer, D.S., Klinman, D.M., Krause, P.R., and Kohn, L.D. (1999). Activation of target-tissue immune-recognition molecules by double stranded polynucleotides. *Proc. Natl. Acad. Sci. USA* 96, 2285–2290.

Takei, M., Tachikawa, E., Hasegawa, H., and Lee, J.-J. (2004). Dendritic cell maturation promoted by M1 and M4, end products of steroidal ginseng saponins metabolized in digestive tracts, drive potent Th1 polarization. *Biochem. Pharmacol.* 68, 441–452.

Tan, M.C.A.A., Mommaas, A.M., Drijfhout, J.W., Jordens, R., Onderwater, J.J.M., Verwoerd, D., Mulder, A.A., Van der Heiden, A.N., Scheidegger, D., Oomen, L.C.J.M., Ottenhoff, T.H.M., Tulp, A., Neefjes, J.J., and Koning, F. (1997). Mannose receptor-mediated uptake of antigens strongly enhances HLA class II-restricted antigen presentation by cultured dendritic cells. *Eur. J. Immunol.* 27, 2426–2435.

Tudor D., Riffault, S., Carrat, C., Lefevre, F., Bernoin, M., and Charley, B. (2001). Type I IFN modulates the immune response induced by DNA vaccination to pseudorabies virus glycoprotein C. *Virology* 286, 197–205.

Walduck, A.K. and OpdeBeeck, J.P. (1997). Effect of the profile of antigen delivery on antibody responses in mice. *J. Controlled Release* 43, 75–80.

Wallin, R.P., Lundqvist, A., More, S.H., von Bonin, A., Kiessling, R., and Ljunggren, H.G. (2002). Heat-shock proteins as activators of the innate immune system. *Trends Immunol.* 23, 130–135.

Weinberg, A.D. (2002). OX40: targeted immunotherapy: implications for tempering autoimmunity and enhancing vaccines. *Trends Immunol.* 23, 102–109.

Westermann, J., Scmetzer, O., Pezzutto, A., Hoai, T.N., and Dorken, B. (2002). Flt-3L as adjuvant in DNA vaccination: expansion of immature DC and induction of a TH2 type T cell response. *Blood* 100, abstr. 4188.

Yamamoto, Y., Klein, T., and Friedman, H. (1997). Involvement of mannose receptor in cytokine interleukin-1-beta (IL-1-B), IL-6, granulocyte-macrophage colony stimulating factor responses, but not in chemokine macrophage inflammatory protein-1 B (MIP-1B), MIP-2, and KC receptors, caused by attachment of *Candida albicans* to macrophages. *Infect. Immun.* 65, 1077–1082.

Zinkernagel, R.M. (2000). Localization dose and time of antigens determine immune reactivity. *Semin. Immunol.* 12, 163–171.

Zinkernagel, R.M., Ehl, S., Aichele, P., Oehen, S., Kundig, T., and Hengarten, H., (1997). Antigen localization regulates immune responses in a dose- and time-dependent fashion: a geographical view of immune reactivity. *Immunol. Rev.* 156, 199–209.

Zurbriggen, R. (2003). Immunostimulating reconstituted influenza virosomes. *Vaccine* 21, 921–924.

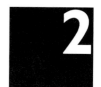

Dendritic cells as targets and tools in vaccines

Imerio Capone, Paola Rizza, and Filippo Belardelli
Istituto Superiore di Sanità, Rome, Italy

Introduction

The recent progress in immunology has revealed the crucial role of dendritic cells (DCs) in the generation of a protective immune response against both infectious diseases and tumors (Banchereau et al., 2000). Today, understanding how to manipulate DCs can be considered as strictly instrumental to the progress in vaccine research. In fact, the development of vaccines has often been hampered by the poor immunogenicity of the relevant antigenic components, which require potent adjuvants in order to promote efficiently a protective immune response. Thus, a critical issue in vaccinology is how to enhance the immune response to defined antigens; addressing this issue means understanding how to exploit the recent knowledge of the interactions between DCs and lymphocytes for the identification of more effective and safe adjuvants for modern vaccines.

DCs are the professional antigen-presenting cells (APCs) playing a fundamental role in linking innate and adaptive immunity (Banchereau et al., 2000). DCs originate from pluripotent stem cells in the bone marrow, enter the blood stream, and localize into almost all organs (Hart, 1997). Typically, circulating immature DCs enter tissues in response to inflammatory chemoactracting cytokines. After having ingested and processed incoming pathogens, they switch their chemokine receptor set and migrate to regional lymph nodes in response to lymphoid chemokines, which also direct their position within lymphoid tissues, so that DCs can efficiently present processed antigens to lymphocytes, priming them for specific immune response (Forster et al., 1999; Sozzani et al., 1999). Some types of DCs and DC precursors have recently attracted major interest from immunologists (for a review, see Liu, 2001). Based on the relative expression of a series of surface markers, different subsets of human DCs or DC precursors can be identified in peripheral blood, including a major CD1a+/CD11c+ and CD1a−/CD11c+ population, expressing the CD13, CD33, and GM-CSF receptor (referred as myeloid DCs), and a CD1a−/CD11c− population expressing high levels of CD123 (IL-3Rα), originally called lymphoid DCs and recently named plasmacytoid DCs, which represent the major type I interferon (IFN) producers upon virus challenge (Cella et al., 1999; Siegal et al., 1999). The myeloid DCs are found in deep interstitial and epithelial tissues, whereas in the skin dermal and epithelial DCs (LC) can be distinguished (Liu, 2001).

DCs are responsible for directing different types of T cell responses, from thymic negative selection to the generation of effector and memory cells as well as to the induction of peripheral tolerance. Recent studies indicate that the extent of DC recruitment into inflamed tissues and migration to lymph nodes as well as the nature of maturation stimuli and the kinetics of activation have a quantitative and qualitative impact on T cell stimulation and response (Gallucci et al., 1999; Figdor et al., 2004; Reis and Sousa, 2004). It is now becoming clear that the phenotype and functions of DCs are regulated by an ensemble of soluble factors (namely cytokines) that can either promote immunity or favor the induction of tolerance (Figure 2.1).

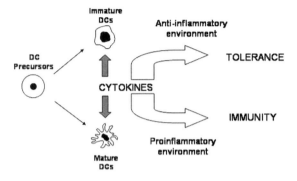

Figure 2.1 A simplified model illustrating the role of DCs in the induction of immunity or tolerance. Typically, circulating or tissue-resident DCs exist in an immature state capable of capturing self or exogenous antigens. If no inflammation occurs in this process, DCs remain immature (i.e., lacking the expression of costimulatory molecules), thus resulting in peripheral tolerance possibly via induction of T cell anergy and/or regulatory T cells. This occurs in the presence of anti-inflammatory cytokines. Alternatively, in the presence of a proinflammatory environment, which is characterized by the production of a defined set of cytokines, DCs undergo a maturation process resulting in the activation of T cells and induction of immunity.

As we have begun to understand the central role played by DCs in "decision making" in terms of immunity vs. tolerance, we can exploit the potential exhibited by this special class of immune cells for improving vaccines. In particular, the recent progress in basic immunology and vaccinology has revealed that DCs can be considered as main targets and tools for the development of modern vaccines (Figure 2.2). In fact, on the one hand, any kind of vaccine has to reach host DCs in a suitable manner and multiple strategies for *in vivo* targeting of antigens to DCs are currently being explored in order to enhance vaccine efficacy. On the other hand, DCs can be considered as ideal tools for the development of therapeutic vaccines against cancer and some severe infectious diseases (Hart, 2001; Steinman and Dhodapkar, 2001; Svane et al. 2003; Figdor et al., 2004) and several clinical studies have recently been performed to evaluate the safety and the possible efficacy of DC-based vaccines in patients.

In this chapter, we provide an overview of the main current strategies for exploiting the recent knowledge of DC biology for developing new and more effective vaccine adjuvants

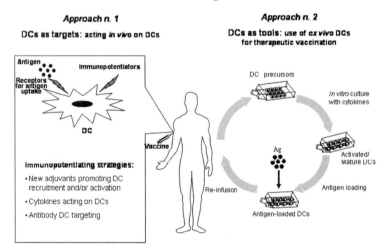

Figure 2.2 The dual approach for exploiting the recent knowledge of DC biology for the development of novel vaccination strategies. Approach I: DCs can be targeted *in vivo* by immunopotentiating agents (TLRs ligands, cytokines, antibodies, etc.), which may enhance their capability to take up and process antigens and/or to promote their activation and migration to lymphoid organs in order to prime efficiently immune responses. Approach 2: DCs can be generated *ex vivo* by culturing DC precursors, obtained from leukapheresis products in cytokine-containing medium and, after antigen loading, are re-injected in patients for therapeutic purposes.

(i.e., DCs as vaccine targets) as well as for using autologous DCs from patients for the preparation of therapeutic vaccines (i.e., DCs as tools for therapeutic vaccination).

■ DCs as targets for modern vaccines

The understanding of the signals necessary to convert DCs into immunostimulatory APCs capable of priming appropriate effector T cells has allowed the identification of key molecules suitable for the development of novel and effective adjuvants in modern vaccines. Among them, certain cytokines and newly developed compounds have shown promise as potentially new adjuvants and are currently being tested in clinical studies. The scope of this section is to provide the reader with newly acquired knowledge on strategies whose ultimate goal is to target DCs, including an overview on immunopotentiators recognized as strong DC activators, as well as on the novel strategies of *in vivo* targeting of DCs. Because of space limitations, we focus on some representative molecules particularly relevant to this topic.

■ New adjuvants and DCs

Originally developed as factors empirically conceived to enhance the immunogenic properties of an antigen, adjuvants are now being redesigned in a more rational way as substances capable of profoundly affecting the magnitude and the type of the adaptive immune response (Schijns, 2003). In fact, the enormous bulk of concepts accumulated over the years in the field of vaccinology and molecular immunology has provided a scientific explanation of the mechanisms of actions of many adjuvants and novel criteria are now being established for defining both traditional and newly developed adjuvants. Thus, according to a functional definition, it has been proposed to divide adjuvants into two main categories: (i) delivery systems; and (ii) immunopotentiators (O'Hagan and Valiante, 2003). Whereas delivery systems act

by promoting the targeting of the antigen to professional APCs (mainly the DCs), immune potentiators exert their effects directly on these cells through specific receptors. It is clear that both represent essential components of successful vaccines, especially for those based on highly purified subunits of pathogens, which are safer but poorly immunogenic. Notably, early vaccines based on live attenuated or killed whole-cell products intrinsically contained both the adjuvant components required. In this view, the search for new adjuvants fits with the need for restoring in the newly designed vaccines those immunopotentiating activities that have been lost along the way of conceiving more selected and pure vaccines.

■ Pathogen-associated molecular pattern-dependent DC targeting

An important impulse to the search for new immune potentiating adjuvants has been provided by the recent discovery of the so-called pathogen-associated molecular patterns (PAMPs), a family of evolutionary conserved structural elements shared by microbial pathogens, such as lypopolysaccharide (LPS) and CpG motifs, which can act as powerful activators of the immune system (Janeway, 1989). These compounds represent signatures of potentially noxious substances and are recognized by specific receptors, collectively termed pattern recognition receptors (PRRs) (Medzhitov et al., 1997). Importantly, these receptors are expressed on DCs that constantly screen the environment by using their PRRs as "sensors" for pathogens and process this information by eliciting distinct functional responses. An increasing number of PRRs have been identified, including the ten recently discovered members of the human Toll-like receptor (TLR) family, and some of their ligand counterparts have been characterized (Takeda et al., 2003). For example, LPS from *E. coli* is now known to interact with TLR4, double-stranded RNA (Poly I:C) is recognized by TLR3, TLR7 can be triggered by the synthetic compounds imidazoquino-lines, and CpG-rich DNA motifs are natural ligands for TLR9 (for a review, see Pulendran, 2004). The recognition of the microbial stimu-lus through the specific receptor expressed by DCs is translated into a biochemical signal inside the cell, which in turn leads to the transcriptional activation of proinflammatory cytokines and chemokines and upregulation of costimulatory molecules, finally resulting in the activation of an adaptive immune response.

The TLRs are differentially expressed by distinct DC subsets (and in distinct cellular compartments) and the trigger of the differ-ent TLRs may mediate distinct Th-polarized responses, or induce T regulatory pathways or CTL responses or antibody production. Thus, it is possible to target selectively functionally distinct DCs through the selection of specific TLR ligands. For example, there is evidence showing that the engagement of TLR7 and TLR9, selectively expressed by plasmacytoid human DCs (PDC), induces strong interleukin (IL)-12 (p70) and IFN-α production, which subsequently stimulate Th1-type immune responses (Pulendran, 2004). Myeloid human DCs have been found to express all TLRs except TLR7 and TLR9 and produce high levels of IL-12 upon TLR2- or TLR4-mediated activation (Pulendran, 2004).

Only some TLRs, particularly TLR3, TLR4, TLR7, and TLR9, can induce type I IFNs, which play an important role in antiviral defense by multiple mechanisms, including autocrine DC activation (reviewed by Santini et al., 2002). The question of whether TLR2 can induce Th2 responses is still controversial. To date, several studies on the signaling triggered by certain TRL2 ligands support a role of this receptor in mediating Th2 biased or T regulatory responses (Pulendran, 2004). The involvement of distinct TLRs in the induction of CTL responses has been demonstrated. Interestingly, TLR3, TLR7, and TLR9 engagement by their relative ligands may induce type I IFN production, which is well known to enhance cross-presentation by

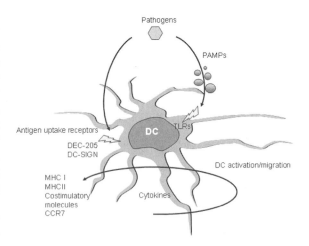

Figure 2.3 Signals involved in DC activation potentially exploitable for the development of novel adjuvants. A family of evolutionary conserved structural elements shared by microbial pathogens, the pathogen-associated molecular patterns (PAMPs), are recognized by specific receptors expressed by DCs (e.g., Toll-like receptors, TLRs) and act as powerful activators of DCs. In addition, antibody-mediated antigen targeting to DCs, by exploiting the receptors for antigen uptake, is considered a valuable approach to improve vaccine design. Finally, conditioning of DCs by cytokines can also lead to maturation and/or activation as well as to improved migratory capacity of DCs.

DCs and strong CTL activation (reviewed by Tough, 2004). This effect is of particular relevance for vaccines facing viral infections, for which CTL responses represent a funda-mental correlate of protection. It is clear that the comprehension of the signaling pathways triggered by microbial stimuli engaged by TLRs on distinct subsets of DCs is fundamental for identifying new candidates to be used as adjuvants to be targeted to DCs (Figure 2.3).

■ *CpG oligonucleotides*

Among the novel adjuvants showing strong immunostimulatory effects on DC activa-tion are the synthetic oligodeoxynucleotides (ODNs) containing unmethylated CpG motifs. CpG motifs are sequences typical of bacterial DNA, 20 times more common than in mam-malian DNA (Krieg et al., 1995; Klinman et al., 2004). The release of bacterial DNA upon infection functions as a "danger signal," alert-ing the innate immune system to react against the microbe. In mice and humans, TLR9 is responsible for the recognition of CpG motifs by immune cells, being B cells and plasmacytoid DCs the predominant human cell types expressing TLR9 (Klinman et al., 2004). It has been shown that CpG is rapidly internalized by immune cells, thus binding to TLR9 inside endocytic vesicles. In fact, unlike most TLRs, TLR9 is not expressed at the cell surface. Since the first report showing immunostimulatory effects on immune cells such as natural killer (NK) cells, a large number of preclinical studies have been performed with CpG motifs in animal models to assess whether CpG ODNs could boost the immune response elicited by vaccines. An ensemble of early experiments showed that the administration of these compounds in combination with or crosslinked to a reference antigen resulted in an antibody immune response enhanced by several orders of magnitude. The requirement for this effect to occur was the close spatial and temporal proximity of injection of both antigen and adjuvant. The antibody isotype profiling correlated with the induction of a Th1-type immune response; this was further supported in a variety of experiments, which indeed confirmed that CpG ODNs are potent inducers of Th1-type responses (Chu et al., 1997). In addition, CpG ODNs have been shown to increase, in a dose-dependent manner, *in vivo* IFN-γ secretion, consistent with a Th1-biased immune response. Subsequent studies established that CpG ODNs induce activation of DCs, implying improved antigen presentation of soluble proteins to class I-restricted T cells and stimulation of CTL responses (Askew et al., 2000; Shirota et al., 2001).

A large number of reports have presented data obtained in animal models using CpG ODNs as adjuvant of conventional antiviral vaccines. The coadministration of CpG ODNs and vaccines against influenza virus, measles virus, lymphocytic choriomeningitis virus, hepatitis B surface antigen, or tetanus toxoid was shown to induce an increase of the antibody titers up to three-fold with respect to vaccine alone, an antibody profile consistent

with IFN-γ production and the development of CTL responses. Of note, protection from virus challenge for some viral models was also observed. Studies in nonhuman primates for evaluating the potential of CpG ODNs to improve immune responses to reference antigens and experimental and conventional vaccines have also been performed (Verthelyi et al., 2002). The ensemble of preclinical data obtained in these animal models confirmed the expectations that selected compounds could boost immunity *in vivo* to otherwise ineffective vaccines. However, these studies have shown that different types of CpG ODNs may have optimal adjuvant activity for different vaccines. Therefore, while accumulating data are suggesting how to design these compounds in a more rational way, only results from relevant clinical studies will provide conclusive evidence on the effectiveness and advantages of using specific CpG ODNs in conjunction with vaccines.

Recently, some CpG ODNs have been developed for clinical use, and clinical trials with these compounds have been started, involving more than 500 subjects. These studies consisted in phase I clinical trials aimed at evaluating the safety and the immunomodulatory activity of CpG ODNs administered alone or in combination with licensed vaccines, antibodies, or allergens, and phase II studies in the field of cancer immunotherapy and allergy (Klinman et al., 2004). The results of a study in which CpG ODNs have been used as adjuvant of hepatitis B vaccine have shown an earlier development of antibody responses and a significant increase of geometric mean titers in recipients receiving vaccine plus ODNs (Halperin et al., 2003). In another study where CpG was administered as adjuvant of influenza vaccine (Klinman et al., 2000), an increase in antibody responses was detected only among subjects with preexisting antiflu antibodies, and PBMCs from these subjects proved to be capable of secreting large amounts of IFN-γ upon *in vitro* restimulation. Even though this ensemble of clinical data represents a proof of concept, further clinical investigation and optimization of the use of CpG ODNs are necessary to validate their use as vaccine adjuvants in humans.

PAMP-independent DC activation

A related though distinct concept for DC activation is the theory recently proposed by Matzinger and co-workers (Gallucci et al., 1999). This group has emphasized that "danger" signals produced by damaged or infected cells, rather than pathogen-derived components, represent major DC activation stimuli driving the immune response (Gallucci et al., 1999). This paradigm implies that the immune system can discriminate dangerous from harmless rather than self from nonself. This theory fits with the notion that the magnitude of the immune response is proportional to the tissue damage evoked by the adjuvant. Notably, the ability to cause danger by local reaction at the injection site seems to be a feature shared by most widely used adjuvants.

It has been suggested that the endogenous signals derived by wound cells may mimic PAMPs and act as ligands for some PRRs. Consistent with this notion, heat-shock proteins (HSPs) released by cells undergoing necrosis have been found to activate DCs via TLR2 and TLR4 in a PAMP-similar fashion. Although some controversy exists on this matter, the documented ability of HSPs to activate DCs through TLRs as well as to bind peptides and promote a MHC class I presentation pathway makes these molecules attractive candidates for peptide-based vaccines against tumors and intracellular pathogens (Srivastava and Amato, 2001).

Small-molecule immune potentiators: Imidazoquinolines

Whereas the study of PAMPs has represented an important impetus for the selection of products to be used as natural adjuvants for boosting DC-driven immunity, many laboratories are also putting their efforts in establishing platforms to develop new small-molecule immune potentiator (SMIP) approaches. This is mainly due to the need for relying on more potent and less toxic molecules. A family of compounds, which may hold promise for the future, is represented by the imidazoquinolines (Hemmi et al., 2002). These molecules have been shown to enhance the antigen-specific immune response in mouse models, by binding to TLR7 and TLR8 expressed on DCs (Jurk et al., 2002). It is clear that SMIP-based adjuvant development offers several advantages such as low-cost manufacturing, high purity, and more standardized chemical profiles. It is expected for the future an intensive investigation on these small compounds to be pursued in the perspective of their use as vaccine adjuvant in humans.

Cytokines and DCs

As highlighted in the previous sections, DCs possess the innate ability to respond to exogenous stimuli directly by using PRRs, which have evolved to recognize conserved structural features shared among potential noxious foreign agents (Pulendran, 2004). In addition, DCs are able to respond to endogenous signals locally produced by other components of the innate immune system and to translate them into an adaptive response (Reis and Sousa, 2004). This cross talk between innate and adaptive response is mediated by cytokines and DCs are the major players involved in this process (Belardelli and Ferrantini, 2002; Smyth et al., 2004). In particular, certain cytokines are produced rapidly in response to pathogens or "danger signals" and can profoundly affect the function of DCs by inducing differentiation, activation, maturation, and migration of these types of cells.

It has become increasingly evident that adjuvants generally act through the induction of cytokines, which are the key mediators of the immune response. This fact has raised the question of whether the direct use of certain selected cytokines as natural adjuvants could be of some advantage with respect to the conventional adjuvants. Attempts to give an answer to this issue have been pursued (Rizza et al., 2003) and here the most relevant preclinical investigation on cytokines potentially valuable as vaccine adjuvants as well as some remarkable clinical results are summarized. In this section, we focus on cytokines known to play an important role in linking innate and adaptive immunity, with special attention paid to GM-CSF, IL-12, and IFN-α, and to their action as vaccine adjuvants. It should be noted, however, that some of the effects induced by these cytokines may be due to the induction of other cytokines. For example, some of the IFN-α-induced effects on differentiation/activation of DCs and expansion/survival of memory CD8+ T cells may be mediated by IL-15, which is produced by DCs in response to IFN-α (Santini et al., 2000). Thus, complex interactions between host cells and cytokines determine the modalities and mechanisms involved in linking innate and adaptive immunity and regulate quality and intensity of the immune response. Because of space limitations, we will not review the role of IL-2 and IFN-γ, two important cytokines typically produced by cells of the adaptive immunity, which have also been used to enhance vaccine efficacy in experimental models.

▪ GM-CSF

The immunomodulatory effects of GM-CSF (Mellstedt et al., 1999) have represented the rationale of its use as adjuvant, especially with regard to the attempts to develop therapeutic cancer vaccines (Borrello and Pardoll, 2002; Weber et al., 2003). Some studies have shown that the use of soluble GM-CSF for vaccination therapy can enhance the induction of a humoral and a type 1 T cell response in cancer patients. In patients with advanced colon carcinoma, the combination of GM-CSF with an anticolon carcinoma monoclonal antibody resulted in a significant response rate. GM-CSF may augment the antibody antitumor effect by enhancing ADCC and by amplifying the induction of a humoral and cellular

idiotypic network response. However, GM-CSF may also induce an impairment of the immune response by virtue of its ability to recruit myeloid suppressor cells (Serafini et al., 2004). Activation vs. suppression of the immune response by GM-CSF may depend on the dose, with high doses promoting release of immunosuppressive factors by macrophages (Mellstedt et al., 1999). GM-CSF has been shown to promote a protective and therapeutic immunity in a variety of mouse tumor models, by using different strategies such as fusion protein vaccines, gene transfection into tumor cells or DCs, and DNA immunization (Warren et al. 2000). The encouraging results of the preclinical studies have prompted the testing of GM-CSF gene-transduced tumor vaccines in phase I and phase II clinical trials for immunotherapy of some malignancies (Borrello and Pardoll, 2002). GM-CSF has also been used as adjuvant of viral vaccines with little or poor success so far (Looney et al., 2001). Further studies are needed to better define the possible optimal modalities for using this cytokine as adjuvant of human vaccines.

▪ IL-12

IL-12 is mostly produced by macrophages and DCs in response to certain pathogens and activation factors and has been considered as a key cytokine in linking innate and adaptive immunity by the induction of a Th1 type of immune response (Colombo and Trinchieri, 2002). However, in spite of the promising results obtained in animal tumor models, the clinical use of IL-12 has been restricted by severe toxicity. In order to minimize the toxic effects associated with systemic administration of IL-12 and to exploit fully the immunomodulatory activities of this cytokine, a large number of studies in preclinical models of cancer have focused on gene therapy approaches (Melero et al., 2001). Overall, the results obtained in a variety of mouse tumor models indicate that IL-12 gene transfer leads to significant antitumor activity and to the development of a potent cellular immune response, with CD8+ T cells playing a major role in most models.

Type I IFN

Originally described for its antiviral activities, type I IFN has recently been shown to exert important effects on the immune system (Belardelli et al., 2002; Tough, 2004), including promotion of cellular and humoral responses by virtue of its adjuvant effects on APCs (Santini et al., 2002). Type I IFN (especially IFN-α) is the most widely used cytokine in patients with cancer and certain viral infections, such as hepatitis C. Recent studies have pointed out the potential interest of using type I IFN as an adjuvant of vaccines against cancer and infectious diseases (Belardelli et al., 2002; Proietti et al., 2002). In fact, these cytokines potently enhance both T cell and antibody responses to a soluble protein and promote immunological memory by acting on DCs (Le Bon et al., 2001). Furthermore, recent studies (Proietti et al., 2002; Bracci et al., 2005) have shown that: (i) endogenous type I IFN is indispensable for the action of several Th1-promoting adjuvants; and (ii) administration of this cytokine as an adjuvant of the human influenza vaccine results in a remarkable enhancement of vaccine immunogenicity in mice, comparable or even superior to that obtained with the most powerful adjuvants. Recent studies have shown that type I IFN is a potent inducer of the differentiation and activation of both mouse and human DCs (for a review, see Santini et al., 2003). Of note, studies in murine models have revealed that type I IFN is a potent enhancer of the cross-priming of CD8+ T cells against exogenous antigens by acting on DCs (Le Bon et al., 2003). The challenge will now be to evaluate whether the remarkable vaccine adjuvant activity observed in mouse models can also be demonstrated in humans.

In vivo targeting of DCs

One crucial issue in vaccination is to deliver efficiently the antigen to DCs in order to induce a protective immune response. Conventional adjuvants, such as aluminum salts or mineral oil emulsions, act by entrapping the antigen, thus allowing antigen stabilization and slow release. Importantly, they also induce a wide spectrum of proinflammatory cytokines and chemokines, which in turn promote the recruitment and activation of immune cells. This reaction may not always be beneficial for the development of the protective immune response. First, this mechanism acts nonspecifically on a broad range of immune cells and does not ensure that the key APCs are selected for stimulation. Second, it does not ensure that the desired cytokine milieu is evoked. Actually, aluminum salts, the currently used adjuvants in human vaccines, have been shown to be potent inducers of Th2-promoting cytokine profile, which does not always mirror the immune correlate of protection for many infectious agents (Gupta, 1998). In addition, failure of efficient antigen presentation or DC stimulation that is not optimal could impair the trigger of the immune response. Hence, a number of delivery systems have been developed for delivering more selectively the antigen to the APCs. These systems act mainly indirectly, by accessing specific endosomal uptake function of APCs and include emulsions, liposomes, immunostimulatory complexes (ISCOMs), virus-like particles, and microparticles. As these approaches are treated in more depth in other more specialized chapters, this section focuses only on the direct approach of *in vivo* targeting of DCs.

Steinman and co-workers have recently provided an important proof of feasibility of the *in vivo* targeting of the antigen directly to the DCs. This group has exploited the property exhibited by the DEC-205 molecule, an endocytic receptor and member of the C-type lectin-like receptor family, which is specifically expressed by DCs within the T cell area of lymphoid tissues and particularly abundant on lymphoid DCs. DEC-205 binding to microbial antigens results in an efficient transfer into the endocytic compartment for antigen processing and loading on MHC class II molecules, thus leading to CD4+ T cell proliferation (Engering et al., 2002). More interestingly, DEC-205 engagement may also induce CD8+ T cell responses, implying that cross-presentation mechanisms are ensured by recognition of antigen through this receptor (Bonifaz et al., 2002). Therefore, DEC-205 provides an efficient receptor-based mechanism for DCs to process proteins for MHC class I presentation *in vivo*.

To assess the potential of this receptor to act as a specific key for introducing antigen into DCs, an ensemble of experiments were performed in mice, by injecting a reference antigen fused to an antibody to DEC-205 (Bonifaz et al., 2002). The first experiments showed that this treatment, in the absence of additional stimuli for DC maturation, induced transient antigen-specific T cell activation followed by T cell deletion and unresponsiveness (Bonifaz et al., 2002). These results demonstrated that DCs play a crucial role in the maintenance of peripheral tolerance and that the state of maturation/activation of DCs does influence the balance of tolerance vs. immunity. Consistent with these results, further experiments did demonstrate that strong CD4+ and CD8+ T cell immunity is induced by the antibody-mediated antigen targeting via the DEC-205 receptor, as long as DC maturation stimulus (agonistic anti-CD40 antibody) was also administered (Bonifaz et al., 2004). Interestingly, this approach was found to generate much stronger immunity than the standard use of the soluble antigen injected with complete Freund's adjuvant. Furthermore, the antigen-coupled antibody rapidly reached distal sites, allowing a systemic delivery of the antigen to a large number of DCs. A prolonged presentation of the antigen in most lymphoid tissues was another feature observed in this model, which implies that antigens gaining access to DCs via this receptor may persist in subcellular compartments for long periods.

These results have major implications in designing vaccines. First, they represent an important proof of efficacy of antigen targeting *in vivo* to DCs, provided that maturation stimuli are also supplied, in inducing T cell-mediated protective immunity. This is of major importance for the development of antimicrobial and therapeutic cancer vaccines. Second, their exploitation could be of value for vaccination strategies aimed at inducing antigen-specific tolerance for the treatment of autoimmune diseases. Third, they provide information relevant for implementing other DC-based vaccination strategies, such as the approach of using *ex vivo* antigen-loaded autologous DCs, which is discussed in the last section of this chapter.

■ DCs as tools for the development of therapeutic vaccines

■ Clinical studies with DC-based vaccines

Over the last few years, much attention has been focused on the attempts to use DCs in the development of therapeutic vaccines against cancer (for recent reviews, see Figdor et al., 2004; Cerundolo et al., 2004). The overall evaluation of the results of clinical trials shows that although DC-based vaccines are superior to other cancer vaccines in inducing an immune response against tumor antigens, the general clinical response is not significantly improved. However, if we consider the continuously emerging knowledge on DC biology and the early phase of clinical experimentation, we can be optimistic about the chances of implementing the efficacy of DC-based cancer vaccines by manipulating DC functions and by identifying effective combination therapies. All this justifies a particular attention on DC-based vaccines. Table 2.1 summarizes the main published clinical trials involving the use of DC-based vaccines in patients. Most of the studies concern immunization protocols with DC-based vaccines in patients with melanoma and prostate and renal cancers. Of interest, a recent study by Lu et al. (2004) has

Table 2.1 Main clinical studies with DCs

Disease	Vaccine	No. of patients	Immune response[a]	Clinical response[a]	Authors
Melanoma	iDC[b] pulsed with tumor peptides or lysate	16	11/16	5/16	Nestle (1998)
Melanoma	mDC[c] pulsed with MAGE-3 peptide	13	8/11	6/11	Thurner (1999)
Melanoma	mDC pulsed with tumor peptides	14	4/14	8/14	Mackensen (2000)
Melanoma	mDC pulsed with tumor peptides	18	16/18	10/17	Banchereau (2001)
Melanoma	mDC pulsed with tumor peptides	28	12/16	9/16	Schuler-Thurner (2002)
Melanoma	mDC pulsed with tumor cells	19	3/10	6/12	O'Rourke (2003)
Melanoma	iDC pulsed with MART peptide	18	18/18	3/18	Butterfield (2003)
Melanoma	iDC pulsed with tumor peptides or lysate	33	5/15	9/33	Hersey (2004)
Prostate cancer	mDC pulsed with PSM-P1/PSM-P2	33	–	9/25	Murphy (1999)
Prostate cancer	mDC pulsed with PAP	21	21/21	6/21	Fong (2001a)
Prostate cancer	mDC pulsed with tumor antigen RNA	13	13/13	7/13	Heiser (2002)
RCC	mDC pulsed with tumor lysate	35	5/6	10/27	Holtl (2002)
RCC	mDC pulsed with tumor RNA	15	6/7	–	Su (2003)
RCC	mDC fused with tumor cells	12	7/12	4/12	Marten (2003)
Colon cancer	mDC pulsed with CEA paptide	12	7/12	5/12	Fong (2001b)
Myeloma	mDC pulsed with idiotype Ig	26	4/26	17/26	Liso (2000)
Follicular lymphoma	mDC pulsed with idiotype Ig	35	23/33	8/28	Timmerman (2002)
Cutaneous T cell lymphoma	mDC pulsed with tumor lysate	10	8/8	4/8	Maier (2003)
Gastrointestinal cancer	iDC pulsed with MAGE-3 peptide	12	4/8	3/8	Sadanger (2001)
Pediatric tumors	iDC pulsed with tumor lysate	15	3/7	6/7	Geiger (2001)
Malignant glioma	mDC fused with glioma cells	10	6/10	2/10	Kikuchi (2001)
Malignant glioma	mDC pulsed with tumor lysate	14	6/10	–	Yu (2004)
Nasopharyngeal cancer	mDC pulsed with EBV peptides	16	9/16	2/16	Lin (2002)
Cervical cancer	mDC pulsed with HPV E7 protein	1	1	1	Santin (2002)
AIDS	mDC pulsed with inactivated HIV	18	18/18	8/18	Lu (2004)

[a] Immune and clinical responses are reported according to the number of patients considered fully evaluable.
[b] iDC, immature dendritic cells.
[c] mDC, mature dendritic cells.

shown the efficacy of an autologous DC-based vaccine (DCs pulsed with inactivated HIV-1) in lowering HIV viremia in HIV-infected patients. In the studies summarized in Table 2.1, different protocols of DC preparations were used, thus rendering often difficult the interpretation of the overall results.

■ Protocols for the preparation of DC-based vaccines

There is no consensus yet on the optimal protocol and type of DCs to be used for the preparation of DC-based vaccines for clinical studies, even though it is widely accepted that DCs need to be subjected to some type of activation/maturation step in order to exert potent adjuvant activity for the generation of a potentially protective immune response. In healthy individuals, blood DCs represent 0.5–1.5% of peripheral blood mononuclear cells, thus rendering it difficult to obtain directly from blood samples clinically relevant DC numbers. However, blood DC counts have been shown to increase following cytokine administration. For example, G-CSF and Flt-3L are used to mobilize blood DCs, with an average increase of 40-fold or 10-fold in myeloid or lymphoid subsets, respectively (Pulendran et al., 2000; Maraskovsky et al., 2000), while G-CSF has been shown to favor selectively expansion of the CD123+ subset over the myeloid population (Arpinati et al., 2000). With regard to possible clinical applications of DC-based vaccines, after pulsing with the appropriate antigen(s) with or without exposure to cytokines, DCs are able to stimulate the host immune system and can be reinfused back into the donor or used for *in vitro* expansion of lymphocyte populations to be injected into patients. Notably, there is also growing evidence indicating that special types of DCs, prepared under particular conditions, can serve to induce and maintain tolerance (Jonuleit et al., 2001). This activity is largely dependent on DC ontogeny, maturation stage, and exposure to different

cytokines such as TGF-β or IL-10. In fact, exposure of immature DCs to IL-10 results in a switch in their phenotype, enabling them to favor the induction of anergic T cells, characterized by reduced IL-2 and IFN-γ production and low CD25 expression (Steinbrink et al., 1997; Steinbrink, et al., 1999), while antigen presentation by immature DCs can induce "regulatory T cells," producing large amounts of IL-10 (Shevach, 2000; Dhodapkar et al., 2001). It has been argued that the induction of regulatory T cells by immature DCs could be therapeutically exploited in patients with autoimmune diseases, while the injection of allogeneic immature DCs could promote tolerance to transplanted organs (Jonuleit et al., 2001; Steinman and Nussenzweig, 2002).

Figure 2.4 illustrates three methods of DC generation from blood progenitor cells.

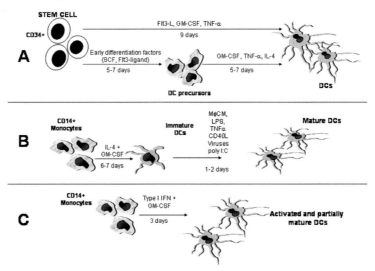

Figure 2.4 Main methods for generation of human DCs for the preparation of DC-based vaccines from precursor cells cultured in the presence of different cytokines. (A) Two main protocols for DC generation from CD34+ progenitor cells are illustrated. Accordingly to the first protocol (Banchereau et al., 2001), CD34+ cells are cultured for 9 days in medium containing GM-CSF, Flt3-L, and TNF-α to generate functionally active CD83^low DCs. According to a second protocol used by several groups, CD34+ cells are first cultured for 5–7 days in the presence of early differentiation factors (SCF, Flt3-L, and/or others) for generating DC precursors, which are then incubated for an additional 5–7 days in the presence of different cytokines, such as GM-CSF, TNF-α, and IL-4, to generate different types of functionally active DCs. (B) Exposure to IL-4 (alternatively IL-13) and GM-CSF drives monocytes to differentiate into immature DCs. This phenotype is lost upon cytokine deprivation or diverted upon exposure to different cytokines. Immature DCs are weak APCs, due to low/moderate surface expression of costimulatory molecules. Their activation/terminal maturation can be promoted by the addition of stimuli such as bacterial or viral components or products, recombinant soluble CD40L, macrophage conditioned medium (MCM), and cytokines, including IL-1β and TNF-α, which induce the expression of the maturation marker CD83 and a marked upregulation of costimulatory molecules. (C) Exposure of monocytes to type I IFN and GM-CSF rapidly induces their differentiation into partially mature DCs (IFN-DCs) expressing higher levels of costimulatory molecules and low to moderate levels of CD83 (Santini et al., 2000; Parlato et al., 2001).

The first one is based on the use of CD34+ stem cells, expanded and differentiated *in vitro* upon exposure to cytokine cocktails, including GM-CSF, IL-4, and TNF-α. Large numbers of immature myeloid DCs are currently generated *in vitro* from CD14+ monocytes exposed to GM-CSF and IL-4 or IL-13. These DCs are weak APCs, due to low/moderate surface expression of costimulatory molecules. However, their activation/maturation can be promoted by exposure to bacterial components, such as LPS, SAC, macrophage conditioned medium (MCM), and cytokines, including IL-1β and TNF-α, or recombinant soluble CD40L, which induce the expression of the maturation marker CD83 and a marked upregulation of costimulatory molecules (Sallusto and Lanzavecchia, 1994; Cella et al., 1997).

Even though the two-step protocol described above (i.e., DC differentiation in the presence of IL-4 or IL-13, and DC activation after exposure to maturation factors) has allowed the performance of the vast majority of clinical studies published so far and the definition of mechanisms of DC activation, it might be argued that DCs generated after several days of *in vitro* exposure of monocytes to high levels of cytokines such as IL-4 or IL-13 hardly reflect the possible scenario of a physiological exposure of monocytes to cytokines induced in the course of a natural infection. We have recently described a new protocol of DC generation from monocytes using type I IFN and GM-CSF (Santini et al., 2000). In particular, highly active partially mature DCs can be generated within 3 days after stimulation of monocytes with type I IFN and GM-CSF (Santini et al., 2000; Parlato et al., 2001). These cells (named IFN-DCs) were characterized by the expression of high levels of the costimulatory molecules CD80, CD86, and CD40 and displayed intermediate levels of CD123 expression. Notably, a variable percentage (12–40%) of the IFN-DCs expressed markers typical of mature DCs, such as CD83 and CD25. Consistent with the appearance of DC activation

markers, IFN-DCs produced significant amounts of IL-15 in culture supernatant without any further stimulus. A remarkable fraction of the IFN-DCs was shown to express CCR7 and showed a migratory response to CCL19 (previously named Mip-3β) (Parlato et al., 2001), a chemokine regulating DC trafficking to secondary lymphoid organs (Forster et al., 1999). Interestingly, IFN-DCs expressed considerable levels of the chemokine CCL19. Subsequent studies also showed that IFN-DCs where capable of inducing a potent CD8+ T cell response against viral (i.e., HIV-1 and EBV) (Lapenta et al., 2003; Santodonato et al., 2003) and tumor antigens (Tosi et al., 2004). When injected intravenously into immunodeficient SCID mice, IFN-DCs exhibited an enhanced migratory behavior with respect to immature DCs generated in the presence of IL-4, rapidly localizing within mouse skin, as demonstrated by the detection of human DNA sequences by RT-PCR (Parlato et al., 2001). Notably, when IFN-DCs pulsed with inactivated HIV-1 were injected into SCID mice reconstituted with autologous PBLs, these APCs proved to be far superior with respect to immature DCs generated in the presence of GM-CSF and IL-4 in inducing the generation of neutralizing anti-HIV-1 antibodies as well as human CD8 T cells reactive against HIV-1 antigens (Lapenta et al., 2003).

The ensemble of these results suggests that partially mature DCs generated from monocytes after a short-term exposure to type I IFN can represent valuable candidates to be used as powerful cellular adjuvants for the preparation of DC-based vaccines in patients with severe chronic infections (e.g., HIV-1, hepatitis C virus (HCV), and human papillomavirus (HPV)) and with certain types of cancer. Only well-designed comparative clinical studies based on the use of DCs generated by different methods will allow us to identify the optimal protocols and the cell phenotype most suitable for the preparation of DC-based vaccines in patients with cancer and different chronic infections.

Final remarks

The recent knowledge of the biology of DCs has opened new perspectives in vaccine research, leading to novel strategies based on either adjuvants selectively acting on DCs (DCs as targets) or on patients' DCs, modulated by cytokines and loaded with defined antigens in order to render them capable of rapidly inducing protective immunity in patients (DCs as tools for therapeutic vaccines). We have learned that new-generation adjuvants mimicking defined pathogen components (e.g., CpG oligos) can greatly enhance the immunogenicity of certain human vaccines and the importance of some cytokines acting on DCs in mediating vaccine adjuvant activity has been revealed. Likewise, we are beginning to understand how to target antigens to DCs and which soluble factors and cell-to-cell interactions need to occur in order to induce long-lasting immunity. There are many questions that still need to be addressed in order to identify optimal strategies for enhancing vaccine immunogenicy by adjuvants. For instance, if the immune-promoting activity induced by typical adjuvants is mediated by cytokines, why not directly use these factors as potentially more selective vaccine adjuvants? Which cytokines or cytokine combinations have a better chance of success? For some cytokines (i.e., type I IFNs, IL-2, and GM-CSF) with a long record of clinical use, their utilization as adjuvants for human vaccines should not pose relevant safety issues; however, we still need to improve our knowledge of how to use these cytokines, alone or in combination with other immune interventions, especially in the case of therapeutic vaccinations. Results from relevant clinical studies are expected to be available in the near future. They will provide the basis for further investigation and will tell us whether some of the remarkable results obtained in mice using cytokines as adjuvants can be translated to humans. It is reasonable to assume that now that we understand much more about the important steps in the initiation and regulation of the immune response, novel and more selective and effective immune adjuvants will be identified in the near future, thus leading to new perspectives for the development of prophylactic and therapeutic vaccines against infectious diseases and cancer.

If we have now good chances of developing novel and more effective strategies for acting on DCs in order to enhance vaccine efficacy, much attention and major expectations are focused on DC-based vaccines to be used in patients with cancer and certain infectious diseases for therapeutic vaccinations. In the light of the complex biology of DCs and in view of an expanding clinical use of DCs for immunotherapy, a requirement for successful clinical immune intervention is the definition of standardized procedures for both DC generation and cell quality controls. Other important issues to be addressed are the definition of the required DC number to be injected to obtain a favorable clinical response and the optimal treatment schedule. The ideal injection route is also far from being identified and systematic comparative studies in clinical trials are needed. The choice of the injection site can be linked to the standardization of the procedures of DC preparation, as DCs obtained by different methods are likely to express different adhesion molecules and chemokine receptors and exhibit various functional characteristics, including the migration activity in response to distinct sets of chemokines. However, in spite of the several still unclear aspects regarding the optimal modalities for preparing and using DC-based vaccines, the research progress in this field is so rapid that we predict that, in the near future, cell therapies based on the use of DCs will represent a valuable treatment option for certain patients with cancer or infectious diseases.

Acknowledgments

The authors are grateful to Cinzia Gasparrini and Anna Ferrigno for excellent secretarial assistance. Work in the authors' laboratory was supported in part by grants from the Italian Association for Cancer Research and from the Italian Ministry of Health (special project entitled "Dendritic Cells and Type I IFN" n°IAE/F)

■ References

Arpinati, M., Green, C.L., Heimfeld, S., Heuser, J.E., and Anasetti, C. (2000). Granulocyte-colony stimulating factor mobilizes T helper 2-inducing dendritic cells. *Blood* 95, 2484–2490.

Askew, D., Chu, R.S., Krieg, A.M., and Harding, C.V. (2000). CpG DNA induces maturation of dendritic cells with distinct effects on nascent and recycling MHC-II antigen-processing mechanisms. *J. Immunol.* 165, 6889–6895.

Banchereau, J., Briere, F., Caux, C., Davoust, J., Lebecque, S., Liu, Y.J., Pulendran, B., and Palucka, K. (2000). Immuno-biology of dendritic cells. *Annu. Rev. Immunol.* 18, 767–811.

Banchereau, J., Palucka, A.K., Dhodapkar, M., Burkeholder, S., Taquet, N., Rolland, A., Taquet, S., Coquery, S., Wittkowski, K.M., Bhardwaj, N., Pineiro, L., Steinman, R., and Fay, J. (2001). Immune and clinical responses in patients with metastatic melanoma to CD34(+) progenitor-derived dendritic cell vaccine. *Cancer Res.* 61, 6451–6458.

Belardelli, F. and Ferrantini, M. (2002). Cytokines as a link between innate and adaptive antitumor immunity. *Trends Immunol.* 23, 201–208.

Belardelli, F., Ferrantini, M., Proietti, E., and Kirkwood, J.M. (2002). Interferon-alpha in tumor immunity and immu-notheraphy. *Cytokine Growth Factor Rev.* 13, 119–134.

Bonifaz, L., Bonnyay, D., Mahnke, K., Rivera, M., Nussenzweig, M.C., and Steinman, R.M. (2002). Efficient targeting of protein antigen to the dendritic cell receptor DEC-205 in the steady state leads to antigen presentation on major histocompatibility complex class I products and peripheral CD8+ T cell tolerance. *J. Exp. Med.* 196, 1627–1638.

Bonifaz, L.C., Bonnyay, D.P., Charalambous, A., Darguste, D.I., Fujii, S., Soares, H., Brimnes, M.K., Moltedo, B., Moran, T.M., and Steinman, R.M. (2004). In vivo targeting of anti-gens to maturing dendritic cells via the DEC-205 receptor improves T cell vaccination. *J. Exp. Med.* 199, 815–824.

Borrello, I. and Pardoll, D. (2002). GM-CSF-based cellular vaccines: a review of the clinical experience. *Cytokine Growth Factor Rev.* 13, 185–193.

Bracci, L., Canini, I., Puzelli, S., Sestili, P., Venditti, M., Spada, M., Donatelli, I., Belardelli, F., and Proietti, E. (2005). Type I IFN is a powerful mucosal adjuvant for a selective intranasal vaccination against influenza virus in mice and affects antigen entrapment at mucosal level. *Vaccine* 23, 2994–3004.

Butterfield, L.H., Ribas, A., Dissette, V.B., Amarnani, S.N., Vu, H.T., Oseguera, D., Wang, H.J., Elashoff, R.M., McBride, W.H., Mukherji, B., Cochran, A.J., Glaspy, J.A., and Economou, J.S. (2003). Determinant spreading associated with clinical response in dendritic cell-based immunotherapy for malignant melanoma. *Clin. Cancer Res.* 9, 998–1008.

Cella, M., Sallusto, F., and Lanzavecchia, A. (1997). Origin, maturation, and antigen-presenting function of dendritic cells. *Curr. Opin. Immunol.* 9, 10–16.

Cella, M., Jarrossay, D., Facchetti, F., Alebardi, O., Nakajima, H., Lanzavecchia, A., and Colonna, M. (1999). Plasmacytoid monocytes migrate to inflamed lymph nodes and produce large amounts of type I interferon. *Nature Med.* 5, 919–923.

Cerundolo, V., Hermans, I.F., and Salio, M. (2004). Dendritic cells: a journey from laboratory to clinic. *Nature Immunol.* 5, 7–10.

Chu, R.S., Targoni, O.S., Krieg, A.M., Lehmann, P.V., and Harding, C.V. (1997). CpG oligodeoxynucleotides act as adjuvants that switch on T helper 1 (Th1) immunity. *J. Exp. Med.* 186, 1623–1631.

Colombo, M.P. and Trinchieri, G. (2002). Interleukin-12 in anti-tumor immunity and immunotherapy. *Cytokine Growth Factor Rev.* 13, 155–168.

Dhodapkar, M.V., Steinman, R.M., Krasovsky, J., Munz, C., and Bhardwaj, N. (2001). Antigen-specific inhibition of effector T cell function in humans after injection of immature dendritic cells. *J. Exp. Med.* 193, 233–238.

Engering, A., Geijtenbeek, T.B., and van Kooyk, Y. (2002). Immune escape through C-type lectins on dendritic cells. *Trends Immunol.* 23, 480–485.

Figdor, C.G., de Vries, I.J., Lesterhuis, W.J., and Melief, C.J. (2004). Dendritic cell immunotherapy: mapping the way. *Nature Med.* 10, 475–480.

Fong, L., Brockstedt, D., Benike, C., Breen, J.K., Strang, G., Ruegg, C.L., and Engleman, E.G. (2001a). Dendritic cell-based xenoantigen vaccination for prostate cancer immu-notherapy. *J. Immunol.* 167, 7150–7156.

Fong, L., Hou, Y., Rivas, A., Benike, C., Yuen, A., Fisher, G.A., Davis, M.M., and Engleman, E.G. (2001b). Altered peptide ligand vaccination with Flt3 ligand expanded dendritic cells for tumor immunotherapy. *Proc. Natl. Acad. Sci. USA* 98, 8809–8814.

Forster, R., Schubel, A., Breitfeld, D., Kremmer, E., Renner-Muller, I., Wolf, E., and Lipp, M. (1999). CCR7 coordinates the primary immune response by establishing function in secondary lymphoid organs. *Cell* 99, 23–33.

Gallucci, S., Lolkema, M., and Matzinger, P. (1999). Natural adjuvants: endogenous activators of dendritic cells. *Nature Med.* 5, 1249–1255.

Geiger, J.D., Hutchinson, R.J., Hohenkirk, L.F., McKenna, E.A., Yanik, G.A., Levine, J.E., Chang, A.E., Braun, T.M., and Mule, J.J. (2001). Vaccination of pediatric solid tumor patients with tumor lysate-pulsed dendritic cells can expand specific T cells and mediate tumor regression. *Cancer Res.* 61, 8513–8519.

Gupta, R.K. (1998). Aluminum compounds as vaccine adjuvants. *Adv. Drug Deliv. Rev.* 32, 155–172.

Halperin, S.A., Van Nest, G., Smith, B., Abtahi, S., Whiley, H., and Eiden, J.J. (2003). A phase I study of the safety and immunogenicity of recombinant hepatitis B surface antigen co-administered with an immunostimulatory phosphorothioate oligonucleotide adjuvant. *Vaccine* 21, 2461–2467.

Hart, D.N. (1997). Dendritic cells: unique leukocyte populations which control the primary immune response. *Blood* 90, 3245–3287.

Hart, D.N. (2001). Dendritic cells and their emerging clinical applications. *Pathology* 33, 479–492.

Heiser, A., Coleman, D., Dannull, J., Yancey, D., Maurice, M.A., Lallas, C.D., Dahm, P., Niedzwiecki, D., Gilboa, E., and Vieweg, J. (2002). Autologous dendritic cells transfected with prostate-specific antigen RNA stimulate CTL responses against metastatic prostate tumors. *J. Clin. Invest.* 109, 409–417.

Hemmi, H., Kaisho, T., Takeuchi, O., Sato, S., Sanjo, H., Hoshino, K., Horiuchi, T., Tomizawa, H., Takeda, K., and Akira, S. (2002). Small anti-viral compounds activate immune cells via the TLR7 MyD88-dependent signaling pathway. *Nature Immunol.* 3, 196–200.

Hersey, P., Menzies, S.W., Halliday, G.M., Nguyen, T., Farrelly, M.L., De Silva, C., and Lett, M. (2004). Phase I/II study of treatment with dendritic cell vaccines in patients with disseminated melanoma. *Cancer Immunol. Immunother.* 53, 125–134.

Holtl, L., Zelle-Rieser, C., Gander, H., Papesh, C., Ramoner, R., Bartsch, G., Rogatsch, H., Barsoum, A.L., Coggin, J.H. Jr., and Thurnher, M. (2002). Immunotherapy of metastatic renal cell carcinoma with tumor lysate-pulsed autologous dendritic cells. *Clin. Cancer Res.* 8, 3369–3376.

Janeway, C.A. Jr. (1989). Approaching the asymptote? Evolution and revolution in immunology. *Cold Spring Harbor Symp. Quant. Biol.* 54 (Pt 1), 1–13.

Jonuleit, H., Schmitt, E., Steinbrink, K., and Enk, A.H. (2001). Dendritic cells as a tool to induce anergic and regulatory T cells. *Trends Immunol.* 22, 394–400.

Jurk, M., Heil, F., Vollmer, J., Schetter, C., Krieg, A.M., Wagner, H., Lipford, G., and Bauer, S. (2002). Human TLR7 or TLR8 independently confer responsiveness to the antiviral compound R-848. *Nature Immunol.* 3, 499.

Kikuchi, T., Akasaki, Y., Irie, M., Homma, S., Abe, T., and Ohno, T. (2001). Results of a phase I clinical trial of vaccination of glioma patients with fusions of dendritic and glioma cells. *Cancer Immunol. Immunother.* 50, 337–344.

Klinman, D.M., Ishii, K.J., Gursel, M., Gursel, I., Takeshita, S., and Takeshita, F. (2000). Immunotherapeutic applications of CpG-containing oligodeoxynucleotides. *Drug News Perspect.* 13, 289–296.

Klinman, D.M., Currie, D., Gursel, I., and Verthelyi, D. (2004). Use of CpG oligodeoxynucleotides as immune adjuvants. *Immunol. Rev.* 199, 201–216.

Krieg, A.M., Yi, A.K., Matson, S., Waldschmidt, T.J., Bishop, G.A., Teasdale, R., Koretzky, G.A., and Klinman, D.M. (1995). CpG motifs in bacterial DNA trigger direct B-cell activation. *Nature* 374, 546–549.

Lapenta, C., Santini, S.M., Logozzi, M., Spada, M., Andreotti, M., Di Pucchio, T., Parlato, S., and Belardelli, F. (2003). Potent immune response against HIV-1 and

protection from virus challenge in hu-PBL-SCID mice immunized with inactivated-virus-pulsed dendritic cells generated in the presence of IFN-α. *J. Exp. Med.* 198, 361–367.

Le Bon, A., Schiavoni, G., D'Agostino, G., Gresser, I., Belardelli, F., and Tough, D.F. (2001). Type I interferons potently enhance humoral immunity and can promote isotype switching by stimulating dendritic cells in vivo. *Immunity* 14, 461–470.

Le Bon, A., Etchart, N., Rossmann, C., Ashton, M., Hou, S., Gewert, D., Borrow, P., and Tough, D.F. (2003). Cross-priming of CD8+ T cells stimulated by virus-induced type I interferon. *Nature Immunol.* 4, 1009–1015.

Lin, C.L., Lo, W.F., Lee, T.H., Ren, Y., Hwang, S.L., Cheng, Y.F., Chen, C.L., Chang, Y.S., Lee, S.P., Rickinson, A.B., and Tam, P.K. (2002). Immunization with Epstein–Barr Virus (EBV) peptide-pulsed dendritic cells induces functional CD8+ T-cell immunity and may lead to tumor regression in patients with EBV-positive nasopharyngeal carcinoma. *Cancer Res.* 62, 6952–6958.

Liso, A., Stockerl-Goldstein, K.E., Auffermann-Gretzinger, S., Benike, C.J., Reichardt, V., van Beckhoven, A., Rajapaksa, R., Engleman, E.G., Blume, K.G., and Levy, R. (2000). Idiotype vaccination using dendritic cells after autologous peripheral blood progenitor cell transplantation for multiple myeloma. *Biol. Blood Marrow Transplant.* 6, 621–627.

Liu, Y.J. (2001). Dendritic cell subsets and lineages, and their functions in innate and adaptive immunity. *Cell* 106, 259–262.

Looney, R.J., Hasan, M.S., Coffin, D., Campbell, D., Falsey, A.R., Kolassa, J., Agosti, J.M., Abraham, G.N., and Evans, T.G. (2001). Hepatitis B immunization of healthy elderly adults: relationship between naive CD4+ T cells and primary immune response and evaluation of GM-CSF as an adjuvant. *J. Clin. Immunol.* 21, 30–36.

Lu, W., Arraes, L.C., Ferreira, W.T., and Andrieu, J.M. (2004). Therapeutic dendritic-cell vaccine for chronic HIV-1 infection. *Nature Med.* 10, 1359–1365.

Mackensen, A., Herbst, B., Chen, J.L., Kohler, G., Noppen, C., Herr, W., Spagnoli, G.C., Cerundolo, V., and Lindemann, A. (2000). Phase I study in melanoma patients of a vaccine with peptide-pulsed dendritic cells generated in vitro from CD34(+) hematopoietic progenitor cells. *Int. J. Cancer* 86, 385–392.

Maier, T., Tun-Kyi, A., Tassis, A., Jungius, K.P., Burg, G., Dummer, R., and Nestle, F.O. (2003). Vaccination of patients with cutaneous T-cell lymphoma using intranodal injection of autologous tumor-lysate-pulsed dendritic cells. *Blood* 102, 2338–2344.

Maraskovsky, E., Daro, E., Roux, E., Teepe, M., Maliszewski, C.R., Hoek, J., Caron, D., Lebsack, M.E., and McKenna, H.J. (2000). In vivo generation of human dendritic cell subsets by Flt3 ligand. *Blood* 96, 878–884.

Marten, A., Renoth, S., Heinicke, T., Albers, P., Pauli, A., Mey, U., Caspari, R., Flieger, D., Hanfland, P., Von Ruecker, A., Eis-Hubinger, A.M., Muller, S., Schwaner, I.,

Lohmann, U., Heylmann, G., Sauerbruch, T., and Schmidt-Wolf, I.G. (2003). Allogeneic dendritic cells fused with tumor cells: preclinical results and outcome of a clinical phase I/II trial in patients with metastatic renal cell carcinoma. *Human Gene Ther.* 14, 483–494.

Medzhitov, R., Preston-Hurlburt, P., and Janeway, C.A. Jr. (1997). A human homologue of the Drosophila Toll protein signals activation of adaptive immunity. *Nature* 388, 323–324.

Melero, I., Mazzolini, G., Narvaiza, I., Qian, C., Chen, L., and Prieto, J. (2001). IL-12 gene therapy for cancer: in synergy with other immunotherapies. *Trends Immunol.* 22, 113–115.

Mellstedt, H., Fagerberg, J., Frodin, J.E., Henriksson, L., Hjelm-Skoog, A.L., Liljefors, M., Ragnhammar, P., Shetye, J., and Osterborg, A. (1999). Augmentation of the immune response with granulocyte-macrophage colony-stimulating factor and other hematopoietic growth factors. *Curr. Opin. Hematol.* 6, 169–175.

Murphy, G.P., Tjoa, B.A., Simmons, S.J., Jarisch, J., Bowes, V.A., Ragde, H., Rogers, M., Elgamal, A., Kenny, G.M., Cobb, O.E., Ireton, R.C., Troychak, M.J., Salgaller, M.L., and Boynton, A.L. (1999). Infusion of dendritic cells pulsed with HLA-A2-specific prostate-specific membrane antigen peptides: a phase II prostate cancer vaccine trial involving patients with hormone-refractory metastatic disease. *Prostate* 38, 73–78.

Nestle, F.O., Alijagic, S., Gilliet, M., Sun, Y., Grabbe, S., Dummer, R., Burg, G., and Schadendorf, D. (1998). Vaccination of melanoma patients with peptide- or tumor lysate-pulsed dendritic cells. *Nature Med.* 4, 328–332.

O'Hagan, D.T., and Valiante, N.M. (2003). Recent advances in the discovery and delivery of vaccine adjuvants. *Nature Rev. Drug Discov.* 2, 727–735.

O'Rourke, M.G., Johnson, M., Lanagan, C., See, J., Yang, J., Bell, J.R., Slater, G.J., Kerr, B.M., Crowe, B., Purdie, D.M., Elliott, S.L., Ellem, K.A., and Schmidt, C.W. (2003). Durable complete clinical responses in a phase I/II trial using an autologous melanoma cell/dendritic cell vaccine. *Cancer Immunol. Immunother.* 52, 387–395.

Parlato, S., Santini, S.M., Lapenta, C., Di Pucchio, T., Logozzi, M., Spada, M., Giammarioli, A.M., Malorni, W., Fais, S., and Belardelli, F. (2001). Expression of CCR-7, MIP-3beta, and Th-1 chemokines in type I IFN-induced monocyte-derived dendritic cells: importance for the rapid acquisition of potent migratory and functional activities. *Blood* 98, 3022–3029.

Proietti, E., Bracci, L., Puzelli, S., Di Pucchio, T., Sestili, P., De Vincenti, E., Venditti, M., Capone, I., Seif, I., De Maeyer, E., Tough, D., Donatelli, I., and Belardelli, F. (2002). Type I interferon as a natural adjuvant for a protective immune response: lessons from the influenza vaccine model. *J. Immunol.* 169, 375–383.

Pulendran, B. (2004). Modulating vaccine responses with dendritic cells and Toll-like receptors. *Immunol. Rev.* 199, 227–250.

Pulendran, B., Banchereau, J., Burkeholder, S., Kraus, E., Guinet, E., Chalouni, C., Caron, D., Maliszewski, C.,

Davoust, J., Fay, J., and Palucka, K. (2000). Flt3-ligand and granulocyte colony-stimulating factor mobilize distinct human dendritic cell subsets in vivo. *J. Immunol.* 165, 566–572.

Reis, E. and Sousa, C. (2004). Activation of dendritic cells: translating innate into adaptive immunity. *Curr. Opin. Immunol.* 16, 21–25.

Rizza, P., Ferrantini, M., Capone, I., and Belardelli, F. (2002). Cytokines as natural adjuvants for vaccine: where are we now? *Trends Immunol.* 23, 381–383.

Sadanaga, N., Nagashima, H., Mashino, K., Tahara K., Yamaguchi, H., Ohta, M., Fujie, T., Tanaka, F., Inoue, H., Takesako, K., Akiyoshi, T., and Mori, M. (2001). Dendritic cell vaccination with MAGE peptide is a novel therapeutic approach for gastrointestinal carcinomas. *Clin. Cancer Res.* 7, 2277–2284.

Sallusto, F. and Lanzavecchia, A. (1994). Efficient presentation of soluble antigen by cultured human dendritic cells is maintained by granulocyte/macrophage colony-stimulating factor plus interleukin 4 and downregulated by tumor necrosis factor alpha. *J. Exp. Med.* 179, 1109–1118.

Santin, A.D., Bellone, S., Gokden, M., Cannon, M.J., and Parham, G.P. (2002). Vaccination with HPV-18 E7-pulsed dendritic cells in a patient with metastatic cervical cancer. *New Engl. J. Med.* 346, 1752–1753.

Santini, S.M., Lapenta, C., Logozzi, M., Parlato, S., Spada, M., Di Pucchio, T., and Belardelli, F. (2000). Type I interferon as a powerful adjuvant for monocyte-derived dendritic cell development and activity in vitro and in Hu-PBL-SCID mice. *J. Exp. Med.* 191, 1777–1788.

Santini, S.M., Di Pucchio, T., Lapenta, C., Logozzi, M., Parlato, S., and Belardelli, F. (2002). The natural alliance between type I IFN and dendritic cells and its role in linking innate and adaptive immunity. *J. Interferon Cytokine Res.* 11, 1071–1080.

Santini, S.M., Di Pucchio, T., Lapenta, C., Parlato, S., Logozzi, M., and Belardelli, F. (2003) A new type I IFN-mediated pathway for the rapid differentiation of monocytes into highly active dendritic cells. *Stem Cells* 21, 357–362.

Santodonato, L., D'Agostino, G., Nisini, R., Mariotti, S., Monque, D. M., Spada, M., Lattanzi, L., Perrone, M.P., Andreotti, M., Belardelli, F., and Ferrantini, M. (2003). Monocyte-derived dendritic cells generated after a short-term culture with IFN-α and granulocyte-macrophage colony-stimulating factor stimulate a potent Epstein-Barr virus-specific CD8+ T cell response. *J. Immunol.* 170, 5195–5202.

Schijns, V.E. (2003). Mechanisms of vaccine adjuvant activity: initiation and regulation of immune responses by vaccine adjuvants. *Vaccine* 21, 829–831.

Schuler-Thurner, B., Schultz, E.S., Berger, T.G., Weinlich, G., Ebner, S., Woerl, P., Bender, A., Feuerstein, B., Fritsch, P.O., Romani, N., and Schuler, G. (2002) Rapid induction of tumor-specific type 1 T helper cells in metastatic melanoma patients by vaccination with mature, cryopreserved, peptide-loaded monocyte-derived dendritic cells. *J. Exp. Med.* 195, 1279–1288.

Serafini, P., Carbley, R., Noonan, K.A., Tan, G., Bronte, V., and Borrello, I. (2004). High-dose granulocyte-macrophage colony-stimulating factor-producing vaccines impair the immune response through the recruitment of myeloid suppressor cells. *Cancer Res.* 64, 6337–6343.

Shevach, E.M. (2000). Regulatory T cells in autoimmunity. *Annu. Rev. Immunol.* 18, 423–449.

Shirota, H., Sano, K., Hirasawa, N., Terui, T., Ohuchi, K., Hattori, T., Shirato, K., and Tamura, G. (2001). Novel roles of CpG oligodeoxynucleotides as a leader for the sampling and presentation of CpG-tagged antigen by dendritic cells. *J. Immunol.* 167, 66–74.

Siegal, F.P., Kadowaki, N., Shodell, M., Fitzgerald-Bocarsly, P.A., Shah, K., Ho, S., Antonenko, S., and Liu, Y.J. (1999). The nature of the principal type I interferon-producing cells in human blood. *Science* 284, 1835–1837.

Smyth, M.J., Cretney, E., Kershaw, M.H., and Hayakawa, Y. (2004). Cytokines in cancer immunity and immunotherapy. *Immunol. Rev.* 202, 275–293.

Sozzani, S., Allavena, P., Vecchi, A., and Mantovani, A. (1999). The role of chemokines in the regulation of dendritic cell trafficking. *J. Leukoc. Biol.* 66, 1–9.

Srivastava, P.K., and Amato, R.J. (2001). Heat shock proteins: the "Swiss Army Knife" vaccines against cancers and infectious agents. *Vaccine* 19, 2590–2597.

Steinbrink, K., Wolfl, M., Jonuleit, H., Knop, J., and Enk, A.H. (1997). Induction of tolerance by IL-10-treated dendritic cells. *J. Immunol.* 159, 4772–4780.

Steinbrink, K., Jonuleit, H., Muller, G., Schuler, G., Knop, J., and Enk, A.H. (1999). Interleukin-10-treated human dendritic cells induce a melanoma-antigen-specific anergy in CD8(+) T cells resulting in a failure to lyse tumor cells. *Blood* 93, 1634–1642.

Steinman, R.M. and Dhodapkar, M. (2001). Active immunization against cancer with dendritic cells: the near future. *Int. J. Cancer* 94, 459–473.

Steinman, R.M., and Nussenzweig, M.C. (2002). Avoiding horror autotoxicus: the importance of dendritic cells in peripheral T cell tolerance. *Proc. Natl. Acad. Sci. USA* 99, 351–358.

Su, Z., Dannull, J., Heiser, A., Yancey, D., Pruitt, S., Madden, J., Coleman, D., Niedzwiecki, D., Gilboa, E., and Vieweg, J. (2003). Immunological and clinical responses in metastatic renal cancer patients vaccinated with tumor RNA-transfected dendritic cells. *Cancer Res.* 63, 2127–2133.

Svane, I.M., Soot, M.L., Buus, S., and Johnsen, H.E. (2003). Clinical application of dendritic cells in cancer vaccination therapy. *APMIS* 111, 818–834.

Takeda, K., Kaisho, T., and Akira, S. (2003). Toll-like receptors. *Annu. Rev. Immunol.* 21, 335–376.

Thurner, B., Haendle, I., Roder, C., Dieckmann, D., Keikavoussi, P., Jonuleit, H., Bender, A., Maczek, C., Schreiner, D., von den Driesch, P., Brocker, E.B., Steinman, R.M., Enk, A., Kampgen, E., and Schuler, G. (1999). Vaccination with mage-3A1 peptide-pulsed mature, monocyte-derived dendritic cells expands specific cytotoxic T cells and induces regression of some metastases in advanced stage IV melanoma. *J. Exp. Med.* 190, 1669–1678.

Timmerman, J.M., Czerwinski, D.K., Davis, T.A., Hsu, F.J., Benike, C., Hao, Z.M., Taidi, B., Rajapaksa, R., Caspar, C.B., Okada, C.Y., van Beckhoven, A., Liles, T.M., Engleman, E.G., and Levy, R. (2002). Idiotype-pulsed dendritic cell vaccination for B-cell lymphoma: clinical and immune responses in 35 patients. *Blood* 99, 1517–1526.

Tosi, D., Valenti, R., Cova, A., Sovena, G., Huber, V., Pilla, L., Arienti, F., Belardelli, F., Parmiani, G., and Rivoltini, L. (2004). Role of cross-talk between IFN-α-induced monocyte-derived dendritic cells and NK cells in priming CD8+ T cell responses against human tumor antigens. *J. Immunol.* 172, 5363–5370.

Tough, D.F. (2004). Type I interferon as a link between innate and adaptive immunity through dendritic cell stimulation. *Leuk. Lymphoma* 45, 257–264.

Verthelyi, D., Kenney, R.T., Seder, R.A., Gam, A.A., Friedag, B., and Klinman, D.M. (2002). CpG oligodeoxynucleotides as vaccine adjuvants in primates. *J. Immunol.* 168, 1659–1663.

Warren, T.L. and Weiner, G.J. (2000). Uses of granulocyte-macrophage colony-stimulating factor in vaccine development. *Curr. Opin. Hematol.* 7, 168–173.

Weber, J., Sondak, V.K., Scotland, R., Phillip, R., Wang, F., Rubio, V., Stuge, T.B., Groshen, S.G., Gee, C., Jeffery, G.G., Sian, S., and Lee, P.P. (2003). Granulocyte-macrophage colony-stimulating factor added to a multipeptide vaccine for resected stage II melanoma. *Cancer* 97, 186–200.

Yu, J.S., Liu, G., Ying, H., Yong, W.H., Black, K.L., and Wheeler, C.J. (2004). Vaccination with tumor lysate-pulsed dendritic cells elicits antigen-specific, cytotoxic T-cells in patients with malignant glioma. *Cancer Res.* 64, 4973–4979.

Host-derived molecules as adjuvants

Tom Barr
University of Edinburgh Institute of Immunology and Infection Research (IIIR), Edinburgh, UK

Jennifer Carlring and Andrew W. Heath
University of Sheffield School of Medicine and Biomedical Sciences, Sheffield, UK

■ Introduction

This chapter covers the use of various host-derived molecules (or antibodies directed against them) as immunological adjuvants for prophylactic and therapeutic vaccines. The use of host-derived molecules rather than materials derived from bacterial cell walls or plants offers advantages in terms of rational design of adjuvants. At least a prediction, if not a full understanding, of the mode of action of the molecule as an adjuvant comes along with knowledge of the biological function of the particular cytokine or host molecule. This is in contrast to adjuvants derived from other sources, where the mode of action has often had to be determined long after efficacy has been proved, and in some cases is still not fully understood. Furthermore, all of the adjuvants described here are proteins, and can therefore be produced often using the same techniques as are used to produce recombinant vaccine antigens. Another advantage of using proteins as adjuvants is that DNA encoding them can easily be incorporated into nucleic acid vaccines along with DNA encoding the antigen. Along with these advantages of host-derived molecules lie some inherent dangers, the most obvious of which is the possibility of generating autoimmune responses against the host molecule used as an adjuvant in the vaccine. Some of the targets of the adjuvants described herein are shown in Figure 3.1.

There is a wealth of literature on the expression of cytokines and other host molecules by live attenuated organisms, or by tumor cells. We have not attempted to cover those applications here. Instead, we have concentrated on nonliving subunit and DNA vaccines.

■ Cytokines as immunological adjuvants

Cytokines were probably the earliest identified host molecules with adjuvant potential. The first cytokines were cloned and produced in recombinant form more than two decades ago. They are, with a few exceptions, small monomers, homodimers, or homotrimers and almost all of them retain biological activity when produced in bacterial expression systems. Hence they offer the prospect of cheap production using the same methods as might be used to produce the vaccine antigens themselves. The biological functions of cytokines are perhaps better understood than those of bacterially derived adjuvants, and in many

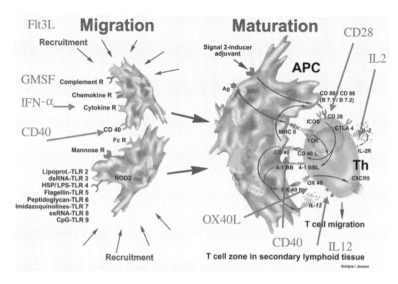

Figure 3.1 Some targets on APCs of the adjuvants discussed within this chapter. (See Color Plate Section.)

cases, clinical safety data are already in the public domain because of a previous history of the use of the cytokine in the therapy of diseases such as cancer. Finally, cytokine-encoding DNA can relatively easily be added into DNA vaccines in an attempt to improve immunogenicity, and this has led to a resurgence in interest in cytokine adjuvants (recently reviewed by Barouch et al., 2004).

The first cytokines to generate interest as potential immunological adjuvants were also, probably not coincidentally, three of the first to be identified and cloned. These were interleukin 1 (IL1), IL2, and interferon gamma (IFNγ). Early work on these three cytokines and their potential as adjuvants has been quite extensively reviewed (Heath and Playfair, 1992; Heath, 1995a; Lin et al., 1995) and we only summarize this early work here.

■ Interferon gamma

IFNγ was probably an early front-runner among these three simply in terms of the practical application of its adjuvant properties. IFNγ was found to be at its most effective mixed with the antigen (Playfair and deSouza, 1987), whereas the other two cytokines in this group presented problems in terms of timing

of administration (see below). Initial studies using a complex murine malaria vaccine were confirmed with purified proteins, and IFNγ was shown to be a more potent adjuvant when administered attached to the antigen (Heath and Playfair, 1990), a finding that was later to be exploited via the use of recombinant fusions between antigen and IFNγ (see below).

IFNγ has been shown to be an effective adjuvant in clinical trials in hepatitis B vaccine nonresponders (Quiroga et al., 1990).

■ Interleukin 2

IL2 was initially found to be an effective adjuvant when administered in a number of different ways. It seems possible that the mode of action varied in each case. The method of administration most studied in early reports was the use of multiple injections after administration of the antigen. The administration of daily IL2 injections for 5 days, 5 days, or 17 days post immunization was able to enhance protection against *Haemophilus pleuropneumoniae*, rabies virus, and herpes simplex virus (HSV), respectively (Anderson et al., 1987; Nunberg et al., 1989; Weinberg and Merigan, 1988). Obviously repeated administration by injection over such prolonged periods has little practical appeal in terms of prophylactic vaccination, although such regimes may well be acceptable in therapeutic vaccination (against cancer for example). There have been attempts to find a more "vaccinee friendly" delivery system. For instance IL2 has been incorporated into liposomes and microparticles and has been shown to add adjuvant effects to both of these delivery systems (Ho et al., 1992; Singh-Hora et al., 1990).

IL2 is of course a Th1 cytokine, and its effects as an adjuvant in models of protection would tend to support the hypothesis that its mode of action is largely by enhancing proliferation of these cells. Multiple doses of IL2 were less effective in a more antibody-dependent system, leptospira-induced septicemia (Nunberg et al., 1989). IL2 has also been shown to be effective as an adjuvant when emulsified along with antigen in oil (Good et al., 1988) and as a single injection given to immunodeficient nonresponders to hepatitis B vaccine (Meuer et al., 1989).

■ Interleukin I

Again, IL1 was one of the early cytokines touted as a potential immunological adjuvant. Both whole recombinant protein (Staruch and Wood, 1983) and an IL1 peptide (Nencioni et al., 1987) were shown to have adjuvant activity. Early studies though produced some confusion over the relative activities of IL1α and β, and regarding the timing of the cytokine dose. Staruch and Wood administered IL1 two hours after antigen, and Boraschi et al. reported that IL1β but not IL1α had adjuvant activity (Boraschi et al., 1990). Subsequently, however, IL1α was shown to be effective as an adjuvant, and was also found to work when administered mixed with the vaccine antigen (Reed et al., 1989; Heath et al., 1989).

■ GM-CSF

Granulocyte macrophage colony-stimulating factor (GM-CSF) was shown to be an immunological adjuvant when administered as a

fusion with a lymphoma idiotype protein (Tao and Levy, 1993) and is now probably the most commonly used cytokine adjuvant, generally given as multiple injections to enhance responses against therapeutic cancer vaccines (Murray et al., 2002; Kunkel, 2004).

■ Interleukin 12 and similar cytokines

IL12 is a heterodimer of p40 and p35 subunits first identified as a proinflammatory IFNγ-inducing cytokine. It has since become recognized as one of the pivotal cytokines involved in the induction of type I immune responses (Romani et al., 1997). Afonso et al. were able to show in 1994 that IL12 had considerable potential as a Th1 generating adjuvant in a *Leishmania major* vaccination system. IL12 has since been shown to have potent Th1 inducing ability as an adjuvant in a range of systems (Romani et al., 1997; Buchanan et al., 2001; Wrightsman et al., 2000; Campos-Neto et al., 2002; Chang et al., 2004) including in humans (Sha et al., 2004; Lee et al., 2001). As mentioned above, IL12 was first identified as an IFNγ-inducing cytokine, and the adjuvant effect of IL12 has been shown to be dependent upon IFNγ induction (Schijns et al., 1995).

IL23 is a cytokine with similar properties to IL12, and indeed is a heterodimer of IL12 p40 subunit with a new partner, p19. IL23 has been shown to be effective in inducing cytotoxic T cell (CTL) responses specific to hepatitis C virus when used as part of a prime-boost regime (Matsui et al., 2004). In another study IL23 was found to be more effective than IL12 in inducing CTL responses and Th1-type responses to HCV (Ha et al., 2004). This group also assessed the effects of a glycosylation mutant of IL23 which resulted in less p40 expression, but similar IL23 expression. The glycosylation mutant was more effective still, and may be an improved adjuvant.

IL12 in some studies has had detrimental effects on protective responses (Chen et al., 2001) and is not without its toxicity problems (Leonard et al., 1997; Huber et al., 2003; Portjiele et al., 2005; Hedlund et al., 2001) and these may limit its use as an adjuvant for prophylactic vaccines, although it is possible that problems may be overcome by careful assessment of the appropriate doses to be used. It is unclear at present whether IL23 will exhibit similar toxicity.

Type I interferon

Type I interferons were of course among the earliest cytokines to be assessed as therapeutic agents, but their use as potential vaccine adjuvants in the 1970s and early 1980s produced contradictory results, with some studies showing a positive and some a negative effect on antibody responses (Braun and Levy, 1972; Chester et al., 1973; Brodeur and Merigan, 1974, 1975; Vignaux et al., 1980). More recently type I IFN has been revived as a potential adjuvant by the work of Le Bon et al. (2001) who have shown that induction of type I IFN is required for the adjuvant effect of complete Freund's adjuvant, and that type I IFN has an adjuvant effect itself on antibody responses. This group has also shown that the adjuvant effects of type I IFN are mediated through inducing maturation of dendritic cells (DCs). Unfortunately three injections of IFN on days 0, 1, and 2 are required, and this timing problem of course reduces the practical applicability of the cytokine as an adjuvant with prophylactic vaccines.

Anti-cytokine antibodies

Cytokines are often classified into pro- and anti-inflammatory groups, and as described in this chapter, there are many examples of successful use, particularly of proinflammatory cytokines (IL12, IFNγ and IFNα) as immunological adjuvants. Type 2 cytokines such as IL4, IL10, and IL13 typically act as a counterbalance to proinflammatory cytokines, and this effect has been utilized in the adjuvant field in the form of antibodies inhibitory to the effects of the type 2 cytokine IL10, which inhibit its antiinflammatory effect, and therefore have an action analogous to a proinflammatory

cytokine. Castro et al. (2000) were able to show using a T cell receptor transgenic model, that anti-IL10 receptor mAb was able to enhance the Th1 recall response to ovalbumin, although this adjuvant effect occurred only in the presence of lipopolysaccharide (LPS). Of course while LPS itself is not generally tolerated in vaccines, molecules acting in a similar way, through toll-like receptors, are either approved as adjuvants or are in the process of approval.

Improvement of cytokine activity: incorporation into liposomes or other carriers

There are a large number of studies on the adjuvant effects of liposome-incorporated cytokines, and these have been reviewed by Lachman et al. (1996). In many cases the question asked has been, "does the cytokine improve the immunogenicity of the liposome preparation?" with the answer often being yes. An important question, however, is "does the liposome incorporation improve the adjuvant effect of the cytokine?" In most studies this question has not been specifically addressed, although there are strong theoretical reasons why incorporation of the cytokine into liposomes or microparticles along with the vaccine antigen might enhance the effect of the cytokine. The major reason that it might is that the cytokine and antigen are co-localized, as described above, simply by coencapsulation. Furthermore the liposome itself may have some targeting effect to antigen-presenting cells (APCs).

Improvement of cytokine activity: fusion to antigen

Cytokines are relatively small molecules, and when administered by injection along with antigen are able to diffuse around the body relatively easily, opening up the possibility that they may exert their effects on immune cells which are irrelevant to the immune response against the vaccine antigen. Some cytokine adjuvants may operate systemically, and this lack of direction to the appropriate immune cells may not be a particular problem. Others, however, such as IFNγ, clearly exert a local effect. Thus IFNγ is ineffective when administered at a site different from the antigen, such as the opposite flank (Heath, unpublished). While the cytokine is clearly effective when simply administered mixed with the antigen, findings such as those above raised the question as to whether cytokine adjuvant effects might be further enhanced by co-localization with the vaccine antigen, ensuring delivery of the cytokine signal to the appropriate APCs (those presenting the vaccine antigen) and minimizing delivery of the cytokine signal to irrelevant APCs expressing other antigens, such as self antigens. Such delivery to irrelevant APCs might in some circumstances have risks such as the initiation of autoimmune responses, but otherwise could still be detrimental simply by diverting the immune response away from the desired direction (Heath and Playfair, 1993).

There are a number of potential methods available for co-localization of cytokine and antigen. These include co-entrapment in particulate vehicles such as liposomes or microparticles, co-emulsification in oil, and co-precipitation on alum. We were able to show using IFNγ that a high affinity attachment to the antigen avidin via biotinylation of the cytokine resulted in a strongly enhanced adjuvant effect, in particular for type I-related antibody responses against avoiding, as assessed by the IgG2a response (Heath and Playfair, 1990). Obviously the ultimate method of co-localization of cytokine and antigen is via their production as a single molecule in the form of a recombinant chimeric fusion protein (Heath and Playfair, 1993). The use of such a method allows a guaranteed 1:1 molar ratio of cytokine:antigen to be achieved, and offers potentially simplified production, as the purification of a fusion protein should not be inherently more difficult than the purification of the original recombinant vaccine antigen. Tao and Levy (1993) showed that a lymphoma idiotype protein fused to GM-CSF was more strongly immunogenic than a mixture of

the two proteins in inducing anti-idiotype antibody responses. Hazama et al. (1993) showed an adjuvant effect of IL2 fused to HSV glycoprotein D, and ourselves and others (McCormick et al., 2001; Faulkner et al., 2003) have been able to show that, consistent with the findings described above, using avidin, a recombinant IFNγ fusion protein induced stronger antibody and T cell responses than a mixture of the cytokine and antigen. As with avidin, there were particularly strongly enhanced Th1-related responses induced. Why the fusion should especially target Th1 responses is not really understood at present, but the finding with IFNγ is consistent, and appears whether the protein itself is delivered, or whether delivery of the fusion is via DNA vaccination (Nimal et al., 2005).

▪ Problems associated with fusion to antigen

There is a major potential problem with the administration of any fusion protein consisting of foreign epitopes and a self-protein such as a cytokine or CD154. The foreign T helper epitopes which are present in all T-dependent protein antigens (such as most vaccine antigens) are potentially able to act as helper epitopes for immune responses against the host protein. The foreign (vaccine) antigen thus can act as a "carrier" for the induction of immune responses against the host protein, in the same way as proteins like KLH are used as carriers to induce anti-Id or antiganglioside responses. Obviously the induction of a strong autoimmune response against a host protein, such as IFNα or CD154, could have potentially serious consequences. For instance anti-CD154 monoclonal antibodies have profound immunosuppressive effects (Foy et al., 1993). At the very least such responses may prevent a second dose of the vaccine from working effectively. Most studies on the use of self-protein/vaccine antigen fusions as vaccines have not addressed this potential problem. However, autoantibody responses against GM-CSF have been found in mice following hyperimmunization with an idiotype-GM-CSF fusion protein. These autoantibodies were able to neutralize GM-CSF *in vitro*, but apparently had no detrimental effects on hematopoiesis in the mice, or on immune responses, except when a similar GM-CSF fusion was used for immunization, in which case the adjuvant effect of GM-CSF was inhibited (Chen and Levy, 1995). The authors found that a single priming immunization with the fusion protein, followed by a boost with Id protein alone, was sufficient to induce a strong anti-Id response without the anti-GM-CSF response, and they proposed such a protocol as a potential solution to the autoimmunity problem.

■ C3d-based adjuvants

To circumvent the local and systemic toxicity typically associated with strong chemical adjuvants or cytokines, components of the innate immune system can be employed. The complement system plays an essential role in host defense against infectious agents and in the inflammatory process. The so-called "complement cascade" is initiated when the first complement molecule, C1, encounters antibody bound to antigen in an antigen–antibody complex. The C3d fragment of the third complement protein (C3) is one of the final degradation products of the complement system pathway. Upon activation, C3 cleavage products form covalent bonds with foreign antigens, thereby generating ligands such as C3dg and C3d (a proteolytic fragment of C3dg) that engage CD21/35 complement receptors expressed by mature B cells and follicular DCs (Haas et al., 2004). Conjugation of C3d to an immunogen may influence every step of the humoral immune response as transport of antigen to secondary lymphoid organs could facilitate interactions between C3d and CD21 on circulating B cells. Additionally, ligation of CD21 and antigen receptors on B cells may lower the concentration and affinity threshold for B-cell activation, increase the level of B-cell activation for a given dose of antigen, increase costimulatory molecule expression, and decrease B-cell apoptosis, all promoting development and maintenance of memory B cells. Interactions between antigen-specific B cells and follicular DCs may therefore be enhanced as a result of increased follicular trapping of antigen.

Complement's potential use as a vaccine adjuvant was realized when Dempsey et al. demonstrated that antihen egg lysozyme (anti-HEL) transgenic mice immunized with HEL fused to three copies of mouse C3d showed a 1000-fold increase in the IgG1 anti-HEL primary antibody response as compared to mice immunized with unmodified HEL (Dempsey et al., 1996). The effectiveness of C3d as a molecular adjuvant has subsequently been demonstrated in a number of systems, and these are reviewed below.

Although some studies have shown an adjuvant effect for single C3 fragments covalently attached to antigen (Villiers et al., 1999; Lou and Kohler. 1998), one study has reported that fusions with one or two copies of C3d with bovine rotavirus VP7 or bovine herpesvirus type 1 glycoprotein D inhibited the specific humoral immune response following DNA immunization and suggested that three or more copies of the C3d molecule may be necessary for an efficient antigen-specific immune response (Suradhat et al., 2001). A recent report has indeed shown that four or more repeats of C3d conjugated to P28, an active peptide corresponding to the CD21 binding site on C3d, may be necessary for an efficient enhancement of antigen-specific immune responses (Wang et al., 2004). Certainly most published studies appear to use three or more copies of C3d in conjugations to antigens in order to attain potent immune responses.

Streptococcus pneumoniae is a major cause of pneumonia in the elderly and of meningitis and bacteremia in children aged 6 to 15 months. As several serotypes of *S. pneumoniae* have been identified, the use of multivalent vaccines is required to provide adequate protection against infection. However, the presence of several antigens in a single vaccine can lead to high total concentration of polysaccharide or carrier protein, which may decrease the antibody response to individual components (Klein et al., 1997). Therefore, there is a need for methods to improve the antibody response to individual pneumococcal polysaccharide components of a multivalent vaccine. One approach has been to use conjugates of C3d with the serotype 14 pneumococcal capsular polysaccharide (PPS14). PPS14-C3d has been shown to enhance significantly serum anti-PPS14 antibody responses in immunized mice, with isotype switching from IgM to IgG1 (Test, 2001). PPS14 (a T cell-independent type 2 antigen) is able to activate the alternative pathway of complement (Griffioen et al., 1991) and its ability to induce an antibody response in BALB/c mice is complement dependent (Markham et al., 1982). PPS14-C3d conjugates showed an efficacy similar to a PPS14-OVA conjugate, a T-dependent protein carrier. This is important, as T-dependent protein carriers have been used in the pneumococcal conjugate vaccines either recently licensed or in clinical trial.

Much effort is being made to improve the efficacy of influenza vaccines. Fusion proteins of viral antigen and host-derived C3d component of complement could be a prophylactic therapy against a number of viral infections. By fusing the secreted form of hemagglutinin (sHA) to C3d (sHA-3C3d), the HA moiety signals through the B-cell receptor by binding anti-HA Ig receptors on the B cell and simultaneously the C3d moiety binds CD21 and signals through CD19. Using this approach in a mouse model resulted in more rapid appearance of HA inhibition activity and protective immunity (Ross et al., 2000). Eight weeks after vaccination, the avidity of the antibody to HA in boosted mice was stronger in sera from mice inoculated with sHA-3C3d than in sera from sHA DNA-inoculated mice. Further evidence has demonstrated that the adjuvant-free intranasal vaccine sHA-mC3d3 produced serum IgA in the nasal area, and intranasal vaccination of the C3d-sHA fusion proteins resulted in complete protection against live influenza virus challenge (Watanabe et al., 2003). It has been argued that as secretory IgA

at the mucosal epithelium elicits more effective cross-protective immunity than IgG, C3d-fused proteins might protect against different subtypes of influenza (Tamura et al., 2003). To support this, a recent study has confirmed that not only can C3d, when coupled to HA, enhance immunity to a homologous strain or subtype of influenza, but also expand and enhance the immunogenicity and protection in mice to a lethal challenge using a strain of influenza from a different subtype (Mitchell et al., 2003). The protective efficacy of intranasally administered C3d fusions is currently under investigation using a variety of viral antigens from viruses that infect primarily the nasal mucosa.

Introduction of DNA induces both humoral and cell-mediated immune responses; however, there is a slower rise in antibody titer, as compared to protein or attenuated viral vaccines. Green et al. (2002) investigated the effect of a measles sH-C3d fusion protein on the neutralizing antibody response. Results from this study showed that vaccination using the sH-C3d fusion resulted in a 7- to 15-fold increase in antibody levels as compared to mice vaccinated with DNA expressing sH alone. A similar approach was used with the HIV-1 envelope (gp120) fused with three copies of C3d. The fusion constructs induced higher Env antibody responses and a faster onset of affinity maturation (Ross et al., 2001). It has further been demonstrated that outbred mice vaccinated with DNA-expressing C3d conjugated to sgp120 elicited similar titers of anti-Env antibodies as vaccinated inbred strains (Toapanta and Ross, 2004), although a mixed T helper response was elicited in the outbred mice, whereas a Th2-biased immune response was seen in the three inbred stains tested. Additionally, as the avidity of the elicited antibody in the outbred mice was enhanced compared to the inbred strains, this may have implications for the use of C3d-conjugated vaccines in outbred primate populations.

C3d has been proposed to function as a molecular adjuvant by efficiently targeting antigens to CD21/35, which interacts with

CD19 to regulate transmembrane signals during B-cell activation (Tedder et al., 1994). A recent study by Haas et al. (2004) confirms that C3d can function as a molecular adjuvant during humoral immune responses to antigens administered as proteins or as DNA vaccines. In this study antigen responses to streptavidin (SA) and gp120 were significantly impaired in CD21/35−/− mice; surprisingly, however, IgG responses to SA-C3dg and gp120-C3d were significantly augmented. This suggested that C3d can function as a molecular adjuvant independent of the CD21/35 pathway. The precise mechanisms through which C3d functions as a molecular adjuvant therefore remain to be determined.

Heat shock proteins

Heat shock proteins (HSPs), also called stress proteins, are among the most highly conserved molecules of the biosphere, and are present in all cells in all known life forms. They are a family of molecular chaperones important in protein synthesis and folding. HSPs are important in the control of protective immunity by participating in the assembly of antibody molecules, stabilizing MHC class I and class II molecules and through their ability to stimulate the synthesis of cytokines (Audibert, 2003). Cell death leads to the release of biologically potent HSPs loaded with peptides. Cross-presentation of the HSP-peptide complexes by DCs allows the activation of professional APCs to induce cytokines and induce expression of costimulatory molecules on the DCs.

The HSP70 subfamily is one of the most important HSP subfamilies. HSP70 is a constitutively expressed cytosolic member of this family, assisting in the folding of newly synthesized polypeptides into their correct conformation by binding to them during protein synthesis. It also assists in the translocation of proteins across membranes into different compartments of the cell. Apart from their properties as chaperones and protein transporters (Ellis and van der Vies, 1991), HSP70

proteins have the ability to bind short peptides (Flynn et al., 1991). HSP70 can bind to CD91, CD14, and TLR2/4 receptors on the surface of APCs, to activate APCs and facilitate the re-presentation of HSP-associated antigen via a TAP-dependent or TAP-independent route. Extremely small quantities of peptides (nano- or picograms) are sufficient for eliciting potent CD8 T cell responses, if the peptides are chaperoned by HSPs (Audibert, 2003). The capacity of HSP70-peptide complexes to induce specific CD4 and CD8 T-cell immune responses to the bound peptide in vivo makes HSP70 an attractive target for specific vaccination against cancers and infectious diseases.

It is now well known that bacterial HSPs stimulate the host immune response, e.g., as a component in Freund's complete adjuvant. Several studies have shown that HSPs can be used as carrier proteins without additional adjuvants in both protein- or DNA-based vaccination strategies using different experimental systems, making HSPs the first adjuvant of mammalian origin. Some of these studies are reviewed in more detail in this chapter.

When chemically conjugated to synthetic peptides or oligosaccharides, mycobacterial HSP70 apply a strong helper activity in vivo (del Guidice, 1992), and evidence for this is plentiful, with both CD4 and CD8 T cell responses elicited. By immunizing mice with mycobacterial HSP70 noncovalently bound to the MHC class II influenza A peptide (pNP 206–229), proliferative CD4 T cell responses were elicited to the HSP70-binding peptide (Roman and Moreno, 1996). Mixing viral peptides from lymphocytic choriomeningitis virus (LCMV) with recombinant human HSP70 in vitro and immunizing mice, successfully induced protective antiviral immunity to LCMV with a low dose of a minimal T cell epitope, without the need of additional adjuvants (Ciupitu et al., 1978). Similarly, a fused mycobacterial HSP70 to HIV-1 gag p24 enhanced the immunogenicity of the p24 Ag and rendered the need for an exogenous adjuvant unnecessary (Suzue et al., 1996).

Both humoral and cellular immune responses against p24 could be elicited; however, physical linkage of HSP70 to p24 was essential for this augmented response. Moreover, a later report by the same group (Suzue et al., 1997) demonstrated that a soluble HSP70 fusion protein having a large fragment of chicken ovalbumin (OVA) as a fusion partner could, in the absence of adjuvants, stimulate H-2^b mice to produce OVA-specific CD8 CTLs that recognize the immunodominant peptide SIINFEKL in association with Kb. Additionally, the immunized mice were protected against a lethal challenge with an OVA-expressing melanoma tumor. These CTLs were as effective in recognizing the SIINFEKL-Kb complex as a CTL clone raised against cells in which OVA is expressed and processed naturally for class I presentation.

Evidence from several publications has shown that HSPs work as adjuvants in the absence of T cell help. Cho et al. (2000) reported that in C57BL/6 mice and CD4-deficient mice, mycrobacterial HSP65 fused to the polypeptide P1, activated DCs but not macrophages, and stimulated the production of P1-specific CTL in the absence of CD4 T cells. A study by Cheng et al. (2001) used HPV-16 E7 as a model Ag for vaccine development as this protein may provide an opportunity to prevent and treat HPV-associated cervical malignancies. Linkage of HSP70 to E7 Ag in a Sindbis virus RNA vector led to an enhancement of E7-specific CD8 T cell-mediated immunity and antitumor effect against HPV-16 E7-expressing murine tumors, which bypassed the CD4 arm. After DNA vaccination of E7 Ag linked to HSP70 via a gene gun, a dramatically increased expansion and activation of E7-specific CD8 T cells was observed (Chen et al., 2000). Depletion of CD4 or NK1.1+ cells did not decrease the antitumor immunity generated by E7-HSP70 DNA, indicating that CD8 T cells are the key players in gene gun-mediated E7-HSP70 DNA vaccination. In a fusion of HSP70 with OVA, results showed that the ability of HSP fusion proteins to elicit CTLs against the fusion partner was not a consequence of the HSPs' chaperone activity. Data from this study supports a model whereby HSP70 directly or indirectly affect the maturation state of the APC in a similar manner to some viruses. The ability of HSP70 fusion proteins to elicit CTL responses in the absence of CD4 cells suggests that HSP70 may be a useful vehicle for the development of prophylaxis and therapy of HIV-1 and its opportunistic infections (Huang et al., 2000), as infection by HIV-1 can lead to a substantial reduction in CD4 T cells, thereby crippling the host's immune response to HIV and other pathogens. The loss of CD4 cells is thought to impair the development and maintenance of CD8 CTL responses.

The capacity of HSPs to directly activate DCs may account for their ability to bypass the requirement for CD4 T cells and added adjuvants. It has been suggested that HSP complexes can enter into professional APCs via receptor-mediated endocytosis, providing a possible explanation for the cross-priming of HSP-peptide complexes where the HSP can lead exogenous proteins to the MHC-I restricted antigen presentation pathway. Bone marrow-derived DCs pulsed with HSP70 fused with a protein effectively induced CTL, where intravenous injection induced a more favorable response than subcutaneous or intradermal injection. This indicates that perhaps splenic DC rather than i.d. Langerhans cells are the primary APC responsible for internalizing HSP70 fusion proteins (Udono et al., 2001). This study demonstrated that vaccination of murine HSP70 fused to CTL epitopes lacking both N- and C-terminal flanking sequences primes CD8 T cells independently of CD4 T cells.

That HSPs mediate their adjuvanticity via DC activation was supported in a recent report, which presented evidence that a novel HSP (HSP70L1) derived from human DCs has potent adjuvant effects that polarize responses toward Th1 (Wan et al., 2004). HSP70L1 is smaller in size than HSP70 but resembles it both structurally and functionally; however, it is more potent than HSP70 in the stimulation of IL-12p70, MIP-1α, MIP-1β, RANTES, CCR7, and CXCR4 expression by DCs, and it was hypothesized that it may therefore polarize Th1 responses more effectively than HSP70. Fused to an $OVA_{257-264}$ hybrid peptide, HSP70L1 strongly induced $OVA_{257-264}$-specific IFNγ- and IL2-secreting Th1 cells, as well as $OVA_{257-264}$-specific CTLs. Additionally, a potent $OVA_{257-264}$-specific antitumor immunity was observed following HSP70L1-$OVA_{257-264}$ immunization in a murine tumor challenge model. To be effectively presented by DCs, the antigenic peptide had to be associated with HSP70L1, as peptide alone or simply mixed with HSP70L1 failed to elicit $OVA_{257-264}$-specific CTL or tumor growth inhibition. These results taken together lead the authors to presume the adjuvant effects of HSP70L1 were mediated via DC activation. Although OVA was used as a model antigen in this study, one might assume that as a member of the HSP70 subfamily, HSP70L1 may bind a variety of viral antigenic peptides or tumor-specific antigens, conferring adjuvant properties to them. Therefore, HSP70L1, as a novel and potent adjuvant of mammalian origin, may be used to induce and enhance immune responses against cancers and infectious diseases such as HIV, human papillomavirus (HPV), and hepatitis B virus (HBV) infection.

Although most studies appear to investigate the adjuvant effect of HSP70, a few studies have focused on using the 60 kDa HSP (HSP60) as an adjuvant. When conjugated to the *Salmonella typhi* capsular polysaccharide Vi, the HSP peptide was able to induce the production of antisalmonella IgG Ab (Konen-Waisman et al., 1995) and induced resistance to lethal bacterial challenge when conjugated to *Streptococcus pneumoniae* (Pn) type 4 (PS4) (Konen-Waisman et al., 1999). Another publication presents evidence that HSP60 peptide conjugated to PS4 induced nearly complete resistance to challenge with high amounts of Pn of both young and old mice. This vaccine protected mice vaccinated at 1 year of age and induced long-lasting serum Ab to PS4, which protected old mice that had been vaccinated 1 year prior to challenge (Amir-Kroll et al., 2003). This is an important consideration as finding a vaccine for the elderly is a critical step toward reducing mortality from Pn infection.

HSPs isolated from tumors have been shown to carry minute amounts of tumor peptides and have been shown to induce CTL responses *in vitro* against a number of antigens expressed in the cells from which the HSPs have been purified. Their use is therefore seriously considered for immunotherapy of tumors. Clinical trials using HSPs (especially gp96) isolated from tumors have successfully been performed in various cancers including melanoma, pancreas, kidney, colon, and lymphoma (Castelli et al., 2001). A vaccine, Oncophage (HSPPC-96, Antigenics), composed by isolating HSPs and antigens from the patient's own cancer cells, is entering phase III clinical trials in both metastatic melanoma and renal cell carcinoma (Caudill and Li, 2001; www.antigenics.com/products/cancer/oncophage/).

◼ Host cell surface proteins

◼ TNFR and TNF superfamiles

The tumor necrosis factor (TNF) and TNF receptor superfamilies (TNFSF and TNFRSF) are two large and expanding families of ligands and receptors which are very important in control of immune responses. The TNFSF are either soluble or membrane-bound type II proteins, and are often trimeric. Their receptors are membrane-bound type I proteins, with some soluble versions. We concentrate here on CD40/CD154 as this system is probably the best studied in terms of adjuvant effects, but various other systems are covered briefly.

◼ CD40–CD154 costimulatory pathway

The CD40–CD154 pathway represents perhaps the most widely studied and well-defined costimulatory pathway. The literature on this pair and their role in the various areas of the immune response is extensive and a full in-depth discussion of pathways involved is beyond the scope of this chapter. Many excellent reviews have been published over the last decade on the CD40 antigen and some points, which are only touched upon in this review, are explored in more depth in these texts (Quezada et al., 2003; Gordon et al., 2000; Grewal et al., 1998; van Kooten and Banchereau, 1996, 1997).

The CD40 antigen was discovered independently by two teams of workers in 1985 and 1986. Paulie et al. identified a novel surface antigen associated with carcinoma cells and B lymphocytes using the monoclonal antibody (mAb) S2C6 (Paulie et al., 1985). Clark et al., using mAb G28-5, showed that its antigen induced costimulatory effects on B lymphocytes (Clark and Ledbetter, 1986). This antigen (formerly p50 and Bp50) was designated as CD40 at the Fourth International Workshop on Leukocyte Antigens in 1989.

CD40 is a member of the TNFRSF and is expressed on many cells of the immune system. It displays a wide range of functions, dependent upon the expressing cell, the quality and quantity of the signal, and the environment in which the signal is encountered. Most notably for those interested in adjuvant development is its constitutive expression on APCs such as DCs, macrophages, and B cells. Ligation of CD40 on these cells is critical for the initiation and development of an effective immune response.

The cognate ligand for CD40 is called CD154 (also known as CD40L and gp39) and is a member of the TNFSF. Expression of CD154 was initially thought to be restricted to CD4+ T helper (Th) lymphocytes, although it is now known to be expressed on other lymphocytes and nonlymphocytic leukocytes. These include natural killer (NK) cells, monocytes, mast cells, basophils, CD8+ T cells, B cells, endothelium, smooth muscle cells, DCs, and platelets. As well as being expressed as a membrane-bound, trimeric form, this molecule is also secreted as a soluble form following proteolytic cleavage. Expression on CD4 T cells is rapid and transient following activation. The molecule can be detected very early after activation (5–10 minutes), peaking at about 6 hours then declining over the next 12–18 hours (Schonbeck et al., 2000).

One defining characteristic of the TNF/TNFR superfamily is the promiscuity of binding displayed by members, with each receptor ligand possessing several counterstructures. In this respect, the CD40 antigen was for some time thought to be unique, in that alternative ligands, although hypothesized, had not been demonstrated. However, several recent reports have shown that CD40 does indeed bind molecules other than CD154, namely HSP70 (Wang et al., 2001) and HSP70-peptide complexes (Becker et al., 2002). There may therefore be a link between some of the adjuvant effects of some HSPs (above) and the effects of CD40 antibodies and CD154.

Ligation of CD40 by the transiently expressed ligand CD154 leads to costimulation of the CD40-expressing cell. In the case of DCs this means maturation from an immature "antigen sampling" state to an activated "antigen presenting" state with associated upregulation of other costimulatory molecules such as CD80/86, MHC class II, and proinflammatory cytokines such as IL-12. In the case of B cells the CD40 molecule represents the major signal for T cell help. Ligation of CD40 by activated T cells, in conjunction with antigen recognition via the B cell receptor (BCR), is essential for T-dependent (TD) immune responses in B cells. Isotype switching, germinal center formation, affinity maturation, and memory – all hallmarks of the adaptive response and essential outcomes of a successful vaccination strategy – require the CD40–CD154 interaction. This fact is highlighted in patients suffering from hyper IgM syndrome. This condition is caused by a mutation in the CD154 molecule resulting in a lack of cognate interaction with the CD40 receptor. As a consequence patients produce elevated levels of IgM and are unable to produce class switched antibodies (Allen et al., 1993; DiSanto et al., 1993). The essential nature of this interaction has been confirmed in CD40 and CD154 "knockout" mice which, like hyper-IgM patients, are unable to mount class switched responses (Kawabe et al., 1994; Xu et al., 1994). In addition to the direct influence of CD40 ligation on the B cell response, ligation of CD40 can also indirectly influence T cell immunity via action on DCs.

Exploiting the CD40–CD154 pathway. Given the critical role that CD40 activation has in the successful priming of APCs, it is not surprising that this molecule has been presented as an ideal target for therapeutic agents. Most adjuvants currently in use have been discovered by an empirical approach, and are dependent upon microbial products inducing "danger" signals via Toll-like receptor (TLR) pathways. This approach to adjuvant development has proven to be successful in one aspect of vaccine development, in that they can be potent adjuvants, stimulating a strong host response against coadministered antigens. However, they do have a possibly insurmountable limitation. TLR-based adjuvants may possess a *de facto* requirement for inflammation and associated side effects, as this is the mechanism by which they exert their effect. As a result most TLR-based adjuvants are unacceptable for human use due to severe inflammatory repercussions. We, and others, propose that effective adjuvants, capable of safely enhancing responses without widespread TLR-mediated inflammatory side effects, can be achieved by exploiting this costimulatory pathway as the CD40 pathway acts "downstream" of TLR signaling.

CD40-based enhancement of T-independent (TI) responses. The first report using the CD40 stimulatory approach was made by Dullforce et al. using agonistic antibodies against murine CD40 (Dullforce et al., 1998). This report illustrated significant enhancement of antibody responses to a coadministered TI-type 2 antigen (capsular polysaccharide (PS) from *Streptococcus pneumoniae*). This work is particularly interesting in that resultant antibody responses were also class switched, a phenomenon not normally observed in responses to TI antigens. The CD40-enhanced, isotype-switched

antibody responses were also shown to be protective against subsequent pneumococcal challenge. The proposed mode of action for this adjuvant effect is that the CD40 stimulation was acting as a surrogate for T cell help lacking in the normal response to a TI antigen. The same system was also to good effect in the enhancement of immune responses against TI-1 antigens (i.e., LPS). Again, enhanced, class-switched, protective antibody responses were observed against a salmonella challenge following intraperitoneal immunization with LPS and anti-CD40 (Barr and Heath, 1999). These studies were performed using high doses of CD40 antibodies administered admixed with the antigen. Enhancement of TI responses using anti-CD40 has also been demonstrated by Garcia de Vinuesa et al., who used large doses of antibody mixed with bacterial capsular polysaccharides (Garcia de Vinuesa et al., 1999). This group observed similarly enhanced protective antibody responses. However, they contest the theory that the CD40 agonist acts as a surrogate form of T cell help in the TI response. They state that the response maintains a distinctive TI profile, despite presenting data showing enhanced responses across the spectrum of Ig isotypes, including those indicative of isotype switched T-dependent-like responses. Garcia de Vinuesa et al. propose that rather than acting as a surrogate form of T cell help, CD40 agonists act via activation of APCs such as DCs and macrophages. Clearly this is an important consideration, as CD40 is a widely expressed costimulatory molecule. Administering large doses of unconjugated antibody would "flood" the immune system with a costimulatory signal which would in no way be preferentially directed to antigen-specific cells. It seems likely that the adjuvant effect of anti-CD40 mAb is at least in part mediated by APCs other than B cells. The relative roles of B cells and other APCs in this system are currently under investigation in this laboratory using a mixed bone marrow chimera system in which the CD40 deficiency is restricted to B cells (manuscript in preparation).

CD40-based enhancement of T cell responses and T-dependent (TD) antigens. In addition to the work on enhancement of antibody responses to TI antigens through CD40 stimulation, we have recently shown that CD40 mAbs can also enhance memory antibody responses and T cell responses. This work also sheds some light on the mode of action of CD40-based adjuvants, as it is possible to transfer the secondary response with T cells rather than with B cells. Therefore, it seems likely that the effects are partly mediated through enhanced antigen presentation by specific B cells (Carlring et al., 2004). Certainly with regard to protocols that involve enhancing responses to TD antigens rather than TI antigens, we have recently shown that despite providing a direct signal to B cells, there remains a requirement for T cells, indicating the mechanism is partially mediated indirectly via other APCs or that other T cell signals to B cells are required (Barr et al., 2005).

Studies into the potential applications of CD40 agonists as immunological adjuvants for the enhancement of B and T cell has also been carried out by several other groups. Ninomiya et al. have effectively used anti-CD40 mAb to induce protective immunity against influenza A infection in mice when administered with antigenic peptide in liposomes (Ninomiya et al., 2002). Another exciting therapeutic potential of the CD40 agonist approach is the use of such therapeutic agents in the enhancement of CTL responses. Diehl et al. and French et al. have shown that high doses of Vanti-CD40 mAb can bypass T cell help, with resultant enhancement of CTL responses (Diehl et al., 1999; French et al. 1999). The most probable mechanism of action in these studies is the activity of CD40 mAb is acting as a surrogate Th cell signal leading to enhanced APC function (Schoenberger et al., 1998; Ridge et al., 1998; Bennett et al., 1998). Enhanced CD8+ T cell responses have also been demonstrated using CD40-based adjuvants, illustrating the potential application of this technology to intracellular pathogens. Ahonen et al. showed enhanced CD8+ responses using a combined CD40/TLR therapy (Ahonen et al., 2004). Rolph et al. have used anti-CD40 mAb as an adjuvant in responses to *Listeria monocytogenes* antigens (Rolph et al., 2001). This group has shown that the coadministration of anti-CD40 mAb effectively enhances T cell responses and reduces bacterial load in the livers and spleens of vaccinated animals.

Refining CD40-based adjuvants. All of the work outlined above has one serious limitation with regards to potential transfer to the clinic, namely the requirement for large doses of anti-CD40 to enhance responses when administered as a mixture with antigen. As already mentioned, CD40 is widely expressed and there is, in all likelihood, the very real possibility of activation of nonantigen-specific cells, or more seriously, potentially self-reactive B cells. Indeed, in our hands, large doses of anti-CD40, though effective immunological adjuvants, do lead to splenomegaly and increased levels of polyclonal Ig. We have recently refined the CD40 mAb as adjuvant approach by conjugating the vaccine antigen to the CD40 agonist (Barr et al., 2003). These antigen–adjuvant conjugates have been shown to be effective against a range of antigens, including avidin and herpes viral glyco-proteins. In this form the CD40-based vaccine can be administered at greatly reduced doses, resulting in effective enhancement against the coupled antigen without the harmful side effects, such as splenomegaly and polyclonal Ig production observed with large doses of CD40 agonist. We propose that the mechanism by which these conjugate vaccines act is two-fold. In the first case, a molecule containing both costimulatory and antigenic motifs could simultaneously provide signal 1 and signal 2 to antigen-specific B cells, thus preferentially activating and expanding B cells specific for the vaccine antigen. Additionally, we envisage that such constructs also act to co-localize antigen to APCs along with a host-derived costimulatory signal (i.e., CD40), with subsequent enhancement of antigen

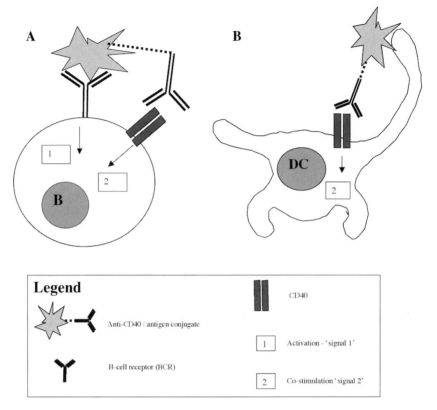

Figure 3.2 Schematic of theoretical modes of action of CD40-based vaccine conjugates. (A) Provision of both the antigenic stimulus (signal I), through the BCR, and costimulatory signal, through CD40, to an antigen-specific B cell. This would lead to activation of vaccine antigen-specific B cells in a manner very similar to the normal B cell response to TD antigens. Subsequent B cell proliferation would result in further expansion of the antigen-specific population, resulting in a robust response. (B) Costimulation of nonantigen-specific APCs, such as DCs, macrophages, via CD40 ligation. As CD40 is constitutively expressed on APCs, ligation of anti-CD40 would lead to activation of these non-antigen-specific cells, with resultant increase in APC effector functions (NO production by macrophages, enhanced antigen presentation by APCs, etc.). Additionally, the cell receiving the costimulatory signal would, by virtue of the conjugate, also encounter antigen in the immediate microenviroment.

presentation to T cells. Schematics of these potential mechanisms are presented in Figure 3.2.

One potential complication with the conjugate approach is the immunogenic nature of the adjuvant itself. As antibodies are traditionally generated in a nonhost animal (e.g., rat anti-mouse CD40 in many studies), the CD40 agonist will be immunogenic in the host. This could potentially limit the application of the adjuvant, as repeated doses would lead to the generation of responses against the adjuvant, with consequent reduction in efficacy (e.g., human anti-mouse or HAMA). We envisage that further refinement of these adjuvants will be required in order to use these therapies in prophylactic vaccination regimes. One obvious way to circumvent this problem would be to engineer the antibody to appear more "human" or less immunogenic through CDR grafting technology. Another potential solution would be the use of different, nonimmunogenic CD40 agonists. This approach has proven to be effective when using DNA constructs containing both antigenic and CD40-stimulating (e.g., CD154) sequences (Harcourt et al., 2003; Manoj et al., 2003). However, these systems have their own inherent implications. Presenting the immune system with a "self" antigen (CD154) coupled to a "nonself" antigen (vaccine candidate) opens up the very real possibility of generating host responses against host CD154, leading to a potentially immunosuppressive autoimmune disorder. Xiang et al. have in fact shown that such a construct can break peripheral T cell tolerance to a coupled antigen in CEA transgenic mice (Xiang et al., 2001). Another CD154-based approach has been described by Manoj et al. (2003). This HSV glycoprotein–CD154 construct led to enhanced and neutralizing antibody responses in sheep. The potential for autoantibody production was not assessed in either of these studies.

A recent report by Hanks et al. has used a subtle modification of the CD40 adjuvant-based system (Hanks et al., 2005). This group have approached the problem from the DC-based vaccine point of view and engineered a drug-inducible form of CD40 (iCD40). iCD40 expressing DCs were found to be more potent inducers of CD8+ T cell responses, presumably through prolonged CD40-mediated activation of DCs. This approach represents a significant improvement on standard DC-based vaccines.

CD134

CD134, or OX40 (TNFRSF), is expressed transiently on activated T cells following TCR ligation, while its ligand (OX40L) is expressed constitutively on various APCs. Both recombinant OX40L and agonistic OX40 antibodies have been investigated as potential immunological adjuvants, and both approaches have proven effective in tumor models (Weinberg et al., 2000; Pan et al., 2002). An OX40L recombinant fusion protein has also recently been shown to be an effective adjuvant in a *Cryptococcus neoformans* model of infection (Grosenbach et al., 2003).

CD137 (4-1BB)

4-1BB or CD137 (TNFRSF) is involved later in the immune response than CD28. Its ligand, CD137L, is expressed on activated T and B cells

and costimulates T cell activation and growth. There appears to be a bidirectional effect in that the binding of CD137L by CD137 also appears to induce B cell costimulation. Diehl et al. (2002) were able to show that four doses of agonistic anti-CD137 antibody were able to enhance strongly CTL responses against a peptide.

CD27/CD70

CD27 is another member of the TNFRSF which is expressed constitutively in T cells. It binds a ligand, CD70 (TNFSF), which is expressed only on activated T and B cells. Recombinant CD70 was used as a vaccine adjuvant in TCR transgenic mice (transgenic for TCR specific for the ovalbumin CTL epitope SIINFEKL). Administration of three doses of 200 µg of the recombinant CD70-Ig protein gave a 300-fold expansion in SIINFEKL-specific CTLs (Rowley et al., 2004).

CD28

CD28 is a member of the immunoglobulin superfamily, as are its two ligands, B7.1 (CD80) and B7.2 (CD86). CD28 is constitutively expressed on most CD4 and a large proportion of CD8 T cells, and signaling through CD28 provides "signal 2" to T cells which have recognized antigen and received "signal 1" through their TCR. CD28 signaling can either be through CD80 or CD86 expressed on activated APCs, or through antibody against CD28. CD80 and CD86 both bind an alternative receptor CTLA-4 or CD152. CD152 expression appears late on activated T cells, and CD152/CD80 binding has a negative regulatory effect on T cell proliferation and cytokine induction. There are a large number of publications in the cancer field wherein exogenous expression of either CD80 or CD86 by tumor cells has been used to enhance T cell responses against the tumor. As the tumor cells express peptide loaded MHC but do not express B7 molecules, ectopic B7 expression turns the tumor cells into mimics of professional APCs. The use of B7 with subunit vaccines would not be predicted to be effective in enhancing immune responses as B7 would naturally be expressed anyway on APCs. We have, however, shown that CD28 antibody conjugated to antigen is able to enhance specific antibody responses by around 1000-fold, and also to enhance strongly T cell, particularly Th1, responses (Carlring et al., 2003). This potent adjuvant effect is seen with very small (10 μg) doses of anti-CD28. It was already known that high doses of anti-CTLA4, sufficient to block all binding, have a modest adjuvant effect of their own (Hurwitz et al., 1998). We believe the major adjuvant effect of CD28 conjugates is mediated through CD28 stimulation, in the absence of CTLA4 downregulation that would normally be seen, because CD28 antibody, unlike B7 molecules, is unable to bind CTLA4 (Carlring et al., 2003).

■ Fms-like tyrosine kinase 3 ligand (Flt3L)

Many tumor therapeutic approaches (therapeutic vaccines) are based upon *in vitro* antigen loading of DCs. Flt3 ligand is a cytokine which is able to induce a potent mobilization of DCs on *in vivo* immunization. Disis et al. (2002) used recombinant Flt3 ligand as an adjuvant with a her2/neu cancer vaccine in humans. Flt3L was shown to strongly increase numbers of antigen-specific T cells expressing IFNγ, but there was no effect on antigen-induced T cell proliferation, and one patient developed autoimmune symptoms such as anti-DNA antibodies.

Evans et al. (2002) used Flt3L as an adjuvant for a hepatitis B vaccine in humans; however, despite the fact that circulating populations of specific B cells were strongly enhanced, there was no effect of Flt3L on hepatitis B antibody responses. Similarly, Chui et al. (2004) found that Flt3L had an enhancing effect on delayed-type hypersensitivity responses of human volunteers to the recall antigen tetanus toxoid, while there was no effect on either T cell proliferation or antibody responses. If Flt3 ligand has an application in vaccination therefore it is likely to be in cases where Th1-type (or perhaps CTL) responses are required, and

is also likely to be restricted to therapeutic vaccines due to the dosing schedule required.

■ Special applications of host-derived adjuvants

The greater understanding of the mode of action of host-derived adjuvants may make them particularly useful in cases where natural signals are lacking or are suppressed. We reviewed some time ago the potential of cytokines as adjuvants in immunodeficient hosts (Heath, 1995b), but this applies potentially to any of the host-derived adjuvants described above. A good example has come to the fore during the writing of this chapter. It is known that elderly people respond less well to vaccination against influenza than their younger counterparts, and it has recently been shown that there may be a deficiency in CD154 expression in the elderly which could explain in part these poor responses. CD40-based adjuvants therefore may have a particular role to play in vaccination of the elderly.

■ Concluding remarks

We have described a number of adjuvant systems based upon host molecules. Some of these have great promise, and of course others will likely be discovered in the coming years. Such rationally designed adjuvants may have a great impact in realizing the enormous potential presented by recombinant and subunit antigens, which in themselves are often poorly immunogenic. This area of rational adjuvant development has provided some highly encouraging results in various animal models to a range of vaccine antigens. Clearly many approaches are still in their infancy and in need of further refinement; however, the progress made in this field is highly encouraging. Perhaps the goal of producing safe and effective adjuvants through a rational approach will be achieved in the near future. It will be of great interest to see how the efficacy of these technologies translates to clinical trials.

Acknowledgments

The work from our own laboratory described here was supported by the Wellcome Trust (061268 and 042251) and by Adjuvantix Ltd.

References

Afonso, L.C.C., Scharton, T.M., Vieira, L.Q., Wysocka M., Trinchieri G., and Scott, P. (1994). The adjuvant effect of interleukin-12 in a vaccine against leishmania-major. *Science* 263, 235–237.

Ahonen, C.L., Doxsee, C.L., McGurran, S.M. et al. (2004). Combined TLR and CD40 triggering induces potent CD8+ T cell expansion with variable dependence on type I IFN. *J. Exp. Med.* 199, 775–784.

Allen. R.C., Armitage, R.J., Conley, M.E., Rosenblatt, H., Jenkins, N.A., Copeland, N.G., Bedell, M.A., Edelhoff, S., Disteche, C.M., and Simoneaux, D.K. (1993). CD40 ligand gene defects responsible for X-linked hyper-IgM syndrome. *Science* 259, 990–993.

Amir-Kroll, H., Mussbaum, G., and Cohen, I.R. (2003). Proteins and their derived peptides as carriers in a conjugate vaccine for Streptococcus pneumoniae: self-heat shock protein 60 and tetanus toxoid. *J. Immunol.* 170, 6165–6171.

Audibert, F. (2003). Adjuvants for vaccines, a quest. *Int. Immunopharmacol.* 3, 1187–1193.

Barouch, D.H., Letvin, N.L., and Seder, R.A. (2004). The role of cytokine DNAs as vaccine adjuvants for optimizing cellular immune responses. *Immunol. Rev.* 266–274.

Barr, T.A. and Heath, A.W. (1999) Enhanced *in vivo* immune responses to bacterial lipopolysaccharide by exogenous CD40 stimulation. *Infect. Immun.* 67, 3637–3640.

Barr, T.A., McCormick, A.L., Carlring, J., and Heath, A.W. (2003). A potent adjuvant effect of CD40 antibody attached to antigen. *Immunology* 109, 87–91.

Barr, T.A., Carlring, J., and Heath, A.W. (2005). CD40 antibody as a potent immunological adjuvant: CD40 antibody provides the CD40 signal to B cells but does not substitute for T cell help in responses against TD antigens. *Vaccine* 23, 3477–3482.

Becker, T., Hartl, F.U., and Wieland, F. (2002). CD40, an extracellular receptor for binding and uptake of Hsp70-peptide complexes. *J. Cell Biol.* 158, 1277–1285.

Bennett, S.R., Carbone, F.R., Karamalis, F., Flavell, R.A., Miller, J.F., and Heath, W.R. (1998). Help for cytotoxic T-cell responses is mediated by CD40 signalling. *Nature* 393, 478.

Boraschi, D., Villa, L., Volpini, G., Bossu, P., Censini, S., Ghiara, P. et al. (1990). Differential activity of interleukin 1α and interleukin 1β in the stimulation of immune responses *in vivo. Eur. J. Immunol.* 20, 317–321.

Braun, W. and Levy, H.B. (1972). Interferon preparations as modifiers of immune responses. *Proc. Soc. Exp. Biol. Med.* 141, 769–773.

Brodeur, B.R. and Merigan, T.C. (1974). Suppressive effect of interferon on the humoral immune response to sheep red blood cells in mice. *J. Immunol.* 113, 1319–1325.

Brodeur, B.R. and Merigan, T.C. (1975). Mechanism of the suppressive effect of interferon on antibody synthesis *in vivo. J. Immunol.* 114, 1323–1328.

Buchanan, R.M., Briles, D.E., Arulanandam, B.P., Westerink, M.A.J., Raeder, R.H., and Metzger, D.W. (2001). IL-12-mediated increases in protection elicited by pneumococcal and meningococcal conjugate vaccines. *Vaccine* 19, 2020–2028.

Campos-Neto, A., Webb, J.R., Greeson, K., Coler, R.N., Skeiky, Y.A.W., and Reed, S.G. (2002). Vaccination with plasmid DNA encoding TSA/LmSTI1 leishmanial fusion proteins confers protection against leishmania major infection in susceptible BALB/c mice. *Infect. Immun.* 70, 2828–2836.

Carlring, J., Barr, T., Buckle, A.M., and Heath, A.W. (2003). Anti-CD28 has a potent adjuvant effect on the antibody response to soluble antigens mediated through CTLA4 by-pass. *Eur. J. Immunol.* 33, 135–142.

Carlring, J., Barr, T.A., McCormick, A.L., and Heath, A.W. (2004). CD40 antibody as an adjuvant induces enhanced T cell responses. *Vaccine* 22, 3323–3328.

Castelli, C., Ciupitu, A.M.T., Rini, F., Rivoltini, L., Mazzocchi, A. et al. (2001). Human heat shock protein 70 peptide complexes specifically activate antimelanoma T cells. *Cancer Res.* 61, 222–227.

Castro, A.G., Neighbors, M., Hurst, S.D., Zonin, F., Silva, R.A., Murphy, E., Liu, Y.J., and O'Garra, A. (2000). Anti interleukin 10 receptor monoclonal antibody is an adjuvant for T helper 1 type responses only in the presence of lipopolysaccharide. *J. Exp. Med.* 192, 1529–1534.

Caudill, M.M. and Li, Z. (2001). HSPPC-96: a personalised cancer vaccine. *Expert Opin. Biol. Ther.* 1, 539–547.

Chang, S.Y., Lee, K.C., Ko, S.Y., Ko, H.J., and Kang, C.Y. (2004). Enhanced efficacy of DNA vaccination against Her-2/neu tumor antigen by genetic adjuvants. *Int. J. Cancer* 111, 86–95.

Chen, C.-H., Wang, T.L., Hung, C.-F., Yang, Y., Young, R.A., Pardoll, D.M., and Wu, T.-C. (2000). Enhancement of DNA vaccine potency by linkage of antigen gene to an HSP70 gene. *Cancer Res.* 60, 1035–1042.

Chen, H.W., Pan, C.H., Huan, H.W., Liau, M.Y., Chiang, J.R., and Tao, M.H. (2001). Suppression of immune response and protective immunity to a Japanese encephalitis virus DNA vaccine by coadministration of an IL-12-expressing plasmid. *J. Immunol.* 166, 7419–7426.

Chen, T.T. and Levy, R. (1995). Induction of autoantibody responses to GMCSF by hyperimmunization with an Id-GMCSF fusion protein. *J. Immunol.* 154, 3105–3117.

Cheng, W.-F., Hung, C.-F., Chai, C.-Y., Hsu, K.-F., He, L., Rice, C.M., Ling, M., and Wu, T.-C. (2001). Enhancement of Sindbis virus self-replicating RNA vaccine potency by linkage of mycobacterium tuberculosis heat shock protein 70 gene to an antigen gene. *J. Immunol.* 166, 6218–6226.

Chester, T.J., Paucker, K., and Merigan, T.C. (1973). Suppression of mouse antibody producing spleen cells by various interferon preparations. *Nature* 246, 92–94.

Cho, B.K., Palliser, D., Guillen, E., Wisniewski, J., Young, R.A., Chen, J., and Eisen, H.N. (2000). A proposed mechanism for the induction of cytotoxic T lymphocyte production by heat shock fusion proteins. *Immunity* 12, 263–272.

Chui, S., Clay, T.M., Mosca, P.J., Hobeika, A.C., Osada, T., Galibert, L., Caron, D., Lyerly, H.K., and Morse, M.A. (2004). Flt3-ligand as a vaccine adjuvant: results in a study of Flt3-ligand plus tetanus toxoid immunization. *J. Appl. Res.* 4, 536–549.

Ciupitu, A.-M.T., Petersson, M., O'Donnell, C.L., Williams, K., Jindal, S., Kiessling, R., and Welsh, R.M. (1998). Immunization with a lymphocytic choriomeningitis virus peptide mixed with heat shock protein 70 results in protective antiviral immunity and specific cytotoxic T lymphocytes. *J. Exp. Med.* 187, 685–691.

Clark, E.A. and Ledbetter, J.A. (1986). Activation of human B cells mediated through two distinct cell surface differentiation antigens, Bp35 and Bp50. *Proc. Natl. Acad. Sci. USA* 83, 4494–4498.

Del Giudice, G. (1992). New carriers and adjuvants in the development of vaccines. *Curr. Opin. Immunol.* 4, 454–459.

Dempsey, P.W., Allison, M.E.D., Akkaraju, S., Goodnow, C.C., and Fearon, D.T. (1996). C3d of complement as a molecular adjuvant: bridging innate and acquired immunity. *Science* 271, 348–350.

Diehl, L., den Boer, A.T., Schoenberger, S.P., van der Voort, E.I., Schumacher, T.N., Melief, C.J., Offringa, R., and Toes, R.E. (1999). CD40 activation *in vivo* overcomes peptide-induced peripheral cytotoxic T-lymphocyte tolerance and augments anti-tumor vaccine efficacy. *Nature Med.* 5, 774.

Diehl, L., van Mierlo, G.J., den Boer, A.T., van der Voort, E., Fransen, M., van Bostelen, L., Krimpenfort, P., Melief, C.J., Mittler, R., Toes, R.E., and Offringa, R. (2002). *In vivo* triggering through 4-1BB enables Th-independent priming of CTL in the presence of an intact CD28 costimulatory pathway. *J. Immunol.* 168, 3755–3762.

DiSanto, J.P., Bonnefoy, J.Y., Gauchat, J.F., Fischer, A., and de Saint Basile, G. (1993). CD40 ligand mutations in X linked immunodeficiency with hyper IgM. *Nature* 361, 541–543.

Disis, M.L., Rinn, K., Knutson, K.L., Davis, D., Caron, D., dela Rosa, C., and Schiffman, K. (2002). Flt3 ligand as a vaccine adjuvant in association with HER-2/neu peptide-based vaccines in patients with HER-2/neu-overexpressing cancers. *Blood* 99, 2845–2850.

Dullforce, P., Sutton, D., and Heath, A.W. (1998). Enhancement of T independent immune responses *in vivo* by CD40 antibodies. *Nature Med.* 4, 88–91.

Ellis, R.J., and van der Vies, S.M. (1991). Molecular chaperones. *Annu. Rev. Biochem.* 60, 321.

Evans, T.G., Hasan, M., Galibert, L., and Caron, D. (2002). The use of Flt3 ligand as an adjuvant for hepatitis B vaccination of healthy adults. *Vaccine* 21, 322–329.

Faulkner, L., Buchan, G., Slobbe, L., Lockhart, E., Wales, J., Wilson, M., and Baird, M. (2003). Influenza hemagglutinin peptides fused to interferon gamma and encapsulated in liposomes protects mice against influenza infection. *Vaccine* 21, 932–939.

Flynn, G.C., Pohl, J., Flocco, M.T., and Rothman, J.E. (1991). Peptide binding specificity of the molecular chaperone BiP. *Nature* 353, 726–730.

Foy, T.M., Shepherd, D.M., Durie, F.H., Aruffo, A., Ledbetter, J.A., and Noelle, R.J. (1993). In-vivo CD40-gp39 interactions are essential for thymus-dependent humoral immunity: 2. Prolonged suppression of the humoral immune-response by an antibody to the ligand for CD40, gp39. *J. Exp. Med.* 178, 1567–1575.

French, R.R., Chan, H.T.C., Tutt A.L., and Glennie, M.J. (1999). CD40 antibody evokes a cytotoxic T-cell response that eradicates lymphoma and bypasses T-cell help. *Nature Med.* 5, 548–553.

Garcia de Vinuesa, C., MacLennan, I.C., Holman, M., and Klaus, GG. (1999). Anti-CD40 antibody enhances responses to polysaccharide without mimicking T cell help. *Eur J. Immunol.* 29, 3216–3224.

Good, M.F., Pombo, D., Lunde, M.N., Maloy, W.L., Halenbeck, R., Koths, K. et al. (1988). Recombinant human IL-2 overcomes genetic nonresponsiveness to malaria sporozoite peptides. *J. Immunol.* 141, 972–977.

Gordon, J. and Pound, J.D. (2000). Fortifying B cells with CD154: an engaging tale of many hues. *Immunology* 100, 269–280.

Green, T.D, Newton, B.R., Rota. P.A., Xu, Y., Robinson, H.L., and Ross, T.M. (2002). C3d enhancement of neutralizing antibodies to measles hemagglutinin. *Vaccine* 20, 242–248.

Griffioen, A.W., Rijkers, G.T., Janssens-Korpela, P., and Zegers, B.J.M. (1991). Pneumococcal polysaccharides complexed with C3d bind to human B lymphocytes via complement receptor type 2. *Infect. Immun.* 29, 1839–1845.

Grosenbach, D.W., Schlom, J., Gritz, L., Gomez Yafal, A., and Hodge, J.W. (2003). A recombinant vector expressing transgenes for four T-cell costimulatory molecules (OX40L, B7-1, ICAM-1, LFA-3) induces sustained CD4+ and CD8+ T-cell activation, protection from apoptosis, and enhanced cytokine production. *Cell Immunol* 222, 45–57.

Ha, S.J., Kim, D.J., Baek, K.H., Yun, Y.D., and Sung, Y.C. (2004). IL-23 induces stronger sustained CTL and Th1 immune responses than IL-12 in hepatitis C virus envelope protein 2 DNA immunization. *J. Immunol.* 172, 525–531.

Haas, K.M., Toapanta, F.R., Oliver, J.A., Poe, J.C., Weis, J.H., Karp, D.R., Bower, J.F., Ross, T.M., and Tedder, T.F. (2004). Cutting edge: C3d functions as a molecular adjuvant in the absence of CD21/35 expression. *J. Immunol* 172, 5833–5837.

Hanks, B.A., Jiang, J., Singh, R.A., Song, W., Barry, M., Huls, M.H., Slawin, K.M., and Spencer, D.M. (2005). Re-engineered CD40 receptor enables potent pharmacological activation of dendritic-cell cancer vaccines *in vivo*. *Nature Med.* 11, 30–137.

Harcourt, J.L., Brown, M.P., Anderson, L.J., and Tripp, R.A. (2003). CD40 ligand (CD154) improves the durability of respiratory syncytial virus DNA vaccination in BALB/c mice. *Vaccine* 21, 2964–2979.

Hazama, M., Mayumiaono, A., Asakawa, N., Kuroda, S., Hinuma, S., and Fujisawa, Y. (1993). Adjuvant independent enhanced immune responses to recombinant herpes simplex virus type 1 fused with biologically active interleukin 2. *Vaccine* 11, 629–639.

Heath, A.W. (1995a). Cytokines as immunological adjuvants. In Powell, M. and Newman, M.J. (Eds) *Vaccine Design the Subunit and Adjuvant Approach*. Plenum Press, New York, pp. 645–655.

Heath, A.W. (1995b). The role of cytokines in the vaccination of immunocompromised hosts. *Int. J. Clin. Lab. Res.* 25, 25–28.

Heath, A.W. and Playfair, J.H.L. (1990). Conjugation of interferon gamma to antigen enhances its adjuvanticity. *Immunology* 71, 454–456.

Heath, A.W. and Playfair, J.H.L. (1992). Cytokines as immunological adjuvants. *Vaccine* 10, 427–434.

Heath, A.W. and Playfair, J.H.L. (1993). Cytokine antigen vaccines. *Nature* 364, 493.

Heath, A.W, Devey, M., Brown, I., Richards, C.E., and Playfair, J.H.L. (1989). Interferon gamma as an adjuvant in immunocompromised mice. *Immunology* 67, 520–524.

Hedlund, J., Langer, B., Konradsen, H.B., Ortqvist, A. (2001). Negligible adjuvant effect for antibody responses and frequent adverse events associated with IL-12 treatment in humans vaccinated with pneumococcal polysaccharide. *Vaccine* 20, 164–169.

Ho, R.J.Y., Burke, R.L., and Merigan, T.C. (1992). Liposome formulated interleukin 2 as an adjuvant of recombinant HSV glycoprotein D for the treatment of recurrent genital herpes in guinea pigs. *Vaccine* 10, 209–213.

Huang, Q., Richmond, J.F.L., Suzue, K., Eisen, H.N., and Young, R.A. (2000). *In vivo* cytotoxic T lymphocyte elicitation by mycobacterial heat shock protein 70 fusion proteins maps to a discrete domain and is CD4 T cell independent. *J. Exp. Med.* 191, 403–408.

Huber, V.C., Arulanandam, B.P., Arnaboldi, P.M, Elmore, M.K., Sheehan, C.E., Kallakury, B.V.S., and Metzger, D.W. (2003). Delivery of IL-12 intranasally leads to reduced IL-12-mediated toxicity. *Int. Immunopharmacol.* 3, 801–809.

Hurwitz, A.A., Yu, T.F.Y., Leach, D.R., and Allison, J.P. (1998). CTLA-4 blockade synergizes with tumor-derived granulocyte-macrophage colony-stimulating factor for treatment of an experimental mammary carcinoma. *Proc. Natl. Acad. Sci. USA* 95, 10067–10071.

Kawabe, T, Naka, T., Yoshida, K., Tanaka, T., Fujiwara, H., Suematsu, S., Yoshida, N., Kishimoto, T., and Kikutani, H. (1994). The immune responses in CD40-deficient mice: impaired immunoglobulin class switching and germinal center formation. *Immunity* 3, 167–178.

Klein, D.L. and Ellis R.W. (1997). Conjugate vaccines against *Streptococcus pneumoniae*. In Levine, M.M., Woodrow, G.C., Kaper, J.B., and Cobon, G.S. (Eds) *New Generation Vaccines*, 2nd edn. Marcel Dekker, New York, pp. 503–525.

Konen-Waisman, S., Fridkin, M., and Cohen, I.R. (1995). Self and foreign 60-kilodalton heat shock protein T cell epitope peptides serve as immunogenic carriers for a T cell-independent sugar antigen. *J. Immunol.* 154, 5977–5985.

Konen-Waisman, S., Cohen, A., Fridkin, M., and Cohen, I.R. (1999). Self heat shock protein (hsp60) peptide serves in a conjugate vaccine against a lethal pneumococcal infection. *J. Infect. Dis.* 179, 403–413.

Kunkel, L.A. (2004). Idiotype vaccines in the treatment of B-cell non-Hodgkin's lymphoma. *Cancer Invest.* 22, 97–105.

Le Bon, A., Schiavoni, G., D'Agostino, G., Gresser, I., Belardelli, F., and Tough, D.F. (2001). Type I interferons potently enhance humoral immunity and can promote class switching by stimulating dendritic cells *in vivo*. *Immunity* 14, 461–470.

Lee, P., Wang, F., Kuniyoshi, J., Rubio, V., Stuges, T., Groshen, S., Gee, C., Lau, R., Jeffery, G., Margolin, K., Marty, V., and Weber, J. (2001). Effects of interleukin-12 on the immune response to a multipeptide vaccine for resected metastatic melanoma. *J. Clin. Oncol.* 19, 3836–3847.

Leonard, J.P., Sherman, M.L., Fisher, G.L., Buchanan, L.J., Larsen, G., Atkins, M.B., Sosman, J.A., Dutcher, J.P., Vogelzang N.J., and Ryan, J.L. (1997). Effects of single-dose interleukin-12 exposure on interleukin-12-associated toxicity and interferon-gamma production. *Blood* 90, 2541–2548.

Lin, R., Tarr, P., and Jones, T.C. (1995). Present status of the use of cytokines as adjuvants with vaccines to protect against infectious diseases. *Clin. Infect. Dis.* 21, 1439–1449.

Lou, D. and Kohler, H. (1998). Enhanced molecular mimicry of CEA using photoaffinity crosslinked C3d peptide. *Nature Biotechnol.* 16, 458–462.

Manoj, S., Griebel, P.J., Babiuk, L.A., and van Drunen Littel-van den Hurk, S. (2003). Targeting with bovine CD154 enhances humoral immune responses induced by a DNA vaccine in sheep. *J. Immunol.* 170, 989–996.

Markham, R.B., Nicholson-Weller, A., Schiffman, G., and Kasper, D.L. (1982). The presence of sialic acid on two related bacterial polysaccharides determines the site of the primary immune response and the effect of complement depletion on the response in mice. *J. Immunol.* 128, 2731–2733.

Matsui, M., Moria, O., Belladonna, M.L., Kamiya, S., Lemonnier, F.A., Yoshimoto, T., and Akatsuka, T. (2004). Adjuvant activities of novel cytokines, interleukin 23 (IL-23) and interleukin 27 (IL27) for induction of hepatitis C virus specific cytotoxic T lymphocytes in HLA A*0201 transgenic mice. *J. Virol.* 78, 9093–9104.

McCormick, A.L., Thomas, M.S., and Heath, A.W. (2001). Immunization with an interferon-γ–gp120 fusion protein induces enhanced immune responses to human immunodeficiency virus gp120. *J. Infect. Dis.* 184, 1423–1430.

Meuer, S.C., Dumann, H., Meyer zum Buschenfelde, K.H., and Kohler, H. (1989). Low-dose interleukin-2 induces systemic immune responses against HBsAg in immuno-deficient non-responders to hepatitis B vaccination. *Lancet* i, 15–17.

Mitchell, J.A., Green, T.D., Bright, R.A., and Ross, T.M. (2003). Induction of heterosubtypic immunity to influenza A virus using a DNA vaccine expressing hemagglutinin-C3d fusion proteins. *Vaccine* 21, 902–914.

Murray, J.L., Gillogly, M.E., Przepiorka, D., Brewer, H., Ibrahim, N.K, Booser, D.J., Hortobagyi, G.N., Kudelka, A.P., Grabstein, K.H., Cheever, M.A., and Ioannides, C.G. (2002). Toxicity, immunogenicity, and induction of E75-specific tumor-lytic CTLs by HER-2 peptide E75 (369-377) combined with granulocyte macrophage colony-stimulating factor in HLA-A2+ patients with metastatic breast and ovarian cancer. *Clin. Cancer Res.* 8, 3407–3418.

Nencioni, L., Villa, L., Tagliabue, A., Antoni, G., Presentini, R., Perin, F. et al. (1987). *In vivo* immunostimulating activity of the 163-171 peptide of human IL-lb. *J. Immunol.* 13, 800–804.

Nimal, S., McCormick, A.L., Thomas, M.S., and Herth, A.W. (2005). An interferon gamma-gp120 fusion delivered as a DNA vaccine induces enhanced priming. *Vaccine* 23, 3984–3990.

Ninomiya, A., Ogasawara, K., Kajino, K., Takada, A., and Kida, H. (2002). Intranasal administration of a synthetic peptide vaccine encapsulated in liposome together with an anti-CD40 antibody induces protective immunity against influenza A virus in mice. *Vaccine* 20, 3123–3129.

Nunberg, J., Doyle, M.V., York, S.M., and York, C.J. (1989). Interleukin 2 acts as an adjuvant to enhance the potency of inactivated rabies virus vaccine. *Proc. Natl. Acad. Sci. USA* 86, 4249–4243.

Pan, P.Y., Zang, Y., Weber, K., Meseck, M.L., and Chen, S.H. (2002). OX40 ligation enhances primary and memory cytotoxic T lymphocyte responses in an immunotherapy for hepatic colon metastases. *Mol. Ther.* 6, 528–536.

Paulie, S., Ehlin-Henriksson, S., Mellstedt, H., Koho, H., Ben-Aissa, H., and Perlmann, P. (1985). A p50 sur-face antigen restricted to human urinary bladder carcino-mas and B lymphocytes. *Cancer Immunol. Immunother.* 20, 23–28.

Quezada, S.A., Jarvinen, L.Z., Lind, E.F., and Noelle, R.J. (2003). CD40/CD154 interactions at the interface of tolerance and immunity. *Annu. Rev. Immunol.* 22, 307–328.

Quiroga, J.A., Castillo, I., Porres, J.C., Casado, S., Saez, F., Gracia Martinez, M. et al. (1990). Recombinant gamma interferon as adjuvant to hepatitis B vaccine in haemodia-lysis patients. *Hepatology* 12, 661–663.

Reed, S.G., Pihl, D.K., Conlon, P.J., and Grabstein, K.H. (1989). IL1 as adjuvant. Role of T cells in the augmentation of specific antibody production by recombinant human IL1α. *J. Immunol.* 142, 3129–3133.

Ridge, J.P., Di Rosa, F., and Matzinger, P. (1998). A conditioned dendritic cell can be a temporal bridge between a CD4 T-helper and a T-killer cell. *Nature* 393, 474.

Rolph, M.S. and Kaufmann, S.H. (2001). CD40 signaling converts a minimally immunogenic antigen into a potent vaccine against the intracellular pathogen Listeria mono-cytogenes. *J. Immunol.* 166, 5115–5121.

Román, E. and Moreno, C. (1996). Synthetic pep-tides noncovalently bound to bacterial hsp70 elicit peptide-specific T-cell responses *in vivo. Immunology.* 88, 487–492.

Romani, L., Puccetti, P., and Bistoni, F. (1997). Interleukin-12 in infectious diseases. *Clin. Micro. Rev.* 10, 611–636.

Ross, T.M., Xu, Y., Bright, R.A., and Robinson, H.L. (2000). C3d enhancement of antibodies to hemagglutinin accelerates protection against influenza challenge. *Nature Immunol*, 1, 127–131.

Ross, T.M., Xu, Y., Green, T.D., Montefiori, D.C., and Robinson, H.L. (2001). Enhanced avidity maturation of antibody to human immunodeficiency virus envelope: DNA vaccination with gp120-C3d fusion proteins. *AIDS Res. Hum. Retrovir.* 17, 829–836.

Rowley, T.F. and Al-Shamkhani, A. (2004). Stimulation by soluble CD70 promotes strong primary and secondary CD8 cytotoxic T cell responses *in vivo J. Immunol.* 172, 6039–6046.

Schijns, V.E.C.J., Haagmans, B.L., and Horzinek, M.C. (1995). IL-12 stimulates an antiviral type-1 cytokine response but lacks adjuvant activity in IFN-gamma-receptor-deficient mice *J. Immunol.* 2525–2532.

Schonbeck, U., Mach, F., and Libby P. (2000). Molecules in focus: CD154 (CD40 ligand). *Int. J. Biochem. Cell Biol.* 32, 687–693.

Schoenberger, S.P., Toes R.E., van der Voort, E.I., Offringa, R., and Melief, C.J. (1998). T-cell help for cytotoxic T lymphocytes is mediated by CD40-CD40L interactions. *Nature* 393, 480.

Sha, B.E., Onorato, M., Bartlett, J.A, Bosch, R.J, Aga, E., Nokta, M., Adams, E.M., Li, X.D., Eldridge, J., and Pollard, R.B. (2004). Safety and immunogenicity of a polyvalent peptide C4-V3HIV vaccine in conjunction with IL-12. *AIDS* 18, 1203–1206.

Singh-Hora, M., Rana, R.K., Nunberg, J.H., Tice, T.R., Gilley, R.M., and Hudson, M.E. (1990). Controlled release of interleukin 2 from biodegradable microspheres. *Biotechnology* 8, 755–758.

Staruch, M.J. and Wood, D.D. (1983). The adjuvanticity of interleukin 1 in vivo. *J. Immunol.* 130, 2191–2194.

Suradhat, S., Braun, R.P., Lewis, P.J., Babiuk, L.A., Little-van den Hurk, S.D., Griebel, P.J., and Abca-Estrada, M.E. (2001). Fusion of C3d molecule with bovine rotavirus VP7 or bovine herpesvirus type 1 glycoprotein D inhibits immune responses following DNA immunization. *Vet. Immunol. Immunopathol.* 83, 79–92.

Suzue, K. and Young, R.A. (1996). Adjuvant-free hsp70 fusion protein elicits humoral and cellular immune responses to HIV-1 p24. *J. Immunol.* 156, 873–879.

Suzue, K., Zhou, X., Eisen, H.N., and Young, R.A. (1997). Heat shock fusion proteins as vehicles for antigen delivery into the major histocompatibility complex class I presentation pathway. *Proc. Natl. Acad. Sci. USA* 94, 13146–13151.

Tamura, S., Ito, Y., Asanuma, H., Hirabnayashi, Y., Suzuki, Y., Nagamine, T., Aizawa, C., Kurata, T., and Oya, A. (2003). Cross-protection against influenza virus infection afforded by trivalent inactivated vaccines inoculated intranasally with cholera toxin B subunit. *J. Immunol.* 149, 981–988.

Tao, M.-H. and Levy, R. (1993). Idiotype/granulocyte-macrophage colony-stimulating factor fusion protein as a vaccine for B-cell lymphoma. *Nature* 362, 755–758.

Tedder, T.F., Zhou, L.-J., and Engel, P. (1994). The CD19/CD21 signal transduction complex by B lymphocytes. *Immunol. Today* 15, 437–442.

Test, S.T., Mitsuyoshij, J., Connolly, C.C, and Lucas, A.H. (2001). Increased immunogenicity and induction of class switching by conjugation of complement C3d to pneumococcal serotype 14 capsular polysaccharide. *Infect. Immun.* 69, 3031–3040.

Toapanta, F.R. and Ross, T.M. (2004). Mouse strain-dependent differences in enhancement of immune responses by C3d. *Vaccine* 22, 1773–1781.

Udono, H., Yamano, T., Kawabata, Y., Ueda, M., and Yui, K. (2001). Generation of cytotoxic T lymphocytes by MHC class I ligands fused to heat shock cognate protein 70. *Int. Immunol.* 13, 1233–1242.

Van Kooten, C. and Banchereau, J. (1996). CD40-CD40 ligand: a multifunctional receptor–ligand pair. *Adv. Immunol.* 61, 1–77.

Van Kooten, C. and Banchereau, L. (1997). Functions of CD40 on B cells, dendritic cells and other cells. *Curr. Opin. Immunol.* 9, 330–337.

Vignaux, F., Gresser, I., and Fridman, W.H. (1980). Effect of virus induced interferon on the antibody response of suckling and adult mice. *Eur. J. Immunol.* 10, 767–772.

Villiers, M.B., Villiers, C.L., Laharie, A.-M., and Marche, P.N. (1999). Amplification of the antibody response by C3b complexed to antigen through an ester link. *J. Immunol.* 162, 3647–3652.

Wan, T., Zhou, X., Chen, G., An, H., Chen, T., Zhang, W., Liu, S., Jiang, Y., Yang, F., Wu, Y., and Cao, X. (2004). Novel heat shock protein Hsp70L1 activated dendritic cells and acts as a Th1 polarizing adjuvant. *Blood* 103, 1747–1754.

Wang, Y., Kelly, C., Kattunen, J., Whitall, T., Lehner, P., Duncan, L., MacAry, P., Younson, J., Singh, M., and Oehlmann, W. (2001). CD40 is a cellular receptor mediating mycobaterial heat shock protein 70 stimulation of CC-chemokines. *Immunity* 15, 971–983.

Wang, L.-X., Xu, W., Guan, Q.-D., Chu, Y.-W., Wang, Y., and Xiong, S.-D. (2004). Contribution of C3d-P28 repeats to enhancement of immune responses against HBV-preS2/S induced by gene immunization. *World J. Gastroenterol.* 10, 2072–2077.

Watanabe, I., Ross, T.M, Tamura, S., Ichinohe, T., Ito, S., Takahashi, H., Sawa, H., Chiba, J., Kurata, T., Sata, T., and Hasegawa, H. (2003). Protection against influenza virus infection by intranasal administration of C3d-fused hemagglutinin. *Vaccine* 21, 4532–4538.

Weinberg, A. and Merigan, T.C. (1988). Recombinant interleukin 2 as an adjuvant for vaccine-induced protection. Immunisation of guinea pigs with herpes simplex virus subunit vaccines. *J. Immunol.* 140, 294–299.

Weinberg, A.D., Rivera, M.M., Prell, R., Morris, A., Ramstad, T., Vetto, J.T., Urba W.J., Alvord, G., Bunce, C., and Shields, J. (2000). Engagement of the OX-40 receptor *in vivo* enhances antitumor immunity. *J Immunol.* 164, 2160–2169.

Wrightsman, R.A. and Manning, J.E. (2000). Paraflagellar rod proteins administered with alum and IL-12 or recombinant adenovirus expressing IL-12 generates antigen-specific responses and protective immunity in mice against Trypanosoma cruzi. *Vaccine* 18, 1419–1427.

Xiang, R., Primus, F.J., Ruehlmann, J.M., Niethammer, A.G., Silletti, S., Lode, H.N., Dolman, C.S., Gillies, S.D., and Reisfeld, R.A. (2001). Dual-function DNA vaccine encoding carcinoembryonic antigen and CD40 ligand trimer induces T cell-mediated protective immunity against colon cancer in carcinoembryonic antigen-transgenic mice. *J. Immunol.* 167, 4560–4565.

Xu, J., Foy, T.M., Laman, J.D., Elliott, E.A., Dunn, J., Waldschmidt, T.J., Elsemore, J., Noelle, R.J., and Flavell, R.A. (1994). Mice deficient for the CD40 ligand. *Immunity* 1, 423–431.

Innate immune mechanisms and the identification of immune potentiators as vaccine adjuvants

Achal Pashine, Jeffrey B. Ulmer, and Nicholas M. Valiante
Chiron Corporation, Emeryville, California

■ Introduction

Vaccines are considered to be one of the most significant medical interventions against infectious diseases (Hilleman, 2000). Despite this success, major obstacles remain in developing vaccines for pathogens against which vaccines do not exist (such as hepatitis C virus, HCV) or against emerging pathogens (such as severe acute respiratory syndrome, SARS) and improving suboptimal vaccines (such as bacille Calmette-Guerin, BCG) (Kieny et al., 2004). Key elements needed to design effective vaccines include (i) identification of protective antigen(s) against which a robust and durable adaptive response must be generated, (ii) compounds that can stimulate the innate immune responses (Hoebe et al., 2004), e.g., bacterial cell wall components, and (iii) optimal delivery systems, which will carry and dispense the antigenic and immunostimulatory cargo to the appropriate cells of the immune system (O'Hagan, 2004). A key gap in our understanding, but an area of significant future gains, centers on issues relating to recent developments in the field of innate immunity, the mechanistic underpinnings of adjuvant activity, and the use of novel immune potentiators in vaccine formulations.

■ Innate immunity: a trigger point for the immune system

Upon interaction with pathogens, the innate immune system provides a first line of defense and reacts within minutes to minimize the immediate threat posed by the pathogen. In addition, the early activation of innate immune components serves to create an inflammatory environment that conditions the host for effective generation of adaptive immune responses (Iwasaki and Medzhitov, 2004). This rapid activation of innate immunity is achieved through the recognition of relatively conserved molecules found associated with pathogens. In essence, the innate immune system has evolved to detect broad and conserved structures associated with infectious agents. Conversely, the adaptive immune system, which is comprised of antigen-specific T and B cells, is more focused on the antigenic epitopes found in the proteins and carbohydrates

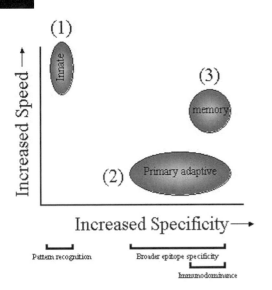

Figure 4.1 Speed and specificity of the immune response. (1)
Cells of the innate immune system, such as macrophages, dendritic
cells, NK cells, and neutrophils, rapidly respond to microbial patterns
through their pattern recognition receptors and are the first line of
defense against invading pathogens. Their early activation also
provides the inflammatory context for antigen recognition by cells of
the adaptive immune response. Despite their ability to respond
quickly, the effectiveness of the innate response is limited due to the
lack of fine specificity. (2) Although slower, adaptive immune
responses are precise because of the incredible diversity of antigen
receptors on the surface of T and B cells. (3) Memory T and B cells are
activated much more rapidly compared to the initiation of primary
adaptive cell responses and their antigen specificity is more focused.
Thus memory responses, the goal of vaccination, provide both speed
and specificity in the recognition and elimination of infectious agents.

derived from pathogens. This focused response is slower due to the time needed to
expand B and T cell clones bearing antigen
receptors with the appropriate specificity. The
ultimate goal of natural host defense and
prophylactic vaccination is to generate adaptive memory responses that are both rapid and
highly focused (Figure 4.1). Targeting of both
the innate and adaptive arms of the immune
systems is critical in achieving this goal.

■ Pathogen-associated molecular patterns and pattern recognition receptors

In 1989 Charles Janeway postulated that the
immune system may be equipped to trigger an
innate immune response using pattern recognition receptors (PRRs) that can be engaged
by pathogen-associated molecular patterns
(PAMPs; Janeway, 1989). At the time it was
known that lipopolysaccharide (LPS), lipo-
techoic acid, double-stranded (ds) RNA, peptidoglycans, and other pathogen components
could nonspecifically stimulate immune cells
and that some of these components functioned
as vaccine adjuvants when added to immunization regimens along with specific antigen.
Thus, the addition of such mircobial components to experimental immunizations leads
to the development of robust and durable
adaptive immune response. The mechanism
behind this potentiation of immune responses
was not very well understood until recently,
when some of the PRRs involved in the innate
immune response to PAMPs were identified
(Table 4.1). Engagement of these PRRs may
lead to the activation of one or more immune
cells, such as macrophages, neutrophils, dendritic cells (DCs), natural killer (NK) cells, and
B cells. Some of the PRRs are also expressed on
nonimmune cells, such as epithelial and endothelial cells, and activate these cells during
infection and possibly vaccination. PRR-
mediated activation of cells leads to secretion
of inflammatory cytokines and chemokines.
In addition, they may lead to maturation and
migration of key antigen-presenting cells
(APCs), such as DCs (Figure 4.2).

While postulating PAMPs, Janeway perhaps
envisioned that the high-order multimeric
patterns (lattices) with precise spatial arrange-
ments of these immunostimulatory compounds
gave rise to pathogen recognition and subsequent innate immune activation. However,
experimental evidence suggests that PRR
specificities are not primarily driven by the
multimeric patterns of well-known PAMPs,
as specific receptor–ligand engagements
appear to be governing recognition of pathogenic signatures or patterns (Beutler, 2003).
This is important to note in the context of the
discovery of novel synthetic compounds that
could stimulate PRRs. Nevertheless, as has been
recently shown with other receptor–ligand

Table 4.1 Pattern recognition receptors (Akira and Takeda, 2004)

Receptor	Ligand
TLR-1[a]	Bacterial lipoproteins from mycobacterium, neisseria
TLR-2[a]	Zymosan yeast particles, peptidoglycan, lipoproteins, glycolipids, lipopolysaccharides
TLR-3	Viral double-stranded RNA, poly (IC)
TLR-4	Bacterial lipopolysaccharides, plant product taxol
TLR-5	Bacterial flagellins
TLR-6[a]	Yeast zymosan particles, lipotechoic acid, lipopeptides from mycoplasma
TLR-7	ssRNA; immiquimod and R848; other synthetic nucleoside analog compounds such as loxoribine and bropirimine
TLR-8[b]	Single-stranded RNA, R848, immiquimod
TLR-9	CpG oligonucleotides[c]
TLR-10	Unknown
TLR11	Bacterial components from uropathogenic bacteria
Nod1, 2	Peptidoglycan
Scavenger receptors	Acetylated/malelylated proteins; modified low-density lipoproteins and other polyanionic ligands
Macrophage mannose receptors and other c-type lectin receptors	Sulfated sugars, mannose, fucose, and galactose modified polysaccharides and proteins
Type 3 complement receptors and dectin type receptors	Zymosan particles, β-glucan

[a] TLR-1 and 6 can form heterodimers with TLR-2 that further changes their specificities.

[b] TLR-8 is found to be active only in humans.

[c] Different CpG oligonucleotide sequences are optimal for murine and human TLR-9.

pairs such as T cell receptor–major histocompatibility complex (TCR-MHC) interactions, the formation of higher order structures of ligand–receptor pairs may be necessary to transmit potent downstream signals.

Janeway's postulate about PRRs was confirmed years later, when the drosophila transmembrane receptor protein, Toll, was shown to regulate antifungal responses (Lemaitre et al., 1996). Soon after this discovery, Medzhitov cloned the first mammalian Toll-like receptor (TLR) that was essential for LPS recognition (Medzhitov et al., 1997). Based on sequence homology, many other mammalian TLRs were subsequently cloned and shown to respond to a multitude of pathogenic ligands (Table 4.1). PRRs can be broadly divided into two classes, one that leads to phagocytosis, such as scavenger receptors, mannose receptors, and β-glucan receptors (Gordon, 2002), and others that are nonphagocytic, such as TLRs and nucleotide binding oligomerizing domain proteins (Nods). However, TLR-induced phagocytosis, which may be due to indirect effects of inflammatory response, has been reported (Doyle et al., 2004). As the name suggests, phagocytic receptors upon engagement with their ligands lead to the engulfment into phagocytic cells, such as macrophages. By contrast, nonphagocytic receptors upon engagement with their respective ligands lead to elaborate signal transduction cascades and distinct cellular activation events.

Some of the PRRs have been shown to bind their ligands directly (Sato et al., 2003; Lien et al., 2000; Rutz et al., 2004), but it remains to be seen whether this is a general rule or whether intermediate protein components are involved. One of the key questions in the biology of PRRs is how to justify a large number of often structurally different ligands being recognized by a limited number of receptors. One way to explain the complexity of ligand recognition is to implicate intermediate proteins which may have conserved sites for PRR binding and other distinct sites that bind different PAMPs. For example, drosophila Toll has been shown to recognize microbial ligands only through its interaction with Spätzle, a host protein that directly interacts with microbial components (Lemaitre et al., 1996). Similarly, mammalian TLR-4 recognizes LPS indirectly through LPS binding protein (LBP) and the surface receptor CD14

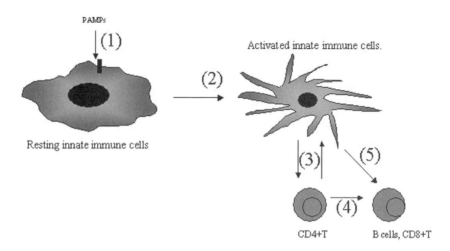

Figure 4.2 Cellular response to PRR-mediated trigger. Upon stimulation through Toll-like receptors (TLRs), tissue resident dendritic cells (I), which bridge innate and adaptive immunity, undergo maturation (2) that leads to their increased expression of costimulatory molecules, increased surface expression of MHC-class II molecules, and their migration to secondary lymphoid tissue, such as spleen and lymph nodes. Priming of antigen-specific naive CD4 T cells (3) takes place in secondary lymphoid organs. Activated CD4+ cells undergo clonal expansion and provide help to antigen-specific B cells to undergo antibody class switching as well as to CD8 T cells (4). In addition, activated dendritic cells may license CD8+ T cells to become cytotoxic. PRR-mediated activation of B cells may contribute to long-term serological memory (Bernasconi et al., 2002).

(Schroder et al., 2000). Moreover, it was shown that LBP also binds to structurally different peptidoglycan moieties from pneumococcal cell wall (PCW) that mainly signal through TLR-2 (Weber et al., 2003). These findings suggests that the addition of a second tier for PAMP recognition by intermediate proteins such as LBP creates greater diversity for ligand recognition by a limited set of receptors like the TLR family.

Innate immunity conditions the host for subsequent adaptive immunity

Goals of innate immune activation are two-fold: to limit the immediate threat by direct action of effector cells such as neutrophils, NK cells, macrophages, etc., and to establish a microenvironment that will be conducive to specific adaptive immunity. Signaling through TLRs as well as Nod proteins results mainly in the activation of transcription factors such as NFkB and IRF3 that provide the inflammatory context for the rapid activation of host defenses

(Akira and Takeda, 2004). The NFkB pathway controls the expression of proinflammatory cytokines such as IL-1β and TNF-α, whereas the IRF3 pathway leads to the production of antiviral type I interferons (IFN-α and IFN-β). Along with these cytokines, various chemokines, such as IL-8, monocyte chemoattractant proteins (MCPs), macrophage inflammatory proteins (MIPs), and RANTES are released and their receptors expressed on the surface of activated cells. As a result, vascular endothelial cells may alter surface expression of selectins and intercellular cell adhesion molecules (ICAMs) leading to the extravasation and selective retention of leukocytes at the inflamed site. This cellular infiltrate consists of activated monocytes, neutrophils, basophils, eosinophils, and NK cells, many of which also express TLRs and subsequently become activated by the presence of their respective ligands and secrete a variety of necessary cytokines and chemokines. As a consequence of this inflammatory microenvironment, monocytes that infiltrate the site can differentiate into macrophages and DCs; the latter being crucial in priming of naive CD4+ helper as well as inducing CD8+ T cell differentiation into killer cells. DC subsets, which express distinct arrays of TLRs, are found at strategic anatomical sites allowing them to respond rapidly to microbial invasion (Kadowaki et al., 2001). Upon capture of antigen and PAMP-induced maturation, DCs migrate to local lymphoid tissues where antigenic peptides are presented to T cells via MHC class I and class II molecules, thus starting the clonal expansion of antigen-specific T cells (Figure 4.2). Besides a direct effect on priming of specific T cells, the innate immune response may have indirect effects, as has been suggested that DCs activated through a TLR may gain an ability to inhibit the suppressive ability of CD4+CD25+ regulatory T cells (Treg) (Pasare and Medzhitov, 2003). Also, it has been suggested that engagement of B cells by some TLRs may be a crucial point in isotype switching as well as antibody secretion capability (Bernasconi et al., 2002; Liu et al., 2003). Hence, innate immune activation is crucial to the robustness of adaptive immunity. Indeed, it has long been the "immunologist's dirty little secret," before the establishment of the PAMP-PRR recognition concept, that the addition of nonspecific microbial components to experimental purified proteins during immunization elicits much stronger specific response (Anderson, 1955). Recent growing knowledge of various components of the mammalian innate immune system can make the process of selection of immune potentiating compounds more informed, thus reducing probable associated toxicity while increasing their usefulness in vaccine formulations.

■ Adjuvants in vaccine research

Adjuvants historically are defined functionally as vaccine components that enhance the immunogenicity of antigen *in vivo*. Adjuvants can be functionally differentiated as immuno-potentiators and delivery vehicles (O'Hagan, 2004). Immune potentiators directly activate the innate immune system (e.g., induction of inflammatory cytokines) whereas delivery systems concentrate and display antigens in repetitive patterns (e.g., cationic microparticles) (O'Hagan et al., 2004), target antigens to APCs, or help co-localize antigens and immune potentiators. Ideal immune potentiators can improve the effectiveness of vaccines by (i) accelerating the generation of robust immune responses, (ii) sustaining responses for a longer duration, (iii) generating antibodies with increased avidity and neutralization capacity, (iv) eliciting cytotoxic T lymphocytes (CTLs), (v) enhancing immune responses in individuals with weakened immune systems (e.g., children and elderly or immunocompromised adults), (vi) increasing a responder to non-responder ratio for a given vaccine, and (vii) reducing the amount of antigen needed, thus reducing the cost of vaccination programs.

Early vaccine research mainly emphasized better humoral responses; as a result currently licensed adjuvants such as aluminum salts are geared towards enhancing antibody responses without significant elicitation of Th1 or CTL responses (Lindblad, 2004). However, the need for effective vaccines that may prevent chronic viral diseases, such as HIV and HCV, has altered a paradigm of vaccination towards the generation of cellular response in addition to neutralizing antibody responses. Moreover, a more detailed and sophisticated understanding of the biology of individual infectious diseases as well as unique characteristics of protective immune responses against them suggests that a few-adjuvants-many-vaccines model will not be an optimal solution. Thus, a battery of specifically tailored adjuvant candidates for next-generation vaccines that can be used to elicit superior (quantitative and qualitative) memory responses is needed. There has been an explosion of information on innate immunity generated in academic research laboratories in the last decade that is slowly being used to generate a new generation of immunopotentiators to tackle conventional as well as emerging infectious diseases. To this end, many new and existing adjuvant formulations are being tested in various clinical and preclinical trials (Table 4.2).

Table 4.2 Adjuvants and delivery systems in preclinical and clinical trials (Aguado et al., 1999; Engers et al., 2003; Kenney et al., 2002; Pink and Kieny, 2004)

Adjuvant category	Representative examples
Mineral salts	Aluminum and calcium salts[a]
Emulsions and surfactant-based formulations	MF59[a], AS02, Montanide ISA-51 and ISA-720, QS21
Particulate delivery vehicles	Microparticles, immunostimulatory complexes; liposomes, virosomes, virus-like particles
Microbial derivatives	Monophosphoryl lipid A, CpG oligonucleotides, cholera toxin and heat labile toxin from *E. coli*, lipoproteins
Cells and cytokines	Dendritic cells; ILl2 and GM-CSF

[a] Currently licensed for human use as adjuvants.

Structure and function of TLRs and Nods

TLRs are the largest and best-studied family of PRRs. They are type I integral membrane glycoproteins with considerable cytoplasmic domain homology to IL-1 receptors. Structurally, TLRs consist of an extracellular domain that contains 19–25 leucine-rich repeat (LRR) motifs. LRR domains have been suggested to form a horseshoe-like concave structure that is thought to interact with their ligands either directly or indirectly through intermediate proteins. Intracellularly a conserved, ~200 amino acid cytoplasmic domain, known as TIR (Toll/IL1 receptor domain), is important for its association with adaptor proteins, thus linking these transmembrane receptors to their downstream signaling pathways (Takeda et al., 2003). Nod proteins consists of three main regions: a LRR domain, which may work similar to LRR domain of TLRs; a nuclear oligomerization domain that is essential for Nod clustering and subsequent signaling; and effector motifs such as the caspase recruitment domain that leads to actual signal transduction through binding to signaling kinases (Chamaillard et al., 2003a). In the absence of a canonical oligomerization domain,

it is not known whether oligomerization of TLRs takes place and whether it is required for signaling. As transmembrane proteins, it is possible that TLR membrane aggregation may occur through other transient structures such as lipid rafts or caveoli.

Ligands of TLRs and Nods

The TLR family is the single most abundant family of proteins identified to date that recognizes molecular signatures, with TLR-1-11 discovered mostly based on homology searches. Ligands to these receptors were either identified with over expression of these receptors in cells lacking them (such as human embryonic kidney (HEK) cells) or by using mouse strains that do not express particular TLRs because of gene targeting or by natural mutations in TLR genes. TLR-1 and TLR-6 share considerable homology and are shown to have qualitatively different functional cooperation with TLR-2 (Takeuchi et al., 1999). For example, in a HeLa cell system coexpression of TLR-1 and TLR-2 resulted in increased reactivity to *Neisseria meningitides* components (Wyllie et al., 2000), whereas TLR-2 and TLR-6 cooperatively recognize peptidoglycan from *Staphylococcus aureus* (Ozinsky et al., 2000). TLR-6-deficient macrophages respond normally to tri-palmitoyl lipopeptides from other bacteria through TLR-2, but do not recognize di-palmitoyl-derived lipopeptides from mycoplasmal origin. The recognition of the latter is only restored when TLR-2 and TLR-6 are coexpressed. This functional cooperation may be due to a physical interaction between individual TLR molecules (Tapping and Tobias, 2003). Interaction of TLR heterodimers, such as the one described above, or their ability to collaborate with other innate immune receptors may also be helpful in generating qualitative differences in microbial component recognition as well as inflammatory outcomes (Mukhopadhyay et al., 2004). This observation could be useful in devising assays to screen for novel TLR agonists.

A specific blocking monoclonal antibody against TLR-3, as well as TLR-3 transfectants of HEK cells, demonstrated that the recognition of poly-I:C sequence and other dsRNA sequences were TLR-3 dependent (Matsumoto et al., 2002). In addition, TLR-3 gene targeted mice have defective responses to viral RNA, indicating that TLR-3 is involved in viral RNA recognition (Alexopoulou et al., 2001). Immunostaining analysis of monocyte-derived DCs as well as transfected B cell lines showed intracellular localization of TLR-3 and the responses were not blockable with anti-TLR-3 monoclonal antibody. Thus, the expression and localization of TLR-3 may be modulated either by TLR-3 or the maturation state type of expressing cells (Matsumoto et al., 2003).

LPS is a major membrane component of Gram-negative bacteria. TLR-4, which is now shown to be the crucial sensor of LPS, was the first mammalian TLR to be cloned based on homology to drosophilla Toll (Medzhitov et al., 1997). Historically, mouse strains such as C3H/HeJ have been known to be LPS hyporesponsive; subsequent to the cloning of TLR-4, a mutation in TLR-4 cytoplasmic region was found in C3H/HeJ mice that explained defective TLR-4-mediated signaling and LPS hyporesponsiveness (Poltorak et al., 1998; Qureshi et al., 1999). Although TLR-4 has been established as an essential receptor for LPS responsiveness, other molecules, such as CD14, LBP, and MD-2, have been identified in aiding LPS recognition (Haziot et al., 2001; Shimazu et al., 1999; Akashi et al., 2003). Moreover, TLR-4 has also been implicated as a sensor for a variety of other structurally divergent pathogen products, suggesting that LPS recognition is one of many functions for this receptor (O'Hagan and Valiante, 2003).

CHO cells expressing TLR-5 were found to respond to culture supernatants from Gram-positive and Gram-negative bacteria. Purification of culture supernatant led to the discovery that bacterial flagellin is a TLR-5 stimulatory component (Hayashi et al., 2001). Since then flagellin proteins from a variety of bacteria have been shown to be TLR-5 agonists.

The life cycles of infectious agents in their hosts can be largely extracellular (e.g., many bacteria), or intracellular where rapid entry into cells is required for survival and continued proliferation (e.g., most viruses and some bacteria like mycobacterium, leishmania, and salmonella). Thus, optimal recognition of some ligands, such as viral RNA and bacterial DNA, requires intracellular receptors, whereas bacterial cell wall components, such as LPS or lipoproteins, are best detected extracellularly. Some other ligands, such as peptidoglycans, appear to be recognized extracellularly as well as intracellularly. TLR-1, 2, 4, 5, 6, and 11, whose ligands are most probably available extracellularly are surface expressed, while TLR-3, 7, 8, and 9 and Nod family proteins are localized in subcellular organelles or in the cytoplasm and are therefore focused on intracellular pathogen ligands. This latter group of sensors also may require acidic compartments for optimal recognition of their natural ligands (Lee et al., 2003). Based on sequence homology and similarity of ligands (purine derivatives), it is suggested that TLR-7, 8, and 9 belong to a common subfamily of TLRs (Du et al., 2000; Chuang and Ulevitch, 2000). The natural ligand for TLR-9 is bacterial DNA. Moreover, species specificity has been observed in optimal ligand recognition; thus human TLR-9 does not optimally recognize CpG oligonucleotide sequences that are best recognized by murine TLR-9 and vice versa (Bauer et al., 2001). These observations on cellular localization of some TLRs and other distinctive features of PRRs should be considered during the experimental screening for novel immune potentiators. TLR-7 gene targeted mice have revealed that it may recognize G+U-rich single-stranded RNA (Lund et al., 2004). TLR-8, which also recognizes G+U-rich single-stranded RNA, is functional in humans but inactive in mice, probably due to amino acid deletions in the extracellular domain of the murine isoform (Jurk et al., 2002). Loxoribine, a low molecular weight guanosine analog that functions as an immune potentiator, is recognized by TLR-7, but not human TLR-8

(Heil et al., 2003). Contrary to this discrimination in ligand recognition, R-848 (resiquimod) stimulates human TLR-7 as well as TLR-8 (Hemmi et al., 2002; Jurk et al., 2002).

Other intracellular regulators of pathogen-induced inflammation include Nod family proteins. Nod1 has been shown to sense peptidoglycan motifs from Gram-negative bacteria (Girardin et al., 2003a; Chamaillard et al., 2003b). It was suggested that Nod1, which is found in the epithelial cells that line the intestinal tract, is thus a sensor of pathogenic Gram-negative bacteria in the gut. Nod2, which has considerable homology to Nod1, specifically recognizes muramyl dipeptide (Girardin et al., 2003b). Nod2 is expressed in cells of the myeloid lineage as well as in muscosal epithelial cells (Gutierrez et al., 2002). Thus, PRRs are expressed extracellularly as well as intracellularly depending on their ligands of choice. After their sensing of ligands, either directly or indirectly through intermediate proteins, specific signal transduction pathways are initiated that lead to inflammatory outcomes.

■ Signaling through PRRs

All TLRs, except TLR-3, share a common signaling pathway that utilizes an adapter protein called MyD88 (myeloid differentiation factor 88). In some cases (e.g., TLR-5, 7, and 9), MyD88 has been shown to bind directly via the TIR domain, whereas in others (e.g., TLR-2 and 4) another intermediate adaptor molecule known as TIRAP (TIR domain-containing adaptor protein) is involved. Through its N-terminal death domain MyD88 binds to another family of signal transducers, known as IRAKs (IL-1 receptor-associated kinase), which in turn bind to TRAF6. Subsequent activation of the transcription factors NFkB and AP-1 by TRAF6 involves yet other adaptor proteins known as TAK1 and TAB2 (Figure 4.3). One of the important questions in TLR biology is how the specificity in signal transduction is achieved given the similarity of the cytoplasmic domains. The multitude of adapter proteins involved in TLR signaling suggests that qualitative differences in signal transduction outcomes can be achieved by

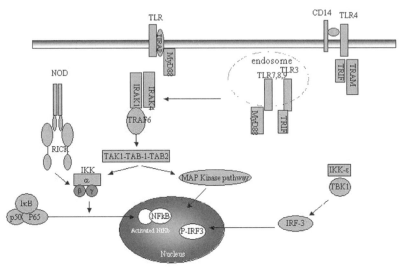

Figure 4.3 Signaling through PRRs. Three kinds of PRRs are shown: cytoplasmic, such as Nod proteins; endosomal, such as TLR-7, 8, and 9; and cell surface receptors, such as TLR-4. Upon interaction with their respective ligands, a signaling cascade is initiated which ultimately leads to the expression of inflammatory genes through activation of transcription factors NFkB or IRF3. A simplified pathway is shown here. Receptors interacting with multiple adapter proteins possibly provide the complexity of outcome. Regulator proteins of PRR signaling pathways provide a rich source of targets for drug discovery.

utilizing various combinations of receptor and adapter proteins (comprehensively reviewed in Akira et al., 2003).

In contrast to TLR signaling pathways, Nod proteins do not signal through a MyD88-dependent pathway. After association with their ligands, Nod1 and 2 activate the NFkB pathway through their CARD domain and the formation of signaling complexes with the receptor-interacting serine/threonine kinase (RICK). Subsequent activation of NFkB and MAPK pathways leads to expression of inflammatory cytokines and chemokines (reviewed in Chamaillard et al., 2003a). Signaling through PRRs thus involves a complex and rapidly growing set of transmembrane and intracellular adaptors and kinases that offer a wide range of potential targets for vaccine adjuvants.

■ Small-molecule immune potentiators: the future of adjuvants?

Given the plethora of natural products capable of activating innate immune mechanisms, research and development efforts to exploit these immune potentiators as vaccine adjuvants and therapeutics have been aggressive. Although *in vivo* proof of concept has been established for the use of many natural PAMPs as adjuvants and therapeutics and a number of these have been advanced into clinical trials, the trend for the future suggests an increased reliance on synthetic analogs. This is due mainly to the lower manufacturing and regulatory hurdles associated with synthetic immune potentiators, as these are highly defined and standardized. In addition, a synthetic platform allows for a more rational approach to the optimization of next-generation compounds possessing greater potency and decreased toxicity. From this perspective, perhaps the most promising immune potentiator platform recently identified is based on a small-molecule approach. The identification of imidizoquinolines as TLR-7- and/or TLR-8-dependent small-molecule immune potentiators (SMIPs) indicates that more traditional pharmaceutical-based or drug-like molecules can be exploited as vaccine adjuvants and immune modulators (Hemmi et al., 2002; Jurk et al., 2002). Indeed, imidizoquinolines have been shown to enhance antigen-specific responses in mouse models and, therefore, have the potential to be developed as adjuvants for humans (Vasilakos et al., 2000). It is important to note that the first-generation imidizoquinoline imiquimod is licensed as an antiviral as well as an anticancer topical therapy (Aldara®) and not a vaccine adjuvant. This indicates that SMIPs offer a flexible platform for use as both vaccine adjuvants and immune therapies.

A SMIP-based platform holds significant potential for the design and development of improved vaccine adjuvants. There are numerous advantages that can be realized throughout the discovery and development pipeline if SMIPs, rather than other natural or synthetic immune potentiators, are chosen as the platform of the future. For discovery efforts the incredible diversity of scaffolds generated through combinatorial chemistry, the ability to target innate immune mechanisms with exceptional selectivity, and the tried and tested drug discovery engines of high-throughput screening (HTS) and hit to lead (HTL) optimization can now be applied to immune potentiators. Moreover, the small-molecule platform opens up new avenues for manipulating the innate immune response by providing new intracellular targets and signaling pathways (Figure 4.3). Later in development and manufacturing a SMIP-based adjuvant provides a low-cost, highly pure, and standardized alternative to all other existing candidate immune potentiators. Given these advantages and the likelihood that more and diverse SMIP families will be discovered, it appears that the TLR-7/8 agonists, imidizaquinolines, represent only the first in a long line of future small-molecule-based adjuvants and therapeutics.

Drug discovery strategies for immune potentiators

Traditionally, efforts have been devoted in vaccine research towards identifying protective antigens rather than optimizing adjuvants able to change qualitatively the immune response. This probably was due to temporally different peaks of research activity in adaptive and innate immunity, with the latter peaking only recently. As a result, only two delivery systems (aluminum salts (Lindblad, 2004) and oil-in-water emulsions, MF59 (Podda, 2004)) and no direct immune potentiators are approved for widespread use in humans as adjuvants for prophylactic vaccines. This lack of progress in approval of immune potentiators as adjuvants is due to perceived toxicity risks and the lack of a comprehensive approach toward adjuvant discovery. Thus, to increase our portfolio of immune potentiator compounds to be used with new subunit vaccines and tailored to the specific requirements of each particular vaccine, a systematic approach towards novel adjuvant discovery is needed. Because of relatively well-understood outcomes of engaging various PRRs, high-throughput assays can be developed to screen large numbers of chemically defined compounds able to trigger them. HTS has been very successfully established in drug discovery research to search for inhibitors of various intracellular proteins and enzymes as well as to search for ligands of orphan receptors. In these drug discovery programs, often diverse chemical libraries were available to screen and the *in vitro* inhibition of a target was predictive of a compound's *in vivo* activity. If these two criteria are satisfied, HTS can become a tool of choice to screen for novel immunopotentiators. The identification of small drug-like chemicals of imidazoquinoline family as TLR-7 and 8 ligands suggests that HTS of large and diverse libraries of small molecules can be applied to novel adjuvant discovery. A general strategy of such a screening is outlined in Figure 4.4. Assays to identify

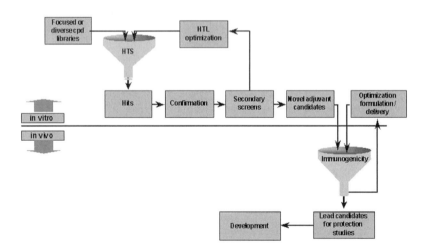

Figure 4.4 Drug discovery approach to immune potentiator discovery and optimization. Libraries of diverse chemical compounds (natural or synthetic) can be mined for immune potentiators using high-throughput screening (HTS). Cell-based assays can be designed to measure general activation of innate immune cells or screens can be targeted towards specific receptors or signaling components of the innate immune system such as Toll-like receptors (TLRs). Active compounds (hits) identified in a primary screen are then confirmed and prioritized based on level of potency and selectivity. In hit-to-lead (HTL) optimization, chemical analogs of the initial hits are generated and tested in an iterative fashion to identify compounds with increased potency and solubility. Secondary screens can be performed to evaluate mechanism of action, toxicity, and other parameters. The HTL-optimized immune potentiators (lead candidates) can then be formulated and tested for increased compatibility with different delivery systems. *In vivo* immunogenicity and toxicity studies using established vaccine candidates are conducted to identify lead immune potentiators, which then are put in development as novel vaccine adjuvants.

compounds can be open ended with functional outcome, such as cytokine secretion, without any bias towards a target as a scoring system. In contrast, well-established assays, such as TLR engagement-driven NFkB activation and cytokine secretion, can be used specifically to identify compounds targeting a particular pathway. Regardless of which approach is used, novel compounds and their analogs identified in HTS will need to be optimized for further development. Again drug discovery engines can be applied to the search for new immune potentiators. HTL optimization is an iterative process of structural modification and creating analogs followed by screening for improved activity to arrive at a lead/optimized compound. Lead compounds, thus identified, may then be tested for their efficacy in experimental vaccine formulations using established animal models and benchmarking against known immune potentiators. The quantity and quality of immune responses can be judged using functional antibodies, CD4+ and CD8+ T cells and protection against an infectious challenge.

■ Random screening based on functional outcome

The observation that most known immune potentiators are capable of inducing the secretion of inflammatory cytokines *in vitro* and that these compounds also act as effective adjuvants in vaccine formulation can be used as a basis of screening compound libraries for families of molecules satisfying these criteria. The methodology for such a screen is straightforward; it relies on established immunological assays, such as ELISA and multiplex cytokine analysis, to measure cytokines and chemokines produced by immune cells such as primary cells or cell lines. Random screening also eliminates any prior assumptions about the mode of action, and thus it can yield compounds for which no known receptors or targets have yet been identified. Because of this unbiased screening approach, once a compound is optimized, a thorough investigation will

need to be carried out to ascertain its target and mode of action. This can be done using available genomics and proteomics approaches, which may aid in identification of previously unknown targets of immunological relevance.

■ Targeted screening

Recent developments in our understanding of PRR-mediated signaling pathways and subsequent molecular outcomes can be used in targeted screening. Thus, libraries of natural (such as pathogen products or peptide sequences) or synthetic compounds can be screened using cells expressing specific TLRs and appropriate reporter genes to identify agonistic compounds. Specifically, cells that do not naturally express TLRs (such as HEK cells) can be cotransfected with an NFkB or IRF-3-driven reporter gene and a TLR cDNA for which a novel agonist is sought. As has been outlined above, TLR ligands can be well-defined immunopotentiators for subunit vaccines. Various TLR ligands, such as CpG (TLR-9 ligand) and imidazoquinolines (TLR-7 and 8 ligands), have been shown to stimulate *in vitro* cytokine production and to activate NFkB-driven reporter genes. Recently, a peptide ALTTE isolated from bacterial fimbriae has been shown to be a TLR-2 ligand (Ogawa and Uchida, 1995). Also, another peptide isolated from insects was able to stimulate NK cells to produce IFN-γ (Chernysh et al., 2002). Thus, immunomodulators can also be based on peptides. Combinatorial peptide libraries, consisting natural or modified amino acids, can be screened in defined TLR-readout assays. Strategies are being explored as to whether linking peptide immunostimulators in frame with antigenic protein will provide a necessary innate immune stimulation along with mounting an adaptive response to the selected antigen (Jackson et al., 2004). Besides selecting agonists for PRR, targeted approaches of identifying inhibitors of known immunological antagonists (such as negative regulators of TLR signaling) or compounds that potentiate positive regulators of the immune system, such as activators of NFkB pathway, can be undertaken.

■ Future directions

Because of intense research activity leading to theoretical and mechanistic understanding of innate immunity, a foundation is provided for systematic approaches towards immuno-potentiator discovery. We envision that the future of vaccine adjuvant research will increasingly employ the tools and platforms of modern drug discovery. The key challenges and opportunities will be found in linking systems biology of the immune system with our growing molecular understanding of adjuvant mechanisms (Figure 4.5). The ultimate goal is to become predictive of how manipulation of the innate immune response at the molecular level gives rise to distinct protective responses in vaccinees. To achieve this goal critical gaps in our understanding of innate immune potentiators will need to be filled. In particular, it will be important to identify the structure–function relationships between innate immune agonists and their molecular targets. The identification of novel and structurally diverse immune potentiators from

small molecule libraries could not only provide a portfolio of vaccine adjuvant candidates but also powerful tools for mechanistic studies of innate immune activation.

Subunit antigens that do not inherently possess structures that stimulate the innate immune system are often shown to be poor immunogens. Vaccines against important but difficult disease targets such as HIV, HCV, herpes simplex virus (HSV), and *Neisseria meningitides* are either in clinical trials or in planning stages. These diseases may need both cellular as well as humoral responses for effective resolution. Also, for some diseases, such as tuberculosis, a greater understanding is available about the quality of T helper responses needed to resolve the infection. These recent breakthroughs in immunology of infectious diseases also allow for a better application of improved antigen discovery and their formulation with novel immune potentiators and delivery systems. Thus, in academic institutions, the vaccine industry, as well as governmental agencies, research and development efforts are converging towards developing next-generation adjuvants. Several of these first-generation candidates (such as CpG, MPL, and imidazoquinolines) have shown some

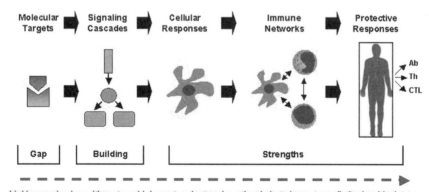

Figure 4.5 Linking molecular mechanisms to systems biology in adjuvant design and development. The long-term goal of adjuvant and immune potentiator research should become increasingly more predictive and rational. Before the appreciation of innate immunity and its mechanistic underpinnings, adjuvant research was almost exclusively empirical. Today, armed with new tools, molecular targets, and platforms, the ability to connect molecular mechanisms to *in vivo* outcomes is possible. The critical gap in our understanding right now lies in the incomplete knowledge surrounding target–ligand binding. However, the overall gaps in connecting each level of interaction (molecular mechanism – signal transduction – cellular responses – immune networks – systems biology) need to be filled to become truly predictive. (See Color Plate Section.)

efficacy in experimental animals and in I clinical studies in humans (Cooper et al., 2004; Mason et al., 2005; Hengge and Cusini, 2003).

Besides use in vaccines to initiate and sustain robust adaptive immune responses, these next-generation immune potentiators may be suitable for use against acute bioterrorism threats, where pathogenic organisms may be modified to have broad antibiotic resistance or evade prophylactic vaccines (Dennis, 2001). In these cases relative toxicity may be acceptable in the face of probable mass casualties because of bioterror weapons. Governmental agencies have a direct stake in the exploration of novel immune potentiators in this national security area. As has been true for most governmental/noncivilian investments in emerging technologies, a byproduct of national security research is usually of use for nongovernmental purposes. Immune potentiator platforms are ideally suited for this dual civilian/governmental use model given their potential utility in prophylactic vaccines, immune-based therapies, and bioweapons countermeasures.

Although there is a heightened acceptance, both by regulatory agencies as well as commercial vaccine manufacturers that improved vaccine adjuvants are needed to meet challenges of the future infectious diseases, there is a skepticism due to new technology carrying unknown risks that are still unevaluated. At present, the safety and regulatory hurdles that will be encountered with the addition of novel immune potentiators and delivery systems to final vaccine formulations may be significant and are still largely ill defined. The key focus should be on separating the potential increases in immune toxicity from improved immunogenicity of adjuvanted vaccines. Currently, our understanding of this "trade-off" is rudimentary but the tools and models are being developed to approach the question rationally. It is likely that improved formulation and controlled release of potent immune potentiators will limit toxicities while increasing efficacy. In addition, the growing number of immune potentiators, targeting

diverse innate immune mechanisms, should allow for the identification of candidates with improved therapeutic indices. Thus, selecting the optimal platform(s) for development and identifying the key cellular and molecular targets of the innate immune system that will trigger the safest and most effective immune responses against diverse pathogens should be the long-term goal. At this early stage, the hurdles appear high and public/private partnerships to fuel research and development may be required to overcome them. Such partnerships have already been established in the areas of HIV and biodefense vaccine research and it is likely that government/industry cooperation on these particularly difficult vaccine problems will lead to breakthroughs in adjuvant development. Overall, despite the aforementioned uncertainties, we are entering a dynamic period in vaccine research driven largely by our increased understanding of innate immunity. The mechanistic understanding and the tools to manipulate this system are growing and it is likely that novel immune potentiators and delivery systems will make a significant impact on vaccine development in the near future.

■ Acknowledgment

The authors would like to thank Nelle Cronen for her help in the preparation of the manuscript.

■ References

Aguado, T., Engers, H., Pang, T., and Pink, R. (1999). Novel adjuvants currently in clinical testing November 2–4, 1998, Fondation Merieux, Annecy, France: a meeting sponsored by the World Health Organization. *Vaccine* 17, 2321–2328.

Akashi, S., Saitoh, S., Wakabayashi, Y., Kikuchi, T., Takamura, N., Nagai, Y., Kusumoto, Y., Fukase, K., Kusumoto, S., Adachi, Y., Kosugi, A., and Miyake, K. (2003). Lipopolysaccharide interaction with cell surface Toll-like receptor 4-MD-2: higher affinity than that with MD-2 or CD14. *J. Exp. Med.* 198, 1035–1042.

Akira, S. and Takeda, K. (2004). Toll-like receptor signalling. *Nature Rev. Immunol.* 4, 499–511.

Akira, S., Yamamoto, M., and Takeda, K. (2003). Role of adapters in Toll-like receptor signalling. *Biochem. Soc. Trans.* 31, 637–642.

Alexopoulou, L., Holt, A.C., Medzhitov, R., and Flavell, R.A. (2001). Recognition of double-stranded RNA and activation of NF-kappaB by Toll-like receptor 3. *Nature* 413, 732–738.

Anderson, J.R. (1955). Iso-immunisation of rabbits by means of Freund-McDermott adjuvants. *Br. J. Exp. Pathol.* 36, 137–142.

Bauer, S., Kirschning, C.J., Hacker, H., Redecke, V., Hausmann, S., Akira, S., Wagner, H., and Lipford, G.B. (2001). Human TLR9 confers responsiveness to bacterial DNA via species-specific CpG motif recognition. *Proc. Natl. Acad. Sci. USA* 98, 9237–9242.

Bernasconi, N.L., Traggiai, E., and Lanzavecchia, A. (2002). Maintenance of serological memory by polyclonal activation of human memory B cells. *Science* 298, 2199–2202.

Beutler, B. (2003). Not "molecular patterns" but molecules. *Immunity* 19, 155–156.

Chamaillard, M., Girardin, S.E., Viala, J., and Philpott, D.J. (2003a). Nods, Nalps and Naip: intracellular regulators of bacterial-induced inflammation. *Cell Microbiol.* 5, 581–592.

Chamaillard, M., Hashimoto, M., Horie, Y., Masumoto, J., Qiu, S., Saab, L., Ogura, Y., Kawasaki, A., Fukase, K., Kusumoto, S., Valvano, M.A., Foster, S.J., Mak, T.W., Nunez, G., and Inohara, N. (2003b). An essential role for NOD1 in host recognition of bacterial peptidoglycan containing diaminopimelic acid. *Nature Immunol.* 4, 702–707.

Chernysh, S., Kim, S.I., Bekker, G., Pleskach, V.A., Filatova, N.A., Anikin, V.B., Platonov, V.G., and Bulet, P. (2002). Antiviral and antitumor peptides from insects. *Proc. Natl. Acad. Sci. USA* 99, 12628–12632.

Chuang, T.H. and Ulevitch, R.J. (2000). Cloning and characterization of a sub-family of human toll-like receptors: hTLR7, hTLR8 and hTLR9. *Eur. Cytokine Netw.* 11, 372–378.

Cooper, C.L., Davis, H.L., Morris, M.L., Efler, S.M., Krieg, A.M., Li, Y., Laframboise, C., Al Adhami, M.J., Khaliq, Y., Seguin, I., and Cameron, D.W. (2004). Safety and immunogenicity of CPG 7909 injection as an adjuvant to Fluarix influenza vaccine. *Vaccine* 22, 3136–3143.

Dennis, C. (2001). The bugs of war. *Nature* 411, 232–235.

Doyle, S.E., O'Connell, R.M., Miranda, G.A., Vaidya, S.A., Chow, E.K., Liu, P.T., Suzuki, S., Suzuki, N., Modlin, R.L., Yeh, W.C., Lane, T.F., and Cheng, G. (2004). Toll-like receptors induce a phagocytic gene program through p38. *J. Exp. Med.* 199, 81–90.

Du, X., Poltorak, A., Wei, Y., and Beutler, B. (2000). Three novel mammalian toll-like receptors: gene structure, expression, and evolution. *Eur. Cytokine Netw.* 11, 362–371.

Engers, H., Kieny, M.P., Malhotra, P., and Pink, J.R. (2003). Third meeting on novel adjuvants currently in or close to clinical testing. World Health Organization-Organization Mondiale de la Sante, Fondation Merieux, Annecy, France, 7–9 January 2002. *Vaccine* 21, 3503–3524.

Girardin, S.E., Boneca, I.G., Carneiro, L.A., Antignac, A., Jehanno, M., Viala, J., Tedin, K., Taha, M.K., Labigne, A., Zahringer, U., Coyle, A.J., DiStefano, P.S., Bertin, J., Sansonetti, P.J., and Philpott, D.J. (2003a). Nod1 detects a unique muropeptide from Gram-negative bacterial peptidoglycan. *Science* 300, 1584–1587.

Girardin, S.E., Boneca, I.G., Viala, J., Chamaillard, M., Labigne, A., Thomas, G., Philpott, D.J., and Sansonetti, P.J. (2003b). Nod2 is a general sensor of peptidoglycan through muramyl dipeptide (MDP) detection. *J. Biol. Chem.* 278, 8869–8872.

Gordon, S. (2002). Pattern recognition receptors: doubling up for the innate immune response. *Cell* 111, 927–930.

Gutierrez, O., Pipaon, C., Inohara, N., Fontalba, A., Ogura, Y., Prosper, F., Nunez, G., and Fernandez-Luna, J.L. (2002). Induction of Nod2 in myelomonocytic and intestinal epithelial cells via nuclear factor-kappa B activation. *J. Biol. Chem.* 277, 41701–41705.

Hayashi, F., Smith, K.D., Ozinsky, A., Hawn, T.R., Yi, E.C., Goodlett, D.R., Eng, J.K., Akira, S., Underhill, D.M., and Aderem, A. (2001). The innate immune response to bacterial flagellin is mediated by Toll-like receptor 5. *Nature* 410, 1099–1103.

Haziot, A., Hijiya, N., Gangloff, S.C., Silver, J., and Goyert, S.M. (2001). Induction of a novel mechanism of accelerated bacterial clearance by lipopolysaccharide in CD14-deficient and Toll-like receptor 4-deficient mice. *J. Immunol.* 166, 1075–1078.

Heil, F., Ahmad-Nejad, P., Hemmi, H., Hochrein, H., Ampenberger, F., Gellert, T., Dietrich, H., Lipford, G., Takeda, K., Akira, S., Wagner, H., and Bauer, S. (2003). The Toll-like receptor 7 (TLR7)-specific stimulus loxoribine uncovers a strong relationship within the TLR7, 8 and 9 subfamily. *Eur. J. Immunol.* 33, 2987–2997.

Hemmi, H., Kaisho, T., Takeuchi, O., Sato, S., Sanjo, H., Hoshino, K., Horiuchi, T., Tomizawa, H., Takeda, K., and Akira, S. (2002). Small anti-viral compounds activate immune cells via the TLR7 MyD88-dependent signaling pathway. *Nature Immunol.* 3, 196–200.

Hengge, U.R. and Cusini, M. (2003). Topical immunomodulators for the treatment of external genital warts, cutaneous warts and molluscum contagiosum. *Br. J. Dermatol.* 149 (Suppl. 66), 15–19.

Hilleman, M.R. (2000). Vaccines in historic evolution and perspective: a narrative of vaccine discoveries. *Vaccine* 18, 1436–1447.

Hoebe, K., Janssen, E., and Beutler, B. (2004). The interface between innate and adaptive immunity. *Nature Immunol.* 5, 971–974.

Iwasaki, A. and Medzhitov, R. (2004). Toll-like receptor control of the adaptive immune responses. *Nature Immunol.* 5, 987–995.

Jackson, D.C., Lau, Y.F., Le, T., Suhrbier, A., Deliyannis, G., Cheers, C., Smith, C., Zeng, W., and Brown, L.E. (2004). A totally synthetic vaccine of generic structure that targets Toll-like receptor 2 on dendritic cells and promotes antibody or cytotoxic T cell responses. *Proc. Natl. Acad. Sci. USA* 101, 15440–15445.

Janeway, C.A., Jr. (1989). Approaching the asymptote? Evolution and revolution in immunology. *Cold Spring Harbor Symp. Quant. Biol.* 54 (Pt 1), 1–13.

Jurk, M., Heil, F., Vollmer, J., Schetter, C., Krieg, A.M., Wagner, H., Lipford, G., and Bauer, S. (2002). Human TLR7 or TLR8 independently confer responsiveness to the antiviral compound R-848. *Nature Immunol.* 3, 499.

Kadowaki, N., Ho, S., Antonenko, S., Malefyt, R.W., Kastelein, R.A., Bazan, F., and Liu, Y.J. (2001). Subsets of human dendritic cell precursors express different toll-like receptors and respond to different microbial antigens. *J. Exp. Med.* 194, 863–869.

Kenney, R.T., Regina Rabinovich, N., Pichyangkul, S., Price, V.L., and Engers, H.D. (2002). Second meeting on novel adjuvants currently in/close to human clinical testing. World Health Organization–Organization Mondiale de la Sante Fondation Merieux, Annecy, France, 5–7 June 2000. *Vaccine* 20, 2155–2163.

Kieny, M.P., Excler, J.L., and Girard, M. (2004). Research and development of new vaccines against infectious diseases. *Am. J. Public Health* 94, 1931–1935.

Lee, J., Chuang, T.H., Redecke, V., She, L., Pitha, P.M., Carson, D.A., Raz, E., and Cottam, H.B. (2003). Molecular basis for the immunostimulatory activity of guanine nucleoside analogs: activation of Toll-like receptor 7. *Proc. Natl. Acad. Sci. USA* 100, 6646–6651.

Lemaitre, B., Nicolas, E., Michaut, L., Reichhart, J.M., and Hoffmann, J.A. (1996). The dorsoventral regulatory gene cassette spatzle/Toll/cactus controls the potent antifungal response in Drosophila adults. *Cell* 86, 973–983.

Lien, E., Means, T.K., Heine, H., Yoshimura, A., Kusumoto, S., Fukase, K., Fenton, M.J., Oikawa, M., Qureshi, N., Monks, B., Finberg, R.W., Ingalls, R.R., and Golenbock, D.T. (2000). Toll-like receptor 4 imparts ligand-specific recognition of bacterial lipopolysaccharide. *J. Clin. Invest.* 105, 497–504.

Lindblad, E.B. (2004). Aluminium adjuvants: in retrospect and prospect. *Vaccine* 22, 3658–3668.

Liu, N., Ohnishi, N., Ni, L., Akira, S., and Bacon, K.B. (2003). CpG directly induces T-bet expression and inhibits IgG1 and IgE switching in B cells. *Nature Immunol.* 4, 687–693.

Lund, J.M., Alexopoulou, L., Sato, A., Karow, M., Adams, N.C., Gale, N.W., Iwasaki, A., and Flavell, R.A. (2004). Recognition of single-stranded RNA viruses by Toll-like receptor 7. *Proc. Natl. Acad. Sci. USA* 101, 5598–5603.

Mason, K.A., Ariga, H., Neal, R., Valdecanas, D., Hunter, N., Krieg, A.M., Whisnant, J.K., and Milas, L. (2005). Targeting Toll-like receptor 9 with CpG oligodeoxynucleotides enhances tumor response to fractionated radiotherapy. *Clin. Cancer Res.* 11, 361–369.

Matsumoto, M., Funami, K., Tanabe, M., Oshiumi, H., Shingai, M., Seto, Y., Yamamoto, A., and Seya, T. (2003). Subcellular localization of Toll-like receptor 3 in human dendritic cells. *J. Immunol.* 171, 3154–3162.

Matsumoto, M., Kikkawa, S., Kohase, M., Miyake, K., and Seya, T. (2002). Establishment of a monoclonal antibody against human Toll-like receptor 3 that blocks double-stranded RNA-mediated signaling. *Biochem. Biophys. Res. Commun.* 293, 1364–1369.

Medzhitov, R., Preston-Hurlburt, P., and Janeway, C.A., Jr. (1997). A human homologue of the Drosophila Toll protein signals activation of adaptive immunity [see comments]. *Nature* 388, 394–397.

Mukhopadhyay, S., Herre, J., Brown, G.D., and Gordon, S. (2004). The potential for Toll-like receptors to collaborate with other innate immune receptors. *Immunology* 112, 521–530.

O'Hagan, D.T. (2004) In Levine, M., Kaper, J.B., Rappuoli, R., Liu, M., and Good, M.F. (Eds) *New Generation Vaccines*, 2nd edn. Marcel-Dekker, New York, pp. 259–270.

O'Hagan, D.T. and Valiante, N.M. (2003). Recent advances in the discovery and delivery of vaccine adjuvants. Nat Rev Drug Discov, 2, 727–735.

O'Hagan, D.T., Singh, M., Dong, C., Ugozzoli, M., Berger, K., Glazer, E., Selby, M., Wininger, M., Ng, P., Crawford, K., Paliard, X., Coates, S., and Houghton, M. (2004). Cationic microparticles are a potent delivery system for a HCV DNA vaccine. *Vaccine* 23, 672–680.

Ogawa, T. and Uchida, H. (1995). A peptide, ALTTE, within the fimbrial subunit protein from Porphyromonas gingivalis, induces production of interleukin 6, gene expression and protein phosphorylation in human peripheral blood mononuclear cells. *FEMS Immunol. Med. Microbiol.* 11, 197–205.

Ozinsky, A., Underhill, D.M., Fontenot, J.D., Hajjar, A.M., Smith, K.D., Wilson, C.B., Schroeder, L., and Aderem, A. (2000). The repertoire for pattern recognition of pathogens by the innate immune system is defined by cooperation between toll-like receptors. *Proc. Natl. Acad. Sci. USA* 97, 13766–13771.

Pasare, C. and Medzhitov, R. (2003). Toll pathway-dependent blockade of CD4+CD25+ T cell-mediated suppression by dendritic cells. *Science* 299, 1033–1036.

Pink, J.R. and Kieny, M.P. (2004). Fourth meeting on novel adjuvants currently in/close to human clinical testing. World Health Organization–Organization Mondiale de la Sante Fondation Merieux, Annecy, France, 23–25 June 2003. *Vaccine* 22, 2097–2102.

Podda, A. and Del Giudice, G. (2004). In Levine, M., Kaper, J.B., Rappuoli, R., Liu, M., and Good, M.F. (Eds) *New Generation Vaccines*. Marcel Dekker, New York, pp. 225–235.

Poltorak, A., He, X., Smirnova, I., Liu, M.Y., Huffel, C.V., Du, X., Birdwell, D., Alejos, E., Silva, M., Galanos, C., Freudenberg, M., Ricciardi-Castagnoli, P., Layton, B., and Beutler, B. (1998). Defective LPS signaling in C3H/HeJ and C57BL/10ScCr mice: mutations in Tlr4 gene. *Science* 282, 2085–2088.

Qureshi, S.T., Gros, P., and Malo, D. (1999). Host resistance to infection: genetic control of lipopolysaccharide responsiveness by TOLL-like receptor genes. *Trends Genet.* 15, 291–294.

Rutz, M., Metzger, J., Gellert, T., Luppa, P., Lipford, G.B., Wagner, H., and Bauer, S. (2004). Toll-like receptor 9 binds single-stranded CpG-DNA in a sequence- and pH-dependent manner. *Eur. J. Immunol.* 34, 2541–2550.

Sato, M., Sano, H., Iwaki, D., Kudo, K., Konishi, M., Takahashi, H., Takahashi, T., Imaizumi, H., Asai, Y., and Kuroki, Y. (2003). Direct binding of Toll-like receptor 2 to zymosan, and zymosan-induced NF-kappa B activation and TNF-alpha secretion are down-regulated by lung collectin surfactant protein A. *J. Immunol.* 171, 417–425.

Schroder, N.W., Opitz, B., Lamping, N., Michelsen, K.S., Zahringer, U., Gobel, U.B., and Schumann, R.R. (2000). Involvement of lipopolysaccharide binding protein, CD14, and Toll-like receptors in the initiation of innate immune responses by Treponema glycolipids. *J. Immunol.* 165, 2683–2693.

Shimazu, R., Akashi, S., Ogata, H., Nagai, Y., Fukudome, K., Miyake, K., and Kimoto, M. (1999). MD-2, a molecule that confers lipopolysaccharide responsiveness on Toll-like receptor 4. *J Exp. Med.* 189, 1777–1782.

Takeda, K., Kaisho, T., and Akira, S. (2003). Toll-like receptors. *Annu. Rev. Immunol.* 21, 335–376.

Takeuchi, O., Kawai, T., Sanjo, H., Copeland, N.G., Gilbert, D.J., Jenkins, N.A., Takeda, K., and Akira, S. (1999). TLR6: a novel member of an expanding toll-like receptor family. *Gene* 231, 59–65.

Tapping, R.I. and Tobias, P.S. (2003). Mycobacterial lipoarabinomannan mediates physical interactions between TLR1 and TLR2 to induce signaling. *J. Endotoxin Res.* 9, 264–268.

Vasilakos, J.P., Smith, R.M., Gibson, S.J., Lindh, J.M., Pederson, L.K., Reiter, M.J., Smith, M.H., and Tomai, M.A. (2000). Adjuvant activities of immune response modifier R-848: comparison with CpG ODN. *Cell. Immunol.* 204, 64–74.

Weber, J.R., Freyer, D., Alexander, C., Schroder, N.W., Reiss, A., Kuster, C., Pfeil, D., Tuomanen, E.I., and Schumann, R.R. (2003). Recognition of pneumococcal peptidoglycan: an expanded, pivotal role for LPS binding protein. *Immunity* 19, 269–279.

Wyllie, D.H., Kiss-Toth, E., Visintin, A., Smith, S.C., Boussouf, S., Segal, D.M., Duff, G.W., and Dower, S.K. (2000). Evidence for an accessory protein function for Toll-like receptor 1 in anti-bacterial responses. *J. Immunol.* 165, 7125–7132.

CpG oligodeoxynucleotides as vaccine adjuvants

Michael J. McCluskie and Risini D. Weeratna
Coley Pharmaceutical Group, Ottawa, Ontario, Canada

Introduction

In recent decades the development and widespread use of vaccines has had a tremendous impact on mortality and morbidity worldwide. Mass immunization programs have met with great success, including the eradication of smallpox worldwide, the near eradication of polio, as well as drastic reductions in the incidence of measles and other viral infections. Nevertheless, infectious diseases still account for more than 13 million deaths annually, and an estimated 30 million children born each year have no access to immunization (World Health Organization, 2001). In order to help correct infectious disease vaccination inequities, a need exists for the improvement of existing vaccines such that fewer boosts or reduced antigen doses are needed, or for the development of novel vaccines. In addition to their traditional role in the prevention of infectious disease, vaccination strategies are also being developed to control an increasing number of other diseases including cancer and asthma/allergies. For the improvement of existing vaccines or for the development of novel vaccines, safe and effective vaccine adjuvants are critical.

It has recently been recognized that the vertebrate innate immune system uses pattern recognition receptors, including the Toll-like receptors (TLRs), specifically to detect pathogen-associated molecular patterns (PAMPs) present in infectious agents. To date, ten different human TLRs have been identified (Akira et al., 2001; Chuang and Ulevitch, 2000, 2001; Rock et al., 1998; Takeuchi et al., 1999), as well as a number of naturally occurring TLR ligands. These include lipoproteins and peptidoglycans (TLR2 ligands) (Schwandner et al., 1999; Yoshimura et al., 1999); double-stranded RNA of viral origin (TLR3) (Alexopoulou et al., 2001); lipopolysaccharide (LPS) from Gram-negative bacteria and lipoteichoic acid from Gram-positive bacteria (TLR4) (An et al., 2002; Chow et al., 1999; Lien et al., 2000; Rhee and Hwang 2000); flagellin, a protein found in bacterial flagella (TLR5) (Gewirtz et al., 2001; Hayashi et al., 2001); single-stranded viral RNA (TLR7 and 8) (Heil et al., 2004); and unmethylated CpG motifs found in bacterial DNA (TLR9) (Hemmi et al., 2000; Krug et al., 2001; Takeshita et al., 2001).

Synthetic TLR ligands have also been identified, including imidazoquinoline compounds such as Imiquimod and Resiquimod (R-848), which activate human TLR7 and 8 (Gibson et al., 2002; Hemmi et al., 2002); oligodeoxynucleotides (ODN) containing CpG motifs (CpG ODN), which are TLR9 agonists (Bauer et al., 2001; Hemmi et al., 2000); and LPS derivatives, such as monophosphoryl lipid A (MPL), which can interact with TLR4 (Baldridge et al., 2004). Many of these ligands can modulate innate as well as adaptive immune responses and have been evaluated as potential vaccine adjuvants. For example, synthetic ligands for TLR7/8 (R-848) (Thomsen et al., 2004; Vasilakos et al., 2000), TLR4 (MPL) (Baldridge et al., 2004), and TLR9 (CpG ODN) (Cooper et al., 2004a; Halperin et al., 2003) have all been demonstrated to possess an adjuvant effect when coadministered with antigen.

In this review chapter, we focus on the TLR9 agonist CpG ODN as an immune adjuvant for infectious disease, cancer, and asthma/allergy.

CpG oligodeoxynucleotides

Mechanism of action of CpG ODN

Most cell types have the capacity to take up CpG ODN via endocytosis (Krieg et al., 1995); however, only those cells expressing the TLR9 receptor are activated. In human immune cells, TLR9 expression immune cells is limited to B cells and plasmacytoid dendritic cells (pDCs), whereas in mice TLR9 is also found on myeloid dendritic cells (mDCs), macrophages, and monocytes (Hemmi et al., 2000; Hornung et al., 2002; Kadowaki et al., 2001; Krug et al., 2001). Within minutes after exposure of these cell types to CpG ODN, it is taken up into an endosomal compartment where interaction with TLR9 occurs (Ahmad-Nejad et al., 2002). This leads to the activation of cell signaling pathways which results in the expression of costimulatory molecules (e.g., MHC II and B7), resistance to apoptosis, upregulation of the chemokine receptor CCR7 that causes cell trafficking to the T cell zone of lymph nodes, as well as secretion of predominantly Th1-type chemokines and cytokines such as macrophage inflammatory protein-1, interferon-inducible protein-10 (IP-10), and type I interferons (Krieg 2002; Krieg 2003). The CpG-induced induction of chemokines and cytokines triggers a cascade of secondary immune events including natural killer (NK) cell activation, maturation of pDCs into potent antigen-presenting cells, enhanced Fc receptor expression on effector cells such as polymorphonuclear (PMN) cells with a consequent increase in antibody-dependent cellular cytotoxicity (ADCC), as well as enhanced

PMN migration in response to inflammatory signals (Krieg, 2002, 2003). The Th1-like pattern of cytokine induction induced by CpG ODN has recently been confirmed in a human clinical trial in which a single subcutaneous injection of CpG ODN was shown to induce the expression of interleukin (IL)-6, IL-12p40, interferon (IFN)-α, and IFN-inducible chemokines (Krieg et al., 2004).

In addition to innate immune activation, in the presence of an antigen CpG can promote the induction of strong Th1-biased antigen-specific immune responses. Stimulation of B cells by CpG in the presence of antigen can selectively enhance the development of antigen-specific antibodies, especially of the isotype associated with Th1-like immune responses (e.g., IgG2a in mice). Following CpG stimulation, both B cells and DCs can effectively present antigen to T cells. Antigen presentation taking place in a Th1-like cytokine milieu can lead to induction of strong Th1-biased immune responses consisting of cellular (antigen-specific cytotoxic T cell responses) as well as humoral immunity (Davis et al., 1998; Sparwasser et al., 2000). It has been reported that, in mice injected with CpG ODN, the Th1-like cytokine milieu and lymphadenopathy in the draining lymph node (LN) peaks at 7–10 days (Kobayashi et al., 1999; Lipford et al., 2000), and is sustained for at least several weeks since CpG-primed mice respond to an antigen injection with a Th1-biased response even five weeks later (Kobayashi et al., 1999; Lipford et al., 2000).

Classes of CpG ODN

Three different classes of CpG ODN have been described so far based on structure and their immune activation profile (Hartmann et al., 2003; Marshall et al., 2003; Vollmer et al., 2004). All three classes (A, B, and C) interact with TLR9 (Hartmann et al., 2003; Marshall et al., 2003; Vollmer et al., 2004).

CpG ODN of the A class can induce the production of high levels of IFN-α from pDCs, and cause marked NK cell activation. However, they are relatively poor in stimulating B cells and contain palindromic CpG phosphodiester sequences with phosphorothioate G-rich ends that result in the formation of high-order secondary structures (Schetter and Vollmer, 2004). In contrast, B-class CpG ODN are strong B cell activators with a weaker capacity to induce IFN-α and activate NK cells (Krug et al., 2001). C-class ODN combine the immune effects of A and B classes (Hartmann et al., 2003; Marshall et al., 2003; Vollmer et al., 2004), and possess unique structural characteristics that provide excellent *in vivo* stability and ease of formulation.

Most animal studies to date using CpG ODN as a vaccine adjuvant have used B-class CpG ODN on account of their strong B cell activation and capacity to induce potent Th1-type immune responses. B-class CpG ODN have also been shown to be safe and efficacious vaccine adjuvants in humans with a number of different antigens (Cooper et al., 2004a, 2004b, 2005; Krieg et al., 2004). To date, relatively little has been published regarding the adjuvant activity or other *in vivo* immune effects of other classes of CpG ODN. However, a C-class ODN, Actilon™ (CPG 10101; Coley Pharmaceutical Group), has recently been shown to produce high levels of IFN-α *in vitro* from cells of individuals infected with hepatitis C virus (HCV) whose DCs would otherwise be functionally impaired as a result of HCV infection (Davis, H.L., Efler, S., and Krieg, A.M., unpublished observations). It is likely that C-class ODN will induce strong long-lasting innate and adaptive antiviral immunity and may prove of great use in the therapy of viral infection. A phase I safety trial in healthy and HCV infected patients with Actilon™ began in 2004 and preliminary results indicate that Actilon™ is well tolerated over a wide range of doses, and that subcutaneous doses induce measurable, dose-related activation of markers of innate immunity, and in some patients significant reduction (>1 log) of serum viral levels.

■ CpG as a vaccine adjuvant

The ability of CpG ODN to activate innate and enhance adaptive Th1-type immune responses has led to their use as vaccine adjuvants against peptide antigens, as well as numerous bacterial and viral proteins. The strong adjuvant effect of CpG ODN is most likely due to a number of factors: (i) purified B cells show strong synergistic responses when they are stimulated by CpG DNA in the presence of antigen, indicating crosstalk between the B cell receptor and CpG signaling pathways (Krieg et al., 1995); (ii) CpG DNA inhibits B cell apoptosis, contributing to the generation of a sustained immune response (Yi et al., 1996, 1998); and (iii) the CpG-induced activation of DCs provides an environment in the secondary lymphoid organs where T cells are exposed to highly activated antigen-presenting cells in the presence of increased levels of Th1-like cytokines such as IL-12 (Lipford et al., 2000; Sparwasser et al., 2000).

While most marketed vaccines are designed for prophylactic purposes and as such are administered to healthy individuals, there is also great potential for therapeutic vaccines particularly in the case of viral infections. Control of viral infection is mediated by broad multispecific Th1-type responses involving both CD4+ and CD8+ T cell responses that depend on the induction of IFN-γ. These mechanisms appear to result in control of viral replication with clearance of virus from the blood, but rarely lead to complete viral eradication. Rather such responses lead to long-term nonlytic control of the virus with no adverse health sequelae. With chronic infections, it appears that the inability of the immune system to control viral replication is due to weak or absent T cell responses, which in turn fail to develop due to DC dysfunction that in turn is due to direct immunosuppressive effects by the virus, which can directly infect DCs. Indeed, DC dysfunction has been shown to play a central role in the pathology of a number of viruses including hepatitis B virus (HBV) (Beckebaum et al., 2003),

HCV (Tsubouchi et al., 2004), HIV (Fantuzzi et al., 2004), vaccinia (Engelmayer et al., 1999), herpes simplex virus (HSV) (Kruse et al., 2000), and measles (Grosjean et al., 1997). It is likely that the ability of CpG ODN to strongly stimulate DCs via TLR9 may help overcome this dysfunction and thereby stimulate the strong Th1-type immune responses required for viral clearance. Therapeutic vaccines may also have potential in cancer applications whereby CpG ODN would either be administered with a tumor antigen, or alternatively would be administered as monotherapy in which case tumor antigens present in tumors would act as *in situ* vaccine antigens.

The use of CpG ODN as prophylactic and therapeutic vaccine adjuvants in the development of novel vaccines against infectious disease, allergy, or cancer is discussed below.

Infectious disease vaccines

Th1-type immune responses

The development of the appropriate type of immune response is essential for successful vaccination. In general, strong cell-mediated immunity that is associated with Th1 responses is thought to be essential for the control of intracellular pathogens whereas strong humoral immunity, which can be associated with both Th1 and Th2 responses, appears necessary for the control of extracellular pathogens. Th1-type responses are characterized by the production of Th1-type cytokines (IFN-γ, TNF-α, and IL-12), opsonizing antibodies, such as those of the IgG2a isotype in mice, and strong cytotoxic T cell (CTL) induction, whereas Th2 responses are characterized by secretion of Th2-type cytokines (IL-4, IL-5) and the generation of IgG1 and IgE antibodies with only weak or absent CTL responses. The requirement of Th1 responses to clear intracellular infection has been demonstrated in murine *Leishmania major* and *Schistosoma mansoni* infection models where resistance or susceptibility to infection is linked to Th1 or Th2 responses, respectively (Heinzel et al., 1989; Sher, 1992). Likewise

Th1 responses have also been shown to be necessary for control of certain viral infections, such as with the hepatitis B virus (Chisari and Ferrari, 1995).

CpG ODN as vaccine adjuvant for infectious disease

Numerous studies have demonstrated the efficacy of CpG ODN as a potent Th1 vaccine adjuvant in a range of species, including mice (Chu et al., 2000; Davis et al., 1998; Freidag et al., 2000; Jones et al., 1999; Walker et al., 1999), nonhuman primates (Davis et al., 2000), and humans (Cooper et al., 2004a, 2004b, 2005; Halperin et al., 2003). When compared with a number of different adjuvants currently used in animal research (Freund's complete adjuvant, FCA, Freund's incomplete adjuvant, FIA, Titermax® Gold), licensed for human use (alum), or in clinical testing for humans (MPL) for their ability to augment humoral responses to hepatitis B surface antigen (HBsAg), CpG DNA was shown to give the highest ratio of IgG2a to IgG1 antibodies, an indirect marker for Th1-biased responses, of any adjuvant used alone (Weeratna et al., 2000). A similar strong Th1 bias of CpG ODN with parenteral delivery in the mouse has also been demonstrated by Kim et al., who compared 19 different immunological adjuvants with KLH conjugate vaccines containing two human cancer antigens (MUC1 peptide and GD3 ganglioside) and demonstrated CpG ODN to induce the most Th1-biased immune responses as demonstrated by highest levels of IFN-γ secretion in antigen restimulated splenocytes (Kim et al., 2000).

The use of CpG ODN as vaccine adjuvant may allow for the use of lower doses of antigen. In a recent phase Ib blinded, randomized, controlled clinical trial, administration of 1 mg CPG 7909 with a one-tenth dose of a commercial trivalent killed split influenza vaccine (Fluarix®), resulted in similar levels of IFN-γ secretion from restimulated peripheral blood mononuclear cells as were obtained with the full-dose vaccine administered without CpG ODN (Cooper et al., 2004b).

■ *CpG ODN may be effective in the very young and elderly*

There are age-related differences in the immune systems in both animals and humans. In the very young, the immune system has not yet fully developed whereas in the elderly there is a decrease in efficacy of innate and adaptive immune responses. Thus in both age groups there is an increased risk of infection and a decreased response to conventional vaccines. This has been associated with a bias towards Th2 immune responses in both age groups. It may be possible to overcome this by the use of strong Th1-promoting vaccine adjuvants such as CpG ODN.

In very young mice CpG ODN has the ability to augment antigen-specific immune responses, with enhanced CTL responses that are even stronger than those obtained with a DNA vaccine (Brazolot Millan et al., 1998). CpG ODN has also been shown to revert preestablished Th2 responses to antigen in adult (Barrios et al., 1996; Serebrisky et al., 2000) and in neonatal mice (Weeratna et al., 2001). Furthermore, CpG ODN has also been shown to skew a neonatally primed Th2 response away from its Th2 bias (Weeratna et al., 2001). For some diseases (i.e., viral diseases), the difficulty or inability to induce Th1-type responses in early life can severely limit the protective efficacy of the vaccine (Arulanandam et al., 2000). However, several reports have shown the ability of either CpG ODN alone or in combination with alum to induce Th1-biased immune responses in young mice following immunization with HBsAg (Brazolot Millan et al., 1998), live measles virus, live recombinant canary pox virus expressing measles viral hemagglutinin, and tetanus toxoid peptide (Kovarik et al., 1999). The ability of CpG ODN to stimulate Th1-biased immune responses has been demonstrated in aged mice by both parenteral (Maletto et al., 2002; Manning et al., 2001) and mucosal routes (Alignani et al., 2005). In these studies similar Th1-type immune responses were induced when CpG ODN was used as an adjuvant in aged compared to young mice. These studies highlight the potential of CpG ODN as a vaccine adjuvant in infants as well as elderly populations.

■ *CpG ODN can overcome vaccine hyporesponsiveness*

A study by Davis et al. reported the potential of CpG ODN to induce immune responses against a commercial hepatitis B vaccine, Engerix-B®, in orangutans which are otherwise hyporesponsive to this vaccine (Davis et al., 2000). The ability of CpG ODN to augment immune responses to vaccines in subjects that would be otherwise hyporesponsive or immunocompromised has also been demonstrated in a human clinical trial, where HIV-positive individuals who were previously nonresponsive to the Engerix-B vaccine were capable of rapidly developing sero-protective antibody titers following immunization with the same vaccine with the addition of CpG ODN and remarkably for this population, titers were maintained at protective levels for up to three years after immunization. In addition, those individuals receiving CpG ODN as adjuvant with HBV vaccine showed significantly enhanced antigen-specific lymphocyte proliferation for at least two years compared to those receiving vaccine alone (Cooper et al., 2005).

■ *Combination of CpG ODN with other adjuvants*

In animal models, CpG ODN has been shown to have some form of synergy with a wide variety of other adjuvants after both parenteral and mucosal delivery. For parenteral delivery, these include particulate adjuvants (e.g., cationic and anionic microparticles, nanoparticles, virus-like particles), emulsions (e.g., Emulsigen®, Montanide ISA51 and ISA720, and MF-59), mineral salts (e.g., aluminum hydroxide), saponins (e.g., QS21, Quill A), liposomes and cationic peptides, polycationic antibiotics (e.g., Polymyxin B), and polysaccharides. For mucosal vaccines, these include both native and genetically detoxified bacterial toxins such as cholera toxin and the *Escherichia coli* heat-labile enterotoxin, liposomes, and microparticles. The strong Th1 bias of CpG ODN also is able to dominate the Th2 bias associated with adjuvants such as alum or FIA (Davis et al., 1998; Weeratna et al., 2000).

It is likely that the synergy between CpG ODN and other adjuvants is due to a number of different factors depending on the adjuvant used.

First, it is possible that by using formulations, antigen and/or ODN that would normally be rapidly degraded or have low immunogenicity may become more immunostimulatory. While most ODN used *in vivo* are synthesized with a phosphorothioate (PS) backbone and hence are resistant to nuclease degradation, ODN synthesized with the native phosphodiester (PO) backbone rapidly degrade *in vivo* and have little or no biological activity and so may benefit from protection. Indeed, it has been demonstrated that encapsulation of PO ODN into liposomes can make them more immunostimulatory than an equivalent dose of PS ODN, perhaps due to a higher affinity of PO ODN to the TLR9 binding site (Mui et al., 2001). Formulation of ODN may also be beneficial for nonparenteral delivery of ODN where bioavailability is lower than with parenteral delivery (Nicklin et al., 1998).

A second mechanism by which formulations may improve efficacy of CpG ODN is through a depot effect which may result in an extended period during which both antigen and CpG ODN are available. This likely explains the synergy seen between CpG ODN and various emulsions as well as aluminum hydroxide. Formulations such as lipid-based or particulate adjuvants may also lead to an enhanced uptake of antigen and/or ODN into antigen-presenting cells.

CpG ODN has been used in humans with the depot-forming adjuvants, aluminum hydroxide, and Freund's incomplete adjuvant (Cooper et al., 2004a; Speiser et al., 2005). In a randomized, double-blind phase I/II dose escalation study, healthy volunteers were immunized at 0, 4, and 24 weeks by intramuscular (IM) injection of VaxImmune™ (CPG 7909) (0.125, 0.5, or 1.0 mg), a B-class CpG ODN, with a commercial HBV vaccine

containing alum-absorbed yeast-derived recombinant HBsAg (Cooper et al., 2004a). The use of VaxImmune as adjuvant resulted in the induction of HBsAg-specific antibody (anti-HBs) responses significantly earlier and at significantly higher levels at all time-points up to and including 24 weeks in VaxImmune recipients compared to control subjects. Surprisingly, a high proportion of vaccinated subjects receiving VaxImmune developed protective levels of anti-HBs IgG within just two weeks of the priming vaccine dose. In addition, there was a trend towards higher rates of positive CTL responses noted in the two higher dose groups of VaxImmune compared to controls. In this study, CPG 7909 not only increased the levels of HBsAg-specific antibodies but was also shown to enhance the late affinity maturation process, thus increasing the pool of high-avidity antibodies (Siegrist et al., 2004).

It is not possible to say what synergy may have existed between the CpG ODN and alum in these studies since studies were not controlled with a vaccine formulation containing antigen plus CpG ODN without alum. Nevertheless, in a separate study, a dose-dependent enhanced immunogenicity of a non-alum absorbed commercial HBV vaccine has been demonstrated with 1018 ISS (immune stimulatory sequence), also a B-class CpG ODN, albeit at higher doses (0.3, 0.65, 1.0, and 3.0 mg) (Halperin et al., 2003). When responses obtained in these studies at four weeks postprime are compared, it appears that higher doses of non-alum absorbed ODN (1018) were required to detect significant antibody titers compared to alum-absorbed VaxImmune. It is not clear what the relative contributions of the CpG sequence or the presence of alum were to this increased response.

CpG ODN as a mucosal vaccine adjuvant

The vast majority of infectious agents enter the body through the mucosal surfaces of the gastrointestinal, genitourinary, and respiratory tracts, where the primary source of protection is the mucosal immune system. For the induction of mucosal immune responses, it is generally required to administer vaccines at a mucosal surface. However, most current vaccines are designed for parenteral delivery, and as such are effective at inducing systemic immune responses, but generally do not induce mucosal immune responses. In contrast, mucosal immunization can lead to efficient mucosal and systemic responses (McGhee et al., 1992). In addition, mucosal vaccines are generally considered easier, less expensive, and safer to administer than parenteral vaccines. Furthermore, since there is no requirement for needles, there is no risk of needle stick injury or cross contamination through repeated use of the same needle. One of the major impediments to the development of mucosal vaccines has been the lack of safe and effective adjuvants. A number of mucosal adjuvants and/or delivery systems are being developed including derivatives of bacterial toxins, microparticles, immunostimulatory complexes (ISCOMs), lipid A derivatives, liposomes, and virus-like particles (Holmgren et al., 2003; Medina and Guzman, 2000; O'Hagan et al., 2001). In addition, we and others have shown CpG DNA to be an effective mucosal adjuvant when coadministered with protein antigens to mice.

CpG ODN has been shown to be an effective mucosal adjuvant in rodents with a number of antigens, including HBsAg (McCluskie et al., 2000; McCluskie and Davis, 1998, 1999), HBsAg–antibody complexes (McCluskie et al., 1998), tetanus toxoid (TT) (McCluskie et al., 2001; McCluskie and Davis, 2000), whole killed influenza virus (McCluskie and Davis, 2000; Moldoveanu et al., 1998), β-galactosidase (Horner et al., 1998; Horner and Raz, 2000), *Mycobacterium bovis* BCG (Freidag et al., 2000), a synthetic measles virus peptide (Olszewska et al., 2000), recombinant glycoprotein B of HSV type-1 (HSV-1) and HSV-2 (Gallichan et al., 2001; Kwant and Rosenthal, 2004), peptide epitopes from HSV-1 glycoprotein D (Nesburn et al., 2005), inactivated gp120-depleted HIV-1 antigen (Dumais et al., 2002; Jiang et al., 2005), recombinant Japanese

encephalitis virus (Rauthan et al., 2004), and respiratory syncytial virus fusion protein (Prince et al., 2003). These immunostimulatory effects of CpG ODN at mucosal surfaces can be seen after delivery of single or multiple antigens (McCluskie and Davis, 2000).

CpG ODN has been shown to be an effective mucosal adjuvant after administration to different mucosal surfaces, such as the respiratory tract (intranasal droplets) (Gallichan et al., 2001; McCluskie and Davis, 1998, 2000), the genitourinary tract (intravaginal) (Kwant and Rosenthal 2004), and the gastrointestinal tract (oral, intrarectal) (Eastcott et al., 2001; McCluskie et al., 2000; McCluskie and Davis, 2000). In most cases, mucosal immune responses, characterized by antigen-specific secretory IgA antibodies, are induced at sites distant to the site of administration. For example, following oral or intranasal administration of tetanus toxoid (TT) with CpG ODN, TT-specific IgA antibodies were detected in lungs, feces, saliva, and nasal, vaginal, and gut washes (McCluskie and Davis, 2000). Intranasal immunization using CpG ODN as mucosal adjuvant has proven effective in the induction of mucosal immunity in the genital tract of mice and in protecting against subsequent intravaginal viral challenge. For example, intranasal vaccination of mice with CpG ODN plus inactivated gp120-depleted HIV-1 elicited strong HIV-specific IgG and IgA antibody responses in serum and genital tract and increased production of β-chemokines and IFN-γ in genital tract compared to mice immunized with antigen alone or with control ODN (Dumais et al., 2002). Furthermore, mice immunized with HIV-1 immunogen plus CpG ODN were protected against intravaginal challenge with a recombinant vaccinia virus expressing HIV-1 gag (Dumais et al., 2002). Similarly, strong mucosal and systemic immune responses as well as protection against vaginal challenge with a lethal dose of HSV-2 has been reported following intranasal immunization using CpG as mucosal adjuvant in association with HSV-1 glycoprotein B (Gallichan et al., 2001).

CpG ODN has also been shown to induce immune responses at the ocular mucosa following immunization at local or distant sites. When administered ocularly with peptide epitopes from the HSV-1 glycoprotein D, CpG ODN has been shown to enhance peptide-specific and virus-neutralizing IgA/IgG in tears and serum as well as local and systemic peptide- and virus-specific T cells (Nesburn et al., 2005). These responses were predominantly of a Th1 type as evidenced by the local production of IFN-γ and IL-2 (Nesburn et al., 2005). In a rat model, intranasal immunization using dinitrophenylated BSA as model antigen was shown to enhance antigen-specific IgA responses in tears (Gill and Montgomery, 2002). While it is generally accepted that, in the absence of hormonal treatment, mucosal immune responses are only induced following mucosal immunization, it has recently been shown that transcutaneous immunization in the lower back region of mice using the major outer membrane protein (MOMP) of *Chlamydia muridarum* with CpG ODN as vaccine adjuvant can result in MOMP-specific IgA and IgG in uterine and vaginal lavage fluid, MOMP-specific IgG in serum, as well as IFN-γ-secreting T cells in reproductive tract draining caudal and lumber lymph nodes (Berry et al., 2004). Moreover, clearance of *C. muridarum* was also enhanced following intravaginal challenge.

When used as a mucosal adjuvant, CpG ODN is capable of inducing equivalent systemic immune responses as those when CpG ODN is used with parenteral vaccines. For example, we have measured equivalent plasma IgG responses in mice after a single immunization of the same dose of antigen (TT) and CpG ODN by oral or intramuscular (IM) routes (McCluskie and Davis, unpublished data). Likewise, equivalent serum IgG, splenic cytokine, and CTL responses can be induced in mice by IN and intradermal (ID) delivery of β-galactosidase with CpG ODN as adjuvant (Horner et al., 1998). However, in these studies, only after IN delivery were mucosal immune responses generated.

In the majority of studies published to date using CpG ODN as a mucosal adjuvant, CpG ODN has been delivered in a simple saline solution. However, similar to what was found with parenteral delivery, CpG ODN as a mucosal adjuvant can have synergistic effects with other mucosal adjuvants. We have seen a strong synergy between CpG and native toxins (CT, LT) when coadministered with tetanus toxoid or HBsAg, but did not see such a strong synergy with their genetically detoxified derivatives (CTB, LTB, LTE112K, LTA69G, LTS61F, LTK63, LTR192G). Thus it is possible that the synergy between CpG ODN and bacterial toxins is dependent, at least in part, on their enzymatic activity. However, it may also be dependent on the particular antigen used, as other groups have demonstrated a synergy between CpG ODN and LTR72 when coadministered with a synthetic peptide immunogen (MAP-M2), containing multiple copies of a peptide mimic of a conformational epitope of the fusion protein of measles virus (Olszewska et al., 2000). Nevertheless, some form of synergy appears to exist between CpG and all CT/LT derivatives, since in all the aforementioned studies CpG ODN combined with bacterial toxin derivatives induced a more Th1-like response than was achieved with the LT-derived adjuvant alone.

For further development of CpG ODN as a potential mucosal adjuvant in humans it may be necessary to evaluate different formulations to protect the antigen and/or CpG ODN, improve uptake by immune cells, and possibly allow lower doses of antigen and/or CpG to be used. Following intranasal administration, a liposomal formulation of CpG ODN has been shown to have a stronger adjuvant effect than unformulated CpG ODN when coadministered with subunit influenza or HBsAg (Joseph et al., 2002). In addition, when used as monotherapy, CpG ODN has been efficacious in protecting against vaginal HSV-2 challenge when coated onto a bio-erodible mucoadhesive film and applied topically to the genital mucosa of mice (Sajic et al., 2003).

Cancer vaccines

The principle of therapeutic cancer vaccines is to stimulate the immune system to induce strong tumor-specific immune responses that would be capable of eradicating established tumors. This would require a strong cellular immune response preferably against multiple tumor targets. Numerous rodent tumor models have now shown that CpG ODN is an effective adjuvant in cancer vaccines as well as in vaccines against infectious disease. In addition, several human trials have tested or are testing CpG ODN as adjuvants in cancer vaccines. Two main strategies have been proposed for the use of CpG in cancer vaccines: (i) in DC vaccines to activate antigen pulsed DC; and (ii) as an adjuvant with tumor antigens.

CpG ODN with DC vaccines

The use of DC vaccines has emerged as a novel therapeutic approach for cancer in recent years. However, one potential drawback of this strategy is that failure to activate properly the antigen-loaded DC can lead to T cell tolerance or T cell anergy rather than the induction of T cell immunity (Kuwana et al., 2001; Martin et al., 2002). It is possible that by using CpG ODN to activate DCs this can be avoided. Indeed, numerous studies have now shown that CpG ODN can efficiently activate antigen pulsed DCs which in turn can productively present antigen to the immune system resulting in strong antitumor immune responses (Heckelsmiller et al., 2002; Kim et al., 2004; Merad et al., 2002; Wang et al., 2002). For example, *in vivo* manipulation of DCs using Flt3 ligand and CpG ODN has been shown to allow effective presentation of tumor antigen by DCs resulting in strong antitumor responses that were capable of rejecting established murine B16 melanoma and CT26 colon carcinoma tumors (Furumoto et al., 2004). Combined DC and CpG ODN therapy has also been shown to cure large chemotherapy-resistant murine renal cell carcinoma and colon carcinoma tumors (Heckelsmiller et al., 2002). Recently it has been shown that the use of CpG

ODN with a DC-tumor fusion cell vaccine could enhance phenotypical maturation of tumor cell fused and unfused DCs, production of Th1 cytokines (i.e. IFN-γ, IL-12), and help induce strong tumor-specific CTLs. Furthermore, vaccinating with fused cells in combination with CpG ODN significantly enhanced survival and decreased lung metastasis as well as protected against tumor re-challenge compared to when vaccine was used alone (Hiraoka et al., 2004). Another approach is the use of DC-derived exosomes expressing MHC molecules that can be loaded with synthetic peptides. DC-derived exosomes have been demonstrated to induce potent anti-tumor responses in animals (Amigorena, 2000), and are currently being tested in humans (Chaput et al., 2004). The antitumor responses generated by DC-derived exosomes can be greatly enhanced by combining with CpG ODN (Chaput et al., 2004).

CpG ODN with tumor antigens

CpG ODN have also been used as adjuvants in classic cancer vaccines using whole cells, cell lysates, tumor antigens, or antigenic peptides as the antigen (Krieg, 2004). In a murine 38C13 B cell lymphoma model, where the idiotype (Id) of the 38C13 surface IgM serves as a highly specific tumor-associated antigen, CpG ODN as an adjuvant enhanced antigen-specific IgG2a antibody titers and resulted in protection against tumor challenge at a level comparable with complete Freund's adjuvant (CFA) but without the toxicity associated with CFA (Weiner et al., 1997). CpG ODN has also been shown to induce faster and stronger immune responses compared to CFA when used with the anti idiotypic antibody 3H1 which functionally mimics carcinoembryonic antigen, a tumor-associated antigen expressed on human colorectal carcinoma and other adenocarcinomas (Baral et al., 2003).

Granulocyte macrophage colony-stimulating factor (GM-CSF)-transduced autologous tumor cells have been used as a cytokine-mediated immunotherapeutic strategy for treatment of cancer in humans (Dummer 2001;

O'Rourke et al., 1997). Combining CpG ODN together with Neuro-2a, murine neuroblastoma cells retrovirally transduced to express murine GM-CSF (GM/Neuro-2a), was shown to enhance significantly tumor-free survival of mice compared to when animals were given GM/Neuro-2a alone. Furthermore, the surviving mice were resistant to tumor re-challenge and demonstrated strong tumor-specific T cell responses (Sandler et al., 2003). CpG ODN has also been shown to augment adjuvant effects of soluble GM-CSF as well as antigen/GM-CSF fusion proteins (Liu et al., 1998). In addition, CpG ODN has shown great promise in enhancing efficacy of other tumor vaccines using autologous tumor cells transduced with genes expressing other cytokines such as IL-12 (Switaj et al., 2004), and immune modulators such as B7.1 (Kochling et al., 2003) and CD154 (Rieger and Kipps, 2003).

Use of synthetic peptides consisting of tumor-associated antigen-derived CTL epitopes as vaccines is theoretically a very simple and effective means of immunotherapy against cancer. However, these peptides are usually not very immunogenic and require strong adjuvants to elicit strong antitumor responses. CpG ODN have been used successfully as adjuvants for such peptide vaccines. For example, immunization of mice with an ovalbumin peptide vaccine together with repeated daily administration of CpG ODN has been shown to promote strong CTL responses and protect mice against tumors expressing ovalbumin (Davila and Celis, 2000). Similar augmentation in CTL responses have been demonstrated using CpG as adjuvant with other peptides including TRP2, a peptide containing CTL epitope from a murine melanoma-specific tumor-associated antigen (Davila et al., 2003), as well as peptide derived from the melanoma-associated differentiation antigen MART-1/Melan-A (Miconnet et al., 2002). In the murine T cell lymphoma RMA model, in which without treatment only weak innate immune system activation and very weak Th1 immune responses are induced such that tumor growth is not controlled,

immunization with the MHC II-restricted tumor peptide H11.1 together with CpG ODN as adjuvant induces protective immunity through CD4-dependent pathways (Stern et al., 2002). When compared to FCA as adjuvant, CpG ODN was shown to induce 2.5-fold higher frequency of H11.1 peptide-specific memory CD4 cells (Stern et al., 2002).

In humans, the ability of CpG ODN to enhance cellular immune responses in a tumor vaccine setting has been demonstrated. In a phase I trial, CPG 7909 (0.5 mg) was administered as 4 monthly vaccinations with Melan-A/MART-1 analog peptide with FIA to eight HLA-A2+ melanoma patients. In all patients, rapid and strong antigen-specific T cell responses were generated with a high frequency of Melan-A-specific T cells (mean value $1.15 \pm 0.93\%$ of circulating CD8+ T cells) which consisted predominantly of effector memory T cells (CD45RA–CCR7–). This was one order of magnitude higher than achieved in eight control patients treated similarly but without CpG ODN as adjuvant, and 1–3 times higher than in previous studies with synthetic vaccines (Speiser et al., 2005).

Use of vaccines for control of cancer resulting from viral infection is another area of potential use for CpG-based adjuvants. For example, vaccines against human papilloma viral infections and viral-associated cervical carcinomas are areas of great promise (Schiller and Davies, 2004). Results of human clinical trials have demonstrated that vaccination of women with HPV-16 vaccine can reduce the incidence of both HPV-16 infection and HPV-16-related cervical intraepithelial neoplasia (Koutsky et al., 2002; Schiller and Davies, 2004). In preclinical studies, both prophylactic and therapeutic immunization of mice with E7 protein of HPV-16 using CpG ODN has been shown to promote the induction of strong E7-specific antibody and T-helper cell proliferative responses and CTL responses compared to when E7 was used alone, and significantly suppress growth of E7-expressing tumors (Kim et al., 2002).

CpG ODN is also effective as monotherapy as demonstrated in numerous animal models of cancer as well as in human clinical trials. When used as monotherapy, CpG ODN induces tumor-specific immune responses, most likely by functioning as an adjuvant to tumor antigens released by necrotic tumors. CpG ODN has also been shown to augment antitumor effects of traditional cancer therapies such as chemotherapy and radiation, both of which are known to cause tumor cell death. Therefore, it is likely that the tumor debulking as a result of chemotherapy or radiation causes the release of tumor-associated antigen resulting in an *in situ* vaccine. When used in combination with CpG ODN, this could lead to the induction of strong tumor-specific immune responses that would be capable of mediating tumor rejection. Numerous studies have reported enhancement of antitumor activity of various chemotherapeutic drugs by CpG ODN including the topoisomerase I inhibitor topotecan (Balsari et al., 2004; Weigel et al., 2003), the alkylating agent cyclophosphamide (Weigel et al., 2003), and the antimetabolite 5-fluorouracil (Wang et al., 2005). For example, when CpG ODN was tested alone or in combination with either cyclophosphamide or topotecan in an orthotopic rhabdomyosarcoma model, the combination therapy using CpG and either of the chemotherapy drugs enabled the long-term survival of 15–40% of the mice whereas neither chemotherapy nor CpG ODN alone has this effect (Weigel et al., 2003). This survival benefit required the presence of T cells, but not NK cells, suggesting that the CpG may have induced the development of an antitumor T cell response, which may have been sufficient to eliminate the residual tumor after chemotherapy. More recently, CpG has also been reported to enhance the antitumor responses to radiation (Milas et al., 2004). The effectiveness of combination therapy using radiation and CpG was diminished in mice that were rendered immunosuppressed by whole body irradiation suggesting the immune-mediated mechanism of the synergy between CpG and radiation.

A number of clinical trials have been undertaken to evaluate ProMune™ in a nonvaccine setting in cancer patients, namely either as a monotherapy or in combination with chemotherapy regimes. ProMune (CPG 7909) has completed phase II clinical studies to treat advanced non small-cell lung cancer (NSCLC), and is currently in phase II testing for malignant melanoma and cutaneous T cell lymphoma (CTCL). Results to date have demonstrated ProMune to be well tolerated and interim results showed significantly enhanced progression-free survival in the NSCLC phase II study (Leichman et al., 2004).

■ Vaccines against asthma and allergy

▓ *Potential of CpG ODN in asthma and allergy*

In industrialized nations the incidence of asthma and allergy has increased steadily over the past century. This has been attributed at least in part to the induction of Th2-type immune responses towards environmental allergens (Cookson and Moffatt, 1997), a lack of early life exposure to bacteria or other infectious agents due to better sanitary conditions, and widespread prophylactic vaccinations using Th2-biased adjuvants such as alum (Davis et al., 1998). While considerable progress has been made in our understanding of asthma and allergies, the current options for treatment remain limited. Corticosteroids are commonly used particularly as inhalants for asthma therapy despite the risk of adverse effects associated with high-dose inhaled steroids, including decrease in growth velocity in children and in sufficient doses bone mineral loss leading to osteoporosis, as well as an increased risk of cataracts, glaucoma, skin atrophy, and vascular changes (Allen et al., 2003).

An alternative to steroid therapy is allergen immunotherapy in which sensitive patients are injected with increasing amounts of allergen to reduce their sensitivity. This is believed to result from the expansion of Th1-type immune responses and a suppression of Th2-type responses resulting in the induction of anergy, probably via the development of allergen-specific regulatory T cells. However, allergen immunotherapy can take months or years to be effective, uses large amounts of allergen, requires frequent medical visits, and can cause severe, in some cases fatal, anaphylactic reactions (Borchers et al., 2004). The use of modified allergens such as T cell reactive peptides or recombinant allergens may help reduce the risk of adverse events, but since they also have reduced immunogenicity will require the use of adjuvants. In addition by using adjuvants it may be possible to further minimize the risk of adverse reactions by reducing the number of injections given as well as the amount of allergen used. The characteristic Th1-type immune responses induced by CpG ODN tend to suppress the cytokine and cellular responses characteristic of asthma and allergies. In addition, CpG ODN has been shown to overcome established Th2 responses in a number of different models (Davis et al., 1998; Weeratna et al., 2000). These findings have led to the investigation of CpG ODN as a novel therapeutic agent for the prevention and treatment of asthma and allergy either as an adjuvant in an allergen vaccine or as monotherapy.

CpG ODN as an allergen vaccine adjuvant

A number of studies have demonstrated the efficacy of CpG ODN as a Th1-type adjuvant when administered prophylactically or therapeutically to mice with allergens. For example, in a mouse model for birch pollen allergy, coadministration of CpG ODN with the major birch pollen allergen Bet v 1 resulted in a Th1-type responses as demonstrated by high serum IgG2a levels and a subsequent reduction in airway inflammation, as well as increased IFN-γ and decreased IL-5 in cell cultures (Jahn-Schmid et al., 1999). In an ovalbumin (OVA)-induced airway disease model, mice were given a course of immunotherapy using low doses of OVA either alone or with CpG ODN. Upon re-challenge, mice that received OVA without CpG ODN developed marked airway eosinophilia and bronchial

hyperresponsiveness, whereas those treated with OVA plus CpG ODN had a significant reduction in airway disease (Kline et al., 2002). Thus CpG ODN immunotherapy was shown effectively to treat established airway disease.

More recently, antigen-conjugated CpG ODN have been tested for their ability to reduce airway eosinophilia and Th2-type cytokine production in response to OVA and to reduce allergenic responses to ragweed antigen Amb a1 using murine models (Shirota et al., 2000; Tighe et al., 2000). These studies have reported that conjugation of CpG ODN to antigen can increase efficacy of CpG administration. For example, in the ovalbumin model, antigen/CpG ODN conjugate was found to be 100-fold more potent than unconjugated CpG ODN and antigen mixture in preventing airway eosinophilia (Shirota et al., 2000). In the Amb a1 model, the antigen/CpG ODN conjugate induced higher levels of IgG2a and lower levels of IgE antibodies and markedly decreased histamine release from basophils than when Amb1 and CpG ODN were admixed together (Tighe et al., 2000).

Initial phase I and II trials in ragweed allergic patients using Amb a 1 as allergen have demonstrated that ragweed allergen/CpG ODN conjugates are well tolerated in humans and induce a rapid increase in allergen-specific IgG but not IgE (Spiegelberg et al., 2002). These studies have shown that allergen-specific IgE levels in patients receiving allergen/CpG ODN conjugates were similar to those in placebo groups, whereas allergen-specific IgG levels after six weekly injections of allergen/CpG ODN conjugates were comparable to titers measured in patients who received immunotherapy for greater than one year with licensed ragweed allergen extracts. In addition, when skin prick tests were done to evaluate local reaction, a mean of 180-fold more allergen/CpG ODN conjugate was necessary to induce the same wheal and skin flare reaction as native Amb a 1 (Spiegelberg et al., 2002). These studies highlight the potential use of CpG ODN as adjuvant in allergen vaccines.

A number of studies have also demonstrated the ability of CpG ODN when administered without allergen to prevent allergen-induced asthmatic responses, including airway eosinophilia, induction of Th2-type cytokine secretion, IgE production, and bronchial hyper activity, by stimulating the innate immune system and redirecting immune responses towards a more Th1-like profile (Banerjee et al., 2004; Broide et al., 1998; Jahn-Schmid et al., 1999; Kline et al., 1998; Shirota et al., 2000; Sur et al., 1999). Studies in a murine model of asthma have shown that CpG ODN can downregulate Th2 responses in IFN-γ and IL-12 knockout mice, suggesting that CpG ODN is capable of generating Th1-like immune responses by multiple mechanisms that involve, but do not require, IL-12 and IFN-γ (Kline et al., 1999). In a murine model of ragweed-induced allergic conjunctivitis, administration of CpG ODN either by systemic (IP injection) or topical (ocular) route was shown to reduce both early and late phase allergic conjunctivitis. CpG ODN also redirected Th2-biased ragweed-specific immune responses towards a more Th1-biased response and protected the animals from allergic inflammation following subsequent challenge with ragweed antigen (Magone et al., 2000).

In humans, when PBMC from allergic patients are stimulated with CpG ODN, there is a considerable increase of polyclonal IgG and IgM synthesis with a suppression of IgE synthesis as well as increased levels of allergen-specific IgG and IgM with no change in IgE levels (Bohle et al., 1999). Furthermore, it has also been shown that CpG ODN can inhibit IgE production by human PBMCs stimulated with IL-4 and anti-CD40 antibodies *in vitro* (Fujieda et al., 2000).

■ Safety of CpG ODN as a vaccine adjuvant

Over the last decade, an increasing number of studies have demonstrated CpG ODN to be a safe and effective vaccine adjuvant in numerous murine and other animal models.

Due to the differential expression of TLR9 in humans and mice, some caution must be made when extrapolating into humans from murine studies. Nevertheless, in recent years several clinical studies have been reported in which CpG ODN has been shown to be an effective and well-tolerated vaccine adjuvant in humans. In the vaccine studies in humans reported to date, the dose of CpG ODN used as has ranged from 0.125 to 3.0 mg. Overall, CpG ODN has been well tolerated, with only mild to moderate adverse events reported (Cooper et al., 2004a, 2004b; Halperin et al., 2003). Adverse events were mainly mild injection site reactions, of short duration and self-limited. In other patients, headache and mild flu-like symptoms have been reported but were also short-lived and did not limit normal daily activities (Cooper et al., 2004a). The events noted are most likely due to the immunostimulatory effects associated with CpG ODN such as the induction of local proinflammatory innate immune responses leading to injection site reaction. It has previously been hypothesized that CpG ODN administration may potentiate autoimmune disease (Krieg, 2003); however, no symptomatic or biochemical evidence of autoimmune disease has been observed in any of the clinical trials using CpG ODN as a vaccine adjuvant to date. No hemodynamic adverse effects were experienced, nor were they expected, since adjuvant doses of CpG ODN are many orders of magnitude lower than the antisense ODN doses previously shown to induce such effects in monkeys (Galbraith et al., 1994).

■ Conclusions

CpG ODN has been demonstrated to be a well-tolerated and effective adjuvant in numerous animal models and humans. These studies indicate that CpG ODN can stimulate strong Th1 responses against a variety of antigens and demonstrate the potential of CpG ODN as an adjuvant in vaccines against infectious disease (both prophylactic and therapeutic), cancer, and asthma/allergy. Clinical data obtained thus far are extremely encouraging, at least for prophylactic vaccines, and a number of trials are ongoing to further evaluate this technology, especially in therapeutic settings. For future development in humans, it may be desirable to further develop formulations (e.g., liposomes, microparticles, emulsions) to protect the antigen, improve uptake by immune cells, allow mucosal delivery, and possibly allow lower doses of antigen or fewer vaccine doses to be used.

References

Ahmad-Nejad, P., Hacker, H., Rutz, M., Bauer, S., Vabulas, R. M., and Wagner, H. (2002). Bacterial CpG-DNA and lipopolysaccharides activate Toll-like receptors at distinct cellular compartments. *Eur. J. Immunol.* 32, 1958–1968.

Akira, S., Takeda, K., and Kaisho, T. (2001). Toll-like receptors: critical proteins linking innate and acquired immunity. *Nature Immunol.* 2, 675–680.

Alexopoulou, L., Holt, A.C., Medzhitov, R., and Flavell, R.A. (2001). Recognition of double-stranded RNA and activation of NF-kappaB by Toll-like receptor 3. *Nature* 413, 732–738.

Alignani, D., Maletto, B., Liscovsky, M., Ropolo, A., Moron, G., and Pistoresi-Palencia, M.C. (2005). Orally administered OVA/CpG-ODN induces specific mucosal and systemic immune response in young and aged mice. *J. Leukoc. Biol.* 77, 898–905.

Allen, D.B., Bielory, L., Derendorf, H., Dluhy, R., Colice, G.L., and Szefler, S.J. (2003). Inhaled corticosteroids: past lessons and future issues. *J. Allergy Clin. Immunol.* 112, (Suppl.), S1–40.

Amigorena, S. (2000). Cancer immunotherapy using dendritic cell-derived exosomes. *Medicina* (Buenos Aires) 60 (Suppl. 2), 51–54.

An, H., Yu, Y., Zhang, M., Xu, H., Qi, R., Yan, X., Liu, S., Wang, W., Guo, Z., Guo, J., Qin, Z., and Cao, X. (2002). Involvement of ERK, p38 and NF-kappaB signal transduction in regulation of TLR2, TLR4 and TLR9 gene expression induced by lipopolysaccharide in mouse dendritic cells. *Immunology* 106, 38–45.

Arulanandam, B.P., Mittler, J.N., Lee, W.T., O'Toole, M., and Metzger, D.W. (2000). Neonatal administration of IL-12 enhances the protective efficacy of antiviral vaccines. *J. Immunol.* 164, 3698–3704.

Baldridge, J.R., McGowan, P., Evans, J.T., Cluff, C., Mossman, S., Johnson, D., and Persing, D. (2004). Taking a Toll on human disease: Toll-like receptor 4 agonists as vaccine adjuvants and monotherapeutic agents. *Expert Opin. Biol. Ther.* 4, 1129–1138.

Balsari, A., Tortoreto, M., Besusso, D., Petrangolini, G., Sfondrini, L., Maggi, R., Menard, S., and Pratesi, G. (2004). Combination of a CpG-oligodeoxynucleotide and a topoisomerase I inhibitor in the therapy of human tumour xenografts. *Eur. J. Cancer* 40, 1275–1281.

Banerjee, B., Kelly, K.J., Fink, J.N., Henderson, J.D., Jr., Bansal, N.K., and Kurup, V.P. (2004). Modulation of airway inflammation by immunostimulatory CpG oligodeoxynucleotides in a murine model of allergic aspergillosis. *Infect. Immunity* 72, 6087–6094.

Baral, R.N., Saha, A., Chatterjee, S.K., Foon, K.A., Krieg, A.M., Weiner, G.J., and Bhattacharya-Chatterjee, M. (2003). Immunostimulatory CpG oligonucleotides enhance the immune response of anti-idiotype vaccine that mimics carcinoembryonic antigen. *Cancer Immunol. Immunother.* 52, 317–327.

Barrios, C., Brandt, C., Berney, M., Lambert, P.H., and Siegrist, C.A. (1996). Partial correction of the TH2/TH1 imbalance in neonatal murine responses to vaccine antigens through selective adjuvant effects. *Eur. J. Immunol.* 26, 2666–2670.

Bauer, S., Kirschning, C.J., Hacker, H., Redecke, V., Hausmann, S., Akira, S., Wagner, H., and Lipford, G.B. (2001). Human TLR9 confers responsiveness to bacterial DNA via species-specific CpG motif recognition. *Proc. Natl. Acad. Sci. USA* 98, 9237–9242.

Beckebaum, S., Cicinnati V.R., Zhang X., Ferencik, S., Frilling, A., Grosse-Wilde, H., Broelsch, C.E., and Gerken, G. (2003). Hepatitis B virus-induced defect of monocyte-derived dendritic cells leads to impaired T helper type 1 response in vitro: mechanisms for viral immune escapes. *Immnology* 109, 487–495.

Berry, L.J., Hickey, D.K., Skelding, K.A., Bao, S., Rendina, A.M., Hansbro, P.M., Gockel, C.M., and Beagley, K.W. (2004). Transcutaneous immunization with combined cholera toxin and CpG adjuvant protects against Chlamydia muridarum genital tract infection. *Infect. Immunity* 72, 1019–1028.

Bohle, B., Jahn-Schmid, B., Maurer, D., Kraft, D., and Ebner, C. (1999). Oligodeoxynucleotides containing CpG motifs induce IL-12, IL-18 and IFN-gamma production in cells from allergic individuals and inhibit IgE synthesis in vitro. *Eur. J. Immunol.* 29, 2344–2353.

Borchers, A.T., Keen, C.L., and Gershwin, M.E. (2004). Fatalities following allergen immunotherapy. *Clin. Rev. Allergy Immunol.* 27, 147–158.

Brazolot Millan, C.L., Weeratna, R., Krieg, A.M., Siegrist, C.A., and Davis, H.L. (1998). CpG DNA can induce strong Th1 humoral and cell-mediated immune responses against hepatitis B surface antigen in young mice. *Proc. Natl. Acad. Sci. USA* 95, 15553–15558.

Broide, D., Schwarze, J., Tighe, H., Gifford, T., Nguyen, M.D., Malek, S., Van Uden, J., Martin-Orozco, E., Gelfand, E.W., and Raz, E. (1998). Immunostimulatory DNA sequences inhibit IL-5, eosinophilic inflammation, and airway hyperresponsiveness in mice. *J. Immunol.* 161, 7054–7062.

Chaput, N., Schartz, N.E., Andre, F., Taieb, J., Novault, S., Bonnaventure, P., Aubert, N., Bernard, J., Lemonnier, F.,

Merad, M., Adema, G., Adams, M., Ferrantini, M., Carpentier, A.F., Escudier, B., Tursz, T., Angevin, E., and Zitvogel, L. (2004). Exosomes as potent cell-free peptide-based vaccine: II. Exosomes in CpG adjuvants efficiently prime naive Tc1 lymphocytes leading to tumor rejection. *J. Immunol.* 172, 2137–2146.

Chisari, F.V. and Ferrari, C. (1995). Hepatitis B virus immunopathogenesis. *Annu. Rev. Immunol.* 13, 29–60.

Chow, J.C., Young, D.W., Golenbock, D.T., Christ, W.J., and Gusovsky, F. (1999). Toll-like receptor-4 mediates lipopolysaccharide-induced signal transduction. *J. Biol. Chem.* 274, 10689–10692.

Chu, R.S., McCool, T., Greenspan, N.S., Schreiber, J.R., and Harding, C.V. (2000). CpG oligodeoxynucleotides act as adjuvants for pneumococcal polysaccharide-protein conjugate vaccines and enhance antipolysaccharide immunoglobulin G2a (IgG2a) and IgG3 antibodies. *Infect. Immunity* 68, 1450–1456.

Chuang, T. and Ulevitch, R.J. (2001). Identification of hTLR10: a novel human Toll-like receptor preferentially expressed in immune cells. *Biochim. Biophys. Acta* 1518, 157–161.

Chuang, T.H. and Ulevitch, R.J. (2000). Cloning and characterization of a sub-family of human toll-like receptors: hTLR7, hTLR8 and hTLR9. *Eur. Cytokine Netw.* 11, 372–378.

Cookson, W.O. and Moffatt, M.F. (1997). Asthma: an epidemic in the absence of infection?. *Science* 275, 41–42.

Cooper, C.L., Davis H.L., Angel, J.B., Morris, M.L., Efler, S.M., Sequin I., Krief, A.M., and Cameron, D.W. (2005). CpG 7909 is safe and highly effective as an adjuvant to HBV vaccine in HIV seropositive adults. *AIDS*, in press.

Cooper, C.L., Davis, H.L., Morris, M.L., Efler, S.M., Adhami, M.A., Krieg, A.M., Cameron, D.W., and Heathcote, J. (2004a). CPG 7909, an immunostimulatory TLR9 agonist iligodeoxynucleotide, as adjuvant to Engerix-B((R)) HBV vaccine in healthy adults: a double-blind phase I/II study. *J. Clin. Immunol* 24, 693–701.

Cooper, C.L., Davis, H.L., Morris, M.L., Efler, S.M., Krieg, A.M., Li, Y., Laframboise, C., Al Adhami, M.J., Khaliq, Y., Seguin, I., and Cameron, D.W. (2004b). Safety and immunogenicity of CPG 7909 injection as an adjuvant to Fluarix influenza vaccine. *Vaccine* 22, 3136–3143.

Davila, E. and Celis, E. (2000). Repeated administration of cytosine-phosphorothiolated guanine-containing oligonucleotides together with peptide/protein immunization results in enhanced CTL responses with anti-tumor activity. *J. Immunol.* 165, 539–547.

Davila, E., Kennedy, R., and Celis, E. (2003). Generation of antitumor immunity by cytotoxic T lymphocyte epitope peptide vaccination, CpG-oligodeoxynucleotide adjuvant, and CTLA-4 blockade. *Cancer Res.* 63, 3281–3288.

Davis, H.L., Weeratna, R., Waldschmidt, T J., Tygrett, L., Schorr, J., Krieg, A.M., and Weeratna, R. (1998). CpG DNA is a potent enhancer of specific immunity in mice immunized with recombinant hepatitis B surface antigen [published erratum appears in *J. Immunol.* 1999, 162, 3103]. *J. Immunol.* 160, 870–876.

Davis, H.L., Suparto, I.I., Weeratna, R.R., Jumintarto, Iskandriati, D.D., Chamzah, S.S., Ma'ruf, A.A., Nente, C.C., Pawitri, D.D., Krieg, A.M., Heriyanto, Smits, W., and Sajuthi, D.D. (2000). CpG DNA overcomes hyporesponsiveness to hepatitis B vaccine in orangutans. *Vaccine* 18, 1920–1924.

Dumais, N., Patrick, A., Moss, R.B., Davis, H.L., and Rosenthal, K.L. (2002). Mucosal immunization with inactivated human immunodeficiency virus plus CpG oligodeoxynucleotides induces genital immune responses and protection against intravaginal challenge. *J. Infect. Dis.* 186, 1098–1105.

Dummer, R. (2001). GVAX (Cell Genesys). *Curr. Opin. Invest. Drugs* 2, 844–848.

Eastcott, J.W., Holmberg, C.J., Dewhirst, F.E., Esch, T.R., Smith, D.J., and Taubman, M.A. (2001). Oligonucleotide containing CpG motifs enhances immune response to mucosally or systemically administered tetanus toxoid. *Vaccine* 19, 1636–1642.

Engelmayer, J., Larsson, M., Subklewe, M., Chahroudi, A., Cox, W.I., Steinman, R.M., and Bhardwaj, N. (1999). Vaccinia virus inhibits the maturation of human dendritic cells: a novel mechanism of immune evasion. *J. Immunol.* 163, 6762–6768.

Fantuzzi, L., Purificato, C., Donato, K., Belardelli, F., and Gessani, S. (2004). Human immunodeficiency virus type 1 gp120 induces abnormal maturation and functional alterations of dendritic cells: a novel mechanism for AIDS pathogenesis. *J. Virol.* 78, 9763–9772.

Freidag, B.L., Melton, G.B., Collins, F., Klinman, D.M., Cheever, A., Stobie, L., Suen, W., and Seder, R.A. (2000). CpG oligodeoxynucleotides and interleukin-12 improve the efficacy of Mycobacterium bovis BCG vaccination in mice challenged with M. tuberculosis. *Infect. Immunity* 68, 2948–2953.

Fujieda, S., Iho, S., Kimura, Y., Yamamoto, H., Igawa, H., and Saito, H. (2000). Synthetic oligodeoxynucleotides inhibit IgE induction in human lymphocytes. *Am. J. Respir. Crit. Care Med.* 162, 232–239.

Furumoto, K., Soares, L., Engleman, E.G., and Merad, M. (2004). Induction of potent antitumor immunity by in situ targeting of intratumoral DCs. *J. Clin. Invest.* 113, 774–783.

Galbraith, W.M., Hobson, W.C., Giclas, P.C., Schechter, P.J., and Agrawal, S. (1994). Complement activation and hemodynamic changes following intravenous administration of phosphorothioate oligonucleotides in the monkey. *Antisense Res.Dev.* 4, 201–206.

Gallichan, W.S., Woolstencroft, R.N., Guarasci, T., McCluskie, M.J., Davis, H.L., and Rosenthal, K.L. (2001). Intranasal immunization with CpG oligodeoxynucleotides as an adjuvant dramatically increases IgA and protection against herpes simplex virus-2 in the genital tract. *J. Immunol.* 166, 3451–3457.

Gewirtz, A.T., Navas, T.A., Lyons, S., Godowski, P.J., and Madara, J.L. (2001). Cutting edge: bacterial flagellin activates basolaterally expressed TLR5 to induce epithelial proinflammatory gene expression. *J. Immunol.* 167, 1882–1885.

Gibson, S.J., Lindh, J.M., Riter, T.R., Gleason, R.M., Rogers, L.M., Fuller, A.E., Oesterich, J.L., Gorden, K.B., Qiu, X., McKane, S.W., Noelle, R.J., Miller, R.L., Kedl, R.M., Fitzgerald-Bocarsly, P., Tomai, M.A., and Vasilakos, J.P. (2002). Plasmacytoid dendritic cells produce cytokines and mature in response to the TLR7 agonists, imiquimod and resiquimod. *Cell Immunol.* 218, 74–86.

Gill, R.F. and Montgomery, P.C. (2002). Enhancement of rat tear IgA antibody responses following intranasal immunization with antigen and CpG ODN. *Curr. Eye Res.* 24, 228–233.

Grosjean, I., Caux, C., Bella, C., Berger, I., Wild, F., Banchereau, J., and Kaiserlian, D. (1997). Measles virus infects human dendritic cells and blocks their allo-stimulatory properties for CD4+ T cells. *J. Exp. Med.* 186, 801–812.

Halperin, S.A., Van Nest, G., Smith, B., Abtahi, S., Whiley, H., and Eiden, J.J. (2003). A phase I study of the safety and immunogenicity of recombinant hepatitis B surface antigen co-administered with an immunostimulatory phosphorothioate oligonucleotide adjuvant. *Vaccine* 21, 2461–2467.

Hartmann, G., Battiany, J., Poeck, H., Wagner, M., Kerkmann, M., Lubenow, N., Rothenfusser, S., and Endres, S. (2003). Rational design of new CpG oligo-nucleotides that combine B cell activation with high IFN-alpha induction in plasmacytoid dendritic cells. *Eur. J. Immunol.* 33, 1633–1641.

Hayashi, F., Smith, K.D., Ozinsky, A., Hawn, T.R., Yi, E.C., Goodlett, D.R., Eng, J.K., Akira, S., Underhill, D.M., and Aderem, A. (2001). The innate immune response to bacterial flagellin is mediated by Toll-like receptor 5. *Nature* 410, 1099–1103.

Heckelsmiller, K., Beck, S., Rall, K., Sipos, B., Schlamp, A., Tuma, E., Rothenfusser, S., Endres, S., and Hartmann, G. (2002). Combined dendritic cell- and CpG oligonucleotide-based immune therapy cures large murine tumors that resist chemotherapy. *Eur. J. Immunol.* 32, 3235–3245.

Heil, F., Hemmi, H., Hochrein, H., Ampenberger, F., Kirschning, C., Akira, S., Lipford, G., Wagner, H., and Bauer, S. (2004). Species-specific recognition of single-stranded RNA via Toll-like receptor 7 and 8. *Science* 303, 1526–1529.

Heinzel, F.P., Sadick, M.D., Holaday, B.J., Coffman, R.L., and Locksley, R.M. (1989). Reciprocal expression of interferon gamma or interleukin 4 during the resolution or progression of murine leishmaniasis. Evidence for expansion of distinct helper T cell subsets. *J. Exp. Med.* 169, 59–72.

Hemmi, H., Takeuchi, O., Kawai, T., Kaisho, T., Sato, S., Sanjo, H., Matsumoto, M., Hoshino, K., Wagner, H., Takeda, K., and Akira, S. (2000). A Toll-like receptor recognizes bacterial DNA. *Nature* 408, 740–745.

Hemmi, H., Kaisho, T., Takeuchi, O., Sato, S., Sanjo, H., Hoshino, K., Horiuchi, T., Tomizawa, H., Takeda, K., and Akira, S. (2002). Small anti-viral compounds activate immune cells via the TLR7 MyD88-dependent signaling pathway. *Nature Immunol.* 3, 196–200.

Hiraoka, K., Yamamoto, S., Otsuru, S., Nakai, S., Tamai, K., Morishita, R., Ogihara, T., and Kaneda, Y. (2004). Enhanced tumor-specific long-term immunity of hemag-glutinating virus of Japan-mediated dendritic cell-tumor fused cell vaccination by coadministration with CpG oligodeoxynucleotides. *J. Immunol.* 173, 4297–4307.

Holmgren, J., Harandi, A.M., and Czerkinsky, C. (2003). Mucosal adjuvants and anti-infection and anti-immuno-pathology vaccines based on cholera toxin, cholera toxin B subunit and CpG DNA. *Expert Rev. Vaccines* 2, 205–217.

Horner, A.A. and Raz, E. (2000). Immunostimulatory sequence oligodeoxynucleotide: a novel mucosal adjuvant. *Clin. Immunol.* 95 (Pt 2), S19–S29.

Horner, A.A., Ronaghy, A., Cheng, P.M., Nguyen, M.D., Cho, H.J., Broide, D., and Raz, E. (1998). Immunostimu-latory DNA is a potent mucosal adjuvant. *Cell Immunol.* 190, 77–82.

Hornung, V., Rothenfusser, S., Britsch, S., Krug, A., Jahrsdor-fer, B., Giese, T., Endres, S., and Hartmann, G. (2002). Quantitative expression of toll-like receptor 1–10 mRNA in cellular subsets of human peripheral blood mononuclear cells and sensitivity to CpG oligodeoxynucleotides. *J. Immunol.* 168, 4531–4537.

Jahn-Schmid, B., Wiedermann, U., Bohle, B., Repa, A., Kraft, D., and Ebner, C. (1999). Oligodeoxynucleotides contain-ing CpG motifs modulate the allergic TH2 response of BALB/c mice to Bet v 1, the major birch pollen allergen. *J. Allergy Clin. Immunol.* 104, 1015–1023.

Jiang, J.Q., Patrick, A., Moss, R.B., and Rosenthal, K.L. (2005). CD8+ T-cell-mediated cross-clade protection in the genital tract following intranasal immunization with inacti-vated human immunodeficiency virus antigen plus CpG oligodeoxynucleotides. *J. Virol.* 79, 393–400.

Jones, T.R., Obaldia, N., III, Gramzinski, R.A., Charoenvit, Y., Kolodny, N., Kitov, S., Davis, H.L., Krieg, A.M., and Hoffman, S.L. (1999). Synthetic oligodeoxynucleotides containing CpG motifs enhance immunogenicity of a peptide malaria vaccine in Aotus monkeys. *Vaccine* 17, 3065–3071.

Joseph, A., Louria-Hayon, I., Plis-Finarov, A., Zeira, E., Zakay-Rones, Z., Raz, E., Hayashi, T., Takabayashi, K., Barenholz, Y., and Kedar, E. (2002). Liposomal immunostimulatory DNA sequence (ISS-ODN): an efficient parenteral and mucosal adjuvant for influenza and hepatitis B vaccines. *Vaccine* 20, 3342–3354.

Kadowaki, N., Ho, S., Antonenko, S., Malefyt, R.W., Kastelein, R.A., Bazan, F., and Liu, Y.J. (2001). Subsets of human dendritic cell precursors express different toll-like receptors and respond to different microbial antigens. *J. Exp. Med.* 194, 863–869.

Kim, S.K., Ragupathi, G., Musselli, C., Choi, S.J., Park, Y.S., and Livingston, P.O. (2000). Comparison of the effect of different immunological adjuvants on the antibody and T-cell response to immunization with MUC1-KLH and GD3-KLH conjugate cancer vaccines. *Vaccine* 18, 597–603.

Kim, T.G., Kim, C.H., Won, E.H., Bae, S.M., Ahn, W.S., Park, J.B., and Sin, J.I. (2004). CpG-ODN-stimulated dendritic cells act as a potent adjuvant for E7 protein delivery to induce antigen-specific antitumour immunity in a HPV 16 E7-associated animal tumour model. *Immunology* 112, 117–125.

Kim, T.Y., Myoung, H.J., Kim, J.H., Moon, I.S., Kim, T.G., Ahn, W.S., and Sin, J.I. (2002). Both E7 and CpG-oligodeoxy-nucleotide are required for protective immunity against challenge with human papillomavirus 16 (E6/E7) immor-talized tumor cells: involvement of CD4+ and CD8+ T cells in protection. *Cancer Res.* 62, 7234–7240.

Kline, J.N., Waldschmidt, T.J., Businga, T.R., Lemish, J.E., Weinstock, J.V., Thorne, P.S., and Krieg, A.M. (1998). Modulation of airway inflammation by CpG oligodeoxy-nucleotides in a murine model of asthma. *J. Immunol.* 160, 2555–2559.

Kline, J.N., Krieg, A.M., Waldschmidt, T.J., Ballas, Z.K., Jain, V., and Businga, T.R. (1999). CpG oligodeoxynucleotides do not require TH1 cytokines to prevent eosinophilic airway inflammation in a murine model of asthma. *J. Allergy Clin. Immunol.* 104, 1258–1264.

Kline, J.N., Kitagaki, K., Businga, T.R., and Jain, V.V. (2002). Treatment of established asthma in a murine model using CpG oligodeoxynucleotides. *Am. J. Physiol. Lung Cell Mol. Physiol.* 283, L170–L179.

Kobayashi, H., Horner, A.A., Takabayashi, K., Nguyen, M.D., Huang, E., Cinman, N., and Raz, E. (1999). Immuno-stimulatory DNA pre-priming: a novel approach for prolonged Th1-biased immunity. *Cell Immunol.* 198, 69–75.

Kochling, J., Konig-Merediz, S.A., Stripecke, R., Buchwald, D., Korte, A., Von Einsiedel, H.G., Sack, F., Henze, G., Seeger, K., Wittig, B., and Schmidt, M. (2003). Protection of mice against Philadelphia chromosome-positive acute lymphoblastic leukemia by cell-based vaccination using nonviral, minimalistic expression vectors and immuno-modulatory oligonucleotides. *Clin. Cancer Res.* 9, 3142–3149.

Koutsky, L.A., Ault, K.A., Wheeler, C.M., Brown, D.R., Barr, E., Alvarez, F.B., Chiacchierini, L.M., and Jansen, K.U. (2002). A controlled trial of a human papillomavirus type 16 vaccine. *N. Engl. J. Med.* 347, 1645–1651.

Kovarik, J., Bozzotti, P., Love-Homan, L., Pihlgren, M., Davis, H.L., Lambert, P.H., Krieg, A.M., and Siegrist, C.A. (1999). CpG oligodeoxynucleotides can circumvent the Th2 polarization of neonatal responses to vaccines but may fail to fully redirect Th2 responses established by neonatal priming. *J. Immunol.* 162, 1611–1617.

Krieg, A.M. (2002). CpG motifs in bacterial DNA and their immune effects. *Annu. Rev. Immunol.* 20, 709–760.

Krieg, A.M. (2003). CpG motifs: the active ingredient in bacterial extracts? *Nature Med.* 9, 831–835.

Krieg, A.M. (2004). Antitumor applications of stimulating toll-like receptor 9 with CpG oligodeoxynucleotides. *Curr. Oncol. Rep.* 6, 88–95.

Krieg, A.M., Yi, A.K., Matson, S., Waldschmidt, T.J., Bishop, G.A., Teasdale, R., Koretzky, G.A., and Klinman, D.M. (1995). CpG motifs in bacterial DNA trigger direct B-cell activation. *Nature* 374, 546–549.

Krieg, A.M., Efler, S.M., Wittpoth, M., Al Adhami, M.J., and Davis, H.L. (2004). Induction of systemic TH1-like innate immunity in normal volunteers following subcutaneous but not intravenous administration of CPG 7909, a synthetic B-class CpG oligodeoxynucleotide TLR9 agonist. *J. Immunother.* 27, 460–471.

Krug, A., Towarowski, A., Britsch, S., Rothenfusser, S., Hornung, V., Bals, R., Giese, T., Engelmann, H., Endres, S., Krieg, A.M., and Hartmann, G. (2001). Toll-like receptor expression reveals CpG DNA as a unique microbial stimulus for plasmacytoid dendritic cells which synergizes with CD40 ligand to induce high amounts of IL-12. *Eur. J. Immunol.* 31, 3026–3037.

Kruse, M., Rosorius, O., Kratzer, F., Stelz, G., Kuhnt, C., Schuler, G., Hauber, J., and Steinkasserer, A. (2000). Mature dendritic cells infected with herpes simplex virus type 1 exhibit inhibited T-cell stimulatory capacity. *J. Virol.* 74, 7127–7136.

Kuwana, M., Kaburaki, J., Wright, T.M., Kawakami, Y., and Ikeda, Y. (2001). Induction of antigen-specific human CD4(+) T cell anergy by peripheral blood DC2 precursors. *Eur. J. Immunol.* 31, 2547–2557.

Kwant, A. and Rosenthal, K.L. (2004). Intravaginal immuniza-tion with viral subunit protein plus CpG oligodeoxy-nucleotides induces protective immunity against HSV-2. *Vaccine* 22, 3098–3104.

Leichman, G., Gravenor, D., Albert G., and Schmalbach, T.A. (2004). TLR9 Cpg Immunomodulator' in combination with chemotherapy as treatment for advanced non-small cell lung cancer (NSCLC), a randomized, controlled phase II study. 41st Annual meeting of the American Society of Clinical Oncology. *J. Clin. Oncol.* 22 (14S) 1726.

Lien, E., Means, T.K., Heine, H., Yoshimura, A., Kusumoto, S., Fukase, K., Fenton, M. J., Oikawa, M., Qureshi, N., Monks, B., Finberg, R.W., Ingalls, R.R., and Golenbock, D.T. (2000). Toll-like receptor 4 imparts ligand-specific recognition of bacterial lipopolysaccharide. *J. Clin. Invest* 105, 497–504.

Lipford, G.B., Sparwasser, T., Zimmermann, S., Heeg, K., and Wagner, H. (2000). CpG-DNA-mediated transient lympha-denopathy is associated with a state of Th1 predisposition to antigen-driven responses. *J. Immunol.* 165, 1228–1235.

Liu, H.M., Newbrough, S.E., Bhatia, S.K., Dahle, C.E., Krieg, A.M., and Weiner, G.J. (1998). Immunostimulatory CpG oligodeoxynucleotides enhance the immune response to vaccine strategies involving granulocyte-macrophage colony-stimulating factor. *Blood* 92, 3730–3736.

Magone, M.T., Chan, C.C., Beck, L., Whitcup, S.M., and Raz, E. (2000). Systemic or mucosal administration of immuno-stimulatory DNA inhibits early and late phases of murine allergic conjunctivitis. *Eur. J. Immunol.* 30, 1841–1850.

Maletto, B., Ropolo, A., Moron, V., and Pistoresi-Palencia, M.C. (2002). CpG-DNA stimulates cellular and humoral immu-nity and promotes Th1 differentiation in aged BALB/c mice. *J. Leukoc. Biol.* 72, 447–454.

Manning, B.M., Enioutina, E.Y., Visic, D.M., Knudson, A.D., and Daynes, R.A. (2001). CpG DNA functions as an effective adjuvant for the induction of immune responses in aged mice. *Exp. Gerontol.* 37, 107–126.

Marshall, J.D., Fearon, K., Abbate, C., Subramanian, S., Yee, P., Gregorio, J., Coffman, R.L., and Van Nest, G. (2003). Identification of a novel CpG DNA class and motif that optimally stimulate B cell and plasmacytoid dendritic cell functions. *J. Leukoc. Biol.* 73, 781–792.

Martin, P., Del Hoyo, G.M., Anjuere, F., Arias, C.F., Vargas, H.H., Fernandez, L., Parrillas, V., and Ardavin, C. (2002). Characterization of a new subpopulation of mouse CD8alpha+ B220+ dendritic cells endowed with type 1 interferon production capacity and tolerogenic potential. *Blood* 100, 383–390.

McCluskie, M.J. and Davis, H.L. (1998). CpG DNA is a potent enhancer of systemic and mucosal immune responses against hepatitis B surface antigen with intranasal administration to mice. *J. Immunol.* 161, 4463–4466.

McCluskie, M.J. and Davis, H.L. (1999). CpG DNA as mucosal adjuvant. *Vaccine* 18, 231–237.

McCluskie, M.J. and Davis, H.L. (2000). Oral, intrarectal and intranasal immunizations using CpG and non-CpG oligodeoxynucleotides as adjuvants. *Vaccine* 19, 413–422.

McCluskie, M.J., Wen, Y.M., Di, Q., and Davis, H.L. (1998). Immunization against hepatitis B virus by mucosal administration of antigen-antibody complexes. *Viral Immunol.* 11, 245–252.

McCluskie, M.J., Weeratna, R.D., Krieg, A.M., and Davis, H.L. (2000). CpG DNA is an effective oral adjuvant to protein antigens in mice. *Vaccine* 19, 950–957.

McCluskie, M.J., Weeratna, R.D., Clements, J.D., and Davis, H.L. (2001). Mucosal immunization of mice using CpG DNA and/or mutants of the heat-labile enterotoxin of *Escherichia coli* as adjuvants. *Vaccine* 19, 3759–3768.

McGhee, J.R., Mestecky, J., Dertzbaugh, M.T., Eldridge, J.H., Hirasawa, M., and Kiyono, H. (1992). The mucosal immune system: from fundamental concepts to vaccine development. *Vaccine* 10, 75–88.

Medina, E. and Guzman, C.A. (2000). Modulation of immune responses following antigen administration by mucosal route. *FEMS Immunol. Med. Microbiol.* 27, 305–311.

Merad, M., Sugie, T., Engleman, E.G., and Fong, L. (2002). In vivo manipulation of dendritic cells to induce therapeutic immunity. *Blood* 99, 1676–1682.

Miconnet, I., Koenig, S., Speiser, D., Krieg, A., Guillaume, P., Cerottini, J. C., and Romero, P. (2002). CpG are efficient adjuvants for specific CTL induction against tumor antigen-derived peptide. *J. Immunol.* 168, 1212–1218.

Milas, L., Mason, K.A., Ariga, H., Hunter, N., Neal, R., Valdecanas, D., Krieg, A.M., and Whisnant, J.K. (2004). CpG oligodeoxynucleotide enhances tumor response to radiation. *Cancer Res.* 64, 5074–5077.

Moldoveanu, Z., Love-Homan, L., Huang, W.Q., and Krieg, A.M. (1998). CpG DNA, a novel immune enhancer for systemic and mucosal immunization with influenza virus. *Vaccine* 16, 1216–1224.

Mui, B., Raney, S.G., Semple, S.C., and Hope, M.J. (2001). Immune stimulation by a CpG-containing oligodeoxynucleotide is enhanced when encapsulated and delivered in lipid particles. *J. Pharmacol. Exp. Ther.* 298, 1185–1192.

Nesburn, A.B., Ramos, T.V., Zhu, X., Asgarzadeh, H., Nguyen, V., and Benmohamed, L. (2005). Local and systemic B cell and Th1 responses induced following ocular mucosal delivery of multiple epitopes of herpes simplex virus type 1 glycoprotein D together with cytosine-phosphate-guanine adjuvant. *Vaccine* 23, 873–883.

Nicklin, P.L., Bayley, D., Giddings, J., Craig, S.J., Cummins, L.L., Hastewell, J.G., and Phillips, J.A. (1998). Pulmonary bioavailability of a phosphorothioate oligonucleotide (CGP 64128A): comparison with other delivery routes. *Pharm. Res.* 15, 583–591.

O'Hagan, D.T., MacKichan, M.L., and Singh, M. (2001). Recent developments in adjuvants for vaccines against infectious diseases. *Biomol. Eng* 18, 69–85.

O'Rourke, M.G., Schmidt, C.W., O'Rourke, T.R., and Ellem, K.A. (1997). Immunotherapy, including gene therapy, for metastatic melanoma. *Aust. NZ J. Surg.* 67, 834–841.

Olszewska, W., Partidos, C.D., and Steward, M.W. (2000). Antipeptide antibody responses following intranasal immunization: effectiveness of mucosal adjuvants. *Infect. Immunity* 68, 4923–4929.

Prince, G.A., Mond, J.J., Porter, D.D., Yim, K.C., Lan, S.J., and Klinman, D.M. (2003). Immunoprotective activity and safety of a respiratory syncytial virus vaccine: mucosal delivery of fusion glycoprotein with a CpG oligodeoxynucleotide adjuvant. *J. Virol.* 77, 13156–13160.

Rauthan, M., Kaur, R., Appaiahgari, M.B., and Vrati, S. (2004). Oral immunization of mice with Japanese encephalitis virus envelope protein synthesized in *Escherichia coli* induces anti-viral antibodies. *Microbes. Infect.* 6, 1305–1311.

Rhee, S.H. and Hwang, D. (2000). Murine TOLL-like receptor 4 confers lipopolysaccharide responsiveness as determined by activation of NF kappa B and expression of the inducible cyclooxygenase. *J. Biol. Chem.* 275, 34035–34040.

Rieger, R. and Kipps, T.J. (2003). CpG oligodeoxynucleotides enhance the capacity of adenovirus-mediated CD154 gene transfer to generate effective B-cell lymphoma vaccines. *Cancer Res.* 63, 4128–4135.

Rock, F.L., Hardiman, G., Timans, J.C., Kastelein, R.A., and Bazan, J.F. (1998). A family of human receptors structurally related to Drosophila Toll. *Proc. Natl. Acad. Sci. USA* 95, 588–593.

Sajic, D., Ashkar, A.A., Patrick, A.J., McCluskie, M.J., Davis, H.L., Levine, K.L., Holl, R., and Rosenthal, K.L. (2003). Parameters of CpG oligodeoxynucleotide-induced protection against intravaginal HSV-2 challenge. *J. Med. Virol.* 71, 561–568.

Sandler, A.D., Chihara, H., Kobayashi, G., Zhu, X., Miller, M.A., Scott, D.L., and Krieg, A.M. (2003). CpG oligonucleotides enhance the tumor antigen-specific immune response of a granulocyte macrophage colony-stimulating factor-based vaccine strategy in neuroblastoma. *Cancer Res.* 63, 394–399.

Schetter, C. and Vollmer, J. (2004). Toll-like receptors involved in the response to microbial pathogens: development of agonists for Toll-like receptor 9. *Curr. Opin. Drug Discov. Devel.* 7, 204–210.

Schiller, J.T. and Davies, P. (2004). Delivering on the promise: HPV vaccines and cervical cancer. *Nat. Rev. Microbiol.* 2, 343–347.

Schwandner, R., Dziarski, R., Wesche, H., Rothe, M., and Kirschning, C.J. (1999). Peptidoglycan- and lipoteichoic acid-induced cell activation is mediated by toll-like receptor 2. *J. Biol. Chem.* 274, 17406–17409.

Serebrisky, D., Teper, A.A., Huang, C.K., Lee, S.Y., Zhang, T.F., Schofield, B.H., Kattan, M., Sampson, H.A., and Li, X.M. (2000). CpG oligodeoxynucleotides can reverse Th2-associated allergic airway responses and alter the B7.1/B7.2 expression in a murine model of asthma. *J. Immunol.* 165, 5906–5912.

Sher, A. (1992). Schistosomiasis. Parasitizing the cytokine system. *Nature* 356, 565–566.

Shirota, H., Sano, K., Kikuchi, T., Tamura, G., and Shirato, K. (2000). Regulation of murine airway eosinophilia and Th2 cells by antigen-conjugated CpG oligodeoxynucleotides as a novel antigen-specific immunomodulator. *J. Immunol.* 164, 5575–5582.

Siegrist, C.A., Pihlgren, M., Tougne, C., Efler, S.M., Morris, M.L., Al-Adhami, M.J., Cameron, D.W., Cooper, C.L., Heathcote, J., Davis, H.L., and Lambert, P.H. (2004). Co-administration of CpG oligonucleotides enhances the late affinity maturation process of human anti-hepatitis B vaccine response. *Vaccine* 23, 615–622.

Sparwasser, T., Vabulas, R.M., Villmow, B., Lipford, G.B., and Wagner, H. (2000). Bacterial CpG-DNA activates dendritic cells in vivo: T helper cell-independent cytotoxic T cell responses to soluble proteins. *Eur. J. Immunol.* 30, 3591–3597.

Speiser, D.E., Lienard, D., Rufer, N., Rubio-Godoy, V., Rimoldi, D., Lejeune, F., Krieg, A.M., Cerottini, J.C., and Romero, P. (2005). Rapid and strong human CD8(+) T cell responses to vaccination with peptide, IFA, and CpG oligodeoxynucleotide 7909. *J. Clin. Invest.* 115, 739–746.

Spiegelberg, H.L., Horner, A.A., Takabayashi, K., and Raz, E. (2002). Allergen-immunostimulatory oligodeoxynucleotide conjugate: a novel allergoid for immunotherapy. *Curr. Opin. Allergy Clin. Immunol.* 2, 547–551.

Stern, B.V., Boehm, B.O., and Tary-Lehmann, M. (2002). Vaccination with tumor peptide in CpG adjuvant protects via IFN-gamma-dependent CD4 cell immunity. *J. Immunol.* 168, 6099–6105.

Sur, S., Wild, J.S., Choudhury, B.K., Sur, N., Alam, R., and Klinman, D.M. (1999). Long term prevention of allergic lung inflammation in a mouse model of asthma by CpG oligodeoxynucleotides. *J. Immunol.* 162, 6284–6293.

Switaj, T., Jalili, A., Jakubowska, A.B., Drela, N., Stoksik, M., Nowis, D., Basak, G., Golab, J., Wysocki, P.J., Mackiewicz, A., Sasor, A., Socha, K., Jakobisiak, M.,

and Lasek, W. (2004). CpG immunostimulatory oligodeoxynucleotide 1826 enhances antitumor effect of interleukin 12 gene-modified tumor vaccine in a melanoma model in mice. *Clin. Cancer Res.* 10 (Pt 1), 4165–4175.

Takeshita, F., Leifer, C.A., Gursel, I., Ishii, K.J., Takeshita, S., Gursel, M., and Klinman, D.M. (2001). Cutting edge: role of Toll-like receptor 9 in CpG DNA-induced activation of human cells. *J. Immunol.* 167, 3555–3558.

Takeuchi, O., Kawai, T., Sanjo, H., Copeland, N.G., Gilbert, D.J., Jenkins, N.A., Takeda, K., and Akira, S. (1999). TLR6: a novel member of an expanding toll-like receptor family. *Gene* 231, 59–65.

Thomsen, L.L., Topley, P., Daly, M.G., Brett, S.J., and Tite, J.P. (2004). Imiquimod and resiquimod in a mouse model: adjuvants for DNA vaccination by particle-mediated immunotherapeutic delivery. *Vaccine* 22, 1799–1809.

Tighe, H., Takabayashi, K., Schwartz, D., Van Nest, G., Tuck, S., Eiden, J.J., Kagey-Sobotka, A., Creticos, P.S., Lichtenstein, L.M., Spiegelberg, H.L., and Raz, E. (2000). Conjugation of immunostimulatory DNA to the short ragweed allergen amb a 1 enhances its immunogenicity and reduces its allergenicity. *J. Allergy Clin. Immunol.* 106 (Pt 1), 124–134.

Tsubouchi E, Akbar Sk. Md. Fazle, Horiike, N., and Morikazu, O. (2004). Infection and dysfuncation of circulating blook dendritic cells and their subsets in chronic hepatitis C virus infection. *J. Gastroenterol.* 39, 754–762.

Vasilakos, J.P., Smith, R.M., Gibson, S.J., Lindh, J.M., Pederson, L.K., Reiter, M.J., Smith, M.H., and Tomai, M.A. (2000). Adjuvant activities of immune response modifier R-848: comparison with CpG ODN. *Cell Immunol.* 204, 64–74.

Vollmer, J., Weeratna, R., Payette, P., Jurk, M., Schetter, C., Laucht, M., Wader, T., Tluk, S., Liu, M., Davis, H.L., and Krieg, A.M. (2004). Characterization of three CpG oligodeoxynucleotide classes with distinct immunostimulatory activities. *Eur. J. Immunol.* 34, 251–262.

Walker, P.S., Scharton-Kersten, T., Krieg, A.M., Love-Homan, L., Rowton, E.D., Udey, M.C., and Vogel, J.C. (1999). Immunostimulatory oligodeoxynucleotides promote protective immunity and provide systemic therapy for leishmaniasis via IL-12- and IFN-gamma-dependent mechanisms. *Proc. Natl. Acad. Sci. USA* 96, 6970–6975.

Wang, X.S., Sheng, Z., Ruan, Y.B., Guang, Y., and Yang, M.L. (2005). CpG oligodeoxynucleotides inhibit tumor growth and reverse the immunosuppression caused by the therapy with 5-fluorouracil in murine hepatoma. *World J. Gastroenterol.* 11, 1220–1224.

Wang, Y., Wang, W., Li, N., Yu, Y., and Cao, X. (2002). Activation of antigen-presenting cells by immunostimulatory plant DNA: a natural resource for potential adjuvant. *Vaccine* 20, 2764–2771.

Weeratna, R.D., McCluskie, M.J., Xu, Y., and Davis, H.L. (2000). CpG DNA induces stronger immune responses with less toxicity than other adjuvants. *Vaccine* 18, 1755–1762.

Weeratna, R.D., Brazolot Millan, C.L., McCluskie, M.J., and Davis, H.L. (2001). CpG ODN can re-direct the Th bias of established Th2 immune responses in adult and young mice. *FEMS Immunol. Med. Microbiol.* 32, 65–71.

Weigel, B.J., Rodeberg, D.A., Krieg, A.M., and Blazar, B.R. (2003). CpG oligodeoxynucleotides potentiate the anti-tumor effects of chemotherapy or tumor resection in an orthotopic murine model of rhabdomyosarcoma. *Clin. Cancer Res.* 9, 3105–3114.

Weiner, G.J., Liu, H.M., Wooldridge, J.E., Dahle, C.E., and Krieg, A.M. (1997). Immunostimulatory oligodeoxy-nucleotides containing the CpG motif are effective as immune adjuvants in tumor antigen immunization. *Proc. Natl .Acad. Sci. USA* 94, 10833–10837.

World Health Organization. (2001). *World Health Organization. Global Alliance for Vaccines and Immunization (GAVI).* Fact Sheet No. 169.

Yi, A.K., Hornbeck, P., Lafrenz, D.E., and Krieg, A.M. (1996). CpG DNA rescue of murine B lymphoma cells from anti-IgM-induced growth arrest and programmed cell death is associated with increased expression of c-myc and bcl-xL. *J. Immunol.* 157, 4918–4925.

Yi, A.K., Chang, M., Peckham, D.W., Krieg, A.M., and Ashman, R.F. (1998). CpG oligodeoxyribonucleotides rescue mature spleen B cells from spontaneous apoptosis and promote cell cycle entry. *J. Immunol.* 160, 5898–5906.

Yoshimura, A., Lien, E., Ingalls, R.R., Tuomanen, E., Dziarski, R., and Golenbock, D. (1999). Cutting edge: recognition of Gram-positive bacterial cell wall components by the innate immune system occurs via Toll-like receptor 2. *J. Immunol.* 163, 1–5.

Toll-like receptor 4 agonists as vaccine adjuvants

David H. Persing
Corixa Corporation, Seattle, Washington

Patrick McGowan, Jay T. Evans, and Christopher Cluff
Corixa Corporation, Hamilton, Montana

Sally Mossman
Corixa Corporation, Seattle, Washington

David Johnson and Jory R. Baldridge
Corixa Corporation, Hamilton, Montana

■ Introduction

Lipopolysaccharide (LPS), the major component of the Gram-negative bacterial cell wall, has long been known as a powerful immunomodulator. Over a century ago, a New York physician, William B. Coley, noted that some cancer patients experienced spontaneous tumor regression following episodes of acute bacterial illness. Hypothesizing a correlation between the bacterial infection and tumor regression, Coley went on to treat successfully hundreds of cancer patients with heat-killed bacterial preparations known as Coley's toxins (Nauts et al., 1946; Hall, 1997). We now recognize that Coley's toxins likely contained a mixture of immunodulatory substances including LPS and bacterial DNA; these components collectively served to stimulate innate immune responses in Coley's cancer patients, leading to tumor regression in some cases. Similar results have since been observed in animal models in which increasingly refined microbial extracts have been administered. Meanwhile, other studies showed that antibody responses to exogenous antigens could be enhanced by coadministration of bacteria or bacterial extracts (reviewed in Munoz, 1964). In 1956 Arthur Johnson and colleagues determined that the adjuvant component of Gram-negative bacteria was LPS (Johnson et al., 1956).

Despite its well-known ability to enhance immune responses, LPS is considered too toxic by current standards to be clinically useful because of the induction of excessive amounts of inflammatory cytokines which provoke a sepsis-like syndrome. In efforts to unlink its extreme toxicity from its potentially beneficial immunological characteristics, Edgar Ribi and colleagues systematically evaluated modifications to LPS. Via sequential steps of acid and base hydrolysis, an immunoactive lipid A fraction containing a single phosphate moiety was eventually isolated.

This monophosphoryl lipid A (MPL) preparation exhibited significantly reduced toxicity and pyrogenicity compared to the parent LPS but retained much of its intrinsic immunomodulatory activity, leading to the development of MPL adjuvant for use in human vaccines (Figure 6.1A) (Ribi, 1979; Myers et al., 1990; Ulrich and Myers, 1995).

Toll-like receptors: the missing link between innate and adaptive immunity

In 1999 Beutler and colleagues used positional cloning studies of LPS hyporesponsive mice to identify the critical cellular target of LPS as a Toll-like receptor (TLR) (Poltorak et al., 1998, 2000; Ulevitch, 1999). This important work served to provide a thematic link to the seminal work in drosophila by Jules Hoffman and colleagues, in which the functional characteristics of the Toll developmental mutant included extreme susceptibility to fungal infections (reviewed in Imler and Hoffmann, 2000). Bolstered by rapid advances in the human genome project, a total of ten potentially functional human TLRs were identified on the basis of sequence homology, and a flurry of scientific effort within laboratories across the world led to the identification of microbial products from bacteria, fungi, and viruses that interact with these receptors (Hoebe et al., 2004; Takeda and Akira, 2004). As of this writing, the microbial ligand class for only one putatively functional TLR, TLR10, remains unidentified.

Over the past few years, interest in targeting TLRs for intervention against infectious and inflammatory diseases has grown rapidly. TLRs are important gateway receptors for the induction of both the innate and adaptive immune responses, often working synergistically in the inevitable immunological confrontations between humans and infectious agents (reviewed in Akira, 2003). Toll receptors are a family of pattern recognition receptors that detect highly conserved microbial components common to classes of pathogens, such as LPS (TLR4), viral double-stranded RNA (TLR3), viral single-stranded RNA (TLR7 and 8), bacterial DNA (TLR9), bacterial flagellin (TLR5), and bacterial lipopeptide motifs (TLR1, 2, and 6). Strategically and selectively expressed within distinct anatomical compartments and on a variety of cell types, TLRs monitor the environment for signs of infection. Upon activation, TLRs instantly marshal a broad array of defense mechanisms aimed at elimination of invading pathogens. Phagocytic cells become activated leading to enhanced phagocytosis and secretion of antimicrobial molecules, including defensins and reactive oxygen intermediates. The innate immune responses triggered by TLR agonists limit the initial spread of infection, while other TLR-mediated events promote the development of subsequent acquired immune responses. A cascade of proinflammatory cytokines and chemokines, including interleukin (IL)-1, IL-8, IL-12, tumor necrosis factor (TNF)-α, and interferon (IFN)-γ, leads to the recruitment and activation of antigen-presenting cells as well as effector B and T lymphocytes. Within this setting, increased expression of adhesion and costimulatory molecules on cell surfaces leads to heightened cooperation among cells of the immune system resulting in enhanced humoral and cellular responses. Whereas the innate response serves to reduce pathogen burden to survivable levels during the first few days following pathogen exposure, antigen-specific acquired immune responses are often required to eliminate all final traces of the infection. Moreover, unlike innate responses, acquired responses are retained in immunologic memory and are effectively recommissioned upon subsequent infection. Thus, the TLRs serve to link the innate and adaptive responses and comprise important pharmaceutical targets for development of adjuvants and immunomodulators.

MPL and AGPs: TLR4 agonists as vaccine adjuvants

Like LPS, the immunomodulatory activity of MPL adjuvant is mediated via interactions

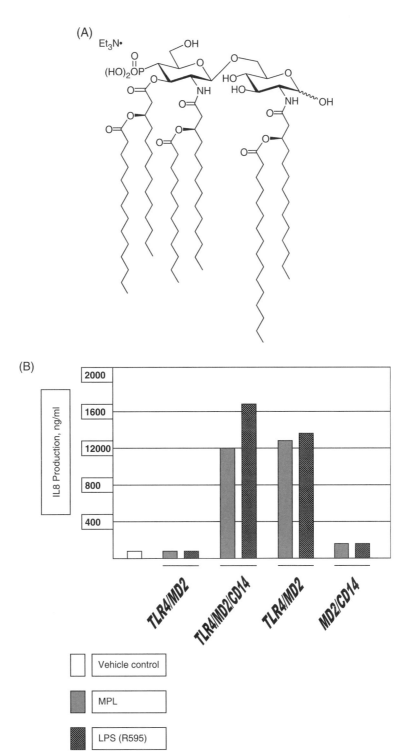

Figure 6.1 (A) The structure of the principal biologically active component in MPL® adjuvant. (B) Hela cells were transfected with human TLR4, MD2, and CD14 cDNAs according to the methods described in Stover et al. (2004).

with TLR4. C3H/HEJ mice harbor a single point mutation resulting in an amino acid change in TLR4 and thus are hyporesponsive to LPS and lipid A (Poltorak et al., 1998). In contrast to wild-type mice, C3H/HEJ mice treated with MPL produce no IFN-γ. Similarly, B cells from wild-type but not C3H/HEJ mice proliferate in response to MPL exposure (Persing et al., 2002). More recently, we have used an *in vitro* system in which Hela cells (which do not express TLRs on their surface) are transfected with expression constructs that direct to express specific TLRs on their surface (da Silva et al., 2001). Using this approach, we have been able to demonstrate both the requirement for and specificity of TLR4 (and the associated MD-2 molecule, in the response to MPL) (Figure 6.1B). Using blocking antibodies specific for TLR4 or TLR2, we have also observed that the response to MPL in human monocytes and human monocytic cells lines is dependent on TLR4, but not TLR2 (unpublished observations). Our findings are not entirely inconsistent with the results from a recent report suggesting that MPL adjuvant can signal via TLR4 and TLR2 (Martin et al., 2003), but the aforementioned experiments in C3H/HEJ mice (which have normal TLR2 signaling) suggest that the vast majority of the immunomodulatory activity of MPL is mediated by TLR4.

Extensive clinical studies with MPL® adjuvant demonstrated that it is a safe and effective vaccine adjuvant (reviewed in Baldridge et al., 2004). To date, over 273,000 doses have been administered in human clinical studies. In vaccine trials intended in support of regulatory approval, an overall safety profile equivalent to alum, which has been used as a vaccine adjuvant for over 60 years, has been documented. Collectively, these studies have indicated significant advantages of including MPL® adjuvant in vaccine formulations; reduced numbers of doses and/or reduced antigen requirements are often cited as significant benefits (Evans et al., 2003). In light of recent concerns that ligands for TLRs other than TLR4 may potentiate autoimmune disease

(Viglianti et al., 2003; Sacher et al., 2002), it has been reassuring that TLR4 agonists have enjoyed a sterling safety profile. Indeed, a European regulatory filing for the first TLR agonist-containing vaccine (Glaxo-Smithkline's Fendrix hepatitis B vaccine, which contains MPL) has been approved.

Recently, scientists at Corixa Corporation developed synthetic lipid A mimetics that are chemically unique, acylated monosaccharides called aminoalkyl glucosaminide 4-phosphates (AGPs) (Figure 6.2) (Johnson et al., 1999). In contrast to the complex family of lipid A congeners found in MLA, the synthetic AGPs represent mimetics of lipid A that are created as highly pure, single chemical entities. The AGPs were designed to accommodate molecular changes for improved biologic and pharmacologic activities. This unique family of molecules, which are chemically and biologically distinct from "natural" TLR4 agonists such as LPS and MPL, may comprise unique characteristics as vaccine adjuvants and as stand-alone therapeutic immunomodulators (Stover et al., 2004; Cluff et al., 2005).

In addition to their use as vaccine adjuvants, MPL and the AGPs can mediate an immunoprophylactic effect in mice against tumors and a variety of infectious organisms through their ability to stimulate TLR4 (Ulrich, 1988; Madonna, 1988; Persing et al., 2002; Baldridge et al., 2002) (Table 6.2). Although the specific mechanisms mediating the protective effect have not been completely elucidated, the principal innate immune effectors probably overlap extensively with those induced by LPS (or lipid A). LPS exposure results in production of defensins, which comprise several distinct families of antibacterial, antifungal, and antiviral peptides (Ayabe et al., 2000). In addition to activation of the MyD88-dependent signaling pathway that results in the production of multiple cytokines and chemokines, TLR4 agonists also activate the so-called MyD88-independent pathway, which results in production of inducible nitric oxide synthetase (iNOS) and type I interferons (Toshchakov et al., 2002), activation of MAP

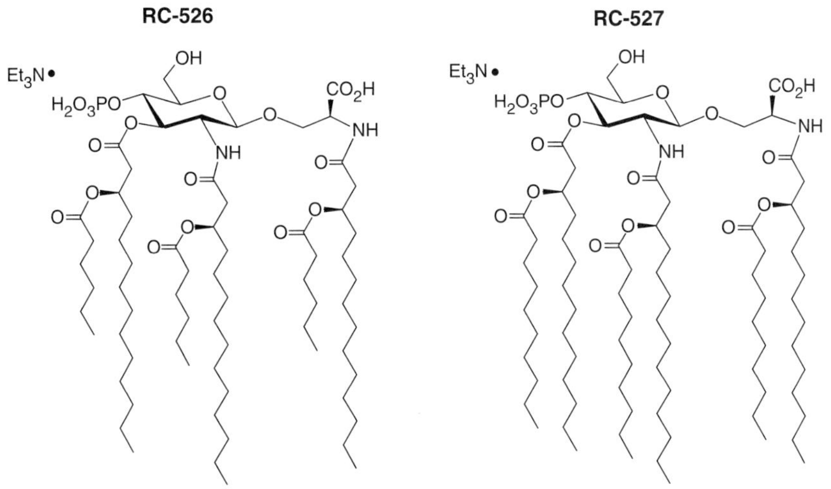

Figure 6.2 The structures of the synthetic AGPs, RC-526, a TLR4 antagonist, and RC527, a TLR4 agonist. The molecules are structurally identical except for the length of the secondary acyl chains.

kinases and NF-kB (Kawai et al., 1999), and functional maturation of dendritic cells (Akira, 2003). Thus, TLR4 activation results in short-term antimicrobial effects, which are observed within hours of receptor ligation, as well as long-term effects on the adaptive immune response as dictated by the tenor of the cytokine and cellular microenvironment in which antigens are presented. The latter effect is thought to play the greatest role in determining the adjuvant effects of TLR agonists (Kaisho and Akira, 2002).

Preclinical experience with TLR4 agonists.

MPL® adjuvant and the AGPs have been studied extensively in preclinical animal models as vaccine adjuvants. In this respect, these molecules have been shown to be potent immunomodulators, capable of enhancing both humoral and cell-mediated immune responses to a wide variety of polysaccharide and protein antigens (Ulrich and Myers, 1995; Evans et al., 2003). In most cases, the inclusion of either class of TLR4 agonist produced a qualitative shift in the immune response, such that IgG2a antibody titers were boosted significantly, providing a more balanced Th1/Th2 response to coadministered vaccine antigens when compared to alum alone. These studies provided an indication that both MPL® adjuvant and the AGPs have the capacity to upregulate Th1 responses and to induce strong cell-mediated immune (CMI) responses. Additional studies have since confirmed this concept, demonstrating the ability of these adjuvants to promote CMI responses in the form of T helper cells and cytotoxic T lymphocytes (CTLs) (De Becker et al., 2000; Baldridge et al., 2000a).

The ability of MPL to serve as a Th1 adjuvant in the context of an established Th2 immune response was recently tested in an allergy model by Wheeler et al. (2001). IgE responses were induced in brown Norway rats (high IgE responders) by immunization with KLH/alum adsorbates plus *Bordetella pertussis* bacteria. The rise in IgE titers following subsequent vaccinations with KLH was blocked by the addition of MPL to the vaccines. In a related experiment, the ratio of ragweed-specific Th2- to Th1-associated antibody isotypes was dramatically decreased from 16:1 to 2:1 in the sera of mice vaccinated with a ragweed vaccine (Pollinex R; Allergy Therapuetics, Ltd) formulated with MPL compared to sera from mice receiving only the Pollinex vaccine (Wheeler et al., 2001). Taken together, these results suggest that MPL preferentially enhances a Th1-biased response that can attenuate an existing Th2 response.

Presumably due to the strategic expression of TLR4 in the airways (Claeys et al., 2003), MPL adjuvant and the AGPs are also active when delivered via intranasal and oral routes, promoting immune responses at local and distal mucosal sites, including enhanced antigen-specific IgA. When applied in vaccine formulations to intranasal (Baldridge et al., 2000b; VanCott et al., 1998) or oral (Doherty et al., 2002) mucosal surfaces, MPL promotes antigen-specific immune responses at local and distal mucosal sites as well as systemic immune responses. These responses are characterized by enhanced antigen-specific IgA both locally and at distal mucosal sites. Importantly, the mucosal vaccination strategy with MPL also induced systemic humoral and cell-mediated immune responses, including induction of CTL, and (most importantly) protection against lethal challenge (Baldridge et al., 2000b; Persing et al., 2002). The ability of MPL to mediate actively mucosal and systemic immunity may be important for the development of protective immunity against a wide range of infectious diseases where the infectious process is initiated at mucosal sites.

The synthetic AGP adjuvant RC-529 has demonstrated comparable adjuvant activity to MPL in preclinical studies. When RC-529 is formulated with hepatitis B surface antigen (HBsAg) significant improvement in both antibody titers and CTL responses were observed (Evans et al., 2003). Similar to the effects seen with MLA, the incorporation of RC-529 into the hepatitis vaccine significantly shifted the response from one dominated by antibodies of the IgG1 isotype to a response that also contained high levels of complement-fixing IgG2a antibodies. As a result of its desirable safety profile and effective adjuvant activity, RC-529 (now called Ribi.529) has emerged as one of Corixa's lead synthetic vaccine adjuvants for clinical evaluation.

■ Clinical experience with TLR4 agonists as adjuvants

MPL® adjuvant has been studied extensively in human clinical trials for a variety of indications spanning the fields of infectious disease, cancer immunotherapy, and allergy immunotherapy. Within the context of these studies, more than 273,000 doses been administered to human subjects, and acceptable safety and efficacy profiles have been established (Table 6.1). Several clinical trials demonstrated that the inclusion of MPL® adjuvant with a hepatitis B vaccine resulted in higher geometric mean antibody titers, enhanced cell-mediated immunity, and increased rates of seroprotection compared to the alum-adsorbed hepatitis B vaccine alone (Figure 6.3) (Thoelen et al., 1998, 2001). Interestingly, a majority of subjects in these studies attained protective levels after a single dose, suggesting that suboptimal vaccination schedules, as might occur in developing countries, would enjoy increased efficacy by the addition of MPL.

A candidate herpes vaccine formulated with MPL® adjuvant was demonstrated to provide significant protection against genital herpes in women who were seronegative for both herpes simplex virus (HSV)-1 and HSV-2 prior to vaccination (Stanberry et al., 2002). The vaccine elicited both binding and neutralizing antibodies against HSV, as well as cellular responses as indicated by lymphoproliferation and IFN-γ secretion. Protection was documented in women who were previously seronegative for HSV, in which a substantial attenuation of HSV-2 seroconversion was observed in previously seronegative subjects. These results are highly significant, since other nearly identical vaccines which lacked TLR4 agonist activity failed to prevent genital infection with HSV (Corey et al., 1999).

A dose-dependent effect of MPL® adjuvant on antigen-specific cellular immune responses was reported in response to a candidate *Streptococcous pneumonia* vaccine in healthy toddlers (Vernacchio et al., 2002). The results demonstrate that MPL® adjuvant stimulated

Table 6.1 Summary of clinical trials with MPL® adjuvant and Ribi.529

Clinical indication	Adjuvant system	Trial highlights and/or immune parameters	Reference
Hepatitis B	MPL + alum (SBAS-4)	Enhanced seroconversion; higher GMT; enhanced cell-mediated immunity	Thoelen et al. (2001, 1998); Desombere et al. (2002); Jacques et al. (2002)
Malaria	MPL +QS21 oil-in-water emulsion (SBAS-2)	Resistance to parasitemia	Alonso et al. (2004); Stoute et al. (1997)
Herpes type 2	MPL + alum (SBAS-4)	Enhanced binding and neutralizing antibody; enhanced cell proliferation; enhanced IFNγ	Stanberry et al. (2002)
Streptococcus pneumoniae	MPL ± alum	Neonate patient population; enhanced cell proliferation; enhanced IFNγ	Vernacchio et al. (2002)
Melanoma	MPL +CWS (Detox)	Extended survival	Sosman et al. (2002)
Grass pollen allergy	MPL + tyrosine	Reduced nasal and ocular symptoms; reduced skin-prick sensitivity	Drachenberg et al. (2001); Mothes et al. (2003)
Hepatitis B	Ribi.529	Enhanced seroconversion; higher GMT. Synthetic adjuvant	Dupont, (2002)

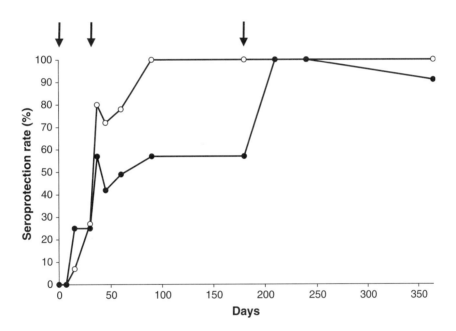

Figure 6.3 Seroprotection rates in groups receiving three doses of SBAS4-HBV (open circles) or HBV (filled circles) vaccines at the time points indicated by the arrows. The HBV vaccine contains 20 μg rHBsAg adsorbed to 0.5 mg alum. The SBAS4-HBV vaccine contains identical components plus MPL® adjuvant. All values are the means of 9–15 subjects at each time point. (Reprinted from Thoelen et al. (1998). Safety and immunogenicity of a hepatitis B vaccine formulated with a novel adjuvant system. *Vaccine* 16, 708–714. Copyright 1998, with permission from Elsevier.)

Th1 responses to the carrier protein in a dose-dependent fashion, and supported the idea that MPL® adjuvant is sufficiently safe for use in children. More importantly, they suggest that MPL adjuvant may be useful for enhancing immune responses to polysaccharide antigens, which are already quite intrinsically antigenic. This data confirms earlier preclinical studies in mice, in which it was shown that MPL adjuvant, even when administered separately from the antigen itself, may be able to boost effective immune responses (Baker et al., 1988; Baker, 1990).

Clinical data accumulated to date indicate that the AGPs, when used as vaccine adjuvants, appear to be safe and effective. The synthetic TLR4 agonist Ribi.529 has been tested in 138 adults as part of a phase III clinical study to develop a more efficacious and faster acting hepatitis B vaccine (Table 6.1). The HBsAg vaccine formulated with Ribi.529 mediated four-fold higher geometric mean antibody titers and increased levels of seroprotection compared to the hepatitis B vaccine adsorbed to alum alone (Dupont, 2002). These data show that like MPL® adjuvant, synthetic TLR4 agonists can be used safely and successfully as vaccine adjuvants in humans. Moreover, they show that the AGPs, as TLR4 agonists, though chemically and biologically distinct from natural products or their derivatives, are able to produce human vaccine responses that are similar to those of MPL.

Recent results of an MPL-containing vaccine for prevention of malaria were reported for a study of over 2000 children (ages 1–4 years) from malaria-endemic areas of Mozambique (Alonso et al., 2004). The study comprised two cohorts of children living in two separate areas which underwent different follow-up protocols. Participants were randomly allocated three doses of either candidate malaria vaccine or control vaccines. The primary endpoint, determined in cohort 1 ($n = 1605$), was time to first clinical episode of *P. falciparum* malaria over a 6-month surveillance period. Efficacy for prevention of new infections was determined in cohort 2 ($n = 417$). Analysis was per protocol. Vaccine efficacy for prevention of first clinical episodes was 29.9%. At the end of the 6-month observation period, prevalence of *P. falciparum* infection was 37% lower in the vaccine group compared with the control group (11.9% vs. 18.9%; $p = 0.0003$). Vaccine efficacy for severe malaria, the most life-threatening form of the disease, was 57.7%. In cohort 2, vaccine efficacy for extending time to first infection was 45.0%. Arguably, one

explanation for the difference in outcome of this vaccine trial compared to previous failures was the inclusion of a TLR4 agonist.

■ Safety of TLR agonists as vaccine adjuvants

A significant concern regarding the use of any TLR agonist to enhance immunological performance revolves around the safety of such an approach. To at least some extent, the safety of TLR agonists probably depends on the cell type that expresses a particular TLR target. Most of these recent safety concerns have centered on the use of agonists of TLR9 (Viglianti et al., 2003; Sacher et al., 2002). Serial administration of CpG oligonucleotides to animal models has shown that TLR9 activation triggers autoimmune disease, presumably since TLR9 is expressed on plasmacytoid dendritic cells which play a critical role in controlling immunological peripheral tolerance. Autoimmune inflammatory infiltrates can also be induced in animal models by LPS. Breaking of peripheral tolerance may someday become an important approach to immunotherapy of cancer and chronic viral infections, but in otherwise healthy individuals the risk/benefit ratio may be unacceptably high. A presumably low but indefinite risk of developing a serious autoimmune disease, such as systemic lupus erythematosis, must not outweigh the potential benefits of protection against uncertain or unpredictable pathogen exposure.

Notwithstanding the potential risks of modulating innate immune responses, there is still considerable interest in applying TLR agonists for the treatment and prevention of human disease, and substantial human safety data already exist in this regard. Imiquimod, a topically administered TLR7 agonist, has been evaluated in over 4000 patients in clinical trials of patients with skin diseases such as external genital warts, skin cancer, and actinic keratoses. Since only a tiny percentage of the drug is taken up systemically in these studies, the risk of triggering systemic symptoms or autoimmune disease appears to be minimal.

Despite the concerns raised by experiments performed in inbred mouse strains, it is quite possible that TLR agonists of any type will be reasonably well tolerated, at least on a short-term basis. After all, the human immune system has learned over time to become tolerant to a variety of acute and chronic infectious insults, some of which establish themselves on a life-long basis. Nonetheless, in light of the safety concerns raised by the use of TLR agonists as vaccine adjuvants, there is no reasonable substitute for human clinical data.

■ Regulatory approval of the first TLR agonist as a vaccine adjuvant

Corixa's MPL® is the most widely tested of any TLR agonist as a vaccine adjuvant in studies of human subjects. To date, more than 273,000 doses of MPL® adjuvant containing vaccines have been administered by injection. The extensive safety record of MPL® adjuvant in humans, combined with its demonstrated efficacy, led to regulatory approval for human use in February 2005. Now that this important milestone has been achieved, it is expected that other regulatory filings will follow in the US and elsewhere. Thus, one of the critical concerns about the use of TLR agonists as vaccine adjuvants has been significantly addressed for the TLR4 agonists, paving the way for the use of these agonists for treatment and prophylaxis of infectious diseases.

■ Mechanism(s) of action of TLR4 agonists

MPL® adjuvant and Ribi.529 adjuvant act as TLR4 agonists to initiate both innate and adaptive immune responses. After contact with cells expressing the TLR4/MD2 receptor complex, both agonists stimulate production of soluble mediators, including cytokines and chemokines. By virtue of secretion of these effector molecules, recruitment and activation of immune effector cells occurs, which enhances cellular interactions and promotes adaptive immunity (antibodies and antigen-specific T cells). Human whole blood or PBMC cultures stimulated with MPL® adjuvant and AGPs produce a number of chemokines, including IL-8 and MIP-1β (Stover et al., 2004; Evans et al., 2003). Early production of these chemokines accelerates the immune response to coadministered antigens through the recruitment of neutrophils, macrophages, dendritic cells, and natural killer (NK) cells (Luster, 2002). Additionally, macrophages exposed to MPL® adjuvant elaborate TNF-α and IL-1β, both of which induce activation and maturation of dendritic cells (Ulrich and Myers, 1995; Belardelli and Ferrantini, 2002). In turn, dendritic cells exposed to MPL produce IL-12, IFN-γ, and IL-5, cytokines that direct development of Th1 and Th2 adaptive responses (Ismaili et al., 2002). Taken together, these results support findings from vaccine studies which indicate that MPL stimulates both Th1 and Th2 responses.

The local production of these chemokines and cytokines leads to enhanced recruitment and cross-communication of immune cells that are important in the development of acquired immunity to coadministered vaccine antigens. From microarray data generated from primary human macrophages, we know that in addition to cytokines, a multitude of intracellular and cell surface markers are upregulated following TLR4 stimulation by MPL and AGPs (Stover et al., 2004). Evaluation of these cell surface markers provides further evidence of immune system activation achieved directly and/or indirectly after TLR4 stimulation. For example, in a series of experiments described previously (Evans et al., 2003), the cell surface expression of various activation and adhesion markers was measured following stimulation of human PBMC with the AGP RC-527 in vitro (Table 6.2). PBMC were stimulated with RC-527, RC-526 (Figure 6.2), or E. coli LPS for 4 hours or 24 hours and immediately stained with fluorochrome conjugated antibodies to various lineage and

Table 6.2 Lineage-specific activation following a 24-hour treatment of peripheral blood mononuclear cells with AGPs or LPS[a]

Group	Marker	Upregulation of cell surface markers (%)[b]			
		None	LPS	RC-527	RC-526
T cells	CD69	3	8	10	2
B cells	CD69	15	49	66	22
	CD25	5	35	34	9
	CD86	17	40	51	22
	CD95	14	71	73	15
Mono/macs	CD69	5	18	22	2
	CD25	1	90	70	1
	CD80	1	18	36	1
NK cells	CD69	4	42	50	4
NK T cells	CD69	2	11	16	2

[a]PBMC were isolated from normal human donors and treated *in vitro* with 10 ng/ml LPS, 10 µg/ml RC-527 (TLR4 agonist), or 10 µg/ml RC-526 (structurally related negative control) for 24 hours. Cells were harvested and immediately stained for lineage and activation markers. Data were acquired using a Becton Dickinson FACSCalibur flow cytometer.
[b]Percentage of cells positive within each lineage for the indicated marker 24 hours following AGP treatment.

activation markers. RC-526 was included as an AGP control because it is structurally identical to RC-527 with the exception of a secondary acyl chain length modification that renders this molecule inactive as a TLR4 agonist (Stover et al., 2004). The lineage markers used in these studies were CD3 for T cells, CD19 for B Cells, CD56 for NK cells, CD56 and CD3 for NK-T cells, and CD14 for monocytes and macrophages. Significant increases in the cell surface expression of the early activation marker CD69 was detected within 4 hours in all lineages tested. By 24 hours, additional cell surface receptors and adhesion markers could easily be detected on CD14+ monocytes and CD19+ B cells activated with RC-527 or LPS. In addition to CD69, these markers included CD25 (low-affinity IL2Rα) and CD80 (B7.1) on both lineages and CD86 (B7.2) and CD95 (FAS, Apo-1) on B cells (Table 6.2 and Figure 6.4). Increased cell surface expression of the B7 molecules on antigen-presenting cells and B cells demonstrates a mechanism of action whereby AGPs can function as adjuvants by providing the costimulatory signals required

for the development of antigen-specific immune responses. In conjunction with these costimulatory responses, increased expression of CD25 (IL2Rα) on monocytes and CD95 (Fas) on B cells provides a regulatory control by which polyclonal T cell and B cell activation is kept in check, thus preventing the stimulation and expansion of autoreactive T and B cells. The increased expression of these cell surface markers demonstrates the profound effects TLR4 agonists have on a variety of relevant hematopietic lineages, resulting in the direct and/or indirect activation of cells involved in both innate (monocytes, macrophages, NK cells) and adaptive (B cells and T cells) immune responses. Taken together, the demonstration that MPL and AGPs can stimulate cellular activation, cytokine production, and enhanced expression of costimulatory molecules provides a clearer picture of how TLR4 agonists work as vaccine adjuvants. The data also highlight potential opportunities to use these molecules as standalone immunomodulators for promoting innate resistance against an array of infectious challenges.

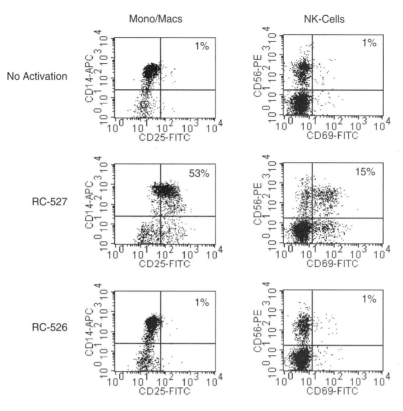

Figure 6.4 AGP and LPS treatment of primary human PBMC causes an increase in the cell surface expression of CD25 on CD14+ monocytes and CD69 on CD56+ NK cells. PBMC were isolated from normal donors and activated *in vitro* with 10 ng/ml LPS, 10 μg/ml RC-527, or 10 μg/ml RC-526. Cells were harvested at 24 hours following treatment, immediately stained with fluorochrome conjugated monoclonal antibodies for the indicated markers and analyzed by flow cytometry. The number in each upper right quadrant indicates the percentage of cells in that quadrant (dual positive cells).

TLR4 agonists as nonspecific immunomodulators

For several years it has been known that administration of sublethal quantities of purified LPS confers protection against bacterial or viral challenge in various animal models, presumably via stimulation of innate immune effector molecules such as defensins and interferons (Berger, 1967; Neter, 1969). Similarly, by using TLR4 agonists, most recently the AGPs, we have demonstrated protection against infectious challenge by a variety of bacterial, viral, and eukaryotic pathogens in murine models of infectious challenge (Table 6.3). These studies highlight an opportunity for using TLR4 agonists against an

increasing variety of clinically relevant pathogens. Treatment of infections caused by pathogens resistant to current antimicrobial agents represents an increasing challenge for clinicians. Unlike the targets of antibiotics, the sheer multiplicity of microbial targets of the innate immune response make it extremely unlikely that microbes will simultaneously amass the requisite mutations that would be require for resistance. Ultimately, some combination of antimicrobials and innate immune stimulation might be necessary to achieve maximal therapeutic effect.

To demonstrate the efficacy of prophylactic antiinfective monotherapy with an AGP we developed a preclinical model for respiratory

Table 6.3 MPL or AGP pretreatment increases resistance to infectious challenge

Type of pathogen	Specific pathogen	Reference
Gram-negative bacteria	Escherichia coli	Rudbach (1994)
	Salmonella enteriditis	Ulrich (1988)
	Klebsiella pneumoniae	Madonna (1988)
	Non-typeable Haemophilus influenzae	U[a]
Gram-positive bacteria	Listeria monocytogenes	Ulrich (1988)
	Staphylococcus aureus	Rudbach (1994)
Viruses	Influenza A	Persing et al. (2002)
	Respiratory syncytial virus (RSV)	Baldridge et al. (2004)
Parasites	Toxoplasma gondii	Madonna (1988)
	Leishmania major	Persing et al. (2002)

[a]U = unpublished observation.

syncytial virus (RSV), a significant human pathogen. RSV is a negative strand RNA virus that causes severe pathology in the lungs of infants, immunocompromised patients (such as transplant patients), and the elderly (Collins, 2001). In children less than 1 year of age, RSV is the leading cause of hospitalizations for bronchiolitis (Collins, 2001). Neonatal infections with RSV that result in hospitalization have been linked to long-term pulmonary dysfunction such as asthma and wheezing (Culley et al., 2002). RSV is also considered a viral trigger of acute exacerbations of asthma and of chronic obstructive pulmonary disease (COPD), the fourth leading cause of death worldwide (Rohde et al., 2003). We recently evaluated the effect of treatment with an AGP, RC-527, on the replication of RSV in a murine model of pulmonary infection (Baldridge et al., 2004). Our data indicated that RC-527 is effective at inhibiting RSV replication when compared to a vehicle control. Similar numbers of copies of RSV were evident in the lungs of all mice within 2 hours postchallenge but within 24 hours a significant difference in viral load was evident, and this difference was greater still at a 96-hour timepoint. The failure of RC-527 to

exhibit antiviral activity against RSV in a TLR4-defective strain of mice provides direct evidence for the requirement of TLR4 signaling to induce protection with this compound (data not shown).

Rapid-acting vaccines

Combining the mucosal adjuvant activity of AGPs with their ability to induce nonspecific resistance could conceivably result in a vaccine capable of providing continuous protection within a few hours of the first dose. Cluff et al. (2004) showed that intranasal administration of an AGP-containing influenza virus vaccine protected mice against lethal infectious challenge two days after the first dose. Weekly administration of two additional doses maintained protection throughout the dosing regimen. Moreover, mucosal and systemic immune responses (IgA and IgG) were observed at the completion of the series which provided durable protection at one month after the last dose. Since the immunoprophylactic effect of the AGP would presumably be gone by 7 days after the last dose, the long-term protection was attributed to the adaptive immune response. Thus, by harnessing features of both innate and adaptive immunity it may be possible to shorten dramatically the time to protection. This feature may be useful in settings of epidemic outbreaks of influenza and other viral respiratory infections in which rapid protection is desirable.

Concluding remarks

After an incubation period of nearly two decades, TLR agonists have finally "come of age" as vaccine adjuvants and show promise as standalone immunomodulators in the treatment of infectious and atopic diseases. Of the TLR agonists currently under development as vaccine adjuvants, MPL® adjuvant has been the first to attain regulatory approval in a vaccine intended for human use. Resting substantially on its strong safety record, MPL® adjuvant is slated for inclusion in a variety of prophylactic and therapeutic vaccines. The synthetic TLR4 agonists, the AGPs, also appear to have potent adjuvant activity and are currently being evaluated in human vaccine trials.

In general, vaccine adjuvants should adhere to the Hippocratic standard to "First do no harm." In this respect MPL® adjuvant is proving to be a highly effective vaccine adjuvant that appears to be sufficiently safe to use in adults and children. In contrast to alum, which tends to drive primarily Th2-type immune responses, MPL® adjuvant drives a more balanced Th1/Th2 response that is essential for the generation of effective immunity to many pathogens. The Th2-inducing properties of alum that some have suggested may contribute to rising atopic disease rates and other potential side effects (Malakoff, 2000). Indeed, the Th1-biasing characteristic of MPL® adjuvant is currently being exploited in allergy vaccines (Pollinex Quattro®) to drive the production of blocking IgG antibodies to allergens resulting in the alleviation of allergy symptoms (Drachenberg et al., 2001; Mothes et al., 2003).

Moving forward, the potential advantages conferred by TLR agonists of improved antibody titers and cell-mediated immune responses, increased duration of protective efficacy, and reversal of atopic responses will be evaluated against a standard of safety that has already been set by alum as a vaccine adjuvant. Of concern is the potential for certain TLR agonists to trigger autoimmune disease (Viglianti et al., 2003) or inflammatory responses (Sacher et al., 2002) which could potentially limit their use in humans; this may be especially of concern when TLR agonists are used in combination. Fortunately, the human experience with TLR4 agonists as vaccine adjuvants is growing, and the experience with MPL® adjuvant to date has been highly promising.

We expect to see an increase in the pharmacologic use of TLR agonists, particularly TLR4 agonists, as vaccine adjuvants in the next few years as next-generation vaccines gain regulatory approval and become available. One population that stands to benefit dramatically is the elderly, for whom current vaccines result in high nonresponder rates and poor vaccine efficacy overall. Addition of TLR agonists may overcome some of the hindrances to achieving protective immunity in this population; TLR agonists, in particular MPL® adjuvant, can induce robust immune responses in aged mice whose immune systems have undergone significant functional decline (Mbawuike et al., 1996). In addition, by combining TLR agonists with sustained release technologies currently used for some drugs, we may be able to develop single-dose vaccines. This would be a boon to the developing and industrialized worlds alike, especially in the area of pediatric immunization. In the latter category, the trend toward combining vaccines into a single multidose regimen will likely continue; as antigen concentrations for each target organism fall, adjuvants may be required to compensate for inherently lower immunogenicity of combined products.

We also anticipate novel uses of TLR agonist-containing vaccines, in which the innate and adaptive immune responses are exploited sequentially to develop vaccines that are continuously active from the first few hours of administration (vs. weeks to months for current vaccines). Since activation of innate immune responses by intranasal MPL® adjuvant can provide protection against airway challenge by influenza virus within hours of administration, a period of reduced susceptibility could be maintained if intranasal booster doses of a vaccine containing antigen plus TLR4 agonist are administered weekly (Cluff et al., 2004). The nonspecific protective effect could theoretically be maintained until durable protection develops via an antigen-specific mucosal immune response against the protein component of the vaccine.

Finally, it is likely that TLR agonists and antagonists will enter clinical trials in the next few years as standalone immunomodulators. Intranasal administration of TLR4 agonists may protect the airways against natural infection by viruses for which there are no effective vaccines or antiviral drugs; the RSV example provided above is a case in point. The transient protection afforded by weekly or biweekly doses of an immunomodulatory nasal spray might prove beneficial for emerging viral infections, such as SARS and avian influenza. The broad protective ability of TLR4 agonists relative to viral and bacterial challenges make them especially well-suited for complex, multifactorial diseases such as asthma and COPD, in which exacerbations are most often triggered by upper respiratory viral infection. Indeed, within the immunological epiphany created by the discovery of the TLRs and their respective ligands, a new generation of designer adjuvants, therapeutic and prophylactic vaccines, and immunomodulatory therapies may be close at hand.

References

Akira, S. (2003). *Curr. Opin. Immunol.* 15, 5–11.

Alonso, P.L., Sacarlal, J., Aponte, J.J., Leach, A., Macete, E., Milman, J., Mandomando, I., Spiessens, B., Guinovart, C., Espasa, M., Bassat, Q., Aide, P., Ofori-Anyinam, O., Navia, M.M., Corachan, S., Ceuppens, M., Dubois, M.C., Demoitie, M.A., Dubovsky, F., Menendez, C., Tornieporth, N., Ballou, W.R., Thompson, R., and Cohen, J. (2004). *Lancet* 364, 1411–1420.

Ayabe, T., Satchell, D.P., Wilson, C.L., Parks, W.C., Selsted, M.E., and Ouellette, A.J. (2000). *Nature Immunol.* 1, 113–118.

Baker, P.J. (1990). *Infect. Immun.* 58, 3465–3468.

Baker, P.J., Hiernaux, J.R., Fauntleroy, M.B., Stashak, P.W., Prescott, B., Cantrell, J.L., and Rudbach, J.A. (1988). *Infect. Immun.* 56, 3064–3066.

Baldridge, J.R., Yorgensen, Y., Ward, J.R., and Ulrich, J.T. (2000a). *Vaccine* 18, 2416–2425.

Baldridge, J.R., Yorgensen, Y., Ward, J.R., and Ulrich, J.T. (2000b). *Vaccine* 18, 2416–2425.

Baldridge, J.R., Cluff, C.W., Evans, J.T., Lacy, M.J., Stephens, J.R., Brookshire, V.G., Wang, R., Ward, J.R., Yorgensen, Y.M., Persing, D.H., and Johnson, D.A. (2002). *J. Endotoxin Res.* 8, 453–458.

Baldridge, J.R., McGowan, P., Evans, J., Cluff, C., Mossman, S., Johnson, D., and Persing, D.H. (2004). *Expert Opin. Biol. Ther.* 4, 1129–1138.

Belardelli, F. and Ferrantini, M. (2002). *Trends Immunol.* 23, 201–208.

Berger, F.M. (1967). *Adv. Pharmacol.* 5, 19–46.

Claeys, S., de Belder, T., Holtappels, G., Gevaert, P., Verhasselt, B., van Cauwenberge, P., and Bachert, C. (2003). *Allergy* 58, 748–753.

Cluff, C.W., Baldridge, J.R., Stöver, A.G., Evans, J.T., Johnson, D.A., Lacy, M.J., Clawson, V.G., Yorgensen, V.M., Johnson, C.L., Livesay, M.T., Hershberg, R.M., and Persing, D.H. (2004). In *2nd Annual ASM Conference on Biodefense*, Washington, DC, in press.

Cluff, C.W., Baldridge, J.R., Stöver, A.G., Evans, J.T., Johnson, D.A., Lacy, M.J., Clawson, V.G., Yorgensen, V.M., Johnson, C.L., Livesay, M.T., Hershberg, R.M., and Persing, D.H. (2005). *Infect Immunity*, in press.

Collins, P.C. and Murphy, B.R. (2001). *Fields Virology*, Lippincott, Williams and Wilkins, Philadelphia.

Corey, L., Langenberg, A.G., Ashley, R., Sekulovich, R.E., Izu, A.E., Douglas, J.M., Jr., Handsfield, H.H., Warren, T., Marr, L., Tyring, S., DiCarlo, R., Adimora, A.A., Leone, P., Dekker, C.L., Burke, R.L., Leong, W.P. and Straus, S.E. (1999). *JAMA* 282, 331–340.

Culley, F.J., Pollott, J., and Openshaw, P.J. (2002). *J. Exp. Med.* 196, 1381–1386.

Da Silva, C.J., Soldau, K., Christen, U., Tobias, P.S., and Ulevitch, R. . (2001). *J. Biol. Chem.* 276, 21129–21135.

De Becker, G., Moulin, V., Pajak, B., Bruck, C., Francotte, M., Thiriart, C., Urbain, J., and Moser, M. (2000). *Int. Immunol.* 12, 807–815.

Desombere, I., Van der Wielen, M., Van Damme, P., Stoffel, M., De Clercq, N., Goilav, C., and Leroux-Roels, G. (2002). *Vaccine* 20, 2597–2602.

Doherty, T.M., Olsen, A.W., van Pinxteren, L., and Andersen, P. (2002). *Infect. Immun.* 70, 3111–3121.

Drachenberg, K.J., Wheeler, A.W., Stuebner, P., and Horak, F. (2001). *Allergy* 56, 498–505.

Dupont, J.-C.A., Sigelchifer, M., Von Eschen, E.B., Timmermans, I., and Wagener, A. (2002). In *ICAAC*, Vol. G-144.

Evans, J.T., Cluff, C.W., Johnson, D.A., Lacy, M.J., Persing, D.H., and Baldridge, J.R. (2003). *Expert Rev. Vaccines* 2, 219–229.

Hall, S.S. (1997). *A Commotion in the Blood*, Henry Holt, New York.

Hoebe, K., Janssen, E., and Beutler, B. (2004). *Nature Immunol.* 5, 971–974.

Imler, J.L. and Hoffmann, J.A. (2000). *Rev. Immunogenet.* 2, 294–304.

Ismaili, J., Rennesson, J., Aksoy, E., Vekemans, J., Vincart, B., Amraoui, Z., Van Laethem, F., Goldman, M., and Dubois, P.M. (2002). *J. Immunol.* 168, 926–932.

Jacques, P., Moens, G., Desombere, I., Dewijngaert, J., Leroux-Roels, G., Wettendorff, M., and Thoelen, S. (2002). *Vaccine* 20, 3644–3649.

Johnson, A.G., Gaines, S., and Landy, M. (1956). *J. Exp. Med.* 103, 225–246.

Johnson, D.A., Sowell, C.G., Johnson, C.L., Livesay, M.T., Keegan, D.S., Rhodes, M.J., Ulrich, J.T., Ward, J.R., Cantrell, J.L., and Brookshire, V.G. (1999). *Bioorg. Med. Chem. Lett.* 9, 2273–2278.

Kaisho, T. and Akira, S. (2002). *Biochim. Biophys. Acta* 1589, 1–13.

Kawai, T., Adachi, O., Ogawa, T., Takeda, K,. and Akira, S. (1999). *Immunity* 11, 115–122.

Luster, A.D. (2002). *Curr. Opin. Immunol.* 14, 129–135.

Madonna, G.L., Funckes, D.C., and Ribi, E.E. (1988). *Adv. Biosci.* 68, 351–356.

Malakoff, D. (2000). *Science* 288, 1323–1324.

Martin, M., Michalek, S.M., and Katz, J. (2003). *Infect. Immun.* 71, 2498–2507.

Mbawuike, I.N., Acuna, C., Caballero, D., Pham-Nguyen, K., Gilbert, B., Petribon, P., and Harmon, M. (1996). *Cell Immunol.* 173, 64–78.

Mothes, N., Heinzkill, M., Drachenberg, K.J., Sperr, W.R., Krauth, M.T., Majlesi, Y., Semper, H., Valent, P., Niederberger, V., Kraft, D., and Valenta, R. (2003). *Clin. Exp. Allergy* 33, 1198–1208.

Munoz, J. (1964). In Dixon, F.J. and Kunkel, H.G. (Eds) *Advances in Immunology.* Academic Press, New York, pp. 397–440.

Myers, K., Truchot, A.T., Ward, J., Hudson, Y., and Ulrich, J.T. (1990). In Nowotny, A., Spitzer, J.J., and Ziegler, E.J. (Eds) *Cellular and Molecular Aspects of Endotoxic Reactions.* Elsevier, Amsterdam, pp. 145–156.

Nauts, H.C., Swift, W.E., and Corley, B.L. (1946). *Cancer Res.* 6, 205–216.

Neter, E. (1969). *Curr. Top. Microbiol. Immunol.* 47, 82–124.

Persing, D.H., Coler, R.N., Lacy, M.J., Johnson, D.A., Baldridge, J.R., Hershberg, R.M., and Reed, S.G. (2002). *Trends Microbiol.* 10, S32–S37.

Poltorak, A., He, X., Smirnova, I., Liu, M.Y., Van Huffel, C., Du, X., Birdwell, D., Alejos, E., Silva, M., Galanos, C., Freudenberg, M., Ricciardi-Castagnoli, P., Layton, B., and Beutler, B. (1998). *Science* 282, 2085–2088.

Poltorak, A., Ricciardi-Castagnoli, P., Citterio, S., and Beutler, B. (2000). *Proc. Natl. Acad. Sci. USA* 97, 2163–2167.

Ribi, E.S., Mizuno, Y., Nowotny, A., Von Eschen, K.B., Cantrell, J.L. et al. (1979). *Cancer Immunol. Immunother.* 7, 43–58.

Rohde, G., Wiethege, A., Borg, I., Kauth, M., Bauer, T.T., Gillissen, A., Bufe, A., and Schultze-Werninghaus, G. (2003). *Thorax* 58, 37–42.

Rudbach, J.M., Rechtman, D.J., and Ulrich, J.T. (1994). In *Bacterial Endotoxins: Basic Science to Anti-Sepsis Strategies.* Wiley-Liss, New York, pp. 107–124.

Sacher, T., Knolle, P., Nichterlein, T., Arnold, B., Hammerling, G. J., and Limmer, A. (2002). *Eur. J. Immunol.* 32, 3628–3637.

Sosman, J.A., Unger, J.M., Liu, P.Y., Flaherty, L.E., Park, M.S., Kempf, R.A., Thompson, J.A., Terasaki, P.I., and Sondak, V.K. (2002). *J. Clin. Oncol.* 20, 2067–2075.

Stanberry, L.R., Spruance, S.L., Cunningham, A.L., Bernstein, D.I., Mindel, A., Sacks, S., Tyring, S., Aoki, F.Y., Slaoui, M., Denis, M., Vandepapeliere, P., and Dubin, G. (2002). *N. Engl. J. Med.* 347, 1652–1661.

Stoute, J.A., Slaoui, M., Heppner, D.G., Momin, P., Kester, K.E., Desmons, P., Wellde, B.T., Garcon, N., Krzych, U., and Marchand, M. (1997). *N. Engl. J. Med.* 336, 86–91.

Stover, A.G., Da Silva Correia, J., Evans, J.T., Cluff, C.W., Elliott, M.W., Jeffery, E.W., Johnson, D.A., Lacy, M.J., Baldridge, J.R., Probst, P., Ulevitch, R.J., Persing, D.H., and Hershberg, R.M. (2004). *J. Biol. Chem.* 279, 4440–4449.

Takeda, K. and Akira, S. (2004). *Semin. Immunol.* 16, 3–9.

Thoelen, S., Van Damme, P., Mathei, C., Leroux-Roels, G., Desombere, I., Safary, A., Vandepapeliere, P., Slaoui, M., and Meheus, A. (1998). *Vaccine* 16, 708–714.

Thoelen, S., De Clercq, N., and Tornieporth, N. (2001). *Vaccine* 19, 2400–2403.

Toshchakov, V., Jones, B.W., Perera, P.Y., Thomas, K., Cody, M.J., Zhang, S., Williams, B.R., Major, J., Hamilton, T.A., Fenton, M.J., and Vogel, S.N. (2002). *Nature Immunol.* 3, 392–398.

Ulevitch, R.J. (1999). *Nature Med.* 5, 144–145.

Ulrich, J.M. and Lange, W. (1988). *Adv. Biosci.* 68, 167–178.

Ulrich, J.T. and Myers, K.R. (1995). *Pharm. Biotechnol.* 6, 495–524.

VanCott, T.C., Kaminski, R.W., Mascola, J.R., Kalyanaraman, V.S., Wassef, N.M., Alving, C.R., Ulrich, J.T., Lowell, G.H., and Birx, D.L. (1998). *J. Immunol.* 160, 2000–2012.

Vernacchio, L., Bernstein, H., Pelton, S., Allen, C., MacDonald, K., Dunn, J., Duncan, D.D., Tsao, G., LaPosta, V., Eldridge, J., Laussucq, S., Ambrosino, D.M., and Molrine, D.C. (2002). *Vaccine* 20, 3658–3667.

Viglianti, G.A., Lau, C.M., Hanley, T.M., Miko, B.A., Shlomchik, M.J., and Marshak-Rothstein, A. (2003). *Immunity* 19, 837–847.

Wheeler, A.W., Marshall, J.S., and Ulrich, J.T. (2001). *Int. Arch. Allergy Immunol.* 126, 135–139.

Immunomodulatory adjuvants from *Quillaja saponaria*

Charlotte Read Kensil

Antigenics, Inc., Lexington, Massachusetts

■ Introduction

Plants produce a wide variety of high molecular weight glycosides known as saponins. Saponins typically have detergent-type properties, including the formation of stable foams and hemolytic activity toward erythrocytes. Hence, the term saponin is derived from the Latin word *sapo* (meaning "soap"). A typical saponin consists of a glycoside or glycosides attached to an aglycone (a steroid or triterpene). There are a wide variety of saponins from different plant sources. These have different biological and pharmacological properties, including fungicidal, bactericidal, antiviral, and antitumor activity, depending upon the specific structure (reviewed in Hostettman and Marston, 1995).

Immunomodulation is an unusual feature, with only a few species of plants producing saponins with this activity. The South American tree *Quillaja saponaria Molina* (Rosaceae family) is the best-known producer of immunomodulatory saponins. The bark of this tree is rich in saponins, up to 10% of the weight of the bark. This tree, an evergreen growing 30–40 feet tall, is found in central Chile from the coast up to a 4800 feet elevation in the mountains (McClintock, 1984). McClintock notes the tree was named by a Chilean Jesuit priest, Juan Ignatius Molina in 1782. "Quillaja" is derived from the Chilean word *quillean*, meaning "to wash"; "saponaria" was chosen because of the soap-like properties of the extracts of this bark. The tree is also known as the soap-bark tree or Panama wood. Commercial uses for saponin extracts from this tree include uses as a surfactant in the production of photosensitized film, as a natural emulsifier for foods, and as a foaming agent for shampoo and for beverages (e.g., root beer) (San Martin and Briones, 1999). The use of *Quillaja saponaria* saponin extracts as a source of vaccine adjuvants represents another potential commercial use.

■ Structure of *Quillaja saponaria* saponins

Although differing in structure, most *Q. saponaria* saponins share similar structural features. Figure 7.1 shows the basic structure of saponins from *Q. saponaria*. These saponins are bidesmosidic, meaning two sugar chains. The chains are attached at carbons 3 and 28 of the triterpene, through acetal and ester bonds, respectively. The sugar attached to carbon 3 is glucuronic acid. Hence, *Q. saponaria* saponins are anionic at physiological pH. The primary aglycone is quillaic acid, an olean-12-en aglycone (3β,16α-dihydroxy-23-oxolean-12-en-28-oic acid, shown in Figure 7.1) (Labriola and Deulofeu, 1968). The aglycones gypsogenin, gypsogenic acid, and a hydroxylated quillaic acid isomer have also been

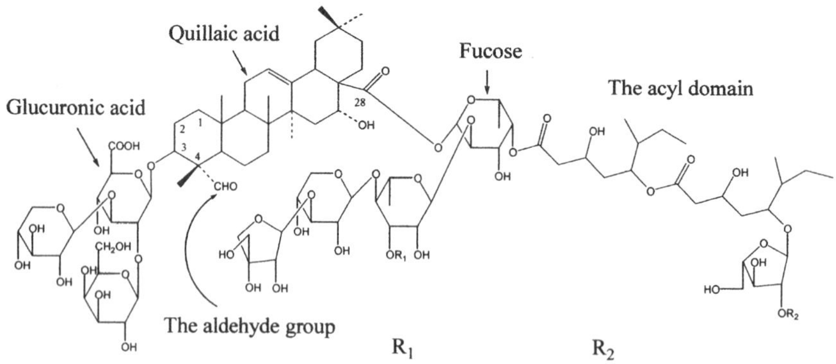

	R_1	R_2
QS-17	glucose	rhamnose
QS-18	glucose	H
QS-21	H	H

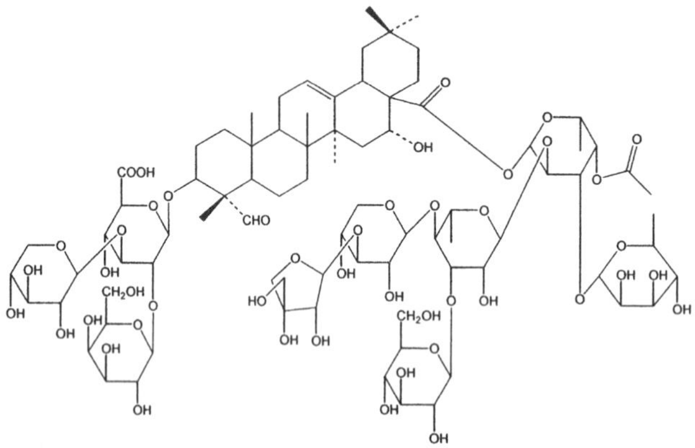

QS-7

Figure 7.1 Structures of selected major saponins from *Quillaja saponaria*, including adjuvant saponins QS-21 and QS-7.

isolated from *Q. saponaria* extracts (van Setten and van de Werken, 1996). A unique feature to quillaic acid is an aldehyde at carbon 23 of the triterpene (a relatively rare feature). Most *Q. saponaria* saponins are ester saponins (acylated on the aglycone or sugar chain). Acylation is a rare feature in saponins in general, although it is possible that the level of acylated saponins is underestimated due to inadvertent hydrolysis during isolation (Hostettman and Marston, 1995). In fact, the deacylated form of *Q. saponaria* saponins was identified first. *Q. saponaria* extracts subjected to mild alkaline hydrolysis produce two major compounds, DS-1 and DS-2, differing only by an additional glucose in DS-2 (Higuchi et al., 1987). Predominant acyl moieties derived from *Q. saponaria* extracts were determined to be 3,5-dihydroxy-6-methyl-octanoic acid, 3,5-dihydroxy-6-methyl-octanoic acid 5-*O*-α-L-arabinofuranoside, and 5-*O*-α-L-rhamnopyranosyl-(1→2)-α-L-arabinofuranoside (Higuchi and Komori, 1987). The first full structure of an acylated *Q. saponaria* saponin, designated QS-III, was published in 1988 (Higuchi et al., 1988). The site of acylation was determined to be at the 3-hydroxyl of the fucose esterified to carbon 28. The structure of another saponin, QS-21, was published in 1996 (Jacobsen et al., 1996).

■ Saponin purification and development

■ Purification

Saponins were first used in foot-and-mouth disease vaccines in cattle (Espinet, 1951). Crude preparations containing a water-extractable mixture of saponins plus plant-derived polyphenolics and tannins were utilized. The whole wood from *Q. saponaria* contains about 8% water-soluble compounds of which about 20% is saponins (San Martin and Briones, 1999). In the early 1970s these preparations were refined to exclude most tannins and polyphenolics. Dialysis, anion exchange, and size exclusion chromatography were used to produce a fraction consisting predominantly of saponin, also known as QuilA (Dalsgaard, 1974). The aqueous separation techniques used were useful to purify the total saponin fraction, but failed to separate individual saponins due to the formation of mixed micelles. High-performance liquid chromatography (HPLC) was used to demonstrate that this product still consisted of a heterogeneous array of related, but structurally unique saponins (Kensil et al., 1991; Kersten et al., 1988; van Setten et al., 1995). This demonstrated that the saponin fraction from *Q. saponaria* consisted of more than 20 different triterpene glycoside saponins. One study estimated up to 50 different saponins in *Q. saponaria* (van Setten et al., 1995).

The diverse QuilA preparation was noted to contain toxic components (Kersten et al., 1988; Kensil et al., 1991). Hence, a further effort was made to separate out individual components to learn if the adjuvant-active component(s) could be separated from toxic components. Individual saponins were separated with HPLC, enabling further characterization of purified molecules (Kensil et al., 1991). More than 20 saponins were isolated by HPLC; the four most prominent (designated QS-7, QS-17, QS-18, and QS-21) were characterized in more detail. Evaluation of toxicity and adjuvant function in mice demonstrated that toxicity and adjuvant function could be separated. QS-7, eluting early on reversed-phase (RP) HPLC, and QS-21, one of the later-eluting peaks, were both found to be adjuvant active and considerably less toxic than the starting QuilA whereas QS-18, an intermediate-eluting peak, was more toxic than QuilA, although it had considerable adjuvant activity. QS-18 is the predominant saponin in *Q. saponaria* extracts, suggesting that it may be the primary source of toxicity in QuilA. A similar observation was made in another study, although on broad fractions rather than individual HPLC peaks. Ronnberg et al. separated *Q. saponaria* saponin into three fractions, an early RP-HPLC-eluting fraction (QH-A), an intermediate fraction (QH-B), and a later-eluting fraction (QH-C) (Ronnberg et al., 1995). The QH-B fraction was toxic to mice whereas the QH-A and QH-C fractions were nontoxic (at doses up to 400 μg).

■ Adjuvants in development

Saponin adjuvants in development for human vaccines include purified saponin QS-21 (Antigenics, Inc., Lexington, MA), ISCOPREP™ 7.0.3 (CSL Limited, Melbourne, Australia), and a semisynthetic saponin, GPI-0100 (Galenica, Birmingham, AL). All are derived from *Q. saponaria* extracts. QS-21 and ISCOPREP contain native saponins in different degrees of purity. QS-21 purified by preparative RP-HPLC consists predominantly of that individual saponin (Kensil, 2000). ISCOPREP 7.0.3 consists of seven parts of QH-A and three parts of QH-C fractions (Cox et al., 1998). GPI-0100 is prepared from a deacylated *Q. saponaria* saponin preparation with dodecylamine conjugated through the glucuronic acid carboxyl as a replacement for the original lipophilic acyl chain, with the goal of improving the stability of the acyl linkage (Marciani et al., 2000).

■ Adjuvant activity of saponins

When discussing the adjuvant activity of *Q. saponaria* saponins, it is important to note that the reports in the literature may discuss unpurified extracts, partially purified extracts, or purified or near-purified individual saponins. In some instances, particularly older studies, the plant source of "saponin" is not defined. Where possible, the discussion in this review is limited to partially purified extracts (such as QuilA or ISCOPREP) or purified saponins such as QS-21. Attributes of the whole extract may not necessarily apply to individual saponins or fractions isolated from that extract.

■ Adjuvants for antibody response

Quillaja saponaria saponins have found broad utility to improve antibody responses to vaccines and have been shown to be among the more effective adjuvants. Unpurified saponin promoted strong IgG2a response and protection in mice immunized with *P. yoelii* blood stage antigen, a response that exceeded many other adjuvants (ten Hagen et al., 1993). QuilA, in simple admixture with antigen, was shown substantially to improve secondary and tertiary serum antibody responses to recombinant HIV-1 gp120 in two strains of mice, inducing earlier responses than aluminum hydroxide, muramyl dipeptide (MDP), and pluronic emulsion (Bomford et al., 1992). The QuilA-adjuvanted vaccine induced a mixed Th1/Th2 response characterized by increased levels of both IgG1 and IgG2a, whereas the vaccine adjuvanted with the known Th2 adjuvant aluminum hydroxide induced only IgG1 titers. Lymph node cells from mice immunized with antigen plus QuilA had a significantly higher interferon (IFN)-γ response to restimulation with antigen than cells from mice immunized with antigen with aluminum hydroxide or a mixture of MDP/pluronic emulsion. One characteristic observed for vaccines formulated with saponin adjuvants is early kinetics of antibody response. An early

antibody response was noted for HIV-1 gp120/QS-21 in guinea pigs when compared to gp120/alum (Powell et al., 1995). In addition, a significant antigen dose sparing effect was observed in the same study (as much as 1000 times more gp120 antigen in aluminum hydroxide was required to achieve the same antibody titers as gp120 in QS-21) (Powell et al., 1995). This was further extended to a clinical study in which a gp120 vaccine (0.3 µg) with QS-21 yielded an equivalent antibody titer to a 100-fold higher dose gp120 vaccine in aluminum hydroxide (Evans et al., 2001).

Saponin adjuvants have been shown to aid in the breadth of the immune response, i.e. in expansion of responding epitopes. In a study in outbred mice, QS-21 was shown to aid in the induction of antibody response to all epitopes included in a recombinant malaria vaccine consisting of 22 identified epitopes with high titers and high responder rates; this contrasted to three other adjuvants which induced a much more selective response pattern (Rafi-Janajreh et al., 2002).

■ Adjuvants for T cell response

Quillaja saponaria saponins are known to be useful in inducing T cell responses. The first indication came from studies with ISCOM (Immune Stimulating Complex) preparations made from the heterogeneous saponin fraction QuilA. ISCOMs prepared from QuilA, lipid, and the HIV-1 envelope protein (Takahashi et al., 1990) or ovalbumin (OVA) (Heeg et al., 1991) were shown to induce CD8+ cytotoxic T lymphocytes (CTL) in mice. The active part of the formulation was the saponin component. QuilA, used in simple admixture with recombinant human papilloma virus (HPV) 16 E7 protein in mice, induced 31% specific lysis against E7-expressing tumors (Fernando et al., 1998a). In contrast, the same protein in aluminum adjuvant or in complete Freund's adjuvant induced just 4.7% and 3.2% lysis. QuilA-containing liposomes, encapsulating various synthetic immunodominant peptides, were shown successfully to adjuvant CTL responses against targets coated with peptides from OVA, cytomegalovirus (CMV), and listeria (Lipford et al., 1994). The ability to stimulate CD8+ T cell-mediated cytotoxic responses has also been confirmed in highly purified *Q. saponaria* saponins. QS-21, used in simple admixture with antigen, has been shown to enhance murine CTL responses against a variety of antigens, including OVA (Newman et al., 1992), HIV envelope (Wu et al., 1992), CMV gB (Britt et al., 1995), and respiratory syncytial virus (RSV) fusion protein (Hancock et al., 1995). Wong et al. (1999) demonstrated that QS-21 boosted the tumor protection yielded by a T cell receptor vaccine against T cell malignancies. Depletion of the CD8+ T cell population eliminated the tumor protection. QS-21 is not the only purified saponin to induce T cell responses. The more polar QS-7 also induces T cell responses. Although higher doses are required for optimal use of QS-7, both these saponins are active as adjuvants for Th1-type responses, indicated by the ability to promote antigen-specific CTL response and IgG2a antibody (Kensil et al., 1991, 1998) as well as IFN-γ production (unpublished: Kensil, C., Anderson, C., Mielcarz, D., Varnovski, A., Scaltreto, H., Lui, G., Burke, J., Antigenics, Inc.).

The adjuvant effect for promotion of Th1 responses appears to be a characteristic of *Q. saponaria* saponins. This is in contrast to alum, which is a known Th2 adjuvant. Saponins and aluminum hydroxide have been mixed and appear to retain the ability to induce Th1 responses. Newman et al. (1992) noted that the saponin QS-21 was still effective at inducing a CTL response to OVA even when it was mixed with aluminum hydroxide. In contrast, the combination of ISCOMATRIX (ISCOM preparation without incorporated antigen) and aluminum hydroxide induced a much lower HPV 16 E7-specific CTL response than a formulation with ISCOMATRIX alone (Stewart et al., 2004). Fernando et al. (1998b) noted that QuilA/E7 given on one flank and an aluminum adjuvant, algammulin/E7, given on the other flank induced a CTL response that

was as strong as QuilA/E7 alone. However, if a Th2 response was set up weeks before by a two-dose immunization with algammulin/E7, then re-immunization with QuilA/ E7 failed to shift the response back to a Th1-type response.

■ Adjuvants for mucosal immune response

Saponins from *Q. saponaria* are effective adjuvants for mucosally administered vaccines. Crude *Q. saponaria* saponin boosted the serum neutralizing titer to orally administered rabies vaccine by 10-fold (Maharaj et al., 1986). Purified saponins also act as mucosal adjuvants. QS-21 increased both serum and mucosal antigen-specific antibody responses when used as an oral adjuvant with tetanus toxoid (Boyaka et al., 2001). Low doses (50 µg and under) were associated with a Th2 type of cytokine response whereas higher doses were associated with a Th1-type response (assessed by antibody isotype and secreted cytokines). QS-21 aided in enhancing serum and mucosal antibody and CTL responses to an intranasal HIV-1 envelope DNA vaccine (Sasaki et al., 1998) plus antibody and CTL to an envelope protein vaccine (Kensil, 2000). QS-21 was shown to be effective in enhancing serum IgG and secretory antibody responses to powdered influenza antigen, administered epidermally; these responses were similar to those invoked by cholera toxin and an LT mutant adjuvant (Chen et al., 2003).

Structure/function studies

Structure/adjuvant function studies have given some insight to certain critical structures in saponins. The aldehyde at carbon 23 is a rare structure in saponins. Insight into the role of this aldehyde has been obtained from structure/function studies on QS-21. The QS-21 triterpene aldehyde was blocked through conjugation to small molecules; the resulting derivatives were evaluated for adjuvant function (Soltysik et al., 1995). The derivatives were inactive for enhancing antibody up to the highest derivative dose tested (40 µg) and were inactive for enhancing CTL at the single derivative dose tested (10 µg, which provides an optimal response with native QS-21). QS-21 (and other *Q. saponaria* saponins) is charged at physiologic pH due to the presence of an anionic sugar, glucuronic acid, attached to triterpene carbon 3. Soltysik et al. (1995) also modified this group to convert the charge to neutral (with ethylamine) or positive (conjugation to ethylenediamine). Although the minimum threshold dose for adjuvant function was shifted to higher saponin doses by these modifications, the resulting derivatives were still adjuvant active. Hence, the anionic charge does not play a role in activity.

Additional studies evaluated the importance of acylation. QS-21 was submitted to mild alkaline hydrolysis, resulting in cleavage of the acyl chain esterified at the 4-hydroxyl of fucose, followed by RP-HPLC isolation of the resulting deacylsaponin, DS-1, and the intact fatty acyl-arabinose fragment (Kensil et al., 1996). DS-1 was evaluated as an adjuvant for OVA at DS-1 doses 10-fold higher than required for an optimal adjuvant effect; it induced low-level anti-OVA IgG serum titers, but the level of enhancement was less than 10-fold, whereas for QS-21, IgG titers were enhanced by over 1000-fold. The fatty acid was ineffective in enhancing responses. Neither fragment induced CTL responses to OVA. DS-1 was evaluated at higher doses (up to 240 µg/mouse) in a later study. It did induce enhanced IgG1 response to OVA in C57BL/6 mice but no IgG2a or CTL response (Liu et al., 2002). In the same study, DS-1 was deacylated and an alternative acyl chain (dodecylamine) was added through conjugation at the glucuronic acid carboxyl. This derivative was not active up to the highest dose evaluated (240 µg). However, it did not rule out that reacylation at a different site or with a different acyl chain might not be effective. These studies suggest that acylation is important but that the activity does not reside in the acyl domain only.

Saponin adjuvants in clinical trials

The refinement and characterization of saponins from *Q. saponaria* has enabled some of these to advance to clinical trials. These include QS-21 and ISCOPREP 7.0.3. QS-21 is the saponin adjuvant that is most advanced in clinical evaluation. Over 5000 subjects have received QS-21 in various experimental vaccines for cancer and infectious diseases as well as neurodegenerative diseases.

QS-21

Cancer vaccines

Table 7.1 summarizes a nonexhaustive list of clinical trials of QS-21 in experimental cancer vaccines. QS-21 was first evaluated in a dose ranging study with a melanoma vaccine, GM2-KLH (Livingston et al., 1994). The goal with this vaccine was to break tolerance to the tumor antigen GM2 since this ganglioside is expressed on some normal tissues. QS-21 doses ranging from 10 to 200 µg were admixed with the vaccine and administered subcutaneously. The injections were associated with local reactions (slight tenderness and transient induration and erythema), which were a median of grade 1 (NCI Common Toxicity Criteria scale) at doses of 50 µg or less, were a median of grade 2 at 100 µg, and more prominent (median grade 3) at 200 µg. For this reason, doses were limited to 100 µg or less for subsequent evaluation. No ulceration, drainage, or subcutaneous nodules were observed. Serological analysis showed enhanced IgG responses against GM2. A further study of 30 subjects receiving GM2-KLH/QS-21 (termed GMK vaccine) showed that QS-21 enhanced IgM and IgG responses (responder rate and titer) to the hapten GM2, with these responses being stronger than subjects receiving GMK in alternative adjuvant formulations (Helling et al., 1995). This antibody was shown to recognize GM2 on tumor cells and to mediate tumor killing through complement and antibody-dependent cellular cytotoxicity (Livingston et al., 1997). Follow-up

Table 7.1 QS-21 in clinical trials in cancer

Indication	Antigen	Comments
Melanoma	GM2-KLH (Livingston et al., 1994; Helling et al., 1995; Kitamura et al., 1995; Kirkwood et al., 2001a, 2001b; Knutson, 2002; Chapman et al., 2000)	QS-21 enhanced responses to hapten GM2 and to carrier KLH (Helling et al., 1995)
	GD2-lactone-KLH (Ragupathi et al., 2003)	Vaccine induced consistent antibody response, including cell binding and ADCC
	BEC-2 antiidiotypic monoclonal antibody (GD3 mimic) (McCaffery et al., 1996)	QS-21 enhanced BEC-2 antibody although not antibody to GD3
	IA7 antiidiotypic antibody mimicking GD2 (Foon et al., 1998, 2000)	Antigen dose ranging study. Forty of 47 subjects developed anti-GD2 response
	Tyrosinase peptide YMDGTMSQV in HLA-A*0201-positive patients (Lewis et al., 2000; Schaed et al., 2002)	Expansion of peptide-specific CD8+ T cells in some subjects. QS-21 induced comparable response to GM-CSF, higher than incomplete Freund's adjuvant
	Gp100 peptide 280-288 YLEPGPVTA (Slingluff et al., 2001)	Montanide or QS-21 used as adjuvants; 14% of subjects had CTL response to peptide
Breast cancer	MUC1-KLH (Adluri et al., 1999; Gilewski et al., 2000; Musselli et al, 2002)	Noted strong T cell response to carrier KLH, but minimal response to MUC1 (Musselli et al, 2002)
	GloboH-KLH (Gilewski et al., 2001)	Tumor-binding IgM antibody in 16 of 27 subjects
Prostate cancer	GloboH-KLH (Slovin et al., 1999)	Immunogenic for IgM against GloboH. Some decline of PSA in a few patients
	α-*N*-acetylgalactosamine-*O*-ser/thr-KLH (Slovin et al., 2003)	Cluster form of antigen, induced IgM and IgG
Chronic myeloid leukemia	Bcr/abl fusion peptide-derived vaccine (Cathcart et al., 2004; Pinilla-Ibarz et al., 2000; Bocchia, 2002)	Fourteen of 14 subjects developed DTH or CD4 proliferative responses; four developed peptide-specific CD8+ IFN-γ elispot responses (Cathcart et al., 2004)

studies of this vaccine include an evaluation in melanoma patients in combination with high-dose IFN-α, confirming that the combination treatment was well tolerated and that IFN-α treatment did not interfere with the immunological response to the GMK vaccine (Kirkwood et al., 2001a). GMK is also under evaluation in patients with resected stage IIB–III melanoma in comparison to high-dose IFN-α (Kirkwood et al., 2001b). The latter trial is continuing, although an early analysis suggested that the high-dose IFN-α treatment benefit was superior to that of the GM2-KLH vaccine; however, there was a trend toward improved outcome for patients with positive IgM and IgG titers to GM2 that suggested that GMK did have some clinical benefit to responding patients (Kirkwood et al., 2001b). This is the most advanced vaccine containing QS-21 in the field of cancer. Clinical studies of GMK are continuing (Knutson, 2002).

Other cancer antigens evaluated with QS-21 include the peptide Muc1 (Gilewski et al., 2000) and the synthetic antigen Globo H in breast cancer (Gilewski et al., 2001) and prostate cancer (Slovin et al., 1999) patients, Lewis[y]-KLH in ovarian cancer patients (Sabbatini et al., 2000), Fucosyl-GM1-KLH in small-cell lung cancer patients (Dickler et al., 1999), bcr-abl fusion peptides in subjects with chronic mylogenous leukemia (Cathcart et al., 2004; Bocchia, 2002), and others (Table 7.1). The aforementioned vaccines were administered with 100 μg QS-21 by subcutaneous route. Toxicities were similar in each trial with local reactions (typically grade 2) and a few mild flu-type symptoms. These vaccines were shown to be immunogenic, although these vaccines have

Table 7.2 QS-21 clinical trials in infectious disease vaccines

Indication	Antigen	Comments
HIV-1	Recombinant soluble gp120 (Evans et al., 2001)	QS-21 had antigen dose-sparing effect although associated with local reactogenicity (pain, tenderness)
	Recombinant gp120 from dualtropic strain (McCormack et al., 2000)	QS-21 used in combination with MPL with or without emulsion. QS-21 formulations induced earlier antibody responses. No CTL noted
	Lipopeptides (envelope, others) (Gahery-Segard et al., 2000, 2003)	B and T cell responses in >85% of volunteers. More sustained responses in QS-21 group
Influenza	Trivalent influenza vaccine (Bouveret Le Cam et al., 1998)	QS-21 enhanced antihemaglutinin titers for A/H3N2 strain post one injection in trial in elderly. Booster effect for two of three strains
Malaria	SPf66 peptide (Kashala et al., 2002)	Addition of QS-21 resulted in high-level antibody titers. Systemic allergic responses in a few volunteers after 3 immunizations
	NANP multiple antigen peptide (Edelman et al., 2002; Nardin et al., 2000; Kublin et al., 2002)	Addition of QS-21 resulted in high antibody titers. Contralateral allergic reactions noted after 3 immunizations
	RTS,S (Doherty et al., 1999; Bojang et al., 2001; Garcon et al., 2003; Alonso et al., 2004)	QS-21 used as part of an adjuvant formulation also including MPL and oil-in-water emulsion. Phase IIb study in children aged 1–4 showed a vaccine efficacy of 29.9% for first clinical episodes and 57.7% for severe malaria

not entered phase III testing to determine clinical utility.

T cell responses have been observed in some of these trials. Immunization with tyrosinase peptide/QS-21 (peptide dose escalation study) induced CD8+ T cell responses in 3 subjects measurable by IFN-γ Elispot (Lewis et al., 2000). In another study of the same peptide, QS-21 and GM-CSF were shown to induce higher IFN-γ Elispot responses than incomplete Freund's adjuvant (Schaed et al., 2002).

▪ HIV vaccines

Table 7.2 provides a summary of trials of QS-21 in infectious disease vaccines, including experimental HIV-1 vaccines. QS-21 was evaluated with recombinant soluble HIV-1$_{MN}$ envelope (rsgp120) in three serial studies in healthy adult volunteers (Keefer et al., 1997; Evans et al., 2001). In this study, pain and tenderness associated with QS-21 was the most common side effect. The majority of subjects receiving QS-21 vaccines reported this in the moderate or severe category after at least one of three scheduled injections. A few vasovagal symptoms were also reported. In the first two protocols, rsgp120 doses of 100 to 600 µg

were tested with doses of 50 and 100 µg QS-21 with or without aluminum hydroxide. It was noted at these doses that QS-21 did not significantly affect binding or neutralizing antibody titers. However, in the third protocol in which rsgp120 doses were dropped to 3 and 30 µg, QS-21 had a significant effect on antibody titers as well as lymphocyte proliferation and delayed type hypersensitivity, suggesting QS-21 was useful as an adjuvant for antigen-dose sparing.

▪ Malaria vaccines

QS-21 has been extensively tested in experimental malaria vaccines. It was evaluated in a phase I trial of a multiantigen peptide vaccine, PfCS-MAP1NYU, which contains an immunodominant B epitope (NANPNANPNANP) and a T cell epitope from the repeat region of the circumsporozoite protein (Nardin et al., 2000). QS-21/aluminum hydroxide was compared to aluminum hydroxide. Both vaccines were administered by subcutaneous route. QS-21 doses of 50 and 100 µg were evaluated in this study. The QS-21-adjuvanted vaccine induced anti-MAP antibody titers in individuals of responder phenotype whereas there was minimal antibody response in the aluminum hydroxide group. Nine of 14 vaccinees with high antibody response also had delayed-type hypersensitivity responses to antigen (Kublin et al., 2002). However, there were immediate-type hypersensitivity reactions (acute systemic urticaria) after three injections in two volunteers; this was correlated with serum anti-MAP IgE (Edelman et al., 2002).

A phase I trial in Columbia evaluated the synthetic peptide SPf66 plus QS-21 (Kashala et al., 2002). This vaccine was administered by intramuscular route. Doses of 50 and 100 µg QS-21 were evaluated with SPf66; in addition, a dose of 50 µg was evaluated on SPf66/aluminum hydroxide. All were compared to a 50 µg QS-21 group (no antigen) and to SPf66/aluminum hydroxide (Kashala et al., 2002). A remarkable adjuvant effect was observed. IgG titers against SPf66 were elevated by from 10- to 1000-fold in QS-21 groups compared to the aluminum hydroxide group. There were a few systemic allergic responses, all occurring in subjects receiving 3 immunizations (primarily contralateral reactions but including two bronchospasm reactions, treatable with corticosteroids and antihistamines). Unlike the MAP vaccine, this was not correlated with IgE response.

A malaria vaccine which is fairly advanced in clinical trials (phase IIb) is the RTS,S vaccine (GlaxoSmithKline). This vaccine is adjuvanted with a complex adjuvant formulation consisting of a proprietary oil-in-water emulsion, MPL, and QS-21 (formulation currently termed AS02). Hence, effects of the adjuvant must be considered in the context of the formulation rather than the saponin alone. This complex formulation was evaluated in a phase I study in comparison to MPL/alum and the proprietary oil-in-water emulsion (no added immunostimulants) (Stoute et al., 1997). In this study, the volunteers received a challenge with bites from *P. falciparum*-infected mosquitoes. The vaccine with QS-21/MPL/oil-in-water protected six of seven subjects in contrast to zero of six control subjects, two of seven subjects receiving the oil-in-water adjuvanted vaccine, and one of eight subjects receiving the

MPL/alum vaccine. This vaccine also protected semiimmune adult men in a field study in Gambia, with protective efficacy initially at 71% in the period immediately after vaccination although this waned with time (Bojang et al., 2001). This vaccine has recently undergone efficacy testing in a pediatric population in a phase IIb study in Mozambique (Alonso et al., 2004). A double-blind, randomized controlled trial in 2022 children (ages 1–4 years) indicated a vaccine efficacy of 29.9% for first clinical episodes of malaria, 57.7% efficacy for severe malaria, and 45% efficacy for extending time to first infection. The children in this study received half the adult dose used in previous studies. The authors noted that the vaccine was more immunogenic in the pediatric population than in adults, which may account for the improved efficacy results. Development is continuing on this vaccine.

Formulation studies with QS-21

Injection pain (in some instances severe) was noted as part of an HIV vaccine trial that included QS-21(Evans et al., 2001). This event was also noted in a few other studies, although not in all. In general, the injection pain was transient. It was also associated more with the intramuscular route of injection than the subcutaneous route. Hence, a series of three clinical studies were carried out to evaluate the effect of QS-21 in different formulations on the frequency and severity of this adverse event (Waite et al., 2001). The studies were designed as randomized, double-blind, cross-over studies. The first study confirmed that intramuscular QS-21 (at a dose of 50 µg) with no other excipients induced a median injection pain that was moderate, although there was a wide variation in reported pain. The pH of the formulation did not affect the response. In the second and third studies, mixtures of QS-21 with certain excipients were found to reduce this injection pain. Excipients that reduced the severity were polysorbate 80, benzyl alcohol, and hydroxypropyl-β-cyclodextrin. The pain responses to the QS-21/cyclodextrin formulation were not statistically different from those to the aluminum hydroxide/saline formulation.

■ Other saponin adjuvants in clinical studies

▨ *Iscoprep 7.03*

Iscoprep 7.0.3 has also been evaluated in clinical studies, primarily in ISCOM-based vaccines. Because ISCOMs are discussed more extensively in another chapter in this book, the discussion here is brief. Iscoprep 7.0.3 has been formulated into ISCOMs (two different formulations, one in which antigen and ISCOM were formulated together and one in which preformed ISCOMs were added to antigen) and used to adjuvant an influenza vaccine in a phase I study (intramuscular injection, healthy adult subjects). Iscoprep was used at a dose of 50 μg saponin; the influenza antigen was adjusted to a standard dose of 15 μg hemagglutinin. The ISCOM formulations induced earlier serum antibody titers than Fluvax for the three serotypes in the vaccine (significant for the two A-strains) (Rimmelzwann et al., 2001). Higher T cell responses were noted if the two ISCOM groups were combined. Iscoprep has also been formulated into ISCOMATRIX (preformed ISCOMs) without antigen and used to adjuvant a recombinant NY-ESO-1 antigen in patients with NY-ESO-1 positive cancers and minimal residual disease (Davis et al., 2004). In this study, ISCOMATRIX was used at a dose of 120 μg. ISCOMATRIX aided in the generation of antibody and T cell responses in these subjects. A few subjects in the ISCOMATRIX groups experienced injection pain that was severe.

■ Conclusions

Saponins from *Quillaja saponaria* are useful vaccine adjuvants, combining the attributes of inducing strong Th1 and Th2 responses to vaccines (preclinical and clinical studies) as well as mucosal responses (preclinical studies).

Their utility for inducing antibody responses and cellular responses in human studies has been demonstrated. Formulation studies have identified excipients to improve tolerability of intramuscular formulations. There are currently no licensed vaccines containing saponin adjuvants. However, experimental vaccines based upon saponin adjuvants continue to be evaluated in the clinic, with malaria and melanoma vaccines adjuvanted with QS-21 in phase IIb and phase III trials, respectively.

■ Acknowledgments

The author thanks Dr. Gui Liu for help in preparing the structure in Figure 7.1 and Laura Cavanaugh for assistance in preparing the manuscript.

■ References

Adluri, S., Gilewski, T., Zhang, S., Ramnath, V., Ragupathi, G., and Livingston, P. (1999). Specificity analysis of sera from breast cancer patients vaccinated with MUC1-KLH plus QS-21. *Br. J. Cancer* 79, 1806–1812.

Alonso, P.L., Sacarlal, J., Aponte, J.J., Leach, A., Macete, E., Milman, J., Mandomando, I., Spiessens, B., Guinovart, C., Espasa, M., Bassat, Q., Aide, P., Ofori-Anyinam, O., Navia, M.M., Corachan, S., Ceuppens, M., Dubois, M.C., Demoitie, M.A., Dubovsky, F., Menendez, C., Tornieporth, N., Ballou, W.R., Thompson, R., and Cohen, J. (2004). Efficacy of the RTS,S/AS02A vaccine against *Plasmodium falciparum* infection and disease in young African children: randomised controlled trial. *Lancet* 364, 1411–1420.

Bocchia, M. (2002). Is there any role left for p210-derived peptide vaccines in chronic myeloid leukemia? *Haematologica* 87, 675–677.

Bojang, K.A., Milligan, P.J., Pinder, M., Vigneron, L., Alloueche, A., Kester, K.E., Ballou, W R., Conway, D.J., Reece, W.H., Gothard, P., Yamuah, L., Delchambre, M., Voss, G., Greenwood, B.M., Hill, A., McAdam, K.P., Tornieporth, N., Cohen, J.D., and Doherty, T. (2001). Efficacy of RTS,S/AS02 malaria vaccine against *Plasmodium falciparum* infection in semi-immune adult men in The Gambia: a randomised trial. *Lancet* 358, 1927–1934.

Bomford, R., Stapleton, M., Winsor, S., McKnight, A., and Andronova, T. (1992). The control of the antibody isotype response to recombinant human immunodeficiency virus gp120 antigen by adjuvants. *AIDS Res. Hum. Retroviruses* 8, 1765–1771.

Bouveret Le Cam, N., Ronco, J., Francon, A., Blondeau, C., and Fanget, B. (1998). Adjuvants for influenza vaccine. *Res. Immunol.* 149, 19–23.

Boyaka, P.N., Marinaro, M., Jackson, R.J., van Ginkel, F.W., Cormet-Boyaka, E., Kirk, K.L., Kensil, C.R., and McGhee, J.R. (2001). Oral QS-21 requires early IL-4 help for induction of mucosal and systemic immunity. *J. Immunol.* 166, 2283–2290.

Britt, W., Fay, J., Seals, J., and Kensil, C. (1995). Formulation of an immunogenic human cytomegalovirus vaccine: responses in mice. *J. Infect. Dis.* 171, 18–25.

Cathcart, K., Pinilla-Ibarz, J., Korontsvit, T., Schwartz, J., Zakhaleva, V., Papadopoulos, E.B., and Scheinberg, D.A. (2004). A multivalent bcr-abl fusion peptide vaccination trial in patients with chronic myeloid leukemia. *Blood* 103, 1037–1042.

Chapman, P.B., Morrissey, D.M., Panageas, K.S., Hamilton, W.B., Zhan, C., Destro, A.N., Williams, L., Israel, R.J., and Livingston, P.O. (2000). Induction of antibodies against GM2 ganglioside by immunizing melanoma patients using GM2-keyhole limpet hemocyanin + QS21 vaccine: a dose-response study. *Clin. Cancer Res.* 6, 874–879.

Chen, D., Endres, R., Maa, Y.F., Kensil, C.R., Whitaker-Dowling, P., Trichel, A., Youngner, J.S., and Payne, L.G. (2003). Epidermal powder immunization of mice and monkeys with an influenza vaccine. *Vaccine* 21, 2830–2836.

Cox, J.C., Sjolander, A., and Barr, I.G. (1998). ISCOMs and other saponin based adjuvants. *Adv. Drug Deliv. Rev.* 32, 247–271.

Dalsgaard, K. (1974). Isolation of a substance from *Quillaja saponaria* Molina with adjuvant activity in foot-and-mouth disease vaccines. *Arch. Gesamte Virusforsch.* 44, 243–254.

Davis, I.D., Chen, W., Jackson, H., Parente, P., Shackleton, M., Hopkins, W., Chen, Q., Dimopoulos, N., Luke, T., Murphy, R., Scott, A.M., Maraskovsky, E., McArthur, G., MacGregor, D., Sturrock, S., Tai, T.Y., Green, S., Cuthbertson, A., Maher, D., Miloradovic, L., Mitchell, S.V., Ritter, G., Jungbluth, A.A., Chen, Y.T., Gnjatic, S., Hoffman, E.W., Old, L.J., and Cebon, J.S. (2004). Recombinant NY-ESO-1 protein with ISCOMATRIX adjuvant induces broad integrated antibody and CD4+ and CD8+ T cell responses in humans. *Proc. Natl. Acad. Sci. USA* 101, 10697–10702.

Dickler, M.N., Ragupathi, G., Liu, N.X., Musselli, C., Martino, D.J., Miller, V.A., Kris, M.G., Brezicka, F.T., Livingston, P.O., and Grant, S.C. (1999). Immunogenicity of a fucosyl-GM1-keyhole limpet hemocyanin conjugate vaccine in patients with small cell lung cancer. *Clin. Cancer Res.* 5, 2773–2779.

Doherty, J.F., Pinder, M., Tornieporth, N., Carton, C., Vigneron, L., Milligan, P., Ballou, W.R., Holland, C.A., Kester, K.E., Voss, G., Momin, P., Greenwood, B.M., McAdam, K.P., and Cohen, J. (1999). A phase I safety and immunogenicity trial with the candidate malaria vaccine RTS,S/SBAS2 in semi-immune adults in The Gambia. *Am. J. Trop. Med. Hyg.* 61, 865–868.

Edelman, R., Wasserman, S.S., Kublin, J.G., Bodison, S.A., Nardin, E.H., Oliveira, G.A., Ansari, S., Diggs, C.L., Kashala, O.L., Schmeckpeper, B.J., and Hamilton, R.G. (2002). Immediate-type hypersensitivity and other clinical reactions in volunteers immunized with a synthetic multi-antigen peptide vaccine (PfCS-MAP1NYU) against *Plasmodium falciparum* sporozoites. *Vaccine* 21, 269–280.

Espinet, R.G. (1951). Nouveau vaccin antiaphteux a complexe glucoviral. *Gac. vet* (Buenos Aires) 13, 268–273.

Evans, T.G., McElrath, M.J., Matthews, T., Montefiori, D., Weinhold, K., Wolff, M., Keefer, M.C., Kallas, E.G., Corey, L., Gorse, G.J., Belshe, R., Graham, B.S., Spearman, P.W., Schwartz, D., Mulligan, M.J., Goepfert, P., Fast, P., Berman, P., Powell, M., and Francis, D. (2001). QS-21 promotes an adjuvant effect allowing for reduced antigen dose during HIV-1 envelope subunit immunization in humans. *Vaccine* 19, 2080–2091.

Fernando, G.J.P., Stewart, T.J., Tindle, R.W., and Frazer, I.H. (1998a). Th2-type CD4$^+$ cells neither enhance nor suppress antitumor CTL activity in a mouse tumor model. *J. Immunol.* 161, 2421–2427.

Fernando, G.J.P., Stewart, T.J., Tindle, R.W., and Frazer, I.H. (1998b). Vaccine-induced Th1-type responses are dominated over Th2-type responses in the short term whereas preexisting Th2 responses are dominant in the longer term. *Scand. J. Immunol.* 47, 459–465.

Foon, K.A., Sen, G., Hutchins, L., Kashala, O.L., Baral, R., Banerjee, M., Chakraborty, M., Garrison, J., Reisfeld, R.A., and Bhattacharya-Chatterjee, M. (1998). Antibody responses in melanoma patients immunized with an anti-idiotype antibody mimicking disialoganglioside GD2. *Clin. Cancer Res.* 4, 1117–1124.

Foon, K.A., Lutzky, J., Baral, R.N., Yannelli, J.R., Hutchins, L., Teitelbaum, A., Kashala, O.L., Das, R., Garrison, J., Reisfeld, R.A., and Bhattacharya-Chatterjee, M. (2000). Clinical and immune responses in advanced melanoma patients immunized with an anti-idiotype antibody mimicking disialoganglioside GD2. *J. Clin. Oncol.* 18, 376–384.

Gahery-Segard, H., Pialoux, G., Charmeteau, B., Sermet, S., Poncelet, H., Raux, M., Tartar, A., Levy, J.P., Gras-Masse, H., and Guillet, J.G. (2000). Multiepitopic B- and T-cell responses induced in humans by a human immunodeficiency virus type 1 lipopeptide vaccine. *J. Virol.* 74, 1694–1703.

Gahery-Segard, H., Pialoux, G., Figueiredo, S., Igea, C., Surenaud, M., Gaston, J., Gras-Masse, H., Levy, J.P., and Guillet, J.G. (2003). Long-term specific immune responses induced in humans by a human immunodeficiency virus type 1 lipopeptide vaccine: characterization of CD8+-T-cell epitopes recognized. *J. Virol.* 77, 11220–11231.

Garcon, N., Heppner, D.G., and Cohen, J. (2003). Development of RTS,S/AS02: a purified subunit-based malaria vaccine candidate formulated with a novel adjuvant. *Expert Rev. Vaccines* 2, 231–238.

Gilewski, T., Adluri, S., Ragupathi, G., Zhang, S., Yao, T.J., Panageas, K., Moynahan, M., Houghton, A., Norton, L., and Livingston, P.O. (2000). Vaccination of high-risk breast cancer patients with mucin-1 (MUC1) keyhole limpet hemocyanin conjugate plus QS-21. *Clin. Cancer Res.* 6, 1693–1701.

Gilewski, T., Ragupathi, G., Bhuta, S., Williams, L. J., Musselli, C., Zhang, X.F., Bornmann, W. G., Spassova, M., Bencsath, K.P., Panageas, K.S., Chin, J., Hudis, C.A., Norton, L., Houghton, A.N., Livingston, P.O., and Danishefsky, S.J. (2001). Immunization of metastatic breast cancer patients with a fully synthetic globo H conjugate: a phase I trial. *Proc. Natl. Acad. Sci. USA* 98, 3270–3275.

Hancock, G.E., Speelman, D.J., Frenchick, P.J., Mineo-Kuhn, M.M., Baggs, R.B., and Hahn, D.J. (1995). Formulation of the purified fusion protein of respiratory syncytial virus with the saponin QS-21 induces protective immune responses in Balb/c mice that are similar to those generated by experimental infection. *Vaccine* 13, 391–400.

Heeg, K., Kuon, W., and Wagner, H. (1991). Vaccination of class I major histocompatibility complex (MHC)-restricted murine CD8+ cytotoxic T lymphocytes towards soluble antigens: immunostimulating-ovalbumin complexes enter the class I MHC-restricted antigen pathway and allow sensitization against the immunodominant peptide. *Eur. J. Immunol.* 21, 1523–1527.

Helling, F., Zhang, S., Shang, A., Adluri, S., Calves, M., Koganty, R., Longenecker, B.M., Yao, T.J., Oettgen, H.F., and Livingston, P.O. (1995). GM2-KLH conjugate vaccine: increased immunogenicity in melanoma patients after administration with immunological adjuvant QS-21. *Cancer Res.* 55, 2783–2788.

Higuchi, R. and Komori, T. (1987). Structures of compounds derived from the acyl moieties of quillajasaponin. *Phytochemistry* 26, 2357–2360.

Higuchi, R., Tokimitsu, Y., Fujioka, T., Komori, T., Kawasaki, T., and Oakenfull, D.G. (1987). Structure of desacylsaponins obtained from the bark of *Quillaja saponaria*. *Phytochemistry* 26, 229–235.

Higuchi, R., Tokimitsu, Y., and Komori, T. (1988). An acylated triterpenoid saponin from *Quillaja saponaria*. *Phytochemistry* 27, 1165–1168.

Hostettman, K. and Marston, A. (1995). *Saponins*, Cambridge University Press, Cambridge.

Jacobsen, N.E., Fairbrother, W.J., Kensil, C.R., Lim, A., Wheeler, D.A., and Powell, M.F. (1996). Structure of the saponin adjuvant QS-21 and its base-catalyzed isomerization product by 1H and natural abundance 13C NMR spectroscopy. *Carbohydr. Res.* 280, 1–14.

Kashala, O., Amador, R., Valero, M.V., Moreno, A., Barbosa, A., Nickel, B., Daubenberger, C.A., Guzman, F., Pluschke, G., and Patarroyo, M.E. (2002). Safety, tolerability and immunogenicity of new formulations of the *Plasmodium falciparum* malaria peptide vaccine SPf66 combined with the immunological adjuvant QS-21. *Vaccine* 20, 2263–2277.

Keefer, M.C., Wolff, M., Gorse, G.J., Graham, B.S., Corey, L., Clements-Mann, M.L., Verani-Ketter, N., Erb, S., Smith, C.M., Belshe, R.B., Wagner, L.J., McElrath, M.J., Schwartz, D.H., and Fast, P. (1997). Safety profile of phase I and II preventive HIV type 1 envelope vaccination: experience of the NIAID AIDS Vaccine Evaluation Group. *AIDS Res. Hum. Retroviruses* 13, 1163–1177.

Kensil, C. R. (2000). In O'Hagan, D.T. (Ed) *Vaccine Adjuvants: Preparation Methods and Research Protocols*. Humana Press, Totawa, NJ, pp. 259–271.

Kensil, C.R., Patel, U., Lennick, M., and Marciani, D. (1991). Separation and characterization of saponins with adjuvant activity from Quillaja saponaria Molina cortex. *J. Immunol.* 146, 431–437.

Kensil, C.R., Soltysik, S., Wheeler, D.A., and Wu, J.Y. (1996). Structure/function studies on QS-21, a unique immunological adjuvant from Quillaja saponaria. *Adv. Exp. Med. Biol.* 404, 165–172.

Kensil, C.R., Wu, J.Y., Anderson, C.A., Wheeler, D.A., and Amsden, J. (1998). QS-21 and QS-7: purified saponin adjuvants. *Dev. Biol. Stand.* 92, 41–47.

Kersten, G.F.A., Teerlink, T., Derks, H.J.G.M., Verkleij, A.J., van Wezel, T.L., Crommelin, D.J.A., and Beuvery, E.C. (1988). Incorporation of the major outer membrane protein of *Neisseria gonorrhoeae* in saponin–lipid complexes (Iscoms): chemical analysis, some structural features, and comparison of their immunogenicity with three other antigen delivery systems. *Infect. Immun.* 56, 432–438.

Kirkwood, J.M., Ibrahim, J., Lawson, D.H., Atkins, M.B., Agarwala, S.S., Collins, K., Mascari, R., Morrissey, D.M., and Chapman, P.B. (2001a). High-dose interferon alfa-2b does not diminish antibody response to GM2 vaccination in patients with resected melanoma: results of the Multicenter Eastern Cooperative Oncology Group Phase II Trial E2696. *J. Clin. Oncol.* 19, 1430–1436.

Kirkwood, J.M., Ibrahim, J.G., Sosman, J.A., Sondak, V.K., Agarwala, S.S., Ernstoff, M.S., and Rao, U. (2001b). High-dose interferon alfa-2b significantly prolongs relapse-free and overall survival compared with the GM2-KLH/QS-21 vaccine in patients with resected stage IIB–III melanoma: results of intergroup trial E1694/S9512/C509801. *J. Clin. Oncol.* 19, 2370–2380.

Kitamura, K., Livingston, P.O., Fortunato, S.R., Stockert, E., Helling, F., Ritter, G., Oettgen, H.F., and Old, L.J. (1995). Serological response patterns of melanoma patients immunized with a GM2 ganglioside conjugate vaccine. *Proc. Natl. Acad. Sci. USA* 92, 2805–2809.

Knutson, K.L. (2002). GMK (Progenics Pharmaceuticals). *Curr. Opin. Invest. Drugs* 3, 159–164.

Kublin, J.G., Lowitt, M.H., Hamilton, R.G., Oliveira, G.A., Nardin, E.H., Nussenzweig, R.S., Schmeckpeper, B.J., Diggs, C.L., Bodison, S.A., and Edelman, R. (2002). Delayed-type hypersensitivity in volunteers immunized with a synthetic multi-antigen peptide vaccine (PfCS-MAP1NYU) against *Plasmodium falciparum* sporozoites. *Vaccine* 20, 1853–1861.

Labriola, R.A. and Deulofeu, V. (1968). The structure of prosapogenin from *Quillaja saponaria*. *Experientia* 25, 124–125.

Lewis, J.J., Janetzki, S., Schaed, S., Panageas, K.S., Wang, S., Williams, L., Meyers, M., Butterworth, L., Livingston, P.O.,

Chapman, P.B., and Houghton, A.N. (2000). Evaluation of CD8(+) T-cell frequencies by the Elispot assay in healthy individuals and in patients with metastatic melanoma immunized with tyrosinase peptide. *Int. J. Cancer* 87, 391–398.

Lipford, G.B., Wagner, H., and Heeg, K. (1994). Vaccination with immunodominant peptides encapsulated in QuilA-containing liposomes induces peptide-specific primary CD8+ cytotoxic T cells. *Vaccine* 12, 73–80.

Liu, G., Anderson, C., Scaltreto, H., Barbon, J., and Kensil, C.R. (2002). QS-21 structure/function studies: effect of acylation on adjuvant activity. *Vaccine* 20, 2808–2815.

Livingston, P., Zhang, S., Adluri, S., Yao, T.J., Graeber, L., Ragupathi, G., Helling, F., and Fleisher, M. (1997). Tumor cell reactivity mediated by IgM antibodies in sera from melanoma patients vaccinated with GM2 ganglioside covalently linked to KLH is increased by IgG antibodies. *Cancer Immunol. Immunother.* 43, 324–330.

Livingston, P.O., Adluri, S., Helling, F., Yao, T.J., Kensil, C.R., Newman, M.J., and Marciani, D. (1994). Phase 1 trial of immunological adjuvant QS-21 with a GM2 ganglioside-keyhole limpet haemocyanin conjugate vaccine in patients with malignant melanoma. *Vaccine* 12, 1275–1280.

Maharaj, I., Froh, K.J., and Campbell, J.B. (1986). Immune responses of mice to inactivated rabies vaccine administered orally: potentiation by *Quillaja* saponin. *Can. J. Microbiol.* 32, 414–420.

Marciani, D.J., Press, J.B., Reynolds, R.C., Pathak, A.K., Pathak, V., Gundy, L.E., Farmer, J.T., Koratich, M.S., and May, R.D. (2000). Development of semisynthetic triterpenoid saponin derivatives with immune stimulating activity. *Vaccine* 18, 3141–3151.

McCaffery, M., Yao, T.J., Williams, L., Livingston, P.O., Houghton, A.N., and Chapman, P.B. (1996). Immunization of melanoma patients with BEC2 anti-idiotypic monoclonal antibody that mimics GD3 ganglioside: enhanced immunogenicity when combined with adjuvant. *Clin. Cancer Res.* 2, 679–686.

McClintock, E. (1984). Trees of Golden Gate Park: three from South America. *Pacific Horticult.* 45, 18–20.

McCormack, S., Tilzey, A., Carmichael, A., Gotch, F., Kepple, J., Newberry, A., Jones, G., Lister, S., Beddows, S., Cheingsong, R., Rees, A., Babiker, A., Banatvala, J., Bruck, C., Darbyshire, J., Tyrrell, D., Van Hoecke, C., and Weber, J. (2000). A phase I trial in HIV negative healthy volunteers evaluating the effect of potent adjuvants on immunogenicity of a recombinant gp120W61D derived from dual tropic R5X4 HIV-1ACH320. *Vaccine* 18, 1166–1177.

Musselli, C., Ragupathi, G., Gilewski, T., Panageas, K.S., Spinat, Y., and Livingston, P.O. (2002). Reevaluation of the cellular immune response in breast cancer patients vaccinated with MUC1. *Int. J. Cancer* 97, 660–667.

Nardin, E.H., Oliveira, G.A., Calvo-Calle, J.M., Castro, Z.R., Nussenzweig, R.S., Schmeckpeper, B., Hall, B.F., Diggs, C., Bodison, S., and Edelman, R. (2000). Synthetic malaria peptide vaccine elicits high levels of antibodies in vaccinees of defined HLA genotypes. *J. Infect. Dis.* 182, 1486–1496.

Newman, M.J., Wu, J.Y., Gardner, B.H., Munroe, K.J., Leombruno, D., Recchia, J., Kensil, C.R., and Coughlin, R.T. (1992). Saponin adjuvant induction of ovalbumin-specific CD8+ cytotoxic T lymphocyte responses. *J. Immunol.* 148, 2357–2362.

Pinilla-Ibarz, J., Cathcart, K., Korontsvit, T., Soignet, S., Bocchia, M., Caggiano, J., Lai, L., Jimenez, J., Kolitz, J., and Scheinberg, D.A. (2000). Vaccination of patients with chronic myelogenous leukemia with bcr-abl oncogene breakpoint fusion peptides generates specific immune responses. *Blood* 95, 1781–1787.

Powell, M.F., Eastman, D.J., Lim, A., Lucas, C., Peterson, M., Vennari, J., Weissburg, R.P., Wrin, T., Kensil, C.R., Newman, M.J. et al. (1995). Effect of adjuvants on immunogenicity of MN recombinant glycoprotein 120 in guinea pigs. *AIDS Res. Hum. Retroviruses* 11, 203–209.

Rafi-Janajreh, A., Tongren, J.E., Kensil, C., Hackett, C., Candal, F., Lal, A., and Udhayakumar, V. (2002). Influence of adjuvants in inducing immune responses to different epitopes included in a multiepitope, multivalent, multistage *Plasmodium falciparum* candidate vaccine (FALVAC-1) in outbred mice. *Exp. Parasitol.* 101, 3–12.

Ragupathi, G., Livingston, P.O., Hood, C., Gathuru, J., Krown, S.E., Chapman, P.B., Wolchok, J.D., Williams, L.J., Oldfield, R.C., and Hwu, W. J. (2003). Consistent antibody response against ganglioside GD2 induced in patients with melanoma by a GD2 lactone-keyhole limpet hemocyanin conjugate vaccine plus immunological adjuvant QS-21. *Clin. Cancer Res.* 9, 5214–5220.

Rimmelzwann, G.F., Nieuwkoop, N., Brandenburg, A., Sutter, G., Beyer, W.E.P., Maher, D., Bates, J., and Osterhaus, A.D.M.E. (2001). A randomized, double blind study in young healthy adults comparing cell mediated and humoral immune responses induced by influenza ISCOM™ vaccines and conventional vaccines. *Vaccine* 19, 1180–1187.

Ronnberg, B., Fekadu, M., and Morein, B. (1995). Adjuvant activity of non-toxic *Quillaja saponaria* Molina components for use in ISCOM matrix. *Vaccine* 13, 1375–1382.

Sabbatini, P.J., Kudryashov, V., Ragupathi, G., Danishefsky, S.J., Livingston, P.O., Bornmann, W., Spassova, M., Zatorski, A., Spriggs, D., Aghajanian, C., Soignet, S., Peyton, M., O'Flaherty, C., Curtin, J., and Lloyd, K.O. (2000). Immunization of ovarian cancer patients with a synthetic Lewis(y)-protein conjugate vaccine: a phase 1 trial. *Int. J. Cancer* 87, 79–85.

San Martin, R. and Briones, R. (1999). Industrial uses and sustainable supply of *Quillaja saponaria* (Rosaceae) saponins. *Economic Botany* 53, 302–311.

Sasaki, S., Sumino, K., Hamajima, K., Fukushima, J., Ishii, N., Kawamoto, S., Mohri, H., Kensil, C.R., and Okuda, K. (1998). Induction of systemic and mucosal immune responses to human immunodeficiency virus type 1 by a DNA vaccine formulated with QS-21 saponin adjuvant via intramuscular and intranasal routes. *J. Virol.* 72, 4931–4939.

Schaed, S.G., Klimek, V.M., Panageas, K.S., Musselli, C.M., Butterworth, L., Hwu, W.J., Livingston, P.O., Williams, L., Lewis, J.J., Houghton, A.N., and Chapman, P.B. (2002). T-cell responses against tyrosinase 368-376(370D) peptide in HLA*A0201+ melanoma patients: randomized trial comparing incomplete Freund's adjuvant, granulocyte macrophage colony-stimulating factor, and QS-21 as immunological adjuvants. *Clin. Cancer Res.* 8, 967–972.

Slingluff, C.L., Jr., Yamshchikov, G., Neese, P., Galavotti, H., Eastham, S., Engelhard, V.H., Kittlesen, D., Deacon, D., Hibbitts, S., Grosh, W.W., Petroni, G., Cohen, R., Wiernasz, C., Patterson, J.W., Conway, B.P., and Ross, W.G. (2001). Phase I trial of a melanoma vaccine with gp100(280-288) peptide and tetanus helper peptide in adjuvant: immunologic and clinical outcomes. *Clin. Cancer Res.* 7, 3012–3024.

Slovin, S.F., Ragupathi, G., Adluri, S., Ungers, G., Terry, K., Kim, S., Spassova, M., Bornmann, W.G., Fazzari, M., Dantis, L., Olkiewicz, K., Lloyd, K.O., Livingston, P.O., Danishefsky, S.J., and Scher, H.I. (1999). Carbohydrate vaccines in cancer: immunogenicity of a fully synthetic globo H hexasaccharide conjugate in man. *Proc. Natl. Acad. Sci. USA* 96, 5710–5715.

Slovin, S.F., Ragupathi, G., Musselli, C., Olkiewicz, K., Verbel, D., Kuduk, S.D., Schwarz, J.B., Sames, D., Danishefsky, S., Livingston, P.O., and Scher, H.I. (2003). Fully synthetic carbohydrate-based vaccines in biochemically relapsed prostate cancer: clinical trial results with alpha-N-acetylgalactosamine-O-serine/threonine conjugate vaccine. *J. Clin. Oncol.* 21, 4292–4298.

Soltysik, S., Wu, J.Y., Recchia, J., Wheeler, D.A., Newman, M.J., Coughlin, R.T., and Kensil, C.R. (1995). Structure/function studies of QS-21 adjuvant: assessment of triterpene aldehyde and glucuronic acid roles in adjuvant function. *Vaccine* 13, 1403–1410.

Stewart, T.J., Drane, D., Malliaros, J., Elmer, H., Malcolm, K.M., Cox, J.C., Edwards, S.J., Frazer, I.H., and Fernando, G.J.P. (2004). ISCOMATRIX™ adjuvant: an adjuvant suitable for use in anticancer vaccines. *Vaccine* 22, 3738–3743.

Stoute, J.A., Slaoui, M., Heppner, D.G., Momin, P., Kester, K.E., Desmons, P., Wellde, B.T., Garcon, N., Krzych, U., and Marchand, M. (1997). A preliminary evaluation of a recombinant circumsporozoite protein vaccine against *Plasmodium falciparum* malaria. RTS,S Malaria Vaccine Evaluation Group. *N. Engl. J. Med.* 336, 86–91.

Takahashi, H., Takeshita, T., Morein, B., Putney, S., Germain, R.N., and Berzofsky, J.A. (1990). Induction of CD8+ cytotoxic T cells by immunization with purified HIV-1 envelope protein in ISCOMs. *Nature* 344, 873–875.

Ten Hagen, T.L.M., Sulzer, A.J., Kidd, M. ., Lal, A.A., and Hunter, R.L. (1993). Role of adjuvants in the modulation of antibody isotype, specificity, and induction of protection by whole blood-stage *Plasmodium yoelii* vaccines. *J. Immunol.* 151, 7077–7085.

Van Setten, D.C. and van de Werken, G. (1996). In Waller, G.R., and Yamasaki, K. (Eds) *Saponins Used in Traditional and Modern Medicine*. Plenum Press, New York, pp. 185–193.

Van Setten, D.C., van de Werken, G., Zomer, G., and Kersten, G.F.A. (1995). Glycosyl compositions and structural characteristics of the potential immuno-adjuvant active saponins in the *Quillaja* saponaria Molina extract QuilA. *Rapid Commun. Mass Spectrom.* 9, 660–666.

Waite, D.C., Jacobson, E.W., Ennis, F.A., Edelman, R., White, B., Kammer, R., Anderson, C., and Kensil, C.R. (2001). Three double-blind, randomized trials evaluating the safety and tolerance of different formulations of the saponin adjuvant QS-21. *Vaccine* 19, 3957–3967.

Wong, C.P., Okada, C.Y., and Levy, R. (1999). TCR vaccines against T cell lymphoma: QS-21 and IL-12 adjuvants induce a protective CD8+ T cell response. *J. Immunol.* 162, 2251–2258.

Wu, J.Y., Gardner, B.H., Murphy, C.I., Seals, J.R., Kensil, C.R., Recchia, J., Beltz, G.A., Newman, G.W., and Newman, M.J. (1992). Saponin adjuvant enhancement of antigen-specific immune responses to an experimental HIV-1 vaccine. *J. Immunol.* 148, 1519–1525.

Microparticles as vaccine delivery systems

Derek T. O'Hagan

Chiron Vaccines, Chiron Corporation, Emeryville, California

Introduction

Vaccines that were developed in the mid to early part of the 20th century mainly consisted of live attenuated pathogens, whole inactivated organisms, or inactivated bacterial toxins. These approaches were successful mainly due to the induction of antibody responses, which neutralized the viruses or toxins, inhibited the binding of microorganisms to cells, or promoted the uptake of microorganisms by phagocytes. In the latter part of the 20th century, additional vaccines were developed based on newer approaches, including recombinant proteins and protein/polysaccharide conjugates. However, these newer vaccines were also effective mainly due to the induction of antibody responses. It has been argued that by the end of the 20th century, all the relatively "easy" vaccines had been developed and that novel approaches would be required for the more "difficult" pathogens. As of today, broadly effective vaccines are not available against a number of important infectious diseases, some of which are caused by pathogens with significant antigenic diversity, e.g., *Neisseria meningitidis* serotype B (bacterial meningitis), or by pathogens that establish chronic infections, e.g., human immunodeficiency virus (HIV), hepatitis C virus (HCV), tuberculosis (TB), and malaria. To combat these pathogens, the induction of more potent immune responses may be required, including the induction of cellular immunity. The cellular immune responses may include the induction of Th1 cytokines from CD4+ T helper cells and CD8+ cytotoxic T lymphocytes (CTL). Of the approaches currently used in licensed vaccines, only live attenuated viruses are able to induce CTL and there is a concern that live attenuated viruses may cause disease in immunosuppressed or immunocompromised individuals. In western societies, the percentage of immunosuppressed individuals is increasing, as medical improvements allow people to live longer, sometimes with chronic conditions that may have killed them at an earlier age in previous decades. In the developing world, the percentage of immunosuppressed people is increasing due to the spread of HIV and due to chronic undernourishment and other consequences of poverty. Moreover, some pathogens cannot be attenuated since they are difficult or impossible to grow in culture (e.g., HCV), while some would present significant safety concerns as a live attenuated vaccine, due to concerns about the possibility of reversion to virulence (e.g., HIV). Since live attenuated approaches are not appropriate for some viruses, novel attenuated vectors are being developed which can be used to deliver heterologous antigens, e.g., adenovirus or vaccinia. However, the safety of these vectors as carriers of heterologous antigens from difficult pathogens needs to be established in widespread studies, including immunosuppressed individuals. In addition, since these vectors have often been used previously as vaccines, preexisting immunity to the vector often limits its ability to induce immune responses to the heterologous antigens.

Several new approaches to vaccine development have emerged in the last couple of decades, which have the potential to allow the development of vaccines against difficult pathogens, including: (1) recombinant protein subunits; (2) protein polysaccharide conjugates, and (3) plasmid DNA. DNA holds significant promise as a means to induce CTL and Th1 cytokine responses, which are difficult to induce with alternative approaches. However, while these newer approaches have a number of advantages over the traditional approaches to vaccine development, including the potential for improved safety, and some have already proven commercially successful (1 and 2), significant improvements will be required if these approaches are to be successful against the most difficult pathogens. A general problem is that these newer vaccine approaches are often poorly immunogenic. This is particularly true for recombinant protein and DNA-based vaccines, but less so for conjugate vaccines, which often use bacterial toxoids as carrier molecules for the chemically conjugated polysaccharides. Traditional vaccines often contained components that could activate the immune system and enhance immune responses against the vaccine antigens, including a variety of bacterial cell components. However, these components have been eliminated from new-generation vaccines to improve safety and reduce reactogenicity. Vaccine adjuvants were included in traditional vaccines to make them more immunogenic and these agents will certainly be required for new-generation vaccines. The most commonly used adjuvants have been insoluble aluminum salts, but these have significant limitations, including their inability to induce CTL or Th1 cytokine responses. Therefore, new-generation adjuvants and vaccine delivery systems will be required to enable the development of vaccines against the most difficult pathogens. In addition, complex prime/boost strategies involving immunization with different modalities may be required for the successful development of some vaccines, e.g., priming with DNA and

boosting with a recombinant protein with an adjuvant.

Immunological adjuvants were originally described by Ramon (1924) as "substances used in combination with a specific antigen that produced a more robust immune response than the antigen alone." This broad definition can encompass a very wide range of materials (Vogel and Powell, 1995). However, despite the extensive evaluation of a large number of candidates over many years, the only adjuvants included in products approved by the US Food and Drug Administration are insoluble aluminum salts, which are generically called alum. Although alum has an excellent safety record, comparative studies show that it is a weak adjuvant for antibody induction to recombinant protein vaccines, is a poor adjuvant for DNA vaccines, and induces Th2 rather than Th1 cytokine responses (Gupta, 1998). In addition, alum is ineffective for the induction of mucosal immunity, and induces IgE antibody responses, which have been associated with allergic reactions in some individuals (Gupta, 1998; Relyveld et al., 1998). Although alum has been used as an adjuvant for many years, its mechanism of action remains poorly defined. It was originally thought to provide a "depot" effect, resulting in persistence of antigen at the injection site. However, studies have suggested that alum does not establish a depot (Gupta et al., 1996), but does appear to upregulate costimulatory signals on human monocytes and promotes the release of interleukin (IL)-4 (Ulanova et al., 2001), a Th2 cytokine. Importantly, alum may contribute to a reduction in toxicity for some multicomponent vaccines, due to the adsorption of contaminating lipopolysaccharide (LPS) (Shi et al., 2001).

A key issue in adjuvant development is toxicity, since safety concerns have predominantly been responsible for restricting the development of adjuvants since alum was first introduced more than 70 years ago (Edelman, 1997). Vaccine safety remains a significant concern, although the perceptions of safety do not always match the realities (O'Hagan and Rappuoli, 2004b) Nevertheless, although many experimental adjuvants have advanced to clinical trials, most have proven too toxic for routine clinical use. For standard prophylactic immunization in healthy individuals, only adjuvants that induce minimal adverse effects will prove acceptable. Additional practical issues that are important for adjuvant development include biodegradability, stability, ease of manufacture, cost, and applicability to a wide range of vaccines.

Role of adjuvants in vaccine development

Adjuvants can be used to improve the immune response to vaccine antigens in a number of different ways, including: (i) increasing the immunogenicity of weak antigens, (ii) enhancing the speed and duration of the immune response, (iii) modulating antibody avidity, specificity, isotype, or subclass distribution, (iv) stimulating cellular immunity, including the desired cytokine profile, (v) promoting the induction of mucosal immunity, (vi) enhancing immune responses in immunologically immature, or senescent individuals, (vii) decreasing the dose of antigen in the vaccine to reduce costs, or (viii) helping to overcome antigen competition in combination vaccines.

Unfortunately, the mechanisms of action of how most adjuvants achieve their effects is complex and often remains poorly understood (see Chapter 1). Nevertheless, significant advances have been made in this area in recent years, following the identification of key receptors on the cells of the innate immune system, which are activated by a variety of adjuvants, including the Toll-like receptor (TLR) family and others (Iwasaki and Medzhitov, 2004). Although adjuvants are notoriously difficult to classify and many examples resist easy definitions, they can be divided into two broad groups based on their principal modes of action (Table 8.1). This classification is a simplistic one, which focuses on whether or not they have direct

Table 8.1 A classification of vaccine adjuvants

Antigen delivery systems	Immunopotentiators
Alum	MPL and synthetic derivatives
Calcium phosphate	MDP and derivatives
Tyrosine	CpG oligos
Liposomes	Alternative PAMPS – flagellin, etc.
Virosomes	Lipopeptides
Emulsions	Saponins
Microparticles	DsRNA
Iscoms	Small-molecule immunopotentiators, e.g., resiquimod
Virus-like particles	

This describes their principal mechanisms of action as antigen delivery systems, which promote antigen uptake by antigen-presenting cells (APC), or immunopotentiators, which activate the APC, mainly through TLR and other receptors of the innate immune system.

immunopotentiating effects on innate immune cells, mostly through TLR or other receptor families, or they function primarily as "delivery systems" to promote antigen uptake into antigen-presenting cells (APC). Adjuvants that have direct immunopotentiating effects are often originally derived from pathogens, or represent synthetic mimics, and are commonly referred to as "pathogen-associated molecular patterns" (PAMPs) (Janeway, 1989; Medzhitov and Janeway, 1997). PAMPs are perceived as "danger signals" by the infected host and induce the release of proinflammatory cytokines from innate immune cells, which triggers and controls the adaptive immune response (Fearon, 1997; Iwasaki and Medzhitov, 2004). Traditional vaccines, including bacterial toxoids and inactivated viruses, contained most of the components of the actual pathogens they were designed to protect against and consequently often induced potent immune responses. In contrast, new-generation antigens are often highly purified, lack many of the features of the original pathogen, and do not evoke strong responses. Therefore, the role of immunopotentiator adjuvants for recombinant vaccines is to ensure that the appropriate components are added to the vaccine to ensure that it sufficiently resembles an infection to induce a protective immune response (Janeway, 1989; Fearon, 1997; Iwasaki and Medzhitov, 2004). Adjuvants that work through a delivery mechanism (Table 8.1) have an alternative, but equally important role to play in the induction of protective immune responses (see also Chapter 1). If one accepts the geographical concept of immune reactivity, in which antigens that do not reach local lymph nodes do not induce responses (Zinkernagel et al., 1997), it becomes easy to appreciate the role of injectable vaccine delivery systems. Key subsets of dendritic cells (DC) circulate in peripheral tissues and act as "sentinels," being responsible for the uptake and transfer of antigens to lymph nodes, where they are presented to T cells. Hence, antigen uptake into DC, the trafficking of DC to lymph nodes, and the triggering of DC maturation are key to the generation of potent immune responses. The role of particulate antigen delivery systems is to promote the uptake of antigens into APC and to enhance their delivery into the local lymph nodes. Particulate delivery systems may also be used to deliver immunopotentiator adjuvants into APC. Formulating immunopotentiators into delivery systems serves two principal purposes: the immunopotentiator effects can be targeted to the APC to enhance potency, while minimizing the potential of the immunopotentiator to induce toxicity, by focusing their effects on the APC and limiting their systemic distribution.

Although this chapter focuses primarily on microparticles as vaccine delivery systems, microparticles have been used as delivery systems for immunopotentiators, and this is also discussed. In addition, we briefly introduce alternative particulate delivery systems, including emulsions, liposomes, and iscoms, which are discussed in more detail in other chapters. More detailed reviews on vaccine adjuvants (Singh and O'Hagan, 2002) and vaccine delivery systems (O'Hagan and Rappuoli, 2004a) have recently been published by the author.

Immunopotentiator adjuvants

A number of immunopotentiators are available for inclusion in vaccines, which are extensively described elsewhere in this book. MPL (monophosphoryl lipid A) is derived from the LPS of the Gram-negative bacteria *Salmonella minnesota* and represents an archetypal PAMP (see Chapters 6 and 10). Like LPS, MPL is thought to interact with TLR4 on APC, resulting in the release of proinflammatory cytokines. In clinical trials, MPL has often been used as a component of complex formulations, including liposomes and emulsions, and has also been used in combination with alum and QS21 (Ulrich, 2000). MPL has been extensively evaluated in the clinic for a range of indications, has shown an acceptable profile of adverse effects, and appears to be moving towards approval as a licensed vaccine adjuvant (see Chapters 6 and 10). MPL is already marketed in Europe for use in combination with allergy vaccines (Wheeler et al., 2001).

In the last few years, a whole new class of immunopotentiator adjuvants based on short sequences of oligonucleotides have been identified (see Chapter 5), following the demonstration that bacterial DNA, but not vertebrate DNA, had direct immunostimulatory effects on immune cells, inducing B cells to proliferate and produce immunoglobulins (Messina et al., 1991; Tokunaga et al., 1984). Unmethylated CpG in conjunction with selective flanking sequences is believed to be recognized by the innate immune system to allow discrimination of pathogen-derived DNA from self DNA (Bird, 1987). Hence, the immunostimulatory effect of oligo-based adjuvants is due to the presence of unmethylated CpG sequences (Krieg et al., 1995), which are under-represented and methylated in vertebrate DNA. It has been shown that responses to CpG are dependent on the presence of TLR9 (Hemmi et al., 2000). CpG DNA has been shown to be particularly potent at stimulating Th1 cytokine responses (see Chapter 5).

A third group of immunopotentiators are the triterpenoid glycosides, or saponins, derived from QuilA, which is extracted from the bark of a Chilean tree, *Quillaja saponaria* (see Chapter 7). Saponins have been widely used as adjuvants for many years and have been included in several veterinary vaccines. QS21, which is a highly purified fraction from QuilA, has been shown to be a potent adjuvant for Th1 cytokines in mice (Kensil, 1996). Saponins have been shown to intercalate into cell membranes, through interaction with structurally similar cholesterol, forming "holes" or pores (Glaueri et al., 1962). However, it is currently unknown if the adjuvant effect of saponins is related to pore formation in cells.

A fourth class of immunopotentiators was recently identified, which have been called small-molecule immunopotentiators (SMIPs) (O'Hagan and Valiante, 2003) of which the first candidate identified was resiquimod, which has also been called an Immune Response Modifier (Hemmi et al., 2002) (see Chapter 4). In contrast to the other immunopotentiators, the SMIP compounds are entirely synthetic, can be cheaply and easily produced, and have physicochemical and toxicological similarities to many related compounds that have already been approved as drugs for use in humans. For example, resiquimod and its closely related analog imiquimod have already been approved for use in humans for several indications (see Chapter 4). This class of compounds are thought to activate innate immune cells through TLR7 and TLR8 (Hemmi et al., 2002) (see Chapter 4).

Immunopotentiators are active primarily as a consequence of their ability to induce immune cells to secrete cytokines. As an alternative to the use of immunopotentiators to activate cytokine release, many cytokines can be used directly to modify and redirect the immune response (see Chapter 3). The cytokines that have been evaluated most extensively as adjuvants include IL-1, IL-2, interferon (IFN)-γ, IL-12, and GM-CSF (Heath, 1995). However, all of these molecules exhibit dose-related toxicity. In addition, since they are proteins, they have stability problems, a short *in vivo* half-life, and are relatively expensive to produce.

■ Particulate vaccine delivery systems

Particulate carriers (e.g., microparticles, emulsions, iscoms, liposomes, virosomes, and virus-like particles) have a similar size to the pathogens which the immune system evolved to combat, and consequently they are efficiently taken up by APC. In addition, particulates can present multiple copies of antigens on their surface, which has been shown to be optimal for B cell activation (Bachmann et al., 1993; Bachmann and Zinkernagel, 1997; Fehr et al., 1998). Therefore, a range of alternative particulate carriers have been widely used as vaccine delivery systems. Immunopotentiators may also be included in the delivery systems to enhance the response by focusing its effects on the APC which take up the particulate carriers. In addition, formulating potent immunopotentiators into delivery systems may limit their potential for adverse events, by restricting their systemic circulation away from the injection site.

A squalene oil-in-water emulsion was developed (MF59), without the presence of additional immunopotentiators, which proved to be a potent adjuvant with an acceptable safety profile (Ott et al., 1995). MF59 is a safe and well-tolerated adjuvant in humans and is effective for the induction of potent antibody responses (see Chapter 9). MF59 is a licensed adjuvant in Europe and has been safely administered to several million people. Similar emulsions have been used as delivery systems for immunostimulatory adjuvants, including MPL and QS21.

Liposomes are phospholipid vesicles which have been evaluated both as adjuvants and as delivery systems for immunopotentiators (Alving, 1992; Gregoriadis, 1990). Unfortunately, liposomes have often been used in complex formulations, which makes it difficult to determine the contribution of the liposome to the overall adjuvant effect. Nevertheless, several liposomal vaccines based on viral membrane proteins (virosomes) without additional immunopotentiators have been extensively evaluated in the clinic and are approved as products in Europe (see Chapter 11).

The immunostimulatory fractions from QuilA have been incorporated into lipid particles comprising cholesterol, phospholipids, and cell membrane antigens, which are called immune stimulating complexes or iscoms (see Chapter 12).

■ Adjuvant effect of synthetic microparticles

The adjuvant effect achieved through linking an antigen to synthetic microparticles has been known for many years and has previously been reviewed in detail (O'Hagan, 1994). However, the particles used in these early studies were mainly nondegradable and therefore were not appropriate for development as vaccine adjuvants for human use. In addition, since antigens were often chemically conjugated to the nondegradable particles (Kovacsovics-Bankowski et al., 1993), this added an extra level of complexity and made commercial development of this concept even less likely. Nevertheless, studies on the use of nondegradable microparticles with conjugated antigens continue to be reported, particularly studies that focus on the potential of microparticles to develop tumor vaccines (Goldberg et al., 2003). A recent paper in this area suggested that nanoparticles were likely to be more effective than microparticles (Fifis et al., 2004). However, it is not easy to control all other parameters in such studies and often it is not only the particle size that is varied when two different particulate formulations are compared. In addition, although we had previously shown that nanoparticles were more potent than microparticles for the delivery of DNA vaccines (Singh et al., 2000), the challenges of manufacturing and processing nanoparticle formulations should not be underestimated.

In general, particulate delivery systems are thought to promote trapping and retention of antigens in local lymph nodes. Moreover, it has been demonstrated that organized arrays of antigens on surfaces are able to efficiently crosslink B cell receptors and constitute a strong activation signal (Bachmann

et al., 1993; Bachmann and Zinkernagel, 1997; Fehr et al., 1998). In addition, recent studies showed that together with the activation of innate immunity, the duration of antigen persistence is important in triggering protective T cell responses (Storni et al., 2003). Antigen persistence is enhanced by association with microparticles, which protect antigens from degradation.

■ Uptake of microparticles into APC

The uptake of microparticles ($<5\,\mu m$) by phagocytic cells has been demonstrated on many occasions and it is assumed that uptake into APC is important in the ability of particles to perform as vaccine adjuvants. The appropriate size for microparticles was defined in an early paper (Kanke et al., 1983), which described the uptake of microparticles of $1–3\,\mu m$ by macrophages, but showed that microparticles of $12\,\mu m$ were not taken up. It was subsequently shown that maximal uptake of microparticles occurred with particles of $<2\,\mu m$ (Tabata and Ikada, 1988, 1990). In addition, the surface charge and hydrophobicity of the microparticles was shown to modify uptake (Tabata and Ikada, 1990). The physicochemical properties of microparticles controlling their uptake into macrophages, including hydrophobicity, surface charge, and particle size, was recently reviewed (Ahsan et al., 2002). It appears that cationic microparticles are optimal for uptake into macrophages and DC (Thiele et al., 2003). It has been reported that macrophages which carry microparticles to lymph nodes can mature into DC (Randolph et al., 1999). In addition, uptake of biodegradable microparticles directly into DC has been demonstrated both *in vitro* (Lutsiak et al., 2002) and *in vivo* (Newman et al., 2002).

■ Microparticles as adjuvants for antibody induction

The biodegradable and biocompatible polyesters, the polylactide-co-glycolides (PLG), are the primary candidates for the development of microparticles as vaccine adjuvants or delivery systems, since they have been used in humans for many years as resorbable suture material and as controlled release drug delivery systems (Okada and Toguchi, 1995; Putney and Burke, 1998). The adjuvant effect achieved through the encapsulation of antigens into PLG microparticles was first demonstrated by several groups in the early 1990s (Eldridge et al., 1991; O'Hagan et al., 1991a, 1991b, 1993b). O'Hagan et al. (1991) and Eldridge et al. (1991) independently showed that microparticles with entrapped antigens had comparable immunogenicity to Freund's adjuvant. Particle size was shown to be an important parameter affecting the immunogenicity of microparticles, since smaller particles ($<10\,\mu m$) were significantly more immunogenic than larger ones (Eldridge et al., 1991; O'Hagan et al., 1993b). The adjuvant effect of microparticles can be further enhanced by their coadministration with additional adjuvants (O'Hagan et al., 1991a, 2000). Early studies in mice suggested that microparticles induced antibodies of predominantly the IgG2a isotype, indicating a Th1 response in this species (Vordermeier et al., 1995).

Unfortunately, the potential of microparticles as vaccine adjuvants has been limited by many reports describing the degradation and denaturation of proteins during microencapsulation (Johnson et al., 1996). Therefore, we developed a novel approach in which antigen encapsulation is avoided, and instead the antigen is adsorbed onto the surface of preformed anionic PLG microparticles (Kazzaz et al., 2000). This approach allowed the induction of significantly enhanced antibody titers in mice with an adsorbed recombinant p55 gag antigen from HIV-1. In a subsequent study, the microparticles with adsorbed p55 gag also induced potent antibody and T cell proliferative responses in nonhuman primates (Otten et al., 2003). Importantly, in a recent study using a recombinant envelope antigen from HIV, we showed that adsorbing the antigen to PLG microparticles allowed retention of the antigenic

Table 8.2 PLG microparticles are an effective delivery system for an adsorbed recombinant antigen from *Neisseria meningitides* serotype B (Men B)

Formulation	ELISA titer	Bactericidal titer
PLG/Men B	227,981	1024
Alum/Men B	50,211	256
PLG/Men B + CpG	382,610	16,384
Alum/Men B + CpG	56,867	4096
Freund's	253,844	8192

PLG microparticles with adsorbed antigen were directly compared with alum, both in the presence and absence of CpG immunopotentiator, for their ability to induce high levels of binding (ELISA) and bactericidal antibodies against a recombinant Men B antigen. Freund's adjuvant was also included as a positive control for comparison. Geometric mean titers for each group ($n = 10$).

structure and good stability, while microencapsulation of the same antigen caused extensive damage to the protein (Singh et al., 2004a). We had shown previously that the anionic microparticles with adsorbed env induced potent antibody responses in mice (Singh et al., 2001). Anionic PLG microparticles with adsorbed recombinant antigens have also been used to induce potent antibody responses against *Neisseria meningitidis* serotype B, including functional titers able to kill effectively the bacteria *in vitro* (Singh et al., 2004b) (Table 8.2). In recent studies, we directly compared anionic PLG microparticles with adsorbed antigens with the more established adjuvant alum (Table 8.3). These studies established that PLG microparticles represent a viable alternative to alum for a range of traditional and new-generation antigens, although PLG appears to work best for recombinant antigens (Tables 8.2 and 8.3).

A related approach to PLG adsorption for vaccine delivery has been described by others (Jung et al., 2002), who used a novel charged polymer to prepare nanoparticles which were able to adsorb tetanus toxoid for mucosal delivery. In addition, nondegradable microparticles for the adsorption of antigens for the development of a HIV vaccine were recently described (Caputo et al., 2004).

Table 8.3 PLG represents a viable alternative to alum for a range of traditional and new-generation vaccines

Formulation	DT ELISA titer	DT neuts (EU/ml)	TT ELISA titer	Men C ELISA titer	Men C BCA titer	HbsAg (MIU/ml)	Men B ELISA titer	Men B BCA titer
Alum	8,568	14.1	31,028	11,117	19,766	9,118	8,143	512
PLG	3,426	9.6	18,052	14,875	28,440	3,641	48,323	8,192

PLG microparticles with adsorbed antigens were compared to alum for their ability to induce binding (ELISA) and functional antibodies (toxin neutralizing or bactericidal antibodies) against a range of vaccine antigens. The antigens evaluated included diphtheria toxoid (DT), tetanus toxoid (TT), *Neisseria meningitides* serotype C conjugate (Men C), hepatitis B surface antigen (HBsAg), and *Neisseria meningitidis* serotype B recombinant antigen (Men B). Geometric mean titers for each group (n = 10).

■ Induction of cell-mediated immunity with microparticles

Several early studies showed that both non-degradable (Kovacsovics-Bankowski et al., 1993) and biodegradable microparticles were able to induce CTL responses in rodents with entrapped proteins and peptides (O'Hagan et al., 1993a; Maloy et al., 1994; Moore et al., 1995; Nixon et al., 1996). Subsequent studies focusing predominantly on nondegradable particles have extensively investigated the mechanisms of how cross presentation is achieved using particulate antigens (Shi and Rock, 2002). Early studies also showed that biodegradable microparticles induced a delayed-type hypersensitivity (DTH) response and potent T cell proliferative responses (Maloy et al., 1994). In a recent study, we evaluated the ability of biodegradable microparticles with adsorbed p55 gag to induce CTL responses in rhesus macaques. Previously, we had shown that the microparticles induced CTL responses in rodents (Kazzaz et al., 2000), which duplicated the earlier work with alternative antigens (O'Hagan et al., 1993a; Maloy et al., 1994; Moore et al., 1995; Nixon et al., 1996). Importantly, we had already shown that the microparticles with adsorbed p55 gag were more potent for CTL induction in rodents than microparticles with the same entrapped antigen (unpublished data). Although the PLG microparticles were not effective for CTL induction in nonhuman primates, they did induce potent antibody and T cell proliferative

responses (Otten et al., 2003). Hence, although biodegradable microparticles appear to be capable of inducing CTL responses in rodents against protein antigens, so far they are ineffective in nonhuman primates. In a recent study in rodents, it was confirmed that biodegradable microparticles with entrapped antigen are able to induce potent CTL, since they were more effective than MPL and were comparable to DNA immunization (Evans et al., 2004a). Nevertheless, early studies highlighted above had established that although microparticles were effective for induction of CTL responses in rodents, iscoms appeared to be more potent (Maloy et al., 1994). In a study in nonhuman primates using a recombinant core antigen from HCV, we established the ability of iscoms formulations to induce potent CTL responses (Polakos et al., 2001). Alternative polymers beyond PLG have been used to prepare microparticles which release entrapped peptide in response to low pH within the phagosomes of DC, and these may prove to have advantages for CTL induction, although this remains to be proven (Haining et al., 2004).

■ Microparticles as delivery systems for DNA vaccines

It has been shown repeatedly that DNA vaccines offer significant potential for the induction of potent CTL responses (Seder and Gurunathan, 1999; Srivastava and Liu, 2003). Nevertheless, the potency of DNA vaccines in humans has so far been disappointing, particularly in relation to their ability to induce antibody responses (Wang et al., 1998; Calarota et al., 1998; Seder and Gurunathan, 1999). This has prompted investigators to work on adjuvants and delivery systems for DNA vaccines and also to use DNA in a prime/boost setting with alternative modalities (Schneider et al., 1998; Sullivan et al., 2000; Amara et al., 2001).

An early study suggested that microparticles with entrapped DNA may have the potential to improve the potency of DNA vaccines, although there was no direct comparison with naked DNA (Hedley et al., 1998). Nevertheless, this approach has moved forward and has generated encouraging clinical data in a trial to assess a microencapsulated DNA vaccine against cervical cancer (Klencke et al., 2002; Luby et al., 2004) However, early studies had made it clear that encapsulating DNA into microparticles had several limitations, which were similar to those previously described for protein antigens. These problems included damage to DNA during microencapsulation, low encapsulation efficiency, and minimal initial release of entrapped DNA (Walter et al., 1999; Ando et al., 1999; Tinsley-Bown et al., 2000). Because of the limitations of PLG microparticles with entrapped DNA, alternative polymers have been investigated with improved characteristics for release of entrapped DNA (Wang et al., 2004; Little et al., 2004). However, as an alternative approach to avoid the problems associated with microencapsulation and release of DNA, we developed a novel cationic PLG microparticle formulation which adsorbed DNA onto the surface (Singh et al., 2000). Importantly, cationic microparticles with adsorbed DNA induced enhanced immune responses in comparison to naked DNA and this enhancement was apparent in all species evaluated, including nonhuman primates (O'Hagan et al., 2001, 2004a; Vajdy et al., 2004a; Otten et al., 2005) (Figure 8.1 and Table 8.4). In addition, the cationic PLG microparticles efficiently adsorbed DNA and could deliver several plasmids simultaneously, at high loading levels (Briones et al., 2001; O'Hagan et al., 2001; Singh et al., 2003). Cationic PLG

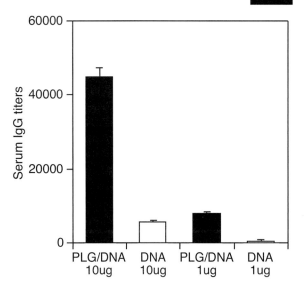

Figure 8.1 Serum IgG antibody responses. These are responses following intramuscular immunization in mice at 0 and 4 weeks with PLG/DNA (encoding HIV p55 gag) at 1 and 10 µg doses, or naked DNA at the same dose levels. Geometric mean titers (± standard error) for each group (n = 10).

microparticles with adsorbed DNA showed protective efficacy in a rodent colon cancer model (Luo et al., 2003a) and enhanced the protective efficacy of a DNA-based tuberculosis vaccine (Mollenkopf et al., 2004). Cationic PLG microparticles with adsorbed DNA are currently being evaluated in a human clinical trial as a delivery system for an HIV vaccine and have also shown significant potential in a nonhuman primate study as a delivery system for an HCV vaccine (O'Hagan et al., 2004a).

Cationic PLG microparticles appear to be effective predominantly as a consequence of the efficient delivery of the adsorbed DNA into DC (Denis-Mize et al., 2000). Following administration, the microparticles are also very effective at recruiting DC to the injection site, and the microparticles also protect adsorbed DNA against degradation *in vivo* (Denis-Mize et al., 2003). The potential of microparticles as delivery systems for DNA vaccines was recently reviewed in detail (O'Hagan et al., 2004b). Cationic emulsions

Table 8.4 The potency of PLG microparticles with adsorbed DNA versus the same plasmids as naked DNA in a nonhuman primate study

Vaccine	Env titer (I mg dose)	Gag titer (0.5 mg dose)	Gag T helper response (mean SI)	Gag T helper (positive responses)	Gag CTL (positive responses)
Naked DNA	49	7	6.4	2/5	1/5
PLG/DNA	11,289	19,256	13.8	5/5	3/5
Fold increase	230	2,750	~2	NA	NA

Cationic PLG microparticles with adsorbed DNA, encoding HIV gag and env antigens, were compared for immunogenicity in rhesus macaques. We evaluated binding antibodies (ELISA) against gag and env, and evaluated gag T helper responses through the mean stimulation indices induced (SI) and the number of responding animals out of five. In addition, we also evaluated gag CTL responses in terms of the numbers of animals responding out of five. Geometric mean titers for each group ($n = 5$).

have also been described, which are able to adsorb DNA onto their surface and to induce enhanced immune responses (Ott et al., 2002). In addition, an alternative approach involving the preparation of cationic microparticles for DNA adsorption and delivery involving an alternative polymer was recently described (Evans et al., 2004b).

■ Microparticles as delivery systems for adjuvants

Simultaneous delivery of antigens and immunopotentiator adjuvants into the same APC population is an attractive concept, which focuses the effect of the immunopotentiator onto the key cells responsible for immune response induction, while limiting the potential of the immunopotentiator to induce adverse events, through inhibiting its systemic distribution and circulation (O'Hagan and Valiante, 2003). Microparticles represent an attractive delivery platform, which can be used simultaneously to deliver both antigens and immunopotentiator adjuvants through their encapsulation or adsorption. For example, we used cationic PLG microparticles to adsorb CpG and induced enhanced antibody responses against a recombinant HIV-1 gp120, which was also adsorbed to microparticles (Singh et al., 2001). Subsequently, this concept of microparticle delivery of adsorbed CpG immunopotentiator has been used to improve the potency of an anthrax vaccine against bacterial challenge in mice (Xie, 2005). Indeed, adsorption to cationic microparticles can be used to make

normally nonactive oligos active as immunopotentiators (Fearon et al., 2003). CpG can also be coentrapped in microparticles with antigens to improve potency (Diwan et al., 2002), or adsorbed to cationic emulsions (O'Hagan et al., 2002). An alternative approach to preparing cationic microparticles for CpG adsorption was recently described, which used polymixin B to construct the microparticles (Marshall et al., 2004).

Tabata and Ikada were the first to entrap an immunopotentiator adjuvant, muramyl dipeptide (MDP), into microspheres (Tabata and Ikada, 1987), and they showed that the pyrogenicity of MDP was reduced by microencapsulation (Tabata and Ikada, 1988). Furthermore, Puri and Sinko independently showed that MDP entrapped in microspheres induced enhanced immune responses (Puri and Sinko, 2000). PLG microparticles have also been used for delivery of coentrapped QS21 immunopotentiator with recombinant gp120 (Cleland et al., 1997). However, the easiest approach with QS21 was to suspend the microparticles containing the antigen in a solution containing the adjuvant, so that it was immediately available to enhance titers (Cleland et al., 1997). Nevertheless, in our own studies, we have shown that codelivery of immunopotentiators in microparticles with adsorbed antigen is an effective way to enhance the potency of immunopotentiators, including MPL (Table 8.5), and with a SMIP synthesized internally within Chiron Vaccines (Table 8.6).

Table 8.5 PLG microparticles improve the potency of an entrapped immunopotentiator, monophosphoryl lipid A, for a Men B antigen, which is coadsorbed to the same particle

Formulation	ELISA titer	Bactericidal titer
PLG/Men B	11,367	512
PLG/Men B + MPL	18,074	2,048
PLG/MPL/Men B	66,493	8,192

The potency of the immunopotentiator monophosphoryl lipid A (MPL) for the induction of binding (ELISA) and bactericidal antibodies is improved by its inclusion into a microparticle formulation to which the recombinant antigen from *Neisseria meningitidis* serotype B is adsorbed. Geometric mean titers for each group ($n = 10$).

Table 8.6 PLG microparticles improve the potency of an entrapped small-molecule immune potentiator (SMIP), for a recombinant HIV env antigen, which is coadsorbed to the same particle

Formulation	Serum IgG titer	Serum IgG2a titer
PLG/gp120	745	25
PLG/gp120 + SMIP	704	10
PLG/SMIP/gp120	11,644	7,039
PLG/gp120 + CpG	8,952	4,163

The SMIP was ineffective as an immunopotentiator for recombinant HIV env gp120 if it was simply coadministered. However, the SMIP was a very effective immunopotentiator for env if it was formulated into the PLG microparticle for codelivery with the recombinant antigen. The SMIP codelivered in PLG microparticles was equally potent with CpG immunopotentiator for the induction of total serum IgG and also IgG2a titers. Geometric mean titers for each group ($n = 10$).

It remains to be determined whether it is more attractive to encapsulate immunopotentiators, to adsorb them onto microparticles, or to simply coadminister them with antigens, and this may vary for different molecules with different mechanisms of action. Encapsulation or adsorption offers the opportunity to minimize the peak local concentrations of the immunopotentiator and to minimize its potential to circulate systemically after diffusing away from the injection site. A reduction in the peak concentration is likely to result in a reduction in adverse events, both locally and systemically.

In addition, delivering the immunopotentiator with a microparticle ensures that it will be taken up efficiently into the APC, the key cells responsible for immune response induction and control. Although both encapsulation and adsorption of immunopotentiators offers the potential for controlled release, the duration of release would be expected to be significantly longer for an entrapped agent. While it may be beneficial to extend the duration of immune activation in some circumstances, in other situations it may be more desirable to have the immunopotentiator available only early in the response induction phase. Hence, simple coadministration might work better for some immunopotentiators, but this might be dependent on their mechanism of action. If the immunopotentiator needs to be internalized into APC to interact with the relevant receptors (TLR, etc.), then association with the microparticle might be preferred. Adsorption might be preferred to ensure maximal availability of adjuvant following uptake into APC. Overall, the optimal delivery formulation for each immunopotentiator is difficult to predict and needs to be determined empirically. Moreover, it is not likely that a single formulation approach will have the optimal delivery characteristics for all immunopotentiators. More likely, the optimal delivery formulation for each immunopotentiator for each application will need to be experimentally determined.

In certain situations, microparticles may also be used in combination with traditional adjuvants, including alum (Singh et al., 1997b, 1998a). In addition, microparticles may also be combined with emulsion-based adjuvants to improve their potency (O'Hagan, 1991; O'Hagan et al., 2002).

Microparticles have also been used as delivery systems for cytokines, including GM-CSF (Pettit et al., 1997) and IL-12 (Egilmez et al., 2000).

■ Microparticles as single-dose vaccines

In the1990s a number of studies were undertaken to evaluate the potential of microparticles with encapsulated antigens for the development of single-dose vaccines, through the controlled release of the entrapped antigen. The objective of these studies was to design a microparticle formulation in which traditional vaccines were entrapped and would be released over time following a single administration, to mimic when booster doses of vaccine would normally be administered. A vaccine that was effective after a single immunization would result in improved vaccine compliance throughout the world, but would be particularly advantageous in the developing world, where access to healthcare personnel can be difficult. The majority of the early work on microencapsulated vaccines focused on tetanus toxoid (TT), although additional work was also performed with diphtheria toxoid (DT), HIV gp120, hepatitis B surface antigen, and human chorionic gonadotrophin (see review of O'Hagan et al., 1998). Controlled-release PLG microparticles had already been developed for a variety of entrapped drugs, including a recombinant protein (Okada and Toguchi, 1995; Putney and Burke, 1998). Hence, there was considerable optimism that PLG microparticles might also prove successful for controlled release of vaccines. However, although microparticles with entrapped antigens were able to induce potent longlasting immune responses in rodent models, it was clear that bacterial toxoid vaccines in particular had significant instability problems following microencapsulation (Schwendeman et al., 1995; Xing et al., 1997). Moreover, although a variety of approaches have been undertaken to attempt to stabilize toxoids entrapped within microparticles, these have generally met with limited success (Johansen et al., 2000; Sasiak et al., 2001; Tamber et al., 2005; Jiang et al., 2005). The formulation modifications applied for the marketed microencapsulated protein product were unique and protein specific, and also required a novel and expensive microencapsulation process (Johnson et al., 1996). Unfortunately, the expense of this process and the limited commercial success of the product resulted in the voluntary removal

of the product from the marketplace in 2004. Recently, it was shown that HBsAg could be entrapped in controlled-release PLG microparticles and induced potent immune responses following a single immunization (Shi et al., 2002), an observation consistent with earlier work on the same antigen (Singh et al., 1997a). The recent study (Shi et al., 2002) also confirmed earlier observations, which showed that controlled-release microparticles work better when they are combined with alum adjuvant (Singh et al., 1997b, 1998b).

In considering the optimal approach for microencapsulation of vaccines, accumulated experience suggests that each protein will present its own distinctive challenges, which may require specific strategies to allow the development of a stable product. Hence, there is unlikely to be a universal formulation approach that can be applied to all vaccine antigens. Moreover, it is unlikely that the vaccine market could support the kind of process that was used to allow the development of the one microencapsulated protein formulation that has reached the market so far. In addition to these significant challenges to the development of microencapsulated vaccines, there are additional problems relating to predevelopment activities, including the suitability of small animal models for assessment of candidate formulations. Although vaccines entrapped in PLG microparticles have induced responses of considerable duration in small animal models, early studies showed that alum formulations could also induce similar longlasting responses (O'Hagan et al., 1993a; Men et al., 1995). Hence, the slow decay kinetics of antibody responses in rodents makes them less than ideal to evaluate the potential of controlled release microparticle formulations, which are designed to provide "pulses" of antigen release, to mimic booster doses of vaccines. Overall, there is little evidence that microparticles can provide *in vivo* boosting of responses, following a single immunization, although many studies confirm that responses can be maintained for extended periods.

An additional problem in the development of microparticles as single-dose vaccines relates to the uncertainty surrounding the question of what is the optimal release profile of antigen to induce long-term responses in larger animals, including humans. Although there have been many claims that a "pulse" of antigen release is preferred, rather than a continuous release profile, the earliest studies on controlled release of vaccines actually showed that continuous antigen release induced high antibody titers (Preis and Langer, 1979). Moreover, many subsequent studies have shown that both continuous and discontinuous antigen release can induce potent immune responses in small animal models (see review of O'Hagan et al., 1998). In our own hands, PLG microparticles with a continuous antigen release profile were as equally immunogenic as microparticle formulations with discontinuous release (McGee et al., 1994). Unfortunately, given their limitations, it seems unlikely that the question of the optimal antigen release profile can be adequately addressed in small animal models. Given these various problems, it is perhaps not surprising that after more than a decade and a half of work, we cannot find any studies in which PLG microparticles with entrapped vaccines have been evaluated in nonhuman primates or humans. In contrast, PLG microparticles with adsorbed DNA vaccines are currently undergoing clinical evaluation and have already been evaluated in nonhuman primates for delivery of a recombinant protein vaccine (Otten et al., 2003).

■ Alternative particulate delivery systems

Several alternative biodegradable polymers, including polyanhydrides, polyorthoesters, hyaluronic acid, chitosan, and starch, have also been used to prepare microparticles for antigen delivery (O'Hagan et al., 1998), as too have polymers that self-assemble into particulates (poloxamers) (Newman et al., 1998), or soluble polymers (polyphosphazenes) (Payne et al., 1998). However, the potency, safety, and tolerability of many of these alternative approaches need further evaluation. Although advantages are often claimed for these approaches over the more established PLG polymers, these are often not clear and are rarely demonstrated in comparative studies. The successful commercial use of PLG in several marketed products and its established safety profile in humans continues to make it an attractive approach, despite some well-documented limitations (O'Hagan et al., 1998).

Recombinant proteins which have the ability naturally to self-assemble into particulate structures are also an attractive approach to enhance the delivery of antigens into APC. The first successful recombinant protein vaccine, against hepatitis B virus (HBV), used hepatitis B surface antigen (HBsAg), which was expressed in yeast as a particulate protein, or a virus-like particle (VLP) (Valenzuela et al., 1982). Subsequently, HBsAg VLP has been used as a carrier protein in a promising malaria vaccine candidate, which recently showed protective efficacy in children (Alonso et al., 2004). A VLP against human papilloma virus also appears highly efficacious as a vaccine candidate, and appears to be moving towards licensure, although like the VLP malaria vaccine, this vaccine also contains additional adjuvants (Harper et al., 2004). Recombinant HBsAg has also been used to prime CTL responses in rodents against HBV epitopes (Schirmbeck et al., 1995) and coexpressed proteins (Gilbert, 2000). Recombinant VLP from the yeast *Saccharomyces cerevisiae* primed CTL responses in mice following a single immunization (Gilbert et al., 1997) and also induced CTL activity in rhesus macaques (Klavinskis et al., 1996). Early clinical trials of yeast-derived VLP had shown them to be safe and immunogenic in humans (Martin et al., 1993).

More recent studies have shown that the potency of an alternative VLP, based on recombinant hepatitis core antigen (HC), could be enhanced by the inclusion of trace amounts of RNA, which binds to the HC protein during its expression (Riedl et al., 2002). Independent studies have also suggested that delivering

CpG with VLP is an attractive way to enhance potency (Storni et al., 2004), an observation which is entirely consistent with the use of microparticles or liposomes to enhance the potency of CpG, which was described earlier. However, the carrier capacity of VLP for coexpressed antigens is often limited to small proteins or peptides, since larger constructs may interfere with VLP particle formation. However, as an alternative approach, larger proteins may be chemically coupled to preformed VLP (Jegerlehner et al., 2002). Large tubular structures have also been described as antigen delivery systems, which comprise a nonstructural protein encoded by bluetongue virus, which can be used to deliver coexpressed protein antigens (Ghosh et al., 2002).

Alternative routes of immunization

Although most vaccines have traditionally been administered by injection with needles and syringe, mucosal administration of vaccines offers a number of important advantages, including easier administration, the potential for self-administration, reduced adverse effects, and the potential for frequent boosting. In addition, local immunization induces mucosal immunity at the sites where most pathogens initially establish infection of hosts. In general, immunization by injection fails to induce mucosal immunity. Oral immunization would be particularly advantageous in isolated communities, where access to healthcare professionals is difficult. Moreover, mucosal immunization would avoid the potential problem of infection due to the reuse of needles. Several orally administered vaccines are commercially available, which are based on live-attenuated organisms, including vaccines against polio virus, rotavirus, *Vibrio cholerae*, and *Salmonella typhi*. In addition, a range of novel approaches are being evaluated for mucosal delivery of vaccines (Levine and Dougan, 1998; Holmgren et al., 2003; Vajdy et al., 2004b), including approaches involving nonliving adjuvants and delivery systems

(see Chapter 14), including microparticles (O'Hagan, 1998; Vajdy and O'Hagan, 2001; Vajdy et al., 2004b).

The most attractive route for mucosal immunization is oral, due to the ease and acceptability of administration through this route. However, due to the presence of low pH in the stomach, an extensive range of digestive enzymes in the intestine, and a protective coating of mucus which limits access to the mucosal epithelium, oral immunization has proved extremely difficult with nonliving antigens. However, novel delivery systems and adjuvants may be used to enhance significantly immune responses following oral immunization.

Mucosal immunization with microparticles

In early studies in mice, it was shown that oral immunization with PLG microparticles could induce potent mucosal and systemic immunity to entrapped antigens (Challacombe et al., 1992, 1997; Eldridge et al., 1990; O'Hagan, 1994). Moreover, early studies involving mucosal immunization in rodents with microparticles also showed the induction of protective immunity against challenge with various pathogens, including *Bordetella pertussis* (Cahill et al., 1995; Jones et al., 1996; Shahin et al., 1995; Conway et al., 2001) *Chlamydia trachomatis* (Whittum-Hudson et al., 1996), *Salmonella typhimurium* (Allaoui-Attarki et al., 1997), *Streptococcus pneumoniae* (Seo et al., 2002), and ricin toxin (Kende et al., 2002). In addition, in early studies in primates, mucosal immunization with microparticles induced protective immunity against challenge with SIV (Marx et al., 1993) and staphylococcal enterotoxin B (Tseng et al., 1995). Moreover, further studies in mice showed that microparticles are one of the most potent adjuvants available for mucosal delivery of vaccines (Ugozzoli et al., 1998). In more recent studies, microparticles have also shown promise for mucosal delivery of DNA vaccines (Jones et al., 1997; Mathiowitz et al., 1997; Singh et al., 2002). Nevertheless, observations in small animal models often do not translate well into studies in larger animals and humans.

The ability of microparticles to perform as adjuvants or delivery systems following mucosal administration is largely a consequence of their uptake into specialized mucosal-associated lymphoid tissue (MALT) (O'Hagan, 1996). Mucosal delivery of vaccines has been undertaken with microparticles prepared from a range of alternative polymers. However, encouraging data with any of these approaches are largely restricted to small animal models, and studies in larger animals have largely been disappointing, including studies in humans (Tacket et al., 1994; Lambert et al., 2001; Katz et al., 2003). Hence, accumulated evidence suggests that simple microencapsulation of vaccines is unlikely to result in the successful development of oral vaccines. Clearly, improvements in the current technology are needed (Brayden, 2001). The overall potential of microparticles and other polymeric delivery systems for mucosal delivery of vaccines has been reviewed previously (O'Hagan, 1998; Vajdy and O'Hagan, 2001).

■ Microparticles as delivery systems for mucosal adjuvants

The most potent mucosal adjuvants currently available are the bacterial toxins from *Vibrio cholerae* and *Escherichia coli*, cholera toxin (CT), and heat-labile enterotoxin (LT) (see Chapter 14). However, since CT and LT are, respectively, the causes of cholera and travelers diarrhea, they are too toxic for mucosal administration in humans. Therefore, these molecules have been genetically manipulated to reduce toxicity (Dickinson and Clements, 1995; Douce et al., 1995, 1997). Single amino acid substitutions in the enzymatically active A subunit of LT allowed the development of mutant toxins that retained adjuvant activity, but showed negligible or dramatically reduced toxicity (Di Tommaso et al., 1996; Giannelli et al., 1997; Giuliani et al., 1998). Oral immunization with recombinant antigens and LT mutants has been shown to induce protective

immunity in mice against *Helicobacter pylori* challenge (Marchetti et al., 1998). More recent studies suggested that optimal immune responses may be induced by combination immunization protocols, involving a variety of different routes (Vajdy et al., 2003). LT mutants have also been used as oral adjuvants for influenza vaccine (Barackman et al., 2001) and model antigens (Douce et al., 1999).

LT mutants have also been extensively evaluated for alternative routes of mucosal immunization, including the intranasal, intravaginal, and intrarectal routes. Of these, intranasal (IN) immunization offers the most promise, since it can be used in all individuals from both genders, induces much more potent responses than oral immunization, and offers easy access using simple commercially available administration devices. On many occasions, the ability of LT mutants to induce potent immune responses following intranasal immunization has been demonstrated (Rappuoli et al., 1999; Peppoloni et al., 2003). Moreover, LT mutants have induced protective immunity against challenge with *B. pertussis* (Ryan et al., 1999), *S. pneumoniae* (Jakobsen et al., 1999), and herpes simplex virus (O'Hagan et al., 1999). In addition, IN immunization with LT mutants also induces potent CTL responses to coadministered antigens (Simmons et al., 1999; Neidleman et al., 2000). We recently showed that the potency of LT mutants for nasal immunization was enhanced by their formulation into a novel bioadhesive microsphere delivery system (Singh et al., 2001) (Figure 8.2). Similar observations were made subsequently, which confirmed the ability of bioadhesive formulations to enhance the potency of LT mutants for coadministered vaccines by the intranasal route (Baudner et al., 2002, 2003). Importantly, we have also shown that the potency of LT mutants as an IN adjuvant for immunization with a second vaccine was not affected by the presence of preexisting immunity to the molecule, which itself is potently immunogenic (Ugozzoli et al., 2001).

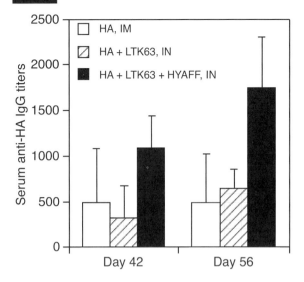

Figure 8.2 Serum IgG antibody responses. These are responses against hemagglutinin (HA) from influenza virus in three groups of pigs immunized at days 0 and 28 with 25 µg HA intramuscularly (IM), HA (25 µg) + LTK63 (100 µg) intranasally (IN), or HA (25 µg) + LTK63 (100 µg) + HYAFF (bioadhesive microspheres) IN. Geometric mean titer (+ standard error) for each group (n = 4).

Adjuvants for therapeutic vaccines

It seems increasingly likely that novel immunopotentiator adjuvants in combination with delivery systems such as microparticles may prove sufficiently potent to allow the development of therapeutic vaccines. Rather than prevent infection, therapeutic vaccines would be designed to eliminate or ameliorate existing diseases, including (i) chronic infectious diseases, including those caused by HSV, HIV, or HCV; (ii) tumors, including melanoma and breast or colon cancer; and (iii) allergic or autoimmune disorders, including multiple sclerosis, type I diabetes, and rheumatoid arthritis.

Generally speaking, the level of toxicity acceptable for an adjuvant to be used in a therapeutic situation is likely to be higher than for a prophylactic vaccine, particularly if the vaccine is designed to treat cancer, or a life-threatening infectious disease. Recently PLG microparticles with encapsulated DNA have been evaluated in humans as a therapeutic cancer vaccine and have shown some evidence of clinical benefit (Klencke et al., 2002; Luby et al., 2004). In addition, cationic microparticles with adsorbed DNA have also shown potency as a cancer vaccine in a preclinical model (Luo et al., 2003b).

Future of microparticles for vaccine delivery

Several recent problems have highlighted the urgent need for the development of new and improved vaccines. These problems include: (i) the lack of success for traditional vaccine approaches in developing vaccines against "difficult" organisms, e.g., HIV, HCV, and *Neisseria meningitides* serotype B; (ii) the emergence of new infectious diseases, e.g., West Nile, SARS, and Hanta viruses; (iii) the reemergence of "old" infections, previously thought to be controlled, e.g., TB; (iv) the continuing spread of antibiotic-resistant bacteria; and (v) the potential use of microorganisms for bioterrorism. The induction of potent CTL responses may be necessary for the successful development of some of these vaccines, but accumulated data show that the induction of CTL is difficult to achieve with protein vaccines. Therefore, DNA remains an attractive approach, which may be used as a priming immunization, in combination with a second vaccine modality, which will be used for boosting, e.g., DNA followed by protein or a viral vector. Nevertheless, DNA needs to be delivered more effectively to improve potency in humans. Preclinical studies suggest that microparticles may have a role to play in improving the potency of DNA vaccines and this is currently being evaluated in a human clinical trial.

Overall, we are entering an exciting and dynamic time in vaccine research in which the principles governing the successful induction of potent and protective immune responses are becoming better understood. At the forefront of this work are discoveries relating to the presence of receptors on innate immune cells, including TLR and others, which recognize the characteristic components present within pathogens. Recognition of the importance of activation of the innate immune system on the eventual induction of antigen-specific immunity has fired enthusiasm to identify the components of pathogens which are recognized by these receptors. Once identified, these components, or synthetic derivatives that mimic their structure, have the potential to be exploited as new-generation immunopotentiator adjuvants. A significant amount of work is underway in this area and almost certainly will result in the development of whole new classes of vaccine adjuvants, which will be able to control and manipulate the immune response in a variety of ways. However, the potency of these immunopotentiator adjuvants needs to be carefully balanced with their potential to overactivate the immune system, which may result in damaging consequences. In this regard, vaccine delivery systems, including microparticles, may have a role to play in limiting the systemic distribution of immunopotentiators following administration. The ability of microparticles to entrap and delay the release of agents may be particularly attractive in this setting and may allow optimal stimulation of the immune response, if the desired release profile for the immunopotentiator being evaluated can be determined. Moreover, the main role of vaccine delivery systems, including microparticles, is to ensure that the antigens and the immunopotentiator adjuvants interact optimally with the appropriate APC to induce the desired responses. Hence the ability of microparticles to perform as a flexible delivery "platform," allowing encapsulation or adsorption of both antigen and immunopotentiator is very appealing. It is likely that optimal combinations of delivery system and immunopotentiator adjuvants may prove sufficiently potent to allow vaccines to be used to treat chronic infectious diseases, autoimmunity, and cancer, but this remains to be proven clinically.

Since the principal problem limiting the use of microparticles for mucosal delivery, particularly the oral route, is the extent of uptake of the particles across the mucosal epithelium, many attempts have been made to specifically target the particles to the MALT to promote uptake (Brayden, 2001; Vajdy and O'Hagan, 2001). However, although this approach has shown some encouraging observations in small animal models, this has not been translated to larger animals or humans. However, novel approaches continue to be applied in attempts to identify the appropriate receptors which can be exploited for vaccine delivery to MALT, including those expressed on M cells (Lo et al., 2002). However, the use of targeting ligands on the surface of microparticles requires the construction of a very complex formulation, which will be required to show dramatic improvements over nontargeted systems to justify scale-up and commercialization. Moreover, the likely expression of different receptors on cells in different animal models makes this concept very difficult realistically to evaluate through a range of species, without changing the formulation significantly in the process. Obviously the inability of small animal models to predict likely outcomes for mucosal delivery studies in larger animals is a serious limitation, making progress in this area very difficult.

■ Acknowledgments

The author would like to acknowledge the contributions of colleagues in Chiron Vaccines to the ideas contained in this chapter. In particular, the author would like to thank all the members of the Vaccine Delivery Group. Thanks are also due to Nelle Cronen for her help in the manuscript preparation.

■ References

Ahsan, F., Rivas, I.P., Khan, M.A., and Torres Suarez, A.I. (2002). Targeting to macrophages: role of physicochemical properties of particulate carriers – liposomes and microspheres – on the phagocytosis by macrophages. *J. Control. Release* 79, 29–40.

Allaoui-Attarki, K., Pecquet, S., Fattal, E., Trolle, S., Chachaty, E., Couvreur, P., and Andremont, A. (1997). Protective immunity against Salmonella typhimurium elicited in mice by oral vaccination with phosphorylcholine encapsulated in poly(D,L-lactide-co-glycolide) microspheres. *Infect. Immun.* 65, 853–857.

Alonso, P.L., Sacarlal, J., Aponte, J.J., Leach, A., Macete, E., Milman, J., Mandomando, I., Spiessens, B., Guinovart, C., Espasa, M., Bassat, Q., Aide, P., Ofori-Anyinam, O., Navia, M.M., Corachan, S., Ceuppens, M., Dubois, M.C., Demoitie, M.A., Dubovsky, F., Mcnendez, C., Tornieporth, N., Ballou, W.R., Thompson, R., and Cohen, J. (2004). Efficacy of the Rts,S/As02a vaccine against *Plasmodium falciparum* infection and disease in young African children: randomised controlled trial. *Lancet* 364, 1411–1420.

Alving, C.R. (1992). Immunologic aspects of liposomes: presentation and processing of liposomal protein and phospholipid antigens. *Biochim. Biophys. Acta* 1113, 307–322.

Amara, R.R., Villinger, F., Altman, J.D., Lydy, S.L., O'Neil, S.P., Staprans, S.I., Montefiori, D.C., Xu, Y., Herndon, J.G., Wyatt, L.S., Candido, M.A., Kozyr, N.L., Earl, P.L., Smith, J.M., Ma, H.L., Grimm, B.D., Hulsey, M.L., Miller, J., McClure, H.M., McNicholl, J.M., Moss, B., and Robinson, H.L. (2001). Control of a mucosal challenge and prevention of Aids by a multiprotein DNA/Mva vaccine. *Science* 292, 69–74.

Ando, S., Putnam, D., Pack, D.W., and Langer, R. (1999). Plga microspheres containing plasmid DNA: preservation of supercoiled DNA via cryopreparation and carbohydrate stabilization. *J. Pharm. Sci.* 88, 126–130.

Bachmann, M.F. and Zinkernagel, R.M. (1997). Neutralizing antiviral B cell responses. *Annu. Rev. Immunol.* 15, 235–270.

Bachmann, M.F., Rohrer, U.H., Kundig, T.M., Burki, K., Hengartner, H., and Zinkernagel, R.M. (1993). The Influence of antigen organization on B cell responsiveness. *Science* 262, 1448–1451.

Barackman, J.D., Ott, G., Pine, S., O'Hagan, D.T. (2001). Oral administration of influenza vaccine in combination with the adjuvants Lt-K63 and Lt-R72 induces potent immune responses comparable to or stronger than traditional intramuscular immunization. *Clin. Diagn. Lab. Immunol.* 8, 652–657.

Baudner, B.C., Balland, O., Giuliani, M.M., Von Hoegen, P., Rappuoli, R., Betbeder, D., and Del Giudice, G. (2002). Enhancement of protective efficacy following intranasal immunization with vaccine plus a nontoxic Ltk63 mutant delivered with nanoparticles. *Infect. Immun.* 70, 4785–4790.

Baudner, B.C., Giuliani, M.M., Verhoef, J.C., Rappuoli, R., Junginger, H.E., and Giudice, G.D. (2003). The concomitant use of the Ltk63 mucosal adjuvant and of chitosan-based delivery system enhances the immunogenicity and efficacy of intranasally administered vaccines. *Vaccine* 21, 3837–3844.

Bird, A.P. (1987). CpG islands as gene markers in the vertebrate nucleus. *Trends Genet.* 3, 342–347.

Brayden, D.J. (2001). Oral vaccination in man using antigens in particles: current status. *Eur. J. Pharm. Sci.* 14, 183–189.

Briones, M., Singh, M., Ugozzoli, M., Kazzaz, J., Klakamp, S., Ott, G., and O'Hagan, D. (2001). The preparation, characterization, and evaluation of cationic microparticles for DNA vaccine delivery. *Pharm. Res.* 18, 709–711.

Cahill, E.S., O'Hagan, D.T., Illum, L., Barnard, A., Mills, K.H., and Redhead, K. (1995). Immune responses and protection against Bordetella pertussis infection after intranasal immunization of mice with filamentous haemagglutinin in solution or incorporated in biodegradable microparticles. *Vaccine* 13, 455–462.

Calarota, S., Bratt, G., Nordlund, S., Hinkula, J., Leandersson, A.C., Sandstrom, E., and Wahren, B. (1998). Cellular cytotoxic response induced by DNA vaccination in HIV-1-infected patients. *Lancet* 351, 1320–1325.

Caputo, A., Brocca-Cofano, E., Castaldello, A., De Michele, R., Altavilla, G., Marchisio, M., Gavioli, R., Rolen, U., Chiarantini, L., Cerasi, A., Dominici, S., Magnani, M., Cafaro, A., Sparnacci, K., Laus, M., Tondelli, L., and Ensoli, B. (2004). Novel biocompatible anionic polymeric microspheres for the delivery of the HIV-1 Tat protein for vaccine application. *Vaccine* 22, 2910–2924.

Challacombe, S.J., Rahman, D., Jeffery, H., Davis, S.S., and O'Hagan, D.T. (1992). Enhanced secretory Iga and systemic Igg antibody responses after oral immunization with biodegradable microparticles containing antigen. *Immunol.* 76, 164–168.

Challacombe, S.J., Rahman, D., and O'Hagan, D.T. (1997). Salivary, gut, vaginal and nasal antibody responses after oral immunization with biodegradable microparticles. *Vaccine* 15, 169–175.

Cleland, J.L., Barron, L., Daugherty, A., Eastman, D., Kensil, C., Lim, A., Weissburg, R.P., Wrin, T., Vennari, J., and Powell, M.F. (1997). Development of a single-shot subunit vaccine for HIV-1: 3. Effect of adjuvant and immunization schedule on the duration of the humoral immune response to recombinant Mn Gp120. *J. Pharm. Sci.* 85, 1350–1357.

Conway, M.A., Madrigal-Estebas, L., McClean, S., Brayden, D.J., and Mills, K.H. (2001). Protection against Bordetella pertussis infection following parenteral or oral immunization with antigens entrapped in biodegradable particles: effect of formulation and route of immunization on induction of Th1 and Th2 cells. *Vaccine* 19, 1940–1950.

Deng, G.M. and Tarkowski, A. (2001). Synovial cytokine mrna expression during arthritis triggered by CpG motifs of bacterial DNA. *Arthritis Res.* 3, 48–53.

Deng, H. and Wolff, J.A. (1994). Self-amplifying expression from the T7 promoter in 3t3 mouse fibroblasts. *Gene* 143, 245–249.

Deng, H., Wang, C., Acsadi, G., and Wolff, J.A. (1991). High-efficiency protein synthesis from T7 RNA polymerase transcripts in 3t3 fibroblasts. *Gene* 109, 193–201.

Denis-Mize, K.S., Dupuis, M., Singh, M., Woo, C., Ugozzoli, D.T., Donnelly, J.J., 3rd, Ott, G., and McDonald, D.M. (2003). Mechanisms of increased immunogenicity for DNA-based vaccines absorbed onto cationic microparticles. *Cell Immunol.* 225(1): 12–20.

Denis-Mize, K.S., Dupuis, M., MacKichan, M.L., Singh, M., Doe, B., O'Hagan, D., Ulmer, J.B., Donnelly, J.J., McDonald, D.M., and Ott, G. (2000). Plasmid DNA adsorbed onto cationic microparticles mediates target gene expression and antigen presentation by dendritic cells. *Gene Ther.* 7, 2105–2112.

Di Tommaso, A., Saletti, G., Pizza, M., Rappuoli, R., Dougan, G., Abrignani, S., Douce, G., and De Magistris, M.T. (1996). Induction of antigen-specific antibodies in vaginal secretions by using a nontoxic mutant of heat-labile enterotoxin as a mucosal adjuvant. *Infect. Immun.* 64, 974–979.

Dickinson, B.L. and Clements, J.D. (1995). Dissociation of Escherichia coli heat-labile enterotoxin adjuvanticity from ADP-ribosyltransferase activity. *Infect. Immun.* 63, 1617–1623.

Diwan, M., Tafaghodi, M., and Samuel, J. (2002). Enhancement of immune responses by co-delivery of a CpG oligodeoxynucleotide and tetanus toxoid in biodegradable nanospheres. *J. Control. Release* 85, 247–262.

Douce, G., Turcotte, C., Cropley, I., Roberts, M., Pizza, M., Domenghini, M., Rappuoli, R., and Dougan, G. (1995). Mutants of *Escherichia coli* heat-labile toxin lacking ADP-ribosyltransferase activity act as nontoxic, mucosal adjuvants. *Proc. Natl. Acad. Sci. USA* 92, 1644–1648.

Douce, G., Fontana, M., Pizza, M., Rappuoli, R., and Dougan, G. (1997). Intranasal immunogenicity and adjuvanticity of site-directed mutant derivatives of cholera toxin. *Infect. Immun.* 65, 2821–2828.

Douce, G., Giannelli, V., Pizza, M., Lewis, D., Everest, P., Rappuoli, R., and Dougan, G. (1999). Genetically detoxified mutants of heat-labile toxin from *Escherichia coli* are able to act as oral adjuvants. *Infect. Immun.* 67, 4400–4406.

Edelman, R. (1997). In Levine, M.M., Woodrow, G.C., Kaper, J.B., and Cobon, G.S. (Eds) *New Generation Vaccines*, Vol. 2. Marcel Dekker, New York, pp. 173–192.

Egilmez, N.K., Jong, Y.S., Sabel, M.S., Jacob, J.S., Mathiowitz, E., and Bankert, R.B. (2000). In situ tumor vaccination with interleukin-12-encapsulated biodegradable microspheres: induction of tumor regression and potent antitumor immunity. *Cancer Res.* 60, 3832–3837.

Eldridge, J.H., Hammond, C.J., Meulbroek, J.A., Staas, J.K., Gilley, R.M., and Tice, T.R. (1990). Controlled vaccine release in the gut-associated lymphoid tissues: I. Orally administered biodegradable microspheres target the Peyer's patches. *J. Control. Release* 11, 205–214.

Eldridge, J.H., Staas, J.K., Meulbroek, J.A., Tice, T.R., and Gilley, R.M. (1991). Biodegradable and biocompatible poly(D,L-lactide-co-glycolide) microspheres as an adjuvant for staphylococcal enterotoxin B toxoid which enhances the level of toxin-neutralizing antibodies. *Infect. Immun.* 59, 2978–2986.

Evans, J.T., Ward, J.R., Kern, J., and Johnson, M.E. (2004a). A single vaccination with protein-microspheres elicits a strong Cd8 T-cell-mediated immune response against Mycobacterium tuberculosis antigen Mtb8.4. *Vaccine* 22, 1964–1972.

Evans, R.K., Zhu, D.M., Casimiro, D.R., Nawrocki, D.K., Mach, H., Troutman, R.D., Tang, A., Wu, S., Chin, S., Ahn, C., Isopi, L.A., Williams, D.M., Xu, Z., Shiver, J.W., and Volkin, D.B. (2004b). Characterization and biological evaluation of a microparticle adjuvant formulation for plasmid DNA vaccines. *J. Pharm. Sci.* 93, 1924–1939.

Fearon, D.T. (1997). Seeking wisdom in innate immunity. *Nature* 388, 323–324.

Fearon, K., Marshall, J.D., Abbate, C., Subramanian, S., Yee, P., Gregorio, J., Teshima, G., Ott, G., Tuck, S., Van Nest, G., and Coffman, R.L. (2003). A minimal human immunostimulatory CpG motif that potently induces IFN-gamma and IFN-alpha production. *Eur. J. Immunol.* 33, 2114–2122.

Fehr, T., Skrastina, D., Pumpens, P., and Zinkernagel, R.M. (1998). T cell-independent type I antibody response against B cell epitopes expressed repetitively on recombinant virus particles. *Proc. Natl. Acad. Sci. USA* 95, 9477–9481.

Fifis, T., Gamvrellis, A., Crimeen-Irwin, B., Pietersz, G.A., Li, J., Mottram, P.L., McKenzie, I.F., and Plebanski, M. (2004). Size-dependent immunogenicity: therapeutic and protective properties of nano-vaccines against tumors. *J. Immunol.* 173, 3148–3154.

Ghosh, M.K., Deriaud, E., Saron, M.F., Lo-Man, R., Henry, T., Jiao, X., Roy, P., and Leclerc, C. (2002). Induction of protective antiviral cytotoxic T cells by a tubular structure capable of carrying large foreign sequences. *Vaccine* 20, 1369–1377.

Giannelli, V., Fontana, M.R., Giuliani, M.M., Guangcai, D., Rappuoli, R., and Pizza, M. (1997). Protease susceptibility and toxicity of heat-labile enterotoxins with a mutation in the active site or in the protease-sensitive loop. *Infect. Immun.* 65, 331–334.

Gilbert, S.C. (2000). In O'Hagan, D. (Ed) *Vaccine Adjuvants: Preparation Methods and Research Protocols*, Vol. 42. Humana Press, Totowa, NJ, pp. 197–210.

Gilbert, S.C., Plebanski, M., Harris, S.J., Allsopp, C.E., Thomas, R., Layton, G.T., and Hill, A.V. (1997). A protein particle vaccine containing multiple malaria epitopes. *Nature Biotechnol.* 15, 1280–1284.

Giuliani, M.M., Del Giudice, G., Giannelli, V., Dougan, G., Douce, G., Rappuoli, R., and Pizza, M. (1998). Mucosal adjuvanticity and immunogenicity of Ltr72, a novel mutant of *Escherichia coli* heat-labile enterotoxin with partial knockout of ADP-ribosyltransferase activity. *J. Exp. Med.* 187, 1123–1132.

Glaueri, A.M., Dingle, J.T., and Lucy, J.A. (1962). Action of saponins on biological membranes. *Nature* 196, 953.

Goldberg, J., Shrikant, P., and Mescher, M.F. (2003). In vivo augmentation of tumor-specific CTL responses by class I/peptide antigen complexes on microspheres (large multivalent immunogen). *J. Immunol.* 170, 228–235.

Gregoriadis, G. (1990). Immunological adjuvants: a role for liposomes. *Immunol. Today* 11, 89–97.

Gupta, R.K. (1998). Aluminum compounds as vaccine adjuvants. *Adv. Drug Del. Rev.* 32, 155–172.

Gupta, R.K., Chang, A.C., Griffin, P., Rivera, R., and Siber, G.R. (1996). In vivo distribution of radioactivity in mice after injection of biodegradable polymer microspheres containing 14C-labeled tetanus toxoid. *Vaccine* 14, 1412–1416.

Haining, W.N., Anderson, D.G., Little, S.R., von Bergwelt-Baildon, M.S., Cardoso, A.A., Alves, P., Kosmatopoulos, K., Nadler, L.M., Langer, R., and Kohane, D.S. (2004). Ph-triggered microparticles for peptide vaccination. *J. Immunol.* 173, 2578–2585.

Harper, D.M., Franco, E.L., Wheeler, C., Ferris, D.G., Jenkins, D., Schuind, A., Zahaf, T., Innis, B., Naud, P., De Carvalho, N.S., Roteli-Martins, C.M., Teixeira, J., Blatter, M.M., Korn, A.P., Quint, W., and Dubin, G. (2004). Efficacy of a bivalent L1 virus-like particle vaccine in prevention of infection with human papillomavirus types 16 and 18 in young women: a randomised controlled trial. *Lancet* 364, 1757–1765.

Heath, A.W. (1995). Cytokines as immunological adjuvants. *Pharm. Biotechnol.* 6, 645–658.

Hedley, M.L., Curley, J., and Urban, R. (1998). Microspheres Containing plasmid-encoded antigens elicit cytotoxic T-cell responses. *Nature Med.* 4, 365–368.

Hemmi, H., Takeuchi, O., Kawai, T., Kaisho, T., Sato, S., Sanjo, H., Matsumoto, M., Hoshino, K., Wagner, H., Takeda, K., Akira, S., and Moingeon, P. (2000). A Toll-like receptor recognizes bacterial DNA. *Nature* 408, 740–745.

Hemmi, H., Kaisho, T., Takeuchi, O., Sato, S., Sanjo, H., Hoshino, K., Horiuchi, T., Tomizawa, H., Takeda, K., and Akira, S. (2002). Small anti-viral compounds activate immune cells via the TLR7 Myd88-dependent signaling pathway. *Nature Immunol.* 3, 196–200.

Holmgren, J., Czerkinsky, C., Eriksson, K., and Mharandi, A. (2003). Mucosal immunisation and adjuvants: a brief overview of recent advances and challenges. *Vaccine* 21, S89–S95.

Iwasaki, A. and Medzhitov, R. (2004). Toll-like receptor control of the adaptive immune responses. *Nature Immunol.* 5, 987–995.

Jakobsen, H., Schulz, D., Pizza, M., Rappuoli, R., and Jonsdottir, I. (1999). Intranasal immunization with pneumococcal polysaccharide conjugate vaccines with nontoxic mutants of *Escherichia coli* heat-labile enterotoxins as adjuvants protects mice against invasive pneumococcal infections. *Infect. Immun.* 67, 5892–5897.

Janeway, C.A., Jr. (1989). Approaching the asymptote? Evolution and revolution in immunology. *Cold Spring Harbor Symp. Quant. Biol.* 54 (Pt 1), 1–13.

Jegerlehner, A., Tissot, A., Lechner, F., Sebbel, P., Erdmann, I., Kundig, T., Bachi, T., Storni, T., Jennings, G., Pumpens, P., Renner, W.A., and Bachmann, M.F. (2002). A molecular assembly system that renders antigens of choice highly repetitive for induction of protective B cell responses. *Vaccine* 20, 3104–3112.

Jiang, W., Gupta, R.K., Deshpande, M.C., and Schwendeman, S.P. (2005). Biodegradable poly(lactic-co-glycolic acid)

microparticles for injectable delivery of vaccine antigens. *Adv. Drug Deliv. Rev.* 57, 391–410.

Johansen, P., Gander, B., Merkle, H.P., and Sesardic, D. (2000). Ambiguities in the preclinical quality assessment of microparticulate vaccines. *Trends Biotechnol.* 18, 203–211.

Johnson, O.L., Cleland, J.L., Lee, H.J., Charnis, M., Duenas, E., Jaworowicz, W., Shepard, D., Shahzamani, A., Jones, A.J., and Putney, S.D. (1996). A month-long effect from a single injection of microencapsulated human growth hormone. *Nature Med.* 2, 795–799.

Jones, D.H., McBride, B.W., Thornton, C., O'Hagan, D.T., Robinson, A., and Farrar, G.H. (1996). Orally administered microencapsulated *Bordetella pertussis* fimbriae protect mice from *B. pertussis* respiratory infection. *Infect. Immun.* 64, 489–494.

Jones, D.H., Corris, S., McDonald, S., Clegg, J.C., and Farrar, G.H. (1997). Poly(D,L-lactide-co-glycolide)-encapsulated plasmid DNA elicits systemic and mucosal antibody responses to encoded protein after oral administration. *Vaccine* 15, 814–817.

Jung, T., Kamm, W., Breitenbach, A., Klebe, G., and Kissel, T. (2002). Loading of tetanus toxoid to biodegradable nanoparticles from branched poly(sulfobutyl-polyvinyl alcohol)-g-(lactide-co-glycolide) nanoparticles by protein adsorption: a mechanistic study. *Pharm. Res.* 19, 1105–1113.

Kanke, M., Sniecinski, I., and DeLuca, P.P. (1983). Interaction of microspheres with blood constituents: I. Uptake of polystyrene spheres by monocytes and granulocytes and effect on immune responsiveness of lymphocytes. *J. Parenter. Sci. Technol.* 37, 210–217.

Katz, D.E., DeLorimier, A.J., Wolf, M.K., Hall, E.R., Cassels, F.J., van Hamont, J.E., Newcomer, R.L., Davachi, M.A., Taylor, D.N., and McQueen, C.E. (2003). Oral immunization of adult volunteers with microencapsulated enterotoxigenic *Escherichia coli* (Etec) Cs6 antigen. *Vaccine* 21, 341–346.

Kazzaz, J., Neidleman, J., Singh, M., Ott, G., and O'Hagan, D.T. (2000). Novel anionic microparticles are a potent adjuvant for the induction of cytotoxic T lymphocytes against recombinant P55 Gag from HIV-1. *J. Control. Release* 67, 347–356.

Kende, M., Yan, C., Hewetson, J., Frick, M.A., Rill, W.L., and Tammariello, R. (2002). Oral immunization of mice with ricin toxoid vaccine encapsulated in polymeric microspheres against aerosol challenge. *Vaccine* 20, 1681–1691.

Kensil, C.R. (1996). Saponins as vaccine adjuvants. *Crit. Rev. Ther. Drug Carrier Syst.* 13, 1–55.

Klavinskis, L.S., Bergmeier, L.A., Gao, L., Mitchell, E., Ward, R.G., Layton, G., Brookes, R., Meyers, N.J., and Lehner, T. (1996). Mucosal or targeted lymph node immunization of macaques with a particulate Sivp27 protein elicits virus-specific CTL in the genito-rectal mucosa and draining lymph nodes. *J. Immunol.* 157, 2521–2527.

Klencke, B., Matijevic, M., Urban, R.G., Lathey, J.L., Hedley, M.L., Berry, M., Thatcher, J., Weinberg, V.,

Wilson, J., Darragh, T., Jay, N., Da Costa, M., and Palefsky, J.M. (2002). Encapsulated plasmid DNA treatment for human papillomavirus 16-associated anal dysplasia: a phase I study of Zyc101. *Clin. Cancer Res.* 8, 1028–1037.

Kovacsovics-Bankowski, M., Clark, K., Benacerraf, B., and Rock, K.L. (1993). Efficient major histocompatibility complex class I presentation of exogenous antigen upon phagocytosis by macrophages. *Proc. Natl. Acad. Sci. USA* 90, 4942–4946.

Krieg, A.M., Yi, A.K., Matson, S., Waldschmidt, T.J., Bishop, G.A., Teasdale, R., Koretzky, G.A., and Klinman, D.M. (1995). CpG motifs in bacterial DNA trigger direct B-cell activation. *Nature* 374, 6546–6549.

Lambert, J.S., Keefer, M., Mulligan, M.J., Schwartz, D., Mestecky, J., Weinhold, K., Smith, C., Hsieh, R., Moldoveanu, Z., Fast, P., Forrest, B., and Koff, W. (2001). A phase I safety and immunogenicity trial of Ubi microparticulate monovalent HIV-1 Mn oral peptide immunogen with parenteral boost in HIV-1 seronegative human subjects. *Vaccine* 19, 3033–3042.

Levine, M.M. and Dougan, G. (1998). Optimism over vaccines administered via mucosal surfaces. *Lancet* 351, 1375–1376.

Little, S.R., Lynn, D.M., Ge, Q., Anderson, D.G., Puram, S.V., Chen, J., Eisen, H.N., and Langer, R. (2004). Poly-beta amino ester-containing microparticles enhance the activity of nonviral genetic vaccines. *Proc. Natl. Acad. Sci. USA* 101, 9534–9539; Epub 2004 Jun 21.

Lo, D., Hilbush, B., Mah, S., Brayden, D., Byrne, D., Higgins, L., and O'Mahony, D.J. (2002). Catching target receptors for drug and vaccine delivery using Toga gene expression profiling. *Adv. Drug Deliv. Rev.* 54, 1213–1223.

Luby, T.M., Cole, G., Baker, L., Kornher, J.S., Ramstedt, U., and Hedley, M.L. (2004). Repeated immunization with plasmid DNA formulated in poly(lactide-co-glycolide) microparticles is well tolerated and stimulates durable t cell responses to the tumor-associated antigen cytochrome P450 1b1. *Clin. Immunol.* 112, 45–53.

Luo, Y., O'Hagan, D., Zhou, H., Singh, M., Ulmer, J., Reisfeld, R.A., James Primus, F., and Xiang, R. (2003). Plasmid DNA encoding human carcinoembryonic antigen (Cea) adsorbed onto cationic microparticles induces protective immunity against colon cancer in Cea-transgenic mice. *Vaccine* 21, 1938–1947.

Lutsiak, M.E., Robinson, D.R., Coester, C., Kwon, G.S., and Samuel, J. (2002). Analysis of poly(D,L-lactic-co-glycolic acid) nanosphere uptake by human dendritic cells and macrophages in vitro. *Pharm. Res.* 19, 1480–1487.

Maloy, K.J., Donachie, A.M., O'Hagan, D.T., and Mowat, A.M. (1994). Induction of mucosal and systemic immune responses by immunization with ovalbumin entrapped in poly(lactide-co-glycolide) microparticles. *Immunology* 81, 661–667.

Marchetti, M., Rossi, M., Giannelli, V., Giuliani, M.M., Pizza, M., Censini, S., Covacci, A., Massari, P., Pagliaccia, C., Manetti, R., Telford, J.L., Douce, G., Dougan, G., Rappuoli, R., and Ghiara, P. (1998). Protection against *Helicobacter pylori* infection in mice by intragastric vaccination with *H. pylori* antigens is achieved using a non-toxic mutant of *E. coli* heat-labile enterotoxin (LT) as adjuvant. *Vaccine* 16, 33–37.

Marshall, J.D., Higgins, D., Abbate, C., Yee, P., Teshima, G., Ott, G., dela Cruz, T., Passmore, D., Fearon, K.L., Tuck, S., and Van Nest, G. (2004). Polymyxin B enhances Iss-mediated immune responses across multiple species. *Cell. Immunol.* 229, 93–105.

Martin, S.J., Vyakarnam, A., Cheingsong-Popov, R., Callow, D., Jones, K.L., Senior, J.M., Adams, S.E., Kingsman, A.J., Matear, P., and Gotch, F.M. (1993). Immunization of human HIV-seronegative volunteers with recombinant P17/P24:Ty virus-like particles elicits HIV-1 P24-specific cellular and humoral immune responses. *AIDS* 7, 1315–1323.

Marx, P.A., Compans, R.W., Gettie, A., Staas, J.K., Gilley, R.M., Mulligan, M.J., Yamschikov, G.V., Chen, D., and Eldridge, J.H. (1993). Protection against vaginal SIV transmission with microencapsulated vaccine. *Science* 260, 1323–1327.

Mathiowitz, E., Jacob, J.S., Jong, Y.S., Carino, G.P., Chickering, D.E., Chaturvedi, P., Santos, C.A., Vijayaraghavan, K., Montgomery, S., Bassett, M., and Morrell, C. (1997). Biologically erodable microspheres as potential oral drug delivery systems. *Nature* 386, 410–414.

McGee, J.P., Davis, S.S., and O'Hagan, D. (1994). The immunogenicity of a model protein entrapped in poly (lactide-co-glycolide) microparticles prepared by a novel phase separation technique. *J. Control. Release* 31, 55–60.

Medzhitov, R. and Janeway, C.A., Jr. (1997). Innate immunity: the virtues of a nonclonal system of recognition. *Cell* 91, 295–298.

Men, Y., Thomasin, C., Merkle, H.P., Gander, B., and Corradin, G. (1995). A single administration of tetanus toxoid in biodegradable microspheres elicits T cell and antibody responses similar or superior to those obtained with aluminum hydroxide. *Vaccine* 13, 683–689.

Messina, J.P., Gilkeson, G.S., and Pisetsky, D.S. (1991). Stimulation of in vitro murine lymphocyte proliferation by bacterial DNA. *J. Immunol.* 147, 1759–1764.

Mollenkopf, H.J., Dietrich, G., Fensterle, J., Grode, L., Diehl, K.D., Knapp, B., Singh, M., O'Hagan, D.T., Ulmer, J.B., and Kaufmann, S.H. (2004). Enhanced protective efficacy of a tuberculosis DNA vaccine by adsorption onto cationic PLG microparticles. *Vaccine* 22, 2690–2695.

Moore, A., McGuirk, P., Adams, S., Jones, W.C., McGee, J.P., O'Hagan, D.T., and Mills, K.H. (1995). Immunization with a soluble recombinant HIV protein entrapped in biodegradable microparticles induces HIV-specific Cd8+ cytotoxic t lymphocytes and Cd4+ Th1 cells. *Vaccine* 13, 1741–1749.

Neidleman, J.A., Ott, G., and O'Hagan, D. (Eds) (2000). *Mutant Heat-Labile Enterotoxins as Adjuvants for CTL Induction*, Humana Press, Totowa, NJ.

Newman, K.D., Elamanchili, P., Kwon, G.S., and Samuel, J. (2002). Uptake of poly(D,L-lactic-co-glycolic acid) microspheres by antigen-presenting cells in vivo. *J. Biomed. Mater. Res.* 60, 480–486.

Newman, M.J., Balusubramanian, M., and Todd, C.W. (1998). Development of adjuvant-active nonionic block copolymers. *Adv. Drug Del. Rev.* 32, 199–223.

Nixon, D.F., Hioe, C., Chen, P.D., Bian, Z., Kuebler, P., Li, M.L., Qiu, H., Li, X.M., Singh, M., Richardson, J., Mcgee, P., Zamb, T., Koff, W., Wang, C.Y., and O'Hagan, D. (1996). Synthetic peptides entrapped in microparticles can elicit cytotoxic T cell activity. *Vaccine* 14, 1523–1530.

O'Hagan, D. (1998). Microparticles and polymers for the mucosal delivery of vaccines. *Adv. Drug Deliv. Rev.* 34, 305–320.

O'Hagan, D. and Rappuoli, R. (2004a). Novel approaches to vaccine delivery. *Pharm. Res.* 9, 1519–1530.

O'Hagan, D., Goldbeck, C., Ugozzoli, M., Ott, G., and Burke, R.L. (1999). Intranasal immunization with recombinant Gd2 reduces disease severity and mortality following genital challenge with herpes simplex virus type 2 in guinea pigs. *Vaccine* 17, 2229–2236.

O'Hagan, D., Singh, M., Ugozzoli, M., Wild, C., Barnett, S., Chen, M., Otten, G.R., and Ulmer, J.B. (2001). Induction of potent immune responses by cationic microparticles with adsorbed HIV DNA vaccines. *J. Virol.* 75, 9037–9043.

O'Hagan, D.T. (1991). HIV and mucosal immunity. *Lancet* 337, 1289.

O'Hagan, D.T. (1994). In O'Hagan, D.T. (Ed) *Novel Delivery Systems for Oral Vaccines*. CRC Press, Boca Raton, FL, pp. 175–205.

O'Hagan, D.T. (1996). The intestinal uptake of particles and the implications for drug and antigen delivery. *J. Anat.* 189 (Pt 3), 477–482.

O'Hagan, D.T. and Rappuoli, R. (2004b). The safety of vaccines. *Drug Discov. Today* 9, 846–854.

O'Hagan, D.T., and Valiante, N.M. (2003). Recent advances in the discovery and delivery of vaccines and adjuvants. *Nature Rev. Drug Discov.* 2, 727–735.

O'Hagan, D.T., Jeffery, H., Roberts, M.J., McGee, J.P., and Davis, S.S. (1991a). Controlled release microparticles for vaccine development. *Vaccine* 9, 768–771.

O'Hagan, D.T., Rahman, D., McGee, J.P., Jeffery, H., Davies, M.C., Williams, P., Davis, S.S., and Challacombe, S.J. (1991b). Biodegradable microparticles as controlled release antigen delivery systems. *Immunology* 73, 239–242.

O'Hagan, D.T., Jeffery, H., and Davis, S.S. (1993a). Long-term antibody responses in mice following subcutaneous immunization with ovalbumin entrapped in biodegradable microparticles. *Vaccine* 11, 965–969.

O'Hagan, D.T., Jeffery, H., and Davis, S.S. (1993b). Long-term antibody responses in mice following subcutaneous immunization with ovalbumin entrapped in biodegradable microparticles. *Vaccine* 11, 965–969.

O'Hagan, D.T., Singh, M., and Gupta, R.K. (1998). Poly(lactide-co-glycolide) microparticles for the development of single-dose controlled-release vaccines. *Adv. Drug Del. Rev.* 32, 225–246.

O'Hagan, D.T., Ugozzoli, M., Barackman, J., Singh, M., Kazzaz, J., Higgins, K., VanCott, T.C., and Ott, G. (2000). Microparticles in Mf59, a potent adjuvant combination for a recombinant protein vaccine against HIV-1. *Vaccine* 18, 1793–1801.

O'Hagan, D.T., Singh, M., Kazzaz, J., Ugozzoli, M., Briones, M., Donnelly, J., and Ott, G. (2002). Synergistic adjuvant activity of immunostimulatory DNA and oil/water emulsions for immunization with HIV P55 Gag antigen. *Vaccine* 20, 3389–3398.

O'Hagan, D.T., Singh, M., Dong, C., Ugozzoli, M., Berger, K., Glazer, E., Selby, M., Wininger, M., Ng, P., Crawford, K., Paliard, X., Coates, S., and Houghton, M. (2004a). Cationic microparticles are a potent delivery system for a HCV DNA vaccine. *Vaccine* 23, 672–680.

O'Hagan, D.T., Singh, M., and Ulmer, J.B. (2004b). Microparticles for the delivery of DNA vaccines. *Immunol. Rev.* 199, 191–200.

Okada, H. and Toguchi, H. (1995). Biodegradable Microspheres in drug delivery. *Crit. Rev. Ther. Drug Carrier Syst.* 12, 1–99.

Ott, G., Barchfeld, G.L., Chernoff, D., Radhakrishnan, R., van Hoogevest, P., and Van Nest, G. (1995). In Powell, M.F. and Newman, M.J. (Eds) *Vaccine Design: The Subunit and Adjuvant Approach*. Plenum Press, New York, pp. 277–296.

Ott, G., Singh, M., Kazzaz, J., Briones, M., Soenawan, E., Ugozzoli, M., and O'Hagan, D.T. (2002). A cationic submicron emulsion (Mf59/Dotap) is an effective delivery system for DNA vaccines. *J. Control. Release* 79, 1–5.

Otten, G., Schaefer, M., Doe, B., Liu, H., Srivastava, I., zur Megede, J., Kazzaz, J., Lian, Y., Singh, M., Ugozzoli, M., Montefiori, D., Lewis, M., Driver, D.A., Dubensky, T.W., Polo, J., Donnelly, J., O'Hagan D, T., Barnett, S., and Ulmer, J. (2005). Enhanced potency of plasmid DNA/ PLG microparticle HIV vaccines in rhesus macaques using a prime-boost regimen with recombinant proteins. *J. Virol.* 79, 8189–8200.

Otten, G.R., Schaefer, M., Greer, C., Calderon-Cacia, M., Coit, D., Kazzaz, J., Medina-Selby, A., Selby, M., Singh, M., Ugozzoli, M., zur Megede, J., Barnett, S., O'Hagan, D., Donnelly, J., and Ulmer, J.B. (2003). Induction of broad and potent anti-HIV immune responses in rhesus macaques by priming with a DNA vaccine and boosting with protein-adsorbed PLG microparticles. *J. Virol.* 77, 6087–6092.

Payne, L.G., Jenkins, S.A., Woods, A.L., Grund, E.M., Geribo, W.E., Loebelenz, J.R., Andrianov, A.K., and Roberts, B.E. (1998). Poly[di(carboxylatophenoxy)phosphazene] (PCPP) is a potent immunoadjuvant for an influenza vaccine. *Vaccine* 16, 92–98.

Peppoloni, S., Ruggiero, P., Contorni, M., Morandi, M., Pizza, M., Rappuoli, R., Podda, A., and Del Giudice, G. (2003). Mutants of the *Escherichia coli* heat-labile enterotoxin as safe and strong adjuvants for intranasal delivery of vaccines. *Expert Rev. Vaccines* 2, 285–293.

Pettit, D.K., Lawter, J.R., Huang, W.J., Pankey, S.C., Nightlinger, N.S., Lynch, D.H., Schuh, J.A.,

Morrissey, P.J., and Gombotz, W.R. (1997). Characterization of poly(glycolide-co-D,L-lactide)/poly(D,L-lactide) microspheres for controlled release of GM-CSF. *Pharm. Res.* 14, 1422–1430.

Polakos, N.K., Drane, D., Cox, J., Ng, P., Selby, M.J., Chien, D., O'Hagan, D.T., Houghton, M., and Paliard, X. (2001). Characterization of hepatitis C virus core-specific immune responses primed in rhesus macaques by a nonclassical iscom vaccine. *J. Immunol.* 166, 3589–3598.

Preis, I. and Langer, R.S. (1979). A single-step immunization by sustained antigen release. *J. Immunol. Methods* 28, 193–197.

Puri, N. and Sinko, P.J. (2000). Adjuvancy enhancement of muramyl dipeptide by modulating its release from a physicochemically modified matrix of ovalbumin microspheres: II. In vivo investigation. *J. Control. Release* 69, 69–80.

Putney, S.D. and Burke, P.A. (1998). Improving protein therapeutics with sustained-release formulations [published erratum appears in *Nature Biotechnol.* (1998), 16, 478]. *Nature Biotechnol.* 16, 153–157.

Ramon, G. (1924). Sur la toxine et surranatoxine diphtheriques. *Ann. Inst. Pasteur* 38, 1.

Randolph, G.J., Inaba, K., Robbiani, D.F., Steinman, R.M., and Muller, W.A. (1999). Differentiation of phagocytic monocytes into lymph node dendritic cells in vivo. *Immunity* 11, 753–761.

Rappuoli, R., Pizza, M., Douce, G., and Dougan, G. (1999). Structure and mucosal adjuvanticity of cholera and Escherichia coli heat-labile enterotoxins. *Immunol. Today* 20, 493–500.

Relyveld, E.H., Bizzini, B., and Gupta, R.K. (1998). Rational approaches to reduce adverse reactions in man to vaccines containing tetanus and diphtheria toxoids. *Vaccine* 16, 1016–1023.

Riedl, P., Stober, D., Oehninger, C., Melber, K., Reimann, J., and Schirmbeck, R. (2002). Priming Th1 immunity to viral core particles is facilitated by trace amounts of RNA bound to its arginine-rich domain. *J. Immunol.* 168, 4951–4959.

Ryan, E.J., McNeela, E., Murphy, G.A., Stewart, H., O'Hagan, D., Pizza, M., Rappuoli, R., and Mills, K.H. (1999). Mutants of *Escherichia coli* heat-labile toxin act as effective mucosal adjuvants for nasal delivery of an acellular pertussis vaccine: differential effects of the nontoxic AB complex and enzyme activity on Th1 and Th2 cells. *Infect. Immun.* 67, 6270–6280.

Sasiak, A.B., Bolgiano, B., Crane, D.T., Hockley, D.J., Corbel, M.J., and Sesardic, D. (2001). Comparison of in vitro and in vivo methods to study stability of PLGA microencapsulated tetanus toxoid vaccines. *Vaccine* 19, 694–705.

Schirmbeck, R., Bohm, W., Ando, K., Chisari, F.V., and Reimann, J. (1995). Nucleic-acid vaccination primes hepatitis-B virus surface antigen-specific cytotoxic T-lymphocytes in nonresponder mice. *J. Virol.* 69, 5929–5934.

Schneider, J., Gilbert, S.C., Blanchard, T.J., Hanke, T., Robson, K.J., Hannan, C.M., Becker, M., Sinden, R., Smith, G.L., and Hill, A.V. (1998). Enhanced immunogenicity for Cd8+ T cell induction and complete protective efficacy of malaria DNA vaccination by boosting with modified vaccinia virus Ankara. *Nature Med.* 4, 397–402.

Schwendeman, S.P., Costantino, H.R., Gupta, R.K., Siber, G.R., Klibanov, A.M., and Langer, R. (1995). Stabilization of tetanus and diphtheria toxoids against moisture-induced aggregation. *Proc. Natl. Acad. Sci. USA* 92, 11234–11238.

Seder, R.A. and Gurunathan, S. (1999). DNA vaccines: designer vaccines for the 21st century. *N. Engl. J. Med.* 341, 277–278.

Seo, J.Y., Seong, S.Y., Ahn, B.Y., Kwon, I.C., Chung, H., and Jeong, S.Y. (2002). Cross-protective immunity of mice induced by oral immunization with pneumococcal surface adhesin A encapsulated in microspheres. *Infect. Immun.* 70, 1143–1149.

Shahin, R., Leef, M., Eldridge, J., Hudson, M., and Gilley, R. (1995). Adjuvanticity and protective immunity elicited by Bordetella pertussis antigens encapsulated in poly(D,L-lactide-co-glycolide) microspheres. *Infect. Immun.* 63, 1195–1200.

Shi, L., Caulfield, M.J., Chern, R.T., Wilson, R.A., Sanyal, G., and Volkin, D.B. (2002). Pharmaceutical and immunological evaluation of a single-shot hepatitis B vaccine formulated with PLGA microspheres. *J. Pharm. Sci.*, 91, 1019–1035.

Shi, Y. and Rock, K.L. (2002). Cell death releases endogenous adjuvants that selectively enhance immune surveillance of particulate antigens. *Eur. J. Immunol.* 32, 155–162.

Shi, Y., HogenEsch, H., Regnier, F.E., and Hem, S.L. (2001). Detoxification of endotoxin by aluminum hydroxide adjuvant. *Vaccine* 19, 1747–1752.

Simmons, C.P., Mastroeni, P., Fowler, R., Ghaem-maghami, M., Lycke, N., Pizza, M., Rappuoli, R., and Dougan, G. (1999). MHC class I-restricted cytotoxic lymphocyte responses induced by enterotoxin-based mucosal adjuvants. *J. Immunol.* 163, 6502–6510.

Singh, M. and O'Hagan, D.T. (2002). Recent advances in vaccine adjuvants. *Pharm. Res.* 19, 715–728.

Singh, M., Li, X.M., McGee, J.P., Zamb, T., Koff, W., Wang, C.Y., and O'Hagan, D.T. (1997a). Controlled release microparticles as a single dose hepatitis B vaccine: evaluation of immunogenicity in mice. *Vaccine* 15, 475–481.

Singh, M., Li, X.M., Wang, H., McGee, J.P., Zamb, T., Koff, W., Wang, C.Y., and O'Hagan, D.T. (1997b). Immunogenicity and protection in small-animal models with controlled-release tetanus toxoid microparticles as a single-dose vaccine. *Infect. Immun.* 65, 1716–1721.

Singh, M., Carlson, J.R., Briones, M., Ugozzoli, M., Kazzaz, J., Barackman, J., Ott, G., and O'Hagan, D. (1998a). A comparison of biodegradable microparticles and Mf59 as systemic adjuvants for recombinant Gd from HSV-2. *Vaccine* 16, 1822–1827.

Singh, M., Li, X.M., Wang, H., McGee, J.P., Zamb, T., Koff, W., Wang, C.Y., and O'Hagan, D.T. (1998b). Controlled release microparticles as a single dose diphtheria toxoid vaccine: immunogenicity in small animal models. *Vaccine* 16, 346–352.

Singh, M., Briones, M., Ott, G., and O'Hagan, D. (2000). Cationic microparticles: a potent delivery system for DNA vaccines. *Proc. Natl. Acad. Sci. USA* 97, 811–816.

Singh, M., Ott, G., Kazzaz, J., Ugozzoli, M., Briones, M., Donnelly, J., and O'Hagan, D.T. (2001). Cationic microparticles are an effective delivery system for immune stimulatory CpG DNA. *Pharm. Res.* 18, 1476–1479.

Singh, M., Vajdy, M., Gardner, J., Briones, M., and O'Hagan, D. (2002). Mucosal immunization with HIV-1 Gag DNA on cationic microparticles prolongs gene expression and enhances local and systemic immunity. *Vaccine* 20, 594–602.

Singh, M., Ugozzoli, M., Briones, M., Kazzaz, J., Soenawan, E., and O'Hagan, D.T. (2003). The effect of Ctab concentration in cationic PLG microparticles on DNA adsorption and in vivo performance. *Pharm. Res.* 20, 247–251.

Singh, M., Chesko, J., Kazzaz, J., Ugozzoli, M., Kan, E., Srivastava, I., and O'Hagan, D. (2004a). Adsorption of a novel recombinant glycoprotein from HIV (Env Gp120dv2sf162) to anionic PLG microparticles retains the structural integrity of the protein, while encapsulation in PLG microparticles does not. *Pharm. Res.* 21, 2148–2152.

Singh, M., Kazzaz, J., Chesko, J., Soenawan, E., Ugozzoli, M., Giuliani, M., Pizza, M., Rappouli, R., and O'Hagan, D.T. (2004b). Anionic microparticles are a potent delivery system for recombinant antigens from Neisseria meningitidis serotype B. *J. Pharm. Sci.* 93, 273–282.

Srivastava, I.K. and Liu, M.A. (2003). Gene vaccines. *Ann. Intern. Med.* 138, 550–559.

Storni, T., Ruedl, C., Renner, W.A., and Bachmann, M.F. (2003). Innate immunity together with duration of antigen persistence regulate effector T cell induction. *J. Immunol.* 171, 795–801.

Storni, T., Ruedl, C., Schwarz, K., Schwendener, R.A., Renner, W.A., and Bachmann, M.F. (2004). Nonmethylated Cg motifs packaged into virus-like particles induce protective cytotoxic T cell responses in the absence of systemic side effects. *J. Immunol.* 172, 1777–1785.

Sullivan, N.J., Sanchez, A., Rollin, P.E., Yang, Z.Y., and Nabel, G.J. (2000). Development of a preventive vaccine for Ebola virus infection in primates. *Nature* 408, 605–609.

Tabata, Y. and Ikada, Y. (1987). Macrophage activation through phagocytosis of muramyl dipeptide encapsulated in gelatin microspheres. *J. Pharm. Pharmacol.* 39, 698–704.

Tabata, Y. and Ikada, Y. (1988). Macrophage phagocytosis of biodegradable microspheres composed of L-lactic acid/glycolic acid homo- and copolymers. *J. Biomed. Mater. Res.* 22, 837–858.

Tabata, Y. and Ikada, Y. (1990). Phagocytosis of polymer microspheres by macrophages. *Adv. Polym. Sci.* 94, 107–141.

Tacket, C.O., Reid, R.H., Boedeker, E.C., Losonsky, G., Nataro, J.P., Bhagat, H., and Edelman, R. (1994). Enteral immunization and challenge of volunteers given enterotoxigenic E. coli Cfa/II encapsulated in biodegradable microspheres. *Vaccine* 12, 1270–1274.

Tamber, H., Johansen, P., Merkle, H.P., and Gander, B. (2005). Formulation aspects of biodegradable polymeric microspheres for antigen delivery. *Adv. Drug Deliv. Rev.* 57, 357–376.

Thiele, L., Merkle, H.P., and Walter, E. (2003). Phagocytosis and phagosomal fate of surface-modified microparticles in dendritic cells and macrophages. *Pharm. Res.* 20, 221–228.

Tinsley-Bown, A.M., Fretwell, R., Dowsett, A.B., Davis, S.L., and Farrar, G.H. (2000). Formulation of poly(D,L-lactic-co-glycolic acid) microparticles for rapid plasmid DNA delivery. *J. Control. Release* 66, 229–241.

Tokunaga, T., Yamamoto, H., Shimada, S., Abe, H., Fukuda, T., Fujisawa, Y., Furutani, Y., Yano, O., Kataoka, T., and Sudo, T. (1984). Antitumor activity of deoxyribonucleic acid fraction from Mycobacterium bovis BCG: I. Isolation, physicochemical characterization, and antitumor activity. *J. Nat. Cancer Inst.* 72, 955–962.

Tseng, J., Komisar, J.L., Trout, R.N., Hunt, R.E., Chen, J.Y., Johnson, A.J., Pitt, L., and Ruble, D.L. (1995). Humoral immunity to aerosolized staphylococcal enterotoxin B (SEB), a superantigen, in monkeys vaccinated with SEB toxoid-containing microspheres. *Infect. Immun.* 63, 2880–2885.

Ugozzoli, M., O'Hagan, D.T., and Ott, G.S. (1998). Intranasal immunization of mice with herpes simplex virus type 2 recombinant Gd2: the effect of adjuvants on mucosal and serum antibody responses. *Immunology* 93, 563–571.

Ugozzoli, M., Santos, G., Donnelly, J., and O'Hagan, D.T. (2001). Potency of a genetically detoxified mucosal adjuvant derived from the heat-labile enterotoxin of Escherichia coli (Ltk63) is not adversely affected by the presence of preexisting immunity to the adjuvant. *J. Infect. Dis.* 183, 351–354.

Ulanova, M., Tarkowski, A., Hahn-Zoric, M., and Hanson, L.A. (2001). The common vaccine adjuvant aluminum hydroxide up-regulates accessory properties of human monocytes via an interleukin-4-dependent mechanism. *Infect. Immun.* 69, 1151–1159.

Ulrich, J.T. (2000). In O'Hagan, D.T. (Ed) *Vaccine Adjuvants: Preparation Methods and Research Protocols.* Humana Press, Totowa, NJ, pp. 273–282.

Vajdy, M. and O'Hagan, D.T. (2001). Microparticles for intranasal immunization. *Adv. Drug Deliv. Rev.* 51, 127–141.

Vajdy, M., Singh, M., Ugozzoli, M., Briones, M., Soenawan, F., Cuadra, L., Kazzaz, J., Ruggiero, P., Peppoloni, S., Norelli, F., del Giudice, G., and O'Hagan, D. (2003). Enhanced mucosal and systemic immune responses to *Helicobacter pylori* antigens through mucosal priming followed by systemic boosting immunizations. *Immunology* 110, 86–94.

Vajdy, M., Singh, M., Kazzaz, J., Soenawan, E., Ugozzoli, M., Zhou, F., Srivastava, I., Bin, Q., Barnett, S., Donnelly, J., Luciw, P., Lourdes, L., Montefiori, D., and O'Hagan, D. (2004a). Mucosal and systemic anti-HIV responses in rhesus macaques following combinations of intra-nasal and parenteral immunizations. *AIDS Res. Hum. Retroviruses* 20, 1269–1281.

Vajdy, M., Srivastava, I., Polo, J., Donnelly, J., O'Hagan, D., and Singh, M. (2004b). Mucosal adjuvants and delivery systems for protein-, DNA- and RNA-based vaccines. *Immunol. Cell Biol.* 82, 617–627.

Valenzuela, P., Medina, A., Rutter, W.J., Ammerer, G., and Hall, B.D. (1982). Synthesis and assembly of hepatitis B virus surface antigen particles in yeast. *Nature* 298, 347–350.

Vogel, F.R. and Powell, M.F. (1995). In Powell, M.F. and Newman, M.J. (Eds) *Vaccine Design: The Subunit and Adjuvant Approach.* Plenum Press, New York, pp. 141–228.

Vordermeier, H.M., Coombes, A.G., Jenkins, P., McGee, J.P., O'Hagan, D.T., Davis, S.S., and Singh, M. (1995). Synthetic delivery system for tuberculosis vaccines: immunological evaluation of the M. tuberculosis 38 kDa protein entrapped in biodegradable PLG microparticles. *Vaccine* 13, 1576–1582.

Walter, E., Moelling, K., Pavlovic, J., and Merkle, H.P. (1999). Microencapsulation of DNA using poly(D,L-lactide-co-glycolide): stability issues and release characteristics. *J. Control. Release* 61, 361–374.

Wang, C., Ge, Q., Ting, D., Nguyen, D., Shen, H.R., Chen, J., Eisen, H.N., Heller, J., Langer, R., and Putnam, D. (2004). Molecularly engineered poly(ortho ester) microspheres for enhanced delivery of DNA vaccines. *Nature Mater,* 3, 190–196; Epub 2004 Feb 15.

Wang, R., Doolan, D.L., Le, T.P., Hedstrom, R.C., Coonan, K.M., Charoenvit, Y., Jones, T.R., Hobart, P., Margalith, M., Ng, J., Weiss, W.R., Sedegah, M., de Taisne, C., Norman, J.A., and Hoffman, S.L. (1998). Induction of antigen-specific cytotoxic T lymphocytes in humans by a malaria DNA vaccine. *Science* 282, 476–480.

Wheeler, A.W., Marshall, J.S., and Ulrich, J.T. (2001). A Th1-inducing adjuvant, MPL, enhances antibody profiles in experimental animals suggesting it has the potential to improve the efficacy of allergy vaccines. *Int. Arch. Allergy Immunol.* 126, 135–139.

Whittum-Hudson, J.A., An, L.L., Saltzman, W.M., Prendergast, R.A., and MacDonald, A.B. (1996). Oral immunization with an anti-idiotypic antibody to the exoglycolipid antigen protects against experimental *Chlamydia trachomatis* infection. *Nature Med.* 2, 1116–1121.

Xie, H. (2005). CpG oligodeoxynucleotides adsorbed onto polylactide-coglycolide microparticles improve the immunogenicity and protective activity of the licensed anthrax vaccine. *Infect. Immun.* 73, 828–833.

Xing, X., Liu, V., Xia, W., Stephens, L.C., Huang, L., Lopez-Berestein, G., and Hung, M.C. (1997). Safety studies of the intraperitoneal injection of E1a–liposome complex in mice. *Gene Ther.* 4, 238–243.

Zinkernagel, R.M., Ehl, S., Aichele, P., Oehen, S., Kundig, T., and Hengartner, H. (1997). Antigen localisation regulates immune responses in a dose- and time-dependent fashion: a geographical view of immune reactivity. *Immunol. Rev.* 156, 199–209.

MF59: a safe and potent adjuvant for human use

Audino Podda and Giuseppe Del Giudice
Chiron Vaccines, Siena, Italy

Derek T. O'Hagan
Chiron Vaccines, Emeryville, California

■ Introduction

When in 1925 Gaston Ramon (1925), working at the Pasteur Institute in Paris, coined the term "adjuvant" to refer to a family of substances capable of enhancing titers to diphtheria toxin in immunized animals, he could not imagine that at the end of the century this would have become such a prolific field of scientific investigation. Nor could he have predicted that research in this area would represent a crucial interface between practical vaccinology and attempts to understand better the controlling role of the innate immune response (O'Hagan and Valiante, 2003). Ramon also established that although a wide variety of diverse compounds had adjuvant activity, only a few were likely to be used without causing serious adverse events. Indeed, among the various materials he evaluated, including sterilized tapioca, aluminum salts, lanolin, tannin, kaolin, and others, only aluminum salts were established for wide-scale use in humans. Additional work in the United Kingdom by Glenny and co-workers further supported the use of aluminum salts (Glenny, 1926).

However, it has subsequently become widely recognized that aluminum salts are not the most ideal vaccine adjuvants, both in terms of quantitative and qualitative antibody responses induced. Indeed, aluminum salts have limited potency for some antigens, and are not sufficient or appropriate to induce protective titers against many important microorganisms. Nevertheless, despite their limitations and despite many attempts over the years to identify alternative adjuvants, aluminum salts remained the only vaccine adjuvants allowed for human use until the late 1990s. The first alternative adjuvant to gain wide acceptance since aluminum salts were first licensed was MF59 emulsion, which was licensed for human use first in Italy in 1997, then subsequently in more than 20 countries, for use in association with influenza vaccine in elderly subjects. The long period that elapsed between the introduction of aluminum salts and that of MF59 was primarily due to the safety profile that adjuvants must show in order to gain acceptance for licensure in humans. Unlike many previous candidates, MF59 met all the required criteria for safety.

■ Initial development of MF59 adjuvant

In the 1980s a number of groups worldwide were working on novel adjuvant formulations, including iscoms, liposomes, and emulsions. All of these approaches had the potential to be more potent and effective than the established aluminum salt adjuvants. However, often these formulations contained immunopotentiators of natural or synthetic origin, which were included to enhance potency. The inclusion of immunopotentiators often raised concerns about the overall safety of the adjuvant formulation. Based on the long history of the use of emulsions as experimental adjuvants, including the widely used Freund's adjuvants in animal models, several groups investigated the development of improved emulsion formulations, which might prove acceptable for use in humans. For example, scientists at Syntex developed a squalane oil-in-water emulsion formulation as a delivery system for a synthetic immunopotentiator, threonyl muramyl dipeptide (MDP) (Allison and Byars, 1986). The Syntex adjuvant formulation (SAF) was designed to be as potent as Freund's, but used a biocompatible oil, which had the potential to prove acceptable for human use. The immunopotentiator class included in SAF, an MDP derivative, was originally identified as the minimal structure isolated from the peptidoglycan of mycobacterial cell walls, which had adjuvant activity (Ellouz et al., 1974). However, MDP was pyrogenic, and various derivatives were synthesized in an effort to identify a potent molecule with an acceptable toxicology profile. Unlike lipopolysaccharide (LPS) and its synthetic derivatives, which are also used as adjuvants (e.g., monophosphoryl lipid A, MPL), MDP does not activate Toll-like receptor TLR2 or TLR4, suggesting a different mechanism of action (Vidal et al., 2001). More recent studies have suggested that MDP derivatives function through activation of the intracellular NOD signaling cascade (Uehara et al., 2005). SAF also contained a pluronic polymer surfactant (L121), which was included to help bind antigens to the surface of the emulsion droplets.

As an alternative to SAF, Chiron scientists developed a squalene oil-in-water emulsion as a delivery system for another synthetic MDP derivative, lipidated muramyl tripeptide (MTP-PE). MTP-PE was lipidated to reduce toxicity and to allow it to be more easily incorporated into lipid-based adjuvant formulations, including emulsions (Wintsch et al., 1991). Unfortunately, clinical testing showed that emulsions of MTP-PE still showed an unacceptable level of reactogenicity, and were unsuitable for routine clinical use (Keitel et al., 1993; Keefer et al., 1996). Nevertheless, these studies highlighted that MF59 emulsion alone, without an additional immunopotentiator, in combination with a recombinant envelope antigen from HIV was well tolerated and had comparable immunogenicity to the formulation containing MTP-PE (Kahn et al., 1994; Keefer et al., 1996). The small droplet size of MF59, generated through the use of a microfluidizer in the emulsion preparation process, was crucial to potency, but also allowed the formulation to be sterile filtered and enhanced stability. Therefore MF59 alone, without the use of additional immunopotentiators, was used in subsequent studies and proved sufficiently potent and safe to allow successful product development (Ott et al., 2000). Hence our early clinical experience with emulsions served to highlight the need for careful selection of immunopotentiators, if it is believed that they need to be included in adjuvant formulations. In addition, the experience with MF59 highlighted that emulsions alone, without additional immunopotentiators, can be highly effective adjuvants for a variety of purposes.

■ Mechanism of action of MF59

Early investigations on the mechanism of action of MF59 focused on the possibility of a "depot" effect, since there had been suggestions that emulsions may retain antigen at the injection site and promote sustained antigen presentation. However, early studies showed that an antigen depot was not established at the injection site and that the emulsion was cleared rapidly (Ott et al., 1995). The lack of an antigen depot at the injection site of MF59 was confirmed in later studies (Dupuis et al., 1999), which also established that MF59 and antigen were cleared independently. Subsequently, it was thought that perhaps the emulsion acted as a "direct delivery system" and was responsible for promoting the uptake of antigen into antigen-presenting cells (APC). This theory

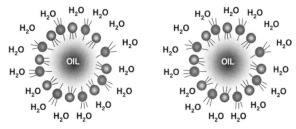

Appearance: milky white oil in water emulsion (o/w emulsion)

Composition: 0.5% Polysorbate 80 – water soluble surfactant
0.5% Sorbitan Triolate – oil soluble surfactant
4.3% Squalene oil
Water for injection
10 nM Sodium citrate buffer

Density: 0.9963 g/ml

Viscosity: close to water, easy to inject

Figure 9.1 The composition of MF59 oil-in-water emulsion adjuvant.

was linked to observations with SAF emulsion, which contained pluronic surfactant, which was claimed to bind antigen to the emulsion droplets (Allison and Byars, 1986). However, studies with recombinant antigens showed that MF59 was an effective adjuvant, despite no evidence of binding of the antigens to the oil droplets. Moreover, an adjuvant effect was still observed if MF59 was injected up to 24 hours before the antigen and up to 1 hour after, confirming that direct association of antigen with the oil droplets was not required (Ott et al., 1995). Nevertheless, administration of MF59 up to 24 hours after the antigen resulted in a much reduced adjuvant effect, suggesting that the emulsion was activating immune cells, which were then able to better process and present the coadministered antigen. Direct effects on cytokine levels *in vivo* have also been observed in independent studies with MF59, confirming the ability of the emulsion to have a direct impact on immune cells (Valensi et al., 1994).

Hence, although the exact mechanism of action of MF59 adjuvant remains to be defined, it appears to function predominantly as a delivery system and promotes the uptake of coadministered vaccine antigens into APC (Dupuis et al., 1998, 2001). However, there does not appear to be a need for the antigen to

be directly associated with the emulsion droplets for them to be taken up. Rather it appears likely that MF59 recruits and activates APC at the injection site, which are then better able to take up, transport, and process coadministered antigens. Nevertheless, further studies are necessary to better define the mechanism of action of MF59.

Composition of MF59

The composition of MF59, which is a low oil content, oil-in-water emulsion, is summarized in Figure 9.1. The oil used for MF59 is squalene, which is a naturally occurring substance found in plants and in the livers of a range of species, including humans. Squalene is an intermediate in the human steroid hormone biosynthetic pathway and is a direct synthetic precursor to cholesterol. Therefore, squalene is biodegradable and biocompatible. Eighty percent of shark liver oil is squalene, and shark liver provides the original natural source of the squalene that is used in MF59. MF59 also contains two nonionic surfactants, polysorbate 80 and sorbitan trioleate 85, with very different hydrophile to lipophile balances, which are designed to stabilize optimally the small emulsion droplets. Citrate buffer is used in MF59 to stabilize pH and the squalene

Table 9.1 MF59 represents a viable alternative to aluminum for a range of traditional and new-generation vaccines

Formulation	DT titer	DT toxin neuts (EU/ml)	TT titer	Men C titer	Men C BCA titer	HBsAg (MIU/ml)	Men B titer	Men B BCA titer
Aluminum	8,568	14.1	31,028	11,117	19,766	9,118	8,143	512
MF59	4,625	4.1	84,922	29,526	32,768	41,211	107,638	4,096

The table shows ELISA and functional titers (toxin neutralization or bacterial cell killing, BCA) for a range of vaccines, including bacterial toxoids (diphtheria toxoid (DT) and tetanus toxoid (TT)), a protein polysaccharide conjugate (Men C), and recombinant proteins (hepatitis B surface antigen and a Men B antigen), evaluated in mice ($n = 10$ per group).

content, since early formulations in water were not sufficiently stable. Although single vial formulations can be developed with vaccine antigens dispersed directly in MF59, MF59 can also be added to antigens immediately prior to their administration. Although a less favorable option, combination prior to administration is often necessary to ensure optimal antigen stability.

■ Manufacturing of MF59

Details of the manufacturing process for MF59 at the 50 liter scale has previously been described (Ott et al., 2000). The process involves dispersing sorbitan trioleate in the squalene phase and polysorbate 80 in the aqueous phase, before high-speed mixing to form a coarse emulsion. The coarse emulsion is then passed repeatedly through a high-energy emulsification step in a microfluidizer, to produce an emulsion of uniform small droplet size (165 nm), which can then be sterile filtered and filled into vials. Methods have also been published previously to allow the preparation of MF59 at small scale for use in research studies, but a microfluidizer is always required (Traquina et al., 1996).

■ Preclinical experience with MF59

Preclinical experience with MF59 is extensive and has been reviewed previously on several occasions (Podda, 2004). MF59 has been shown to be a potent adjuvant in a diverse range of species, in combination with a broad range of vaccine antigens, to include recombinant proteins, isolated viral membrane antigens, bacterial toxoids, protein polysaccharide conjugates, peptides, and virus-like particles. MF59 is particularly effective for inducing high levels of antibodies, including functional titers (neutralizing, bactericidal and opsonophagocytic titers) and is generally more potent than aluminum salt adjuvants. The level of enhancement achieved over aluminum salts is variable and depends upon the antigen and species under evaluation.

In recent studies in small animal models, MF59 was directly compared to aluminum for a range of different vaccines, including bacterial toxoids, recombinant proteins, and protein polysaccharide conjugates. These studies confirmed that MF59 represented a more potent alternative than alum for a wide range of vaccine types (Table 9.1). MF59 has also shown enhanced potency over alum when used in nonhuman primates with protein polysaccharide conjugate vaccines (Table 9.2) (Granoff et al., 1997) and with a recombinant viral antigen (Traquina et al., 1996).

In addition to immunogenicity studies, extensive preclinical toxicology studies have been undertaken with MF59 in combination with a range of different antigens in a number of species. In these studies, it was shown that MF59 is not mutagenic, nor teratogenic, and did not induce sensitization in an established guinea pig model to assess contact hypersensitivity. The favorable toxicological profile established for MF59 in a range of species was used to justify clinical testing for MF59 with a number of different vaccine candidates. There is a general concern that adjuvants and

Table 9.2 Evaluation of MF59 with MenC and Hib protein polysaccharide conjugate vaccines in infant baboons (*n* = 5 per group)

| | Geometric mean anticapsular antibody responses | | | | | |
| | Hib (μg/ml) | | | Men C (IgG titer) | | |
Adjuvant	Post-1	Post-2	Post-3	Post-1	Post-2	Post-3
PBS	0.07	0.10	0.15	25	47	131
Aluminum	0.32	4.7	5.0	111	1,432	923
MF59	0.75	15.1	37.0	668	3,957	4,548

The table shows ELISA responses post 1, 2, and 3 immunizations for antigens alone, adsorbed to aluminum, or mixed with MF59.

immunopotentiators could be themselves immunogenic, which might result in undesirable consequences in some individuals. For example, it has been postulated that the oils contained in some adjuvants have the potential to induce specific antibody responses. MF59 contains squalene, a natural lipid derived from the shark, which is a precursor of cholesterol, and is easily metabolized by humans. In addition, it is well known that lipids are generally very poor immunogens. In our own internal studies, using a very sensitive and specific assay (Matyas et al., 2000, 2004) we have shown that IgG and IgM antibodies against squalene are detectable at very low levels, in normal subjects, prior to their immunization with MF59-adjuvanted influenza vaccines. Moreover, immunization with MF59-adjuvanted vaccine did not induce any changes in the levels of serum antibodies against squalene. Finally, similar low levels of antisqualene antibodies are detectable in the sera of many normal subjects, including those immunized with vaccines adjuvanted with MF59, and those who have never received such vaccines (Fragapane et al., in preparation). These data serve to further reinforce the safety profile of MF59 adjuvant.

■ Clinical experience with MF59 adjuvant

The MF59 adjuvant has been extensively evaluated in clinical trials with several subunit antigens, including those derived from

influenza virus, herpes simplex virus 2 (HSV), human immunodeficiency virus (HIV), cytomegalovirus (CMV), hepatitis B virus (HBV), hepatitis C virus (HCV), and others. Approximately 20,000 subjects have received IM injections of MF59 in the context of Chiron-sponsored clinical trials (Podda and Del Giudice, 2003; Podda, 2004).

The largest clinical experience has been gathered with the adjuvanted influenza vaccine Fluad®, which, after its initial licensure in Italy in 1997, is now licensed in more than 20 countries and more than 15 million doses have been distributed. The adjuvanted influenza vaccine was initially targeted for immunization of the elderly, since conventional vaccines do not provide optimal protection in this age group (Strassburg et al., 1986). For this reason, most of the Fluad® clinical trials have been performed in elderly subjects (Podda, 2001). The adjuvant effect of MF59 resulted in a significant increase of antibody titers against flu antigens compared to conventional non-adjuvanted vaccines (Podda, 2001). The increased immunogenicity was shown to be particularly important in subsets of the elderly population, which have a higher risk of developing influenza and its most severe complications, including subjects with a low preimmunization titer and subjects affected by chronic respiratory, cardiovascular, and metabolic diseases (Podda, 2001; Banzhoff et al., 2003). Additionally, immunogenicity against heterovariant flu viruses was enhanced by MF59, a feature that is particularly beneficial

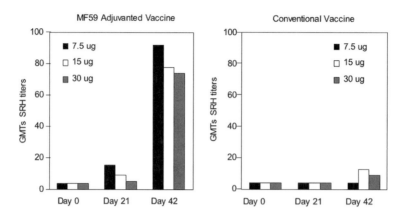

Figure 9.2 Enhanced immunogenicity of MF59-adjuvanted H5N3 (potential pandemic) flu vaccine in humans.

when the vaccine antigens do not match completely those of the circulating viruses (De Donato et al., 1999; Podda, 2001). The increased immune response against flu with MF59 was achieved without affecting the safety profile of the vaccine that, despite a higher rate of mild local reactions, was very well tolerated (Podda, 2001). As expected, given the potent immunogenicity of conventional influenza vaccines in younger adults, the adjuvant effect of MF59 in younger age groups was less than that in the elderly. Again, the adjuvant was shown to be well tolerated, but not necessary in interpandemic periods (Frey et al., 2003). In contrast, immunization of unprimed naive subjects, even young adults, with recently emerged, potentially pandemic viral antigens does not result in good immunogenicity. Hence, it appears likely that the addition of an adjuvant will be required to induce stronger immune responses against potential pandemic strains. For this reason, MF59 was evaluated as a potential adjuvant for pandemic influenza vaccines and was shown to induce a highly significant increase in antibody titers (Nicholson et al., 2001; Stephenson et al., 2003) (Figure 9.2). It is very interesting to note that with the potential pandemic strain, MF59 also allowed a significant reduction in the antigen concentration, a finding that might be very important to increase the production capacity

in case of a real pandemic (Nicholson et al., 2001). Notably, 7.5 µg of MF59-adjuvanted H5 hemagglutinin was significantly more immunogenic than 30 µg of plain H5 hemagglutinin (Nicholson et al., 2001) (Figure 9.2). As already shown for the interpandemic vaccine, broader cross neutralization against heterovariant pandemic strains is also an additional benefit of a MF59-adjuvanted vaccine (Stephenson, 2005) (Table 9.3). This is an important observation, which might favor the use of MF59-adjuvanted pandemic vaccines for stockpiling purposes.

The clinical testing of other MF59-adjuvanted vaccine candidates, including HSV and HBV, provided additional evidence on the safety and adjuvanticity of MF59 in adults (Heineman et al., 1999; Langenberg et al., 1995; Corey et al., 1999). Particularly impressive was the performance of MF59 in combination with HBV vaccine (Figure 9.3). Comparative clinical studies demonstrated an 89% seroconversion rate after a single dose of the MF59-adjuvanted vaccine, compared to a 12% seroconversion rate after one dose of the licensed recombinant vaccine adsorbed to aluminum, with a 100-fold higher geometric mean titer after the full three-shot course (Heineman et al., 1999).

Important clinical data on the use of MF59 as a potential adjuvant for pediatric vaccines

Table 9.3 Cross reactivity of a H5N3 vaccine against different H5NI pathogenic isolates (seroconversion) following vaccination of humans with a plain H5N3 vaccine, or one combined with MF59

Antigen and doses of vaccine received	Frequency of seroconversions (no. and %)		
	MF59 (n = 14)	Plain (n = 11)	P value
A/Dk/Singapore/97 (H5N3) Prevaccination			
2	9 (64)	0 (0)	0.0013
3	14 (100)	2 (18)	<0.0001
A/Hong Kong/156/97 (H5NI) Prevaccination			
2	13 (93)	1 (9)	0.7543
3	14 (100)	3 (27)	0.0001
A/Hong Kong/213/03 (H5NI) Prevaccination			
2	2 (14)	1 (9)	0.7543
3	14 (100)	3 (27)	0.0001
A/Vietnam/1203/04 (H5NI) Prevaccination			
2	1 (7)	0 (0)	0.388
3	6 (43)	0 (0)	0.0128
A/Thailand/16/04 (H5NI) Prevaccination			
2	2 (14)	0 (0)	0.2119
3	10 (71)	0 (0)	0.0004

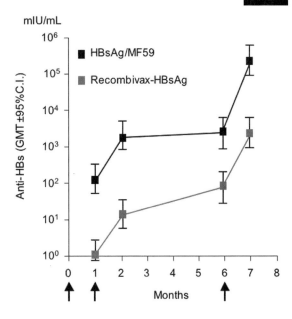

Figure 9.3 Serum titers in humans for HBsAg in MF59 vs. alum-adsorbed product.

have also been obtained, with CMV and HIV vaccines. Seronegative toddlers immunized with three doses of an MF59-adjuvanted CMV gB vaccine produced antibody titers higher than those found in adults naturally infected with CMV. Additionally, the MF59-adjuvanted vaccine was very well tolerated in this age group (Mitchell et al., 2002). The MF59-adjuvanted HIV vaccine was evaluated in newborns, born to HIV-positive mothers, who received four vaccine doses (at birth, and then at 4, 12, and 20 weeks later) (Borkowsky et al., 2000; Cunningham et al., 2001; McFarland et al., 2001). The vaccine was very well tolerated and, despite the presence of maternal antibodies, which might reduce the immunogenicity of a vaccine given so early in life, induced a specific antibody response in 87% of the immunized infants (Cunningham et al., 2001; McFarland et al., 2001). Additionally, the vaccine formulated with MF59 was significantly more immunogenic than an aluminum-adsorbed comparator, as measured by cell-mediated immune responses (proliferative T cell responses) against homologous and heterologous strains (Borkowsky et al., 2000).

In summary, clinical testing of MF59 as a vaccine adjuvant has not only led to the registration in more than 20 countries of an efficacious and well-tolerated influenza vaccine for use in the elderly, but has clearly demonstrated that MF59 can be safely administered with a range of antigens, to diverse age groups, including the pediatric population.

Combination of MF59 with immunopotentiators

Although MF59 is a more potent adjuvant than aluminum salts (Ott et al., 1995), it cannot be expected to be effective or suitable for all vaccines. MF59 works particularly well to

Table 9.4 MF59 in combination with an immunopotentiator, CpG, and E1E2 (HCV) in mouse induces a qualitatively different response to MF59 alone, without CpG ($n = 10$ per group)

Adjuvant	Total IgG	IgG1	IgG2a
MF59	3,475	31,262	3,801
Mf59 + CpG	5,260	3,846	46,747

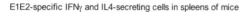

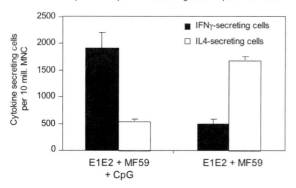

E1E2-specific IFNγ and IL4-secreting cells in spleens of mice

Figure 9.4 MF59 and CpG induces a Th1 response in mice against E1E2 from HCV, while MF59 alone induces a more Th2 response.

enhance antibody and T cell proliferative responses (Ott et al., 1995, 2000). However, it is generally poor for the induction of Th1 responses, which may be required to provide protective immunity against some intracellular pathogens. Nevertheless, Th1 immunopotentiators, including CpG, have been successfully added to MF59 to improve its potency and to alter qualitatively the kind of response induced, Th2 to Th1 shift (O'Hagan et al., 2002). Although MF59 can be modified to promote the association of the CpG immunopotentiator with the emulsion droplets, more recent data suggest that this may not actually be necessary, and similar effects may be achieved by simple addition of CpG to MF59 (Table 9.4 and Figure 9.4). However, careful choice is needed in considering which immunopotentiators to add to the MF59 emulsion and how best to formulate them. Our early experience in the clinic showed that MTP-PE

added to MF59 gave an unacceptable level of reactogenicity (Keitel et al., 1993; Keefer et al., 1996). Fortunately, clinical data showed that the inclusion of MTP-PE was not necessary to enhance the immunogenicity of antigens combined with MF59. Nevertheless, preclinical studies had shown that the potency of MF59 could be enhanced by the inclusion of MTP-PE (Burke et al., 1994).

In addition to immunopotentiators, alternative delivery systems, including microparticles, can also be added to MF59 to enhance potency (O'Hagan et al., 2000). However, the level of enhancement achieved would need to be highly significant, and probably enabling for vaccine efficacy, to justify the development of such a complex formulation.

■ Use of MF59 in prime/boost settings

MF59 can be used as a booster vaccine with recombinant proteins once a Th1 response has already been established by immunization with DNA (Cherpelis et al., 2001). Recently, this strategy has been shown to be highly promising for the development of a vaccine against HIV, since all arms of the immune response, including cytotoxic T lymphocyte (CTL) responses, T helper responses, and neutralizing antibodies, are induced by this combination approach (Otten et al., 2003, 2004). A similar approach of DNA prime and protein boost in MF59 has also shown significant promise in nonhuman primates as a vaccine strategy against HCV (O'Hagan et al., 2004). Alternatively, protein in MF59 can also be used as a boost in animals primed through immunization with attenuated viral vectors. The concept of attenuated virus vector prime followed by MF59 boost has been established in the clinic using canary pox vectors as a strategy for both HIV (AIDS, 2001) and CMV (Bernstein et al., 2002) vaccines. Current studies are also showing encouraging preclinical data with alternative viral vectors, including alphaviruses and adenoviruses (unpublished data).

Future perspectives on the use of MF59

In conclusion, in a very extensive set of clinical studies MF59 has proven to be a safe and potent vaccine adjuvant, resulting in the licensure of an MF59-adjuvanted influenza vaccine in more than 20 countries. In addition, the highly promising clinical data generated using an influenza pandemic vaccine adjuvanted with MF59 have shown that this adjuvant represents an attractive option for the development of an effective vaccine against a potential influenza pandemic.

In addition, the encouraging safety and immunogenicity profiles of MF59 in the clinic suggest that this adjuvant is appropriate for use in pediatric populations. For example, the stronger adjuvanticity for MF59 as compared to alum in newborn infants receiving HIV vaccines could set the basis for further development of MF59-adjuvanted vaccines in this population.

Finally, the large set of preclinical data already available clearly shows the versatility of MF59, which can be successfully combined with immunopotentiators, if required, to enable the successful development of more complex vaccines, e.g., against HCV and/or HIV, which may also require the use of a prime with DNA or viral vectors.

References

AIDS (2001). Vaccine Evaluation Group 022 Protocol Team: cellular and humoral immune responses to a canarypox vaccine containing human immunodeficiency virus type 1 Env, Gag, and Pro in combination with rgp120. *J. Infect. Dis.* 183, 563–570.

Allison, A.C. and Byars, N.E. (1986). An adjuvant formulation that selectively elicits the formation of antibodies of protective isotypes and of cell-mediated immunity. *J. Immunol. Methods* 95, 157–168.

Banzhoff, A., Nacci, P., and Podda, A. (2003). A new MF59-adjuvanted influenza vaccine enhances the immune response in the elderly with chronic diseases: results from an immunogenicity meta-analysis. *Gerontology* 49, 177–184.

Bernstein, D.I., Schleiss, M.R., Berencsi, K., Gonczol, E., Dickey, M., Khoury, P., Cadoz, M., Meric, C., Zahradnik, J., Duliege, A.M., and Plotkin, S. (2002).

Effect of previous or simultaneous immunization with canarypox expressing cytomegalovirus (CMV) glycoprotein B (gB) on response to subunit gB vaccine plus MF59 in healthy CMV-seronegative adults. *J. Infect. Dis.* 185, 686–690; Epub 2002 Feb 2006.

Borkowsky, W., Wara, D., Fenton, T., McNamara, J., Kang, M., Mofenson, L., McFarland, E., Cunningham, C., Duliege, A.M., Francis, D., Bryson, Y., Burchett, S., Spector, S.A., Frenkel, L.M., Starr, S., Van Dyke, R., and Jimenez, E. (2000). Lymphoproliferative responses to recombinant HIV-1 envelope antigens in neonates and infants receiving gp120 vaccines. AIDS Clinical Trial Group 230 Collaborators. *J. Infect. Dis.* 181, 890–896.

Burke, R.L., Goldbeck, C., Ng, P., Stanberry, L., Ott, G., and Van Nest, G. (1994). The influence of adjuvant on the therapeutic efficacy of a recombinant genital herpes vaccine. *J. Infect. Dis.* 170, 1110–1119.

Cherpelis, S., Srivastava, I., Gettie, A., Jin, X., Ho, D.D., Barnett, S.W., and Stamatatos, L. (2001). DNA vaccination with the human immunodeficiency virus type 1 SF162DeltaV2 envelope elicits immune responses that offer partial protection from simian/human immunodeficiency virus infection to CD8(+) T-cell-depleted rhesus macaques. *J. Virol.* 75, 1547–1550.

Corey, L., Langenberg, A.G., Ashley, R., Sekulovich, R.E., Izu, A.E., Douglas, J.M., Jr., Handsfield, H.H., Warren, T., Marr, L., Tyring, S., DiCarlo, R., Adimora, A.A., Leone, P., Dekker, C.L., Burke, R.L., Leong, W.P., and Straus, S.E. (1999). Recombinant glycoprotein vaccine for the prevention of genital HSV-2 infection: two randomized controlled trials. Chiron HSV Vaccine Study Group [see comments]. *JAMA* 282, 331–340.

Cunningham, C.K., Wara, D.W., Kang, M., Fenton, T., Hawkins, E., McNamara, J., Mofenson, L., Duliege, A.M., Francis, D., McFarland, E.J. and Borkowsky, W. (2001). Safety of 2 recombinant human immunodeficiency virus type 1 (HIV-1) envelope vaccines in neonates born to HIV-1-infected women. *Clin. Infect. Dis.* 32, 801–807.

De Donato, S., Granoff, D., Minutello, M., Lecchi, G., Faccini, M., Agnello, M., Senatore, F., Verweij, P., Fritzell, B., Podda, A., Sjolander, A., Cox, J.C., and Barr, I.G. (1999). Safety and immunogenicity of MF59-adjuvanted influenza vaccine in the elderly; ISCOMs: an adjuvant with multiple functions. *Vaccine* 17, 3094–3101.

Dupuis, M., Murphy, T.J., Higgins, D., Ugozzoli, M., Van Nest, G., Ott, G., and McDonald, D.M. (1998). Dendritic cells internalize vaccine adjuvant after intramuscular injection. *Cell. Immunol.* 186, 18–27.

Dupuis, M., McDonald, D.M., and Ott, G. (1999). Distribution of adjuvant MF59 and antigen gD2 after intramuscular injection in mice. *Vaccine* 18, 434–439.

Dupuis, M., Denis-Mize, K., LaBarbara, A., Peters, W., Charo, I.F., McDonald, D.M., and Ott, G. (2001). Immunization with the adjuvant MF59 induces macrophage trafficking and apoptosis. *Eur. J. Immunol.* 31, 2910–2918.

Ellouz, F., Adam, A., Ciorbaru, R., and Lederer, E. (1974). Minimal structural requirements for adjuvant activity of bacterial peptidoglycan derivatives. *Biochem. Biophys. Res. Commun.* 59, 1317–1325.

Frey, S., Poland, G., Percell, S., and Podda, A. (2003). Comparison of the safety, tolerability, and immunogenicity of a MF59-adjuvanted influenza vaccine and a non-adjuvanted influenza vaccine in non-elderly adults. *Vaccine* 21, 4234–4237.

Glenny, A., Pope, C., Waddington, H., and Falacce, U. (1926). The antigenic value of toxoid precipitated by potassium alum. *J. Pathol. Bacteriol.* 29, 31–40.

Granoff, D.M., McHugh, Y.E., Raff, H.V., Mokatrin, A.S., and Van Nest, G.A. (1997). MF59 adjuvant enhances antibody responses of infant baboons immunized with Haemophilus influenzae type b and Neisseria meningitidis group C oligosaccharide-CRM197 conjugate vaccine. *Infect. Immun.* 65, 1710–1715.

Heineman, T.C., Clements-Mann, M.L., Poland, G.A., Jacobson, R.M., Izu, A.E., Sakamoto, D., Eiden, J., Van Nest, G.A., and Hsu, H.H. (1999). A randomized, controlled study in adults of the immunogenicity of a novel hepatitis B vaccine containing MF59 adjuvant. *Vaccine* 17, 2769–2778.

Kahn, J.O., Sinangil, F., Baenziger, J., Murcar, N., Wynne, D., Coleman, R.L., Steimer, K.S., Dekker, C.L., and Chernoff, D. (1994). Clinical and immunologic responses to human immunodeficiency virus (HIV) type 1SF2 gp120 subunit vaccine combined with MF59 adjuvant with or without muramyl tripeptide dipalmitoyl phosphatidylethanolamine in non-HIV-infected human volunteers. *J. Infect. Dis.* 170, 1288–1291.

Keefer, M.C., Graham, B.S., McElrath, M.J., Matthews, T.J., Stablein, D.M., Corey, L., Wright, P.F., Lawrence, D., Fast, P.E., Weinhold, K., Hsieh, R.H., Chernoff, D., Dekker, C., and Dolin, R. (1996). Safety and immunogenicity of Env 2-3, a human immunodeficiency virus type 1 candidate vaccine, in combination with a novel adjuvant, MTP-PE/MF59. NIAID AIDS Vaccine Evaluation Group. *AIDS Res. Hum. Retroviruses* 12, 683–693.

Keitel, W., Couch, R., Bond, N., Adair, S., Van Nest, G., and Dekker, C. (1993). Pilot evaluation of influenza virus vaccine (IVV) combined with adjuvant. *Vaccine* 11, 909–913.

Langenberg, A.G., Burke, R.L., Adair, S.F., Sekulovich, R., Tigges, M., Dekker, C.L., and Corey, L. (1995). A recombinant glycoprotein vaccine for herpes simplex virus type 2: safety and immunogenicity [corrected] [published erratum appears in *Ann. Intern. Med.* (1995) 123, 395]. *Ann. Intern. Med.* 122, 889–898.

Matyas, G.R., Wassef, N.M., Rao, M., and Alving, C.R. (2000). Induction and detection of antibodies to squalene. *J. Immunol. Methods* 245, 1–14.

Matyas, G.R., Rao, M., Pittman, P.R., Burge, R., Robbins, I.E., Wassef, N.M., Thivierge, B., and Alving, C.R. (2004). Detection of antibodies to squalene: III. Naturally occurring antibodies to squalene in humans and mice. *J. Immunol. Methods* 286, 47–67.

McFarland, E.J., Borkowsky, W., Fenton, T., Wara, D., McNamara, J., Samson, P., Kang, M., Mofenson, L., Cunningham, C., Duliege, A.M., Sinangil, F., Spector, S.A., Jimenez, E., Bryson, Y., Burchett, S., Frenkel, L.M., Yogev, R., Gigliotti, F., Luzuriaga, K., and Livingston, R.A. (2001). Human immunodeficiency virus type 1 (HIV-1) gp120-specific antibodies in neonates receiving an HIV-1 recombinant gp120 vaccine. *J. Infect. Dis.* 184, 1331–1335; Epub 2001 Oct 1310.

Mitchell, D.K., Holmes, S.J., Burke, R.L., Duliege, A.M., and Adler, S.P. (2002). Immunogenicity of a recombinant human cytomegalovirus gB vaccine in seronegative toddlers. *Pediatr. Infect. Dis. J.* 21, 133–138.

Nicholson, K.G., Colegate, A.E., Podda, A., Stephenson, I., Wood, J., Ypma, E., Zambon, M.C. (2001). Safety and antigenicity of non-adjuvanted and MF59-adjuvanted influenza A/Duck/Singapore/97 (H5N3) vaccine: a randomised trial of two potential vaccines against H5N1 influenza. *Lancet* 357, 1937–1943.

O'Hagan, D.T. and Valiante, N.M. (2003). Recent advances in the discovery and delivery of vaccine adjuvants. *Nature Rev. Drug Discov.* 2, 727–735.

O'Hagan, D.T., Ugozzoli, M., Barackman, J., Singh, M., Kazzaz, J., Higgins, K., VanCott, T.C., and Ott, G. (2000). Microparticles in MF59, a potent adjuvant combination for a recombinant protein vaccine against HIV-1. *Vaccine* 18, 1793–1801.

O'Hagan, D.T., Singh, M., Kazzaz, J., Ugozzoli, M., Briones, M., Donnelly, J., and Ott, G. (2002). Synergistic adjuvant activity of immunostimulatory DNA and oil/water emulsions for immunization with HIV p55 gag antigen. *Vaccine* 20, 3389–3398.

O'Hagan, D.T., Singh, M., Dong, C., Ugozzoli, M., Berger, K., Glazer, E., Selby, M., Wininger, M., Ng, P., Crawford, K., Paliard, X., Coates, S., and Houghton, M. (2004). Cationic microparticles are a potent delivery system for a HCV DNA vaccine. *Vaccine* 23, 672–680.

Ott, G., Barchfeld, G.L., and Van Nest, G. (1995). Enhancement of humoral response against human influenza vaccine with the simple submicron oil/water emulsion adjuvant MF59. *Vaccine* 13, 1557–1562.

Ott, G., Radhakrishnan, R., Fang, J.-H., and Hora, M. (2000). In O'Hagan, D. (Ed) *Vaccine Adjuvants: Preparation Methods And Research Protocols.* Humana Press, Totowa, NJ, pp. 211–228.

Otten, G., Schaefer, M., Doe, B., Liu, H., Srivastava, I., zur Megede, J., O'Hagan, D., Donnelly, J., Widera, G., Rabussay, D., Lewis, M.G., Barnett, S., and Ulmer, J.B. (2004). Enhancement of DNA vaccine potency in rhesus macaques by electroporation. *Vaccine* 22, 2489–2493.

Otten, G.R., Schaefer, M., Greer, C., Calderon-Cacia, M., Coit, D., Kazzaz, J., Medina-Selby, A., Selby, M., Singh, M., Ugozzoli, M., zur Megede, J., Barnett, S., O'Hagan, D., Donnelly, J., and Ulmer, J.B. (2003). Induction of broad and potent anti-HIV immune responses in rhesus macaques by priming with a DNA vaccine and boosting with protein-adsorbed PLG microparticles. *J. Virol.* 77, 6087–6092.

Podda, A. (2001). The adjuvanted influenza vaccines with novel adjuvants: experience with the MF59-adjuvanted vaccine. *Vaccine* 19, 2673–2680.

Podda, A. and Del Giudice, G. (2003). MF59-adjuvanted vaccines: increased immunogenicity with an optimal safety profile. *Expert Rev. Vaccines* 2, 197–203.

Podda, A. and Del Giudice, G. (2004). In Levine, M., Kaper, J.B., Rappuoli, R., Liu, M., and Good, M.F. (Eds) *New Generation Vaccines*. Marcel Dekker, New York, pp. 225–235.

Ramon, G. (1925). Sur l'augmentation anormale de l'antitoxine chez les chevaux producteurs de serum antidiptherique. *Bull. Soc. Centr. Med. Vet.* 101, 227–234.

Stephenson, I., Nicholson, K.G., Colegate, A., Podda, A., Wood, J., Ypma, E., and Zambon, M. (2003). Boosting immunity to influenza H5N1 with MF59-adjuvanted H5N3 A/Duck/Singapore/97 vaccine in a primed human population. *Vaccine* 21, 1687–1693.

Stephenson, I., Nicholson, K.G., Bugarini, R., Podda, A., Wood, J., Zambon, M., and Katz, J. (2005). Cross reactivity to highly pathogenic avian influenza H5N1 viruses following vaccination with non-adjuvanted and MF-59-adjuvanted influezna A/Duck/Singapore/97 (H5N3) vaccine: a potential priming strategy. *J. Infect. Dis.* 191, 1210–1215.

Strassburg, M.A., Greenland, S., Sorvillo, F.J., Lieb, L.E., and Habel, L.A. (1986). Influenza in the elderly: report of an outbreak and a review of vaccine effectiveness reports. *Vaccine* 4, 38–44.

Traquina, P., Morandi, M., Contorni, M., and Van Nest, G. (1996). MF59 adjuvant enhances the antibody response to recombinant hepatitis B surface antigen vaccine in primates. *J. Infect. Dis.* 174, 1168–1175.

Uehara, A., Yang, S., Fujimoto, Y., Fukase, K., Kusumoto, S., Shibata, K., Sugawara, S., and Takada, H. (2005). Muramyldipeptide and diaminopimelic acid-containing desmuramylpeptides in combination with chemically synthesized Toll-like receptor agonists synergistically induced production of interleukin-8 in a NOD2- and NOD1-dependent manner, respectively, in human monocytic cells in culture. *Cell Microbiol.* 7, 53–61.

Valensi, J.P., Carlson, J.R., and Van Nest, G.A. (1994). Systemic cytokine profiles in BALB/c mice immunized with trivalent influenza vaccine containing MF59 oil emulsion and other advanced adjuvants. *J. Immunol.* 153, 4029–4039.

Vidal, V.F., Casteran, N., Riendeau, C.J., Kornfeld, H., Darcissac, E.C., Capron, A., and Bahr, G.M. (2001). Macrophage stimulation with Murabutide, an HIV-suppressive muramyl peptide derivative, selectively activates extracellular signal-regulated kinases 1 and 2, C/EBPbeta and STAT1: role of CD14 and Toll-like receptors 2 and 4. *Eur. J. Immunol.* 31, 1962–1971.

Wintsch, J., Chaignat, C.L., Braun, D.G., Jeannet, M., Stalder, H., Abrignani, S., Montagna, D., Clavijo, F., Moret, P., Dayer, J.M. et al. (1991). Safety and immunogenicity of a genetically engineered human immunodeficiency virus vaccine. *J. Infect. Dis.* 163, 219–225.

Development and evaluation of AS04, a novel and improved adjuvant system containing MPL and aluminum salt

Nathalie Garçon, Marcelle Van Mechelen, and Martine Wettendorff
GlaxoSmithKline Biologicals, Rixensart, Belgium

■ Introduction

Vaccines represent one of the safest and most cost-saving medical products that have ever been developed for healthcare. They have allowed the eradication of an infectious disease, smallpox, and reduced dramatically morbidity and mortality due to other infectious diseases over the past two centuries. First-generation vaccines were based on replicating (e.g., polio, mumps, measles, or rubella vaccines), non-replicating attenuated pathogens, or whole inactivated microorganisms (e.g., cholera, pertussis, influenza, or rabies vaccines). Second-generation vaccines used highly purified pathogen-derived antigens combined with aluminum salts (tetanus, diphtheria, pertussis vaccines). Introduction of improved production methods and attempts to increase the safety profile of vaccines has led to the development of third-generation vaccines using purified subunit antigens (acellular pertussis vaccines) or subunit proteins as vaccine antigens, produced by recombinant technology (hepatitis B vaccine). It appeared quickly, however, that by decreasing the risk of toxicity, some antigens required the presence of adjuvants for the induction of a potent and more complete immune response.

Adjuvants have been developed since the early 1920s with the introduction of aluminum salts which are known to significantly increase the humoral response to vaccine antigens. Formulating antigens with selected adjuvants composed of immunostimulants, vehicles, or a combination thereof is a likely way to achieve the goal of specific targeting of the immune responses. Among those novel

Trademark information: Engerix-B, Fendrix, Simplirix, and Cervarix are trademarks of GlaxoSmithKline Biologicals SA, Rixensart, Belgium; MPL is a trademark of Corixa Inc., MO, USA; Inflexal is a trademark of Berna Biotech AG Bern, Switzerland; Fluad is a trademark of Chiron S.r.l., Siena, Italy.

vaccine adjuvants and antigen delivery systems, some are licensed for specific indications, such as virosomes or MF59 used in certain influenza vaccines (Inflexal, Berna; Fluad, Chiron) or AS04 employed in a new hepatitis B vaccine designed for hemodialysis patients (Fendrix, GlaxoSmithKline Biologicals), while others are awaiting registration or are still in the early development phase.

AS04 adjuvant system

During the past decade, GlaxoSmithKline Biologicals (GSK Bio) has been developing new adjuvant systems (AS) intended to promote a faster, stronger, and longer protection through induction of high and persistent antibody titers and induction of cell-mediated immunity (CMI). One such proprietary adjuvant system, AS04, has been developed for prophylactic vaccines. AS04 is composed of an antigen carrier (aluminum salt) and an immunostimulant, 3'-deacylated monophosphoryl lipid A (MPL, Corixa, MO, USA).

Aluminum salt adjuvant

Until recently, aluminum salts were the only adjuvants approved for use in humans. Adjuvants based on aluminum hydroxide and aluminum phosphate are the most commonly used compounds and are recognized to enhance antibody response and to stimulate a type II cellular response.

Although the fundamental mode of action of aluminum salts has not been established yet, the hypothesis of an aluminum/antigen depot formed at the site of injection followed by slow release is largely accepted. Adsorption of protein antigens to aluminum salt is considered to be a very important mechanism for the function of these adjuvants. Soluble antigens may, after adsorption, be presented to the immunocompetent cells as particulate antigens. Particulate antigens are inherently more immunogenic than soluble molecules and could facilitate antigen targeting and uptake by antigen-presenting cells (APC). This was

first proposed by Glenny who suggested that the function of aluminum salt was to enable slow release of the antigen and allow delay in clearance from the injection site (Glenny et al., 1931). Antigen adsorption to aluminum salt depends on the surface charge of the molecules, anionic ligand exchange (Hem and White, 1984), or other intermolecular binding forces, including hydrophilic/hydrophobic interaction (Al-Shakhshir et al., 1995). Each binding force may play its role in a given antigen/adjuvant combination depending on the nature of the molecule and the chemical environment (pH, ionic strength, presence of surfactants, etc.). The importance of a depot effect induced by aluminum salts was challenged by Holt (1950), who demonstrated that surgical excision of the aluminum from the injection site did not modify the immune response. Similar conclusions have been drawn recently by Hem and co-workers based on the observation that the combination of selected protein with aluminum salt, without adsorption, also increased the humoral response (Iyer et al., 2003), suggesting that *in situ* adsorption may not be critical for the induction of the immune response.

The effect of aluminum adjuvants at the cellular and cytokine level is very complex and not fully understood. Induction of the immune response by recruitment of immunocompetent cells would be the expected reaction to occur following injection (World Health Organization, 1976). It is not clear, however, whether the antigens associated with the aluminum salt are being taken up by APC or whether they freely migrate to the draining lymph nodes. Results obtained with mice suggest that aluminum salts optimize APC function. They induce an immune response presenting a Th2 bias via induction of interleukin (IL)-4 production by myeloid cell population which plays a key role in promoting humoral response (Jordan et al., 2004). There is no clear evidence to date that aluminum adjuvants are capable of inducing major histocompatibility complex (MHC) class I restricted T cells.

| No. of Fatty | Position | | |
Acids	A	B	C
6	$C_{14}(OC_{14})$	$C_{14}(OC_{12})$	$C_{14}(OC_{16})$
5	$C_{14}(OC_{14})$	$C_{14}(OC_{12})$	$C_{14}OH$
	$C_{14}OH$	$C_{14}(OC_{12})$	$C_{14}(OC_{16})$
	$\Delta\text{-}C_{14}$	$C_{14}(OC_{12})$	$C_{14}(OC_{16})$
4	$C_{14}OH$	$C_{14}(OC_{12})$	$C_{14}OH$
	$\Delta\text{-}C_{14}$	$C_{14}(OC_{12})$	$C_{14}(OC_{16})$
	H	$C_{14}(OC_{12})$	$C_{14}(OC_{16})$
3	H	$C_{14}(OC_{12})$	$C_{14}OH$

Figure 10.1 3-Deacylated monophosphoryl lipid A. MPL isolated from bacterial cell walls is a detoxified form of lipid A derived from the lipopolysaccharide of *Salmonella minnesota* R595. It is a mixture of congeners containing a β-1′,6-linked disaccharide of 2-deoxy-2-aminoglucose, phosphorylated at the 4′ position. Fatty hydroxyacyl or acyloxyacyl groups are variably substituted at the 2,2′ and 3′ positions resulting in total fatty acyl groups varying between 3 and 6. The average molecular weight is 1718.
$C_{14}(OC_{16})$ = 3-(R)-hexadecanoyloxytetradecanoic acid; $C_{14}(OC_{14})$ = 3-(R)-tetradecanoyloxytetradecanoic acid; $C_{14}(OC_{12})$ = 3-(R)-dodecanoyloxytetradecanoic acid; $C_{14}OH$ = 3-(R)-hydroxytetradecanoic acid; $\Delta\text{-}C_{14}$ = tetradecanoic acid.

■ Monophosphoryl lipid A adjuvant

MPL is a purified, nontoxic endotoxin derivative of the lipopolysaccharide (LPS) of the R595 strain of *Salmonella minnesota*. LPS are a group of structurally related complex molecules that are located exclusively on the outer leaflet of the outer membrane of Gram-negative bacteria. Lipid A, the lipid domain found in all bacterial LPS, is responsible for their biological properties. LPS and lipid A have long been known for their strong adjuvant effects. Johnson et al. (1956) reported a 30-fold difference in antitoxin titers in rabbits after three intradermal injections of diphtheria toxoid given at a three-day interval with or without LPS. The high toxicity observed, however, excluded its use in a vaccine formulation. It was shown in the late 1980s that detoxification of the molecule was possible through successive treatment of *S. minnesota* strain R595 with acid and basic solutions (Myers et al., 1990). MPL (Figure 10.1), the product of this detoxification process, presents essentially the same immunostimulatory properties as lipid A but is considerably less toxic than the parent molecule. The reduced endotoxicity of MPL compared with LPS has been related to its lower ability to induce proinflammatory cytokines. Higher levels of IL-10 are reported to be induced in mouse peritoneal macrophages by MPL compared to LPS, which might contribute to the reduced production of inflammatory cytokines observed with MPL and hence to its improved tolerance (Henricson et al., 1990; Salkowski et al., 1997). The development of detoxified LPS, which in the final form contains a mixture of closely related MPL species featuring between 3 and 6 fatty acid

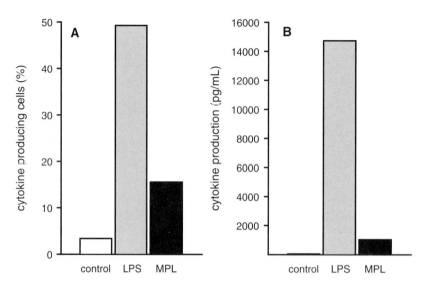

Figure 10.2 Stimulation of TNF-α expression and TNF-α production by MPL or LPS. (A) TNF-α expression was assessed on human CD14 population. PBMC from healthy volunteers were cultured for 6 hours in the presence of MPL (10 μg/ml) or LPS (0.1 μg/ml). The frequency of TNF-α -producing CD14+ cells was measured by intracellular staining and flow cytometry analysis. (B) TNF-α production was measured by the U-937 bioassay. A human U937 monocytic cell line (ATCC, CRL-1593.2) was cultured in 10% FCS-RPMI medium $(5 \times 10^5$ cells/ml) in 24-well culture plates and differentiated into macrophage-like cells in the presence of phorbol myristate acetate (PMA, 30 ng/ml) for 72 hours. Following stimulation, the cells were washed with medium, resuspended in the presence of MPL (10 μg/ml per well) or LPS (100 ng/ml per well), and incubated for 4 hours. Quantitation of TNF-α in the supernatants was performed by ELISA.

moieties (congeners), gave rise to the design of new vaccines based on recombinant antigens. MPL has been employed in many clinical trials, conducted with therapeutic and prophylactic vaccines designed for various diseases, including infectious diseases, cancer, or allergy. MPL-based vaccines demonstrated promising efficacy and a good safety profile.

■ Mechanism of action of MPL

Further understanding of the innate immune mechanisms has allowed the identification of receptors specific for pathogen-associated molecular patterns at the surface of epithelial cells, macrophages, and dendritic cells (DC) that play a key role in the host's first line of defense against infections. Resident macrophages and immature DC have the ability to capture pathogens, process antigen, and express peptide in association with MHC class I and class II molecules. Upon stimulation by pathogen-associated molecules, an immediate cascade of host defense takes place, leading to the activation of APC and the secretion of

inflammatory cytokines by macrophages and DC and to the secretion of chemokines by macrophages. This process allows the maturation of DC into potent APC that migrate to the draining lymph nodes where they stimulate naive T and B lymphocytes of the adaptive immune system. Among the pattern recognition receptors, the Toll-like receptor (TLR) family has been shown to recognize highly conserved microbial components common to large classes of pathogens, such as LPS from Gram-negative bacteria. TLRs play a key role in the stimulation of the innate response required for the induction of an optimal T and B cells response.

LPS and MPL both activate defense mechanisms that involve cells of the monocytic lineage to release a variety of inflammatory mediators such as tumor necrosis factor (TNF)-α and IL-6 (Matsuura et al., 1999). Like LPS, MPL acts through TLR4 binding, leading to an activation pattern similar to the pattern induced by LPS although at a lower level (Figure 10.2). TLR4 involvement in the cellular response to MPL was demonstrated *in vitro* by blocking MPL stimulation of human peripheral blood mononuclear cells (PBMC) in the presence of competing monoclonal antibodies (mAbs) specific to the receptor. In contrast to Martin et al. (2003), several other research groups confirmed that TLR4, but not TLR2, is involved in signalling by LPS or derivatives thereof (Hirschfeld et al., 2000; Tapping et al., 2000).

■ AS04 formulation process

Bulk material of MPL is produced from the lyophilized form of the triethylamine salt. MPL powder is resuspended in water and processed to reach a particle size (as measured by photon correlation light scattering) that allows sterile filtration. The resulting solution is stable over time, both in terms of particle size and chemical composition. Quantification of MPL is performed by HPLC, which allows assessment of the various congener fractions present.

MPL is adsorbed on preformed aluminum salt according to the standard method of adsorption which has almost completely replaced the former coprecipitation method applied in vaccine preparations, where aluminum salt was produced *in situ* in the presence of the antigen. Use of preformed aluminum hydroxide- or aluminum phosphate-hydrated gels has allowed the control of antigen adsorption while limiting/eliminating the risk of heterogeneous protein complex formation observed with the coprecipitation method. Preformed gels can be produced by well-defined and standardized processes with respect to chemical structure and particle size. MPL is mixed with aluminum salt at room temperature (aluminum phosphate or aluminum hydroxide depending on the vaccine considered), and allowed to adsorb. As for LPS (Shi et al., 2001b), the binding affinity to aluminum hydroxide is much stronger than to aluminum phosphate. Due to the high affinity of MPL for the hydroxyl salt, the adsorbed fraction of MPL is quantified without prior desorption from aluminum hydroxide by gas

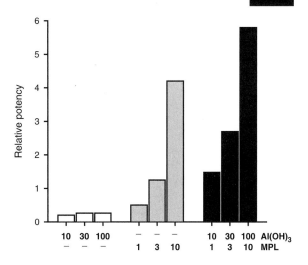

Figure 10.3 Functionality of MPL measured by the U937 cell bioassay. Functionality of MPL was assessed by the U937 cell bioassay coupled with ELISA. U937 cells were cultured as described in the caption to Figure 10.2B. Cells were incubated in the presence of various doses of $Al(OH)_3$, MPL, or both (AS04) for 6 hours. TNF-α secretion by activated cells was induced by the TLR4 agonist MPL in a dose-responsive manner. Response is expressed as a relative potency compared to an internal MPL reference (10 µg/ml).

chromatography/mass spectrometry (GC/MS). Under these conditions, MPL maintains its capacity to act as a TLR4 agonist, as demonstrated in the U937 *in vitro* test, resulting in the same TNF-α secretion profile as with soluble MPL (Figure 10.3).

■ MPL dose selection

Due to its hydrophobic nature, MPL tends to form particles of different sizes in aqueous solution. The optimum size and dose of MPL for its use as vaccine adjuvant, in conjunction with aluminum salt, was determined in preclinical experiments using hepatitis B surface antigen as model antigen. Experiments in mice assessing different doses and various forms of MPL particles ranging from approximately 100 to 500 nm in size revealed that both parameters had an impact on the humoral response. Small-sized particles (100 nm) induced a dose-dependent effect up to 50 µg of MPL, while the antibody response obtained with bigger MPL particles (500 nm) was reduced and was

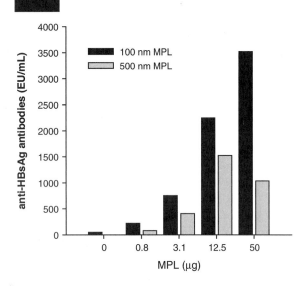

Figure 10.4 Antibody response to HBsAg induced by MPL in mice. Groups of 10 BalbC mice were immunized at day 0 and 15 by the intrafootpad route with 70 μl of the vaccine formulation corresponding to 1/7 of the human dose and different amounts of MPL (the human dose equivalents per 0.5 ml are 500 μg aluminum hydroxide, 20 μg hepatitis B surface antigen (HBsAg), and MPL as indicated in the figure). Anti-HBsAg IgG2a antibodies were measured by ELISA seven days after the second vaccination and are expressed as midpoint titers.

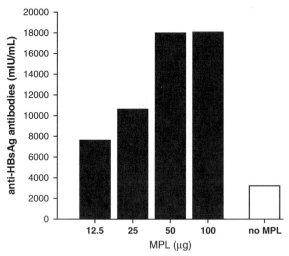

Figure 10.5 Effect of MPL dose on the humoral response in humans. Hepatitis B/AS04 vaccines, containing different concentrations of MPL, 500 μg of aluminum salt, and 20 μg of HBsAg (hepatitis B surface antigen), were administered to healthy adults (18–40 years of age) following a 0, 6 month immunization schedule, and were compared with a hepatitis B vaccine devoid of MPL given in a three-dose regimen (0, 1, 6 months). Anti-HBsAg antibodies were measured by ELISA in postvaccination blood samples at study month 7 and are expressed as geometric mean titers (GMT; mIU/ml).

shown to form a bell-shaped concentration–response curve with a maximum effect at 12.5 μg of MPL (Figure 10.4). These data were confirmed in a guinea pig challenge model of intravaginal herpes simplex virus infection (not shown) where highest protection was induced with MPL at a particle size of <200 nm. The optimal dose of MPL for human AS04-based vaccines was assessed in two open, randomized trials conducted in healthy adults, which compared the immunogenicity of four different hepatitis B formulations. Upon completion of the vaccination course, all subjects were seropositive against hepatitis B and antibody titers obtained with all AS04-based formulations were at least two times higher than with the aluminum salt-based vaccine (Figure 10.5). Moreover, the effect of MPL in the AS04-based vaccine was dose-related, with a maximum antibody response observed at 50 μg MPL (Figure 10.5). Based on the preclinical and clinical evaluations, the AS04 formulations selected for

clinical applications for adults use MPL particles with a maximum size of 200 nm at a concentration of 50 μg per vaccine dose. When assessing the suitability of the two aluminum salts to serve as carrier for MPL and antigen, aluminum hydroxide and aluminum phosphate were both equally effective in inducing the immune response (Figure 10.6).

Safety aspects of adjuvants for use in vaccines

Evaluation of aluminum

Aluminum adjuvants are themselves not immunogenic nor do they act as haptens. Therefore, they are not likely to cause harmful immune complex reactions and contact sensitivity to aluminum is extremely rare (Böhler-Sommeregger and Lindemayr, 1986). The inflammatory reaction induced upon injection of the aluminum is accompanied by a transient swelling, local irritation, and redness. There is

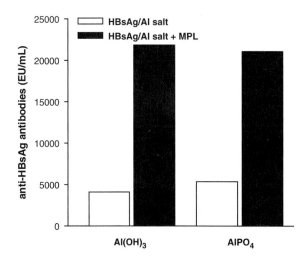

Figure 10.6 Impact of the aluminum species on the humoral response in mice. Groups of 7 BalbC mice were immunized subcutaneously at day 0 and 15 with 1/8 of a human dose of hepatitis B vaccine adjuvanted with or without MPL (the human dose equivalents are 500 μg aluminum hydroxide, 20 μg hepatitis B surface antigen (HBsAg), and 50 μg MPL in 500 μl). Antibody titers were determined by ELISA seven days after the second injection and are expressed as midpoint titers.

no evidence that aluminum adjuvants are pyrogenic by themselves and no carcinogenicity or teratogenicity has been associated with their use. Aluminum hydroxide has, however, a very significant binding affinity to endotoxins which may contribute to reduce the reactogenicity of some adsorbed vaccines containing residual LPS. This applies less to aluminum phosphate, which presents a weaker binding affinity to LPS. Cases of local reactions have occasionally been reported (Gupta et al., 1993), including indurations, swelling, erythemas, and cutaneous nodules that may persist for up to 8 weeks, and occasionally longer. Those cases have been reported to occur during hyposensitization therapy with allergic patients using standard antigenic extracts over extended periods of time.

Mineral adjuvants remain at the site of injection until they are slowly cleared. It can reasonably be assumed that aluminum salt particles containing adsorbed materials follow the same distribution and elimination kinetics as free aluminum particles. Flarend et al. (1997) have described the distribution profile of aluminum hydroxide and aluminum phosphate adjuvants labeled with ^{26}Al after intramuscular (i.m.) administration to New Zealand white rabbits. Part of the formulation was cleared locally by the reticuloendothelial system or was dissolved by the organic acids (citric, lactic, and malic acids) from the interstitial fluid, which drains directly into the lymphatic system. The interstitial fluid is also responsible for eluting the adsorbed molecules from the aluminum particles and for passing them to the lymph fluid (Shi et al., 2001a). Another part of the formulation circulated via the blood to different tissues and was eventually eliminated through the kidney. The most common adjuvant for prophylactic vaccines is aluminum hydroxide which has generally been considered as nontoxic and safe over the past decades.

Despite its 79-year history of safe and effective use in vaccines, the safety of aluminum adjuvants has been challenged in France since the report of a new emerging muscle disorder in 1998, referred to as macrophagic myofasciitis (MMF) (Gherardi et al., 1998). MMF is characterized by histological lesions along with persistent accumulation of macrophages with inclusions of aluminum and evidence of a focal chronic inflammatory reaction. MMF lesions have been suggested to be associated with a syndrome of ascending myalgias, fatigue, and diffuse musculoskeletal pain (Gherardi et al., 1998). However, based on analysis of the data of the case-control study performed in France and animal studies conducted in monkeys and rats, the Global Advisory Committee on Vaccine Safety (GACVS) concluded that the persistence of aluminum-containing macrophages at the site of a previous vaccination is not associated with specific clinical symptoms or disease. The same conclusions were drawn after investigating the epidemiological or clinical characteristics observed in a large panel of studies conducted in humans. At present, although vaccine adjuvant may persist at the injection

Table 10.1 Summary of preclinical safety studies performed with MPL

Study	Species	Route[a]	Dose	Observed outcome
Cardiovascular respiratory	Dog	i.v.	Up to 100 µg/kg	No abnormal effect
Repeat-dose toxicity	Rat	s.c.	Up to 200 µg/kg	No abnormal effect,
	Rabbit	s.c.	Up to 50 µg/kg	no target organ toxicity
	Dog	i.v.	Up to 1200 µg/kg	
Reproduction toxicity (embryo fetal)	Rat	s.c.	Up to 100 µg/kg	No abnormal effect
Reproductive toxicity (pre-/postnatal)	Rat	s.c.	Up to 100 µg/kg	No abnormal effect
Genotoxicity	Reverse mutation	In vitro	Up to 1000 µg/ml	No effect
	CHO cells	In vitro	475 µg/ml	

A series of preclinical safety investigations realized by Corixa and Allergy Therapeutics Ltd (Baldrick, 2002) was performed to support clinical use of MPL in vaccines. Assessments comprised cardiovascular/respiratory testing repeat-dose toxicity, reproduction toxicity, and genotoxicity studies using maximum doses of MPL as indicated.

[a]Route: route of administration; i.v., intravenous; s.c., subcutaneous.

site over years and may induce a local inflammatory response, there is no evidence of a health risk from aluminum-containing vaccines or any justification for changing current vaccination practices (Siegrist, 2005).

■ Preclinical evaluation of MPL

Until the publication of the adopted guidelines of the Committee for Medicinal Products for Human Use (CHMP) on vaccine safety evaluation issued in June 1998, no specific directive was available for vaccine manufacturers to regulate testing of vaccine safety or new adjuvants. Safety evaluations of MPL and AS04, as well as of vaccine candidates, initiated prior to the guidelines taking effect have been completed in compliance with the regulations.

GSK Bio as well as Corixa and Allergy Therapeutics Ltd (Worthing, UK) have thoroughly evaluated the safety profile of MPL according to the intended use. The molecule was subjected to a series of preclinical safety investigations using different routes of administration and various concentrations (Baldrick et al., 2002). Signs of toxicity were observed only during a repeated dose toxicity study and were related to the immunostimulatory

effects of MPL and associated with overstimulation of the immune system (increase in spleen weight and white blood cell count). MPL was shown to induce no adverse effects on cardiovascular/respiratory function, reproduction, or genotoxicity (Table 10.1). The most appropriate route of vaccine administration was the i.m. parenteral injection.

■ Preclinical evaluation of AS04

AS04-based vaccines described in this review are intended for a population ranging from young adolescents to elderly adults. In view of the intended use in vaccine clinical trials, we have evaluated the local and/or systemic toxicity of formulations containing MPL plus aluminum salt after i.m. injection in rabbits and rats (Table 10.2). (i) A repeat-dose toxicity study with rabbits evaluated effects after single and repeated (5 times) administration of a full human dose of the vaccine or adjuvant, equivalent to 30 times the human dose per unit body weight. There was no evidence of systemic toxicity. Symptoms were limited to the injection site but did not extend to the local lymph nodes, and evidence of partial recovery was observed after a one-month washout period. (ii) Pre- and postnatal development

Table 10.2 Preclinical safety studies performed with AS04

Study	Species and strain	Days of administration	Dose	Observed outcome
Local tolerance	NZW rabbit	0	0.5 ml of AS04: 50 µg MPL, 500 µg aluminum salt	Symptoms limited to the injection site and do not extend to the draining lymph node
Repeat-dose toxicity	NZW rabbit	0, 14, 28, 42, 56	0.5 ml of AS04: 50 µg MPL, 500 µg aluminum salt	Symptoms limited to the injection site and do not extend to the draining lymph node. No evidence of systemic toxicity
Reproductive and developmental toxicity	Wistar rat	6, 8, 11, 16 (pregnancy)	0.05 ml of AS04: 5 µg MPL, 50 µg aluminum salt	No treatment-related effects on mothers or offspring. No toxic effect level equivalent of up to 30 times the human dose
Cardiovascular/respiratory function	Wistar rat	0	0.05 ml of AS04: 5 µg MPL, 50 µg aluminum salt	No treatment-related effect. No toxic effect equivalent of up to 60 times the human dose

A series of preclinical safety investigations was performed to support clinical use of AS04 in vaccines. Assessments comprised local tolerance, repeat-dose toxicity, reproduction toxicity, and cardiovascular/respiratory testing using doses of AS04 as indicated. AS04 was administered by the intramuscular route on the indicated days. 0.5 ml of AS04 is equivalent to the full human dose (50 µg of MPL + 0.5 mg of aluminum salt).

studies performed in rats with the adjuvant alone or with an antigen/AS04 formulation have shown that repeated administration of a dose equivalent to 30 times the human dose per unit body weight (up to five injections) did not induce treatment-related effects on mother animals or offspring. (iii) A pharmacology study investigating cardiovascular and respiratory functions in anesthetized Wistar rats revealed no treatment-related effects by AS04-containing vaccines administered i.v. or i.m. at doses up to 60 times the human dose per unit body weight.

Altogether, the preclinical safety data reported here obtained with AS04 alone or AS04-containing vaccines indicate that this adjuvant system represents a safe and well-tolerated addition to vaccines with a high safety margin. Adverse events reported during any study period were not considered to be related to vaccination. AS04-containing vaccines or the AS04 adjuvant by itself failed to indicate evidence of systemic toxicity. The only effects observed were transient, with signs of recovery, and are well expected to occur with formulations that trigger an inflammatory immune response.

■ Clinical safety studies with AS04-containing vaccines

The combination of MPL with aluminum salts has been investigated with various vaccines under development containing antigens as divers as recombinant proteins, glycoproteins, conjugated polysaccharides, or virus-like particles. The most common clinical symptoms reported after administration of AS04-formulated vaccines were injection site reactions such as soreness, redness, and swelling, which were comparable to those seen with other aluminum-based vaccines or aluminum alone. Compared with local (injection site) symptoms, solicited general symptoms were reported somewhat less frequently after vaccination. Of those, fatigue, headache, and malaise were the most frequently noted. The majority of solicited local and general symptoms were reported as mild and moderate in intensity and usually resolved within two to three days after vaccination. The incidence of clinically relevant general symptoms was similar in AS04-containing vaccines and control groups.

From the results obtained in more than 15,000 subjects who received more than 40,000 doses of AS04 combined with the antigen of interest, it can be concluded that the reactogenicity and safety profile of AS04 vaccines is satisfactory and clinically acceptable and that the addition of MPL adjuvant has no clinically relevant impact on the safety profile of these new vaccines compared to classic aluminum-adjuvanted vaccines (Jacques et al., 2002). Clinical studies reported good compliance among the vaccinees for AS04-based vaccines, indicating that AS04 was well tolerated.

■ Examples of AS04-based vaccines

The adjuvant AS04 has been shown to increase the magnitude of the humoral immune response in animals and humans. Compared with aluminum alone, AS04 not only improves the humoral immune response but also induces a balance in favor of a Th1-type immune response in animals, which has been demonstrated to play an important role in clearance of viral infections in general. To date, the AS04 adjuvant has been evaluated in various vaccines intended to protect against distinct viral diseases, such as hepatitis B, and infections with respiratory syncytial virus, herpes simplex virus, human papillomavirus, or Epstein–Barr virus. Major results of preclinical and clinical studies are summarized in the following paragraphs.

■ AS04 improves the kinetics and persistence of the humoral response to hepatitis B antigen

The hepatitis B virus (HBV) can lead to persistent infection of the liver, chronic liver disease, and hepatocellular carcinoma. Hepatitis B infection remains a serious threat to the human population, despite the use of effective prophylactic vaccines over the past 20 years. Although more than 95% of the vaccinated population under 40 years of age responds to the vaccines currently available, there is still need, however, particularly in certain population groups that were found to be low responders, for a vaccine that will induce higher level and faster onset of

antibody response than the current registered vaccines. This applies notably to hemodialysis patients, who require multiple injections on a regular basis to become and remain protected against HBV infection. Also increasing age, male gender, obesity, genetic disposition, and smoking are examples of host factors for low immune response.

Numerous studies in mice using a vaccine that consists of recombinant yeast-derived surface antigen of hepatitis B virus (HBsAg) adjuvanted with aluminum salt and MPL have demonstrated the ability of MPL to mediate an overall increase in antibody titers, both in young and elderly animals (data not shown).

In several clinical trials a hepatitis B vaccine adjuvanted with aluminum salt and MPL (Fendrix) was shown to induce higher antibody titers with longer persistence than the vaccine adjuvanted with aluminum alone (Engerix-B). In those trials, healthy volunteers were seroprotected after two doses (within 90 days). In contrast, volunteers receiving the standard vaccine (adjuvanted with aluminum salt) required three doses and 210 days to reach the same level of protection (Boland et al., 2004). In a further study comparing the HBV vaccine adjuvanted with aluminum alone or with aluminum plus MPL in prehemodialysis/ hemodialysis patients, seroprotection rates in the aluminum/MPL group displayed a faster increase and persisted at a higher level for at least 30 months after the last of four vaccinations (Figure 10.7). The results indicate that by combining MPL with aluminum salts in a hepatitis B vaccine, MPL improves immunogenicity by enhancing the magnitude, kinetics, and persistence of the humoral response to hepatitis B vaccine, which represents a clear advantage for patients with impaired immune function like hemodialyzed patients.

■ AS04 abrogates the enhanced pathology observed with the original formalin-inactivated RSV vaccine

Respiratory syncytial virus (RSV) is the major cause of severe lower respiratory tract

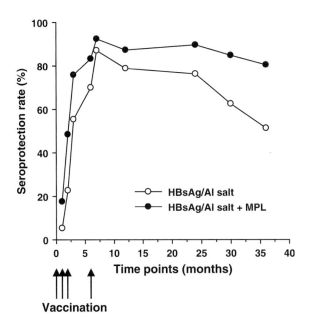

infections in infants and young children and is an important pathogen for adults, particularly immunosuppressed adults and the elderly. Immunity is incomplete and reinfection is common throughout life. At present, no effective antiviral treatment is available to protect people at risk from infections with RSV but control of RSV infection in the general population could be achieved by the development of an effective vaccine. The first vaccine to enter clinical trials contained formalin-inactivated virus (FI-RSV). The vaccine was only moderately antigenic and failed to protect against RSV infection or disease. Moreover, in a number of cases, unexpected enhanced pulmonary disease was observed in infant vaccinees upon subsequent natural infection with RSV (Fulginiti et al., 1969; Kapikian et al., 1969; Kim et al., 1969) requiring hospitalization and occasionally causing death. Induction of an inadequate Th2 profile CMI response to RSV has been suggested as a possible explanation for the vaccine failure, based on murine studies in which predominantly Th2-type cytokines were shown to be induced by the vaccine, in contrast to the predominantly Th1-type response observed during natural infection (Graham, 1995; Waris et al., 1996). In an attempt to develop a safe prophylactic vaccine against RSV disease capable of inducing a Th1-type response, we evaluated the effects of a recombinant subunit vaccine containing the extracellular domain of the F and G surface glycoproteins (FG) of RSV strain A, versus an FI-RSV vaccine, both formulated with AS04. Using the cotton rat challenge model, histological examination of lung specimens of animals immunized with the FI-RSV vaccine and challenged after 49 days with a human strain of RSV (Prince et al., 1999) displayed significantly lower pulmonary viral titers than naive animals but revealed alveolitis and interstitial pneumonitis-like lesions, characteristic of vaccine-enhanced RSV disease. Lungs of animals immunized with FI-RSV vaccine formulated with AS04 showed no significant histological signs of vaccine-enhanced RSV disease. Similar results were observed with the vaccine that contained chimeric FG formulated with AS04 (Prince et al., 2000); following RSV challenge, no enhanced lung histopathology was observed, while only low levels of histopathology were detected in animals previously vaccinated with the FG formulation lacking MPL. The preclinical results demonstrated that the FG/AS04 vaccine formulation was safe and highly effective in reducing viral replication in the lungs, and that AS04 formulation was able to reduce/abrogate the enhanced pathology seen with the original formalin-inactivated vaccine (Prince et al., 2000). It is suggested that the formulation containing MPL induces protection against RSV disease by shifting the cell-mediated immune response towards a Th1 profile as opposed to a profile associated with vaccine-enhanced RSV disease.

■   AS04 affords increased protection compared with aluminum salt alone

■ *Herpes simplex vaccine*

Herpes simplex viruses (HSVs) are among the most common infectious agents of humans. Genital infection with HSV type 1 or 2 is a sexually transmitted disease that has become increasingly prevalent, with painful recurrent mucosal skin lesions as the most common clinical symptom. HSV is transmitted by close sexual contact. Primary infection of the muco-cutaneous surfaces is usually followed by migration via sensory nerves to the trigeminal or spinal ganglia that innervate the oral cavity or genital tract, where life-long latent infection occurs. The clinical implications of a vaccine that would prevent primary and recurrent herpes simplex disease will be significant. Advances in the understanding of pathogenesis of HSV infection have led to the development of many candidate HSV vaccines which have been tested in both animal models and in humans (Stanberry et al., 2000; Stanberry, 2004; Whitley and Megnier, 1990). In view of the potential safety concerns associated with live attenuated vaccines and the poor immunogenicity of previous candidate inactivated vaccines, much research has focused on sub-unit vaccines containing viral proteins but no genetic material. Immunization with artificial mixtures of purified glycoproteins found on the viral envelope has been shown to provide protection against virus challenge in animal models (Burke, 1991). GSK Bio has developed a candidate subunit vaccine (Simplirix) containing glycoprotein D from HSV type 2, designated gD2. This vaccine was formulated with AS04 and was tested for its ability to induce a protective immune response against HSV in preclinical efficacy studies in the guinea pig model (Bourne et al., 2003). The results obtained with this prophylactic model of genital HSV-2 disease have indicated that

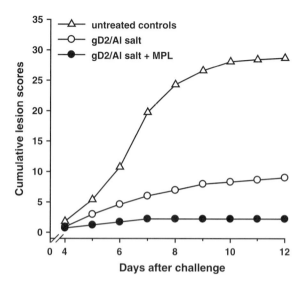

Figure 10.8 Assessment of vaccine efficacy against HSV-2 by *in vivo* virus challenge assay. Groups of 12 female Hartley guinea pigs (200–250 g) were immunized at days 0 and 28 by the subcutaneous route with HSV type 2 glycoprotein D (gD2, 5 μg) formulated in aluminum salt (0.5 mg equivalents Al^{3+}) or aluminum salt plus 50 μg MPL. Injections were given in a 0.5 ml dose. In order to compare the protective immunity induced by both gD2 formulations, all guinea pigs were challenged intravaginally 29 days after the last immunization with 10^5 pfu of HSV-2 strain MS. After challenge, guinea pigs were monitored daily for clinical signs of acute disease (days 4 to 12 postchallenge). The severity of each lesion observed was scored on a scale of 1–16 with 0 for animals with no lesions, 0.5–1 for vaginal lesions, and 2, 4, 8, or 16 for external skin lesions. Cumulative lesion scores (days 4–12) were calculated from the mean daily scores.

addition of MPL to aluminum salt in the formulation improved the prophylactic efficacy according to the lower-to-non lesion index observed after challenge (Figure 10.8). Interestingly, in the same animal model, antibody titers obtained after vaccination were essentially the same whether or not MPL was present in the formulation (data not shown), suggesting that the improved protection afforded by MPL was related to an improved immune response in terms of CMI activation or quality of the antibodies.

Upon vaccination in humans with a gD2-based vaccine, inclusion of MPL in the adjuvant formulation improved both the antibody response to aluminum-adsorbed antigen and

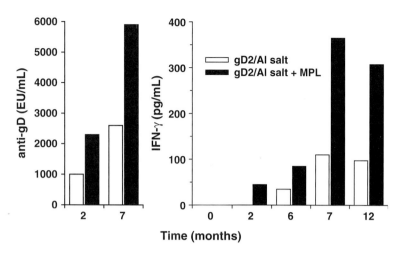

Figure 10.9 Immunogenicity of HSV-2 glycoprotein D formulated with or without MPL. Healthy HSV-negative subjects were immunized twice, a month apart, by the intramuscular route with HSV type 2 glycoprotein D (gD2, 20 µg per dose) formulated in aluminum salt (0.5 mg equivalents Al³⁺) or in aluminum salt plus 50 µg MPL. Whole venous blood samples were taken prior to vaccination, at day 0 (day of administration of the first vaccine dose), and at months 2, 6, 7, and 12. Anti-gD2 antibodies (GMT, EU/ml) were measured by ELISA, IFN-γ (pg/ml) was determined *in vitro* with harvested peripheral blood leucocytes (PBMC) in response to stimulation with purified gD2.

the CMI response as demonstrated by the level of interferon gamma (IFN-γ) secretion (Figure 10.9). In contrast to the vaccine formulated with MPL, another vaccine containing glycoprotein B and D of HSV-2 but combined with MF59 adjuvant was less efficacious giving transient protection of less than 6 months (Corey et al., 1999), even though high titers of neutralizing antibodies were induced. The difference in efficacy of both vaccines may be due to different mechanisms of action. While MF59 adjuvant appears to elicit a Th2-type response, MPL-adjuvanted vaccines have consistently been shown to promote a more Th1-biased cell-mediated immune response.

The protection level initially observed in the animal model with our HSV/AS04 vaccine was confirmed clinically in phase III, double-blind, randomized controlled studies in seronegative subjects whose regular sexual partners had a history of genital herpes (Stanberry et al., 2002). Vaccination elicited both binding and neutralizing antibodies against HSV, as well as a cellular response evidenced by lymphoproliferation and IFN-γ secretion. The vaccine demonstrated significant protection against genital herpes in women that were

seronegative for both HSV-1 and HSV-2 prior to vaccination. The protective mechanism of this formulation is most likely based upon the concomitant induction of an effector cell-mediated immune response by MPL and a potent virus-neutralizing response.

■ *Human papillomavirus vaccine*
Cervical cancer is one of the leading causes of death by cancer in women worldwide. Persistent infection with high-risk (oncogenic) human papillomavirus (HPV) types is the first necessary cause of cervical cancer. Therefore, development of prophylactic vaccines which would prevent persistent HPV infection or decrease its consequences would be of great value in reducing the global burden of cervical cancer.

The most promising approach for a prophylactic HPV vaccine are L1 virus-like particles (VLP) made by genetic engineering techniques, that have been shown to be morphologically and antigenically similar to authentic virions. They have been demonstrated to be effective in various preclinical challenge models to protect against infection and development of lesions. Based on preclinical investigations, an effective VLP-based vaccine designed to prevent cervical cancer would have to induce at least strong and long-lasting humoral responses but also optimal priming of the immune system to allow for long-term protection.

GSK Bio is currently developing an L1 VLP-based prophylactic HPV vaccine (Cervarix) containing HPV-16 and HPV-18 formulated with AS04, in a development alliance with MedImmune (Gaithersburg, MD, USA). In a phase II study conducted in healthy women, superior immunogenicity of the AS04 formulation compared to the vaccine formulated with aluminum salt alone was evidenced by the production of significantly higher neutralizing antibody titers after immunization with L1 VLP/AS04 (S. Giannini, personal communication). The vaccine was further evaluated in a double-blind, multicenter, randomized, placebo-controlled clinical trial that assessed the efficacy of a bivalent HPV-16/18 VLP vaccine against incident and persistent infections with HPV-16 and HPV-18 (Harper et al., 2004). This study demonstrated that the bivalent HPV-16/18 VLP vaccine conferred high (>70%) protection against incident HPV-16/18 infection and full protection against persistent HPV-16/18 infection. Specific antibody titers compared to natural infection were 100 and 80 times greater for HPV-16 and 18, respectively, at 7 months. They remained substantially raised at 18 months and were still 10 and 16 times higher than those seen in women with natural HPV-16 and 18 infection, respectively. The high and persistent antibody titers observed with the AS04-adjuvanted vaccine suggest that the immune response could allow for less frequent booster requirements and enhanced long-term protection from HPV infection. The vaccine appeared to be safe and well tolerated; no serious adverse events due to vaccination were reported. Vaccination against the most prevalent oncogenic HPV types, HPV-16 and HPV-18, could significantly reduce the incidence of cervical cancer worldwide.

■ Summary

Vaccines were some of the most successful medical products of the 20th century with regards to efficacy, cost, and safety. Aluminum has been the adjuvant of choice to generate an improved humoral response to vaccine antigen. Over the past decade GSK Bio has developed new adjuvant systems to provide a faster, stronger, and longer vaccine protection.

The use of an adjuvant in vaccine formulations can facilitate the induction of humoral and/or cellular immune responses which are of more rapid onset, increased magnitude, and/or prolonged duration compared with the unadjuvanted antigen. AS04 is one of GSK Bio's proprietary adjuvant systems which is currently under evaluation in a number of candidate vaccines. The basic components of AS04 are aluminum salts, including aluminum hydroxide or aluminum phosphate, and MPL. The 3-deacylated form of monophosphoryl lipid A is a detoxified derivative of an LPS found in Gram-negative bacteria, which retains the capacity of the natural compound to act as an adjuvant. While aluminum salts are known to improve humoral immune responses, MPL is considered to foster Th1-type cellular immunity, and a combination of both (i.e., AS04) potentially enhances both cellular and humoral immune response, depending on the vaccine antigen. Indeed, extensive preclinical studies conducted by GSK Bio have established that by combining MPL with aluminum salts, the immune responses to antigens are generally enhanced both qualitatively and quantitatively. This was confirmed by observations in human clinical trials showing that MPL can enhance the strength and kinetics of the humoral response.

The safety profile of AS04 has been extensively evaluated according to the intended use. The molecule was subjected to a series of preclinical and clinical safety investigations using different routes of administration and various concentrations. AS04 has proven to be safe and well tolerated, and has been shown to be superior to aluminum salt in terms of antibody response in humans and protection in animal models.

AS04 is currently being used as an adjuvant in several GSK Bio candidate vaccines including vaccines under investigation for the prevention of hepatitis B, genital herpes, and cervical cancer, all close to registration or already registered. Depending on the vaccine considered, the AS04 adjuvant is effective in activating different arms of the immune response. In a new hepatitis B vaccine primarily intended for hepatitis B prophylaxis in hemodialysis patients, this adjuvant induces not only higher antibody titers but most importantly a greater persistence of circulating antibodies. With vaccines designed for other viral diseases such as infection with HSV, distinct parts of the immune system are targeted. In this case, AS04 was shown to improve both the CMI and the antibody response. Finally, with a prophylactic HPV vaccine, AS04 induces a strong and long-lasting antibody response and allows for full protection against persistent virus infection.

■ Abbreviations

APC, antigen presenting cells; AS, adjuvant system; CMI, cell-mediated immunity; DC, dendritic cells; FG, F and G RSV surface glycoproteins; FI-RSV, formalin-inactivated RSV; HBsAg, hepatitis B surface antigen; HBV, hepatitis B virus; HPV, human papillomavirus; HSV, herpes simplex virus; IFN-γ, interferon-γ; IL, interleukin; LPS, lipopolysaccharides; MHC, major histocompatibility complex; MPL, 3'-deacylated monophosphoryl lipid A; PBMC, peripheral blood mononuclear cells; RSV, respiratory syncytial virus; TNF-α, tumor necrosis factor-α; TLR, Toll-like receptor; VLP, virus-like particle; aluminum salt refers to aluminum hydroxide or aluminum phosphate hydrated gels.

■ Acknowledgments

The authors would like to thank the people at GlaxoSmithKline Biologicals who contributed to this work and who provided unpublished data.

■ References

Al-Shakhshir, R.H., Regnier, F.E., White, J.L., and Hem, S.L. (1995). Contribution of electrostatic and hydrophobic interactions to the adsorption of proteins by aluminium-containing adjuvants. *Vaccine* 13, 41–44.

Baldrick, P., Richardson, D., Elliott, G., and Wheeler, A.W. (2002). Safety evaluation of monophosphoryl lipid A (MPL): an immunostimulatory adjuvant. *Regul. Toxicol. Pharmacol.* 35, 398–413.

Böhler-Sommeregger, K. and Lindemayr, H. (1986). Contact sensitivity to aluminium. *Contact Dermatitis* 15, 278–281.

Boland, G., Beran, J., Lievens, M., Sasadeusz, J., Dentico, P., Nothdurft, H., Zuckerman, J.N., Genton, B., Steffen, R., Loutan, L., Van Hattum, J., and Stoffel, M. (2004). Safety and immunogenicity profile of an experimental hepatitis B vaccine adjuvanted with AS04. *Vaccine* 23, 316–320.

Bourne, N., Bravo, F.J., Francotte, M., Bernstein, D.I., Myers, M.G., Slaoui, M., and Stanberry, L.R. (2003). Herpes simplex virus (HSV) type 2 glycoprotein D subunit vaccines and protection against genital HSV-1 or HSV-2 disease in guinea pigs. *J. Infect. Dis.* 187, 542–549.

Burke, R.L. (1991). Development of a herpes simplex virus subunit glycoprotein vaccine for prophylactic and therapeutic use. *Rev. Infect. Dis.* 13 (Suppl. 11), S906–S911.

Corey, L., Langenberg, A.G., Ashley, R., Sekulovich, R.E., Izu, A.E., Douglas, J.M., Jr., Handsfield, H.H., Warren, T., Marr, L., Tyring, S., DiCarlo, R., Adimora, A.A., Leone, P., Dekker, C.L., Burke, R.L., Leong, W.P., and Straus, S.E. (1999). Recombinant glycoprotein vaccine for the prevention of genital HSV-2 infection: two randomized controlled trials. Chiron HSV Vaccine Study Group. *JAMA* 282, 331–340.

Flarend, R.E., Hem, S.L., White, J.L., Elmore, D., Suckow, M.A., Rudy, A.C., and Dandashli, E.A. (1997). *In vivo* absorption of aluminium-containing vaccine adjuvants using 26Al. *Vaccine* 15, 1314–1318.

Fulginiti, V.A., Eller, J.J., Sieber, O.F., Joyner, J.W., Minamitani, M., and Meiklejohn, G. (1969). Respiratory virus immunization: I. A field trial of two inactivated respiratory virus vaccines; an aqueous trivalent parainfluenza virus vaccine and an alum-precipitated respiratory syncytial virus vaccine. *Am. J. Epidemiol.* 89, 435–448.

Gherardi, R.K., Coquet, M., Cherin, P., Authier, F.J., Laforet, P., Belec, L., Figarella-Branger, D., Mussini, J.M., Pellissier, J.F., and Fardeau, M. (1998). Macrophagic myofasciitis: an emerging entity. Groupe d'Etudes et Recherche sur les Maladies Musculaires Acquises et Dysimmunitaires (GERMMAD) de l'Association Francaise contre les Myopathies (AFM). *Lancet* 352, 347–352.

Glenny, A.T., Buttle, G.A.H., and Stevens, M.F. (1931). Rate of disappearance of diphtheria toxoid injected into rabbits and guinea pigs: toxoid precipitated with alum. *J. Pathol.* 34, 267–275.

Graham, B.S. (1995). Pathogenesis of respiratory syncytial virus vaccine-augmented pathology. *Am. J. Respir. Crit. Care Med.* 152, S63–S66.

Gupta, R.K., Relyveld, E.H., Lindblad, E.B., Bizzini, B., Ben Efraim, S., and Gupta, C.K. (1993). Adjuvants: a balance between toxicity and adjuvanticity. *Vaccine* 11, 293–306.

Harper, D.M., Franco, E.L., Wheeler, C., Ferris, D.G., Jenkins, D., Schuind, A., Zahaf, T., Innis, B., Naud, P., De Carvalho, N.S., Roteli-Martins, C.M., Teixeira, J., Blatter, M.M., Korn, A.P., Quint, W., Dubin, G., and GlaxoSmithKline HPV Vaccine Study Group (2004). Efficacy of a bivalent L1 virus-like particle vaccine in prevention of infection with human papillomavirus types 16 and 18 in young women: a randomised controlled trial. *Lancet* 364, 1757–1765.

Hem, S.L. and White, J.L. (1984). Characterization of aluminium hydroxide for use as an adjuvant in parenteral vaccines. *J. Parenter. Sci. Technol.* 38, 2–10.

Henricson, B.E., Benjamin, W.R., and Vogel, S.N. (1990). Differential cytokine induction by doses of lipopolysaccharide and monophosphoryl lipid A that result in equivalent early endotoxin tolerance. *Infect. Immun.* 58, 2429–2437.

Hirschfeld, M., Ma, Y., Weis, J.H., Vogel, S.N., and Weis, J.J. (2000). Cutting edge: repurification of lipopolysaccharide eliminates signaling through both human and murine toll-like receptor 2. *J. Immunol.* 165, 618–622.

Holt, L.B. (1950). *Developments in Diphtheria Prophylaxis*, Heinemann, London, UK.

Iyer, S., HogenEsch, H., and Hem, S.L. (2003). Relationship between the degree of antigen adsorption to aluminum hydroxide adjuvant in interstitial fluid and antibody production. *Vaccine* 21, 1219–1223.

Jacques, P., Moens, G., Desombere, I., Dewijngaert, J., Leroux-Roels, G., Wettendorff, M., and Thoelen, S. (2002). The immunogenicity and reactogenicity profile of a candidate hepatitis B vaccine in an adult vaccine non-responder population. *Vaccine* 20, 3644–3649.

Johnson, A.G., Gaines, S., and Landy, M. (1956). Studies on the O-antigen of *Salmonella typhosa*: V. Enhancement of the antibody response to protein antigens by the purified lipopolysaccharide. *J. Exp. Med.* 103, 246.

Jordan, M.B., Mills, D.M., Kappler, J., Marrack, P., and Cambier, J.C. (2004). Promotion of B cell immune responses via an alum-induced myeloid cell population. *Science* 304, 1808–1810.

Kapikian, A.Z., Mitchell, R.H., Chanock, R.M., Shvedoff, R.A., and Stewart, C.E. (1969). An epidemiologic study of altered clinical reactivity to respiratory syncytial (RS) virus infection in children previously vaccinated with an inactivated RS virus vaccine. *Am. J. Epidemiol.* 89, 405–421.

Kim, H.W., Canchola, J.G., Brandt, C.D., Pyles, G., Chanock, R.M., Jensen, K., and Parrott, R.H. (1969). Respiratory syncytial virus disease in infants despite prior administration of antigenic inactivated vaccine. *Am. J. Epidemiol.* 89, 422–434.

Martin, M., Michalek, S.M., and Katz, J. (2003). Role of innate immune factors in the adjuvant activity of monophosphoryl lipid A. *Infect. Immun.* 71, 2498–2507.

Matsuura, M., Kiso, M., and Hasegawa, A. (1999). Activity of monosaccharide lipid A analogues in human monocytic cells as agonists or antagonists of bacterial lipopolysaccharide. *Infect. Immun.* 67, 6286–6292.

Myers, K.R., Truchot, A.T., Word, J., Hudson, Y., and Ulrich, J.T. (1990). In Nowotny, A., Spitzer, J.J., and Ziegler, E.J. (Eds) *Cellular and Molecular Aspects of Endotoxin Reactions*. Elsevier Science, New York, pp. 145–156.

Prince, G.A., Prieels, J.P., Slaoui, M., and Porter, D.D. (1999). Pulmonary lesions in primary respiratory syncytial virus infection, reinfection, and vaccine-enhanced disease in the cotton rat (Sigmodon hispidus). *Lab. Invest.* 79, 1385–1392.

Prince, G.A., Capiau, C., Deschamps, M., Fabry, L., Garcon, N., Gheysen, D., Prieels, J.P., Thiry, G., Van Opstal, O., and Porter, D.D. (2000). Efficacy and safety studies of a recombinant chimeric respiratory syncytial virus FG glycoprotein vaccine in cotton rats. *J. Virol.* 74, 10287–10292.

Salkowski, C.A., Detore, G.R., and Vogel, S.N. (1997). Lipopolysaccharide and monophosphoryl lipid A differentially regulate interleukin-12, gamma interferon, and interleukin-10 mRNA production in murine macrophages. *Infect. Immun.* 65, 3239–3247.

Shi, Y., HogenEsch, H., and Hem, S.L. (2001a). Change in the degree of adsorption of proteins by aluminum-containing adjuvants following exposure to interstitial fluid: freshly prepared and aged model vaccines. *Vaccine* 20, 80–85.

Shi, Y., HogenEsch, H., Regnier, F.E., and Hem, S.L. (2001b). Detoxification of endotoxin by aluminum hydroxide adjuvant. *Vaccine* 19, 1747–1752.

Siegrist, C.A. (2005). [Vaccine adjuvants and macrophagic myofasciitis]. *Arch. Pediatr.* 12, 96–101.

Stanberry, L.R. (2004). Clinical trials of prophylactic and therapeutic herpes simplex virus vaccines. *Herpes* 11 (Suppl. 3), 161A–169A.

Stanberry, L.R., Cunningham, A.L., Mindel, A., Scott, L.L., Spruance, S.L., Aoki, F.Y., and Lacey, C.J. (2000). Prospects for control of herpes simplex virus disease through immunization. *Clin. Infect. Dis.* 30, 549–566.

Stanberry, L.R., Spruance, S.L., Cunningham, A.L., Bernstein, D.I., Mindel, A., Sacks, S., Tyring, S., Aoki, F.Y., Slaoui, M., Denis, M., Vandepapeliere, P., and Dubin, G. (2002). Glycoprotein-D-adjuvant vaccine to prevent genital herpes. *N. Engl. J. Med.* 347, 1652–1661.

Tapping, R.I., Akashi, S., Miyake, K., Godowski, P.J., and Tobias, P.S. (2000). Toll-like receptor 4, but not toll-like receptor 2, is a signaling receptor for Escherichia and Salmonella lipopolysaccharides. *J. Immunol.* 165, 5780–5787.

Waris, M.E., Tsou, C., Erdman, D.D., Zaki, S.R., and Anderson, L.J. (1996). Respiratory synctial virus infection in BALB/c mice previously immunized with formalin-inactivated virus induces enhanced pulmonary inflammatory response with a predominant Th2-like cytokine pattern. *J. Virol.* 70, 2852–2860.

Whitley, R.J. and Megnier, B. (1990). In Woodrow, C.G. and Levine, M.M. (Eds) *New Generation Vaccines*. Marcel Dekker, New York, pp. 825–854.

World Health Organization (1976). Immunological adjuvants. Technical Report Series 595. Geneva.

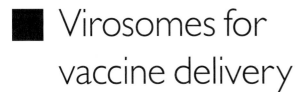

Virosomes for vaccine delivery

Ian C. Metcalfe and Reinhard Glück
Berna Biotech Ltd, Bern, Switzerland

■ Introduction

Next to the availability of clean water, the development of vaccines has had the most dramatic impact on global health. From the initial pioneers, such as Jenner and Pasteur, the last century has seen a marked increase in the effectiveness of vaccination tools and strategies. The eradication of smallpox and the targeting of poliomyelitis for eradication are two excellent examples of the success of vaccinology as a science. The need to further develop vaccines against diseases such as malaria, HIV, hepatitis C virus (HCV), and even cancer is driving the discovery of novel antigens, most of which require adjuvants or delivery vehicles for efficient immunopotentiation. As such, modern vaccines incorporating these new technologies and formulations must face and overcome particular scientific and regulatory hurdles.

This chapter reviews one of the most dynamic and successful modern vaccine concepts: immunopotentiating reconstituted influenza virosomes (IRIVs). Here we present a brief overview of the background behind the IRIV concept; the IRIV mechanism of action; and applications of the IRIV technology.

■ Adjuvants

Adjuvants, a term derived from the Latin *ad* meaning "towards" and *juvare* meaning "help," may be defined as any substance that is added to a vaccine to enhance/target the immune response to an associated antigen. Since initial investigations in the 1920s, traditional adjuvants have been based on alum compounds (Glenny et al., 1926). It is only recently that IRIVs (Moser et al., 2003) and an "oil-in-water emulsion" adjuvant (Ott et al., 1995) have been approved for human use. There have been many investigations made on substances that show potential in terms of adjuvant action. In 1936 Freund developed an emulsion of water and mineral oil containing killed mycobacteria, Freund's complete adjuvant (FCA) (Freund et al., 1937). To this day FCA remains the "gold standard" in terms of immunopotentiation, but is associated with severe local reactions and is not suitable for use in human vaccines.

Despite early developments, the incorporation of novel adjuvants into vaccines is limited by the fact that many adjuvants are only suitable for certain antigens and that in many cases there is a lack of a relevant animal model for demonstration of efficacy. Vaccine design is a complicated issue, particularly with regards to regulatory concerns over safety, as vaccines are generally administered to healthy individuals (Sesardic et al., 2004). However, in order to offer protective disease management covering a broad range of pathogens, modern synthetic and pure recombinant antigens, being far less immunogenic than traditional live or killed whole-organism vaccines, generally require an effective adjuvant for sufficient immunopotentiation.

Delivery vehicles

Vaccine delivery systems are intrinsically adjuvants (see Chapter 1). The artificial separation here acts to highlight the role that modern delivery vehicles play in the protection of encapsulated macromolecules and in targeting the associated antigens to antigen-presenting cells (APC), including macrophages and dendritic cells. Certain delivery systems present antigen to the immune system in a comparable manner to pathogens, in terms of particle size, antigen presentation, or in the facilitation of antigen processing once the particles have been taken up by phagocytic cells of the innate immune system. In many cases delivery systems and immunopotentiating agents are combined in order to achieve the desired responses.

Examples of delivery vehicles that have been thoroughly investigated include microparticles, virus-like particles (VLPs), immunostimulatory complexes (iscoms), liposomes, and virosomes. Each of these has the key function of efficiently delivering associated antigen to immunocompetent cells. In nearly all cases the benefits of delivery vehicles are only fully realized when the selected antigen is either encapsulated within or integrated with the adjuvant in some manner. Difficulties faced in the formulation of these adjuvant–antigen complexes often include problems with efficient encapsulation and instability of entrapped or integrated antigen. However, the potential advantages of a successful vaccine delivery system, especially in terms of the induction of strong cellular immune responses, important against chronic infections such as HCV, malaria, tuberculosis (TB), and HIV, make them a particularly desirable approach.

Routes of administration

Alternative routes of administration are also being investigated for vaccine design (Levine, 2003). Oral, intranasal, and transcutaneous delivery of vaccines may provide benefits through ease of administration, reduced adverse effects, potential for frequent boosting, local mucosal immunity at site of pathogen entry (localized IgA antibody response), and circumvention of disease transmission from reused needles. Further advantages include the expression of a variety of antigens (including proteins, polysaccharides, [glyco]lipids, and nucleic acids); antigens which are only produced under *in vivo* conditions; and the expression of native antigens, their correct postranslational modification, and their long-term expression. However, inactivated vaccines delivered directly to the mucosal surfaces are generally only weakly immunogenic.

One means of eliciting the desired immune response is the use of live attenuated pathogens. Although successful vaccines have been produced, e.g., oral vaccines for cholera (Tacket et al., 1992) and typhoid (Wahdan et al., 1982), and a nasal vaccine for influenza (Medimmune, 2003), the production of a safe and efficacious vaccine relies on the difficult balance between sufficient attenuation for safety and maintaining immunogenicity. The attenuation of certain pathogens for vaccines may also be considered unacceptable, such as HIV or HCV, due to the possibility of reversion to virulence. Hence, relatively few live oral vaccines have been registered (Dietrich et al., 2003).

An alternative may be found in the administration of the less immunogenic, but safer, pure recombinant or synthetic antigens direct to the mucosal surface via an immunopotentiating delivery vehicle. Several groups have researched the potential for the development of an intranasal influenza vaccine using a variety of technologies. These include chitin microparticles (Hasegawa et al., 2005), ISCOMATRIX particles (Coulter et al., 2003), bacterial toxins (Pine et al., 2002) and viral-vector approaches (Van Kampen et al., 2005). However, only one technology platform, IRIVs containing heat-labile toxin from *E. coli* (Glück, 2001), has so far reached the market, but even this was not relicensed due to safety concerns (Mutsch et al., 2004).

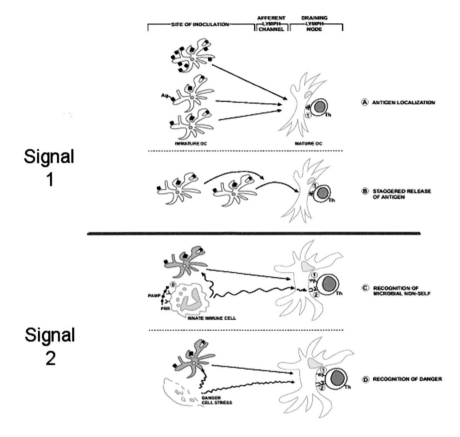

Figure 1.1 Schematic of key events during immune induction. (A) Antigen localization in the lymph node determines immune induction. (B) Staggered release of antigen from the inoculation site facilitates immune induction. (C) Nonself-discrimination by innate immune cells starts an immune response by upregulation of costimulatory signals. (D) Necrotic or stressed cells evoke increased costimulation of antigen-presenting cells. Each step may explain the mechanism underlying a particular type of adjuvant: (0) signal 0, (1) signal 1, (2) signal 2. (After Schijns, V.E.J.C. (2001). *Crit. Rev. Immunol.* 21, 75–85. With permission.)

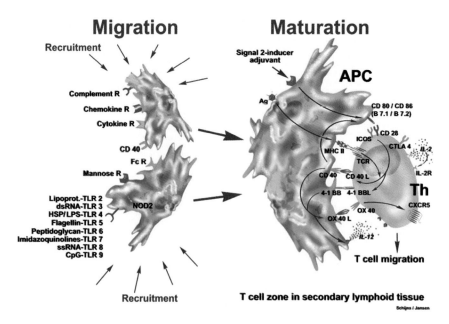

Figure I.2 Adjuvants recruit, target, or activate antigen-presenting dendritic cells (DC). Hence, DC/antigen-presenting cell (APC) migration (signal 1 facilitation) or maturation (signal 2 facilitation) by microbial or nonmicrobial immunopotentiators is key to primary immune induction.

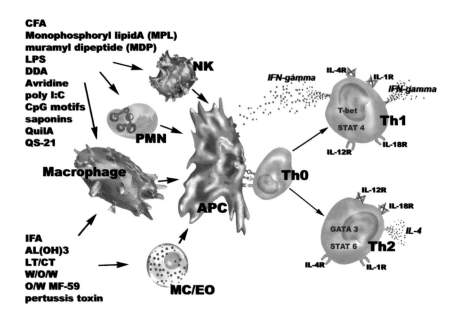

Figure I.3 Immunopotentiators influence the quality of immune reactions. Recognition of adjuvants by innate immune cells generates soluble, secreted, or membrane-bound signals, which shape the direction of downstream Th phenotypes upon priming by activated and conditioned antigen-presenting dendritic cells.

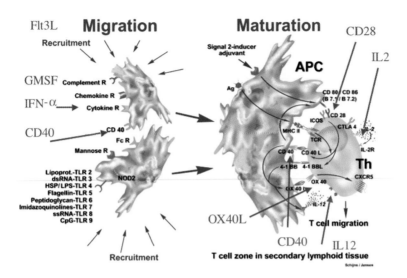

Figure 3.1 Some targets on APCs of the adjuvants discussed in Chapter 3.

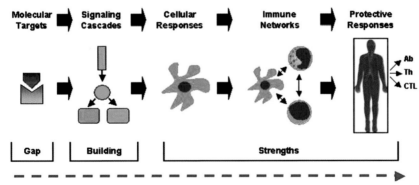

Figure 4.5 Linking molecular mechanisms to systems biology in adjuvant design and development. The long-term goal of adjuvant and immune potentiator research should become increasingly more predictive and rational. Before the appreciation of innate immunity and its mechanistic underpinnings, adjuvant research was almost exclusively empirical. Today, armed with new tools, molecular targets, and platforms, the ability to connect molecular mechanisms to *in vivo* outcomes is possible. The critical gap in our understanding right now lies in the incomplete knowledge surrounding target–ligand binding. However, the overall gaps in connecting each level of interaction (molecular mechanism–signal transduction–cellular responses–immune networks–systems biology) need to be filled to become truly predictive.

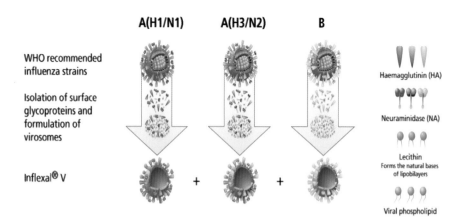

A(H1/N1)   A(H3/N2)   B

WHO recommended
influenza strains

Isolation of surface
glycoproteins and
formulation of
virosomes

Inflexal® V   +   +

Haemagglutinin (HA)

Neuraminidase (NA)

Lecithin
Forms the natural bases
of lipobilayers

Viral phospholipid

Figure II.2 The production of Inflexal V (Berna Biotech, Bern, Switzerland). This is derived from the surface glycoproteins of the three recommended influenza virus strains being isolated and purified prior to reformulation into IRIVs.

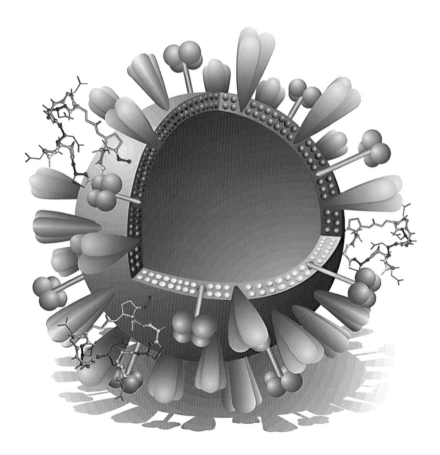

Figure II.3 Malaria vaccine candidate. This is a peptide epitope of the malaria parasite *Plasmodium falciparum* (mimetic PEV302) attached to an IRIV. (Reproduced with the kind permission of Wiley-VCH, from Pfeiffer, B., Peduzzi, E., Moehle, K., Zurbriggen, R., Gluck, R., Pluschke, G., and Robinson, J.A. (2003). A virosome-mimotope approach to synthetic vaccine design and optimisation: synthesis, conformation and immune recognition of a potential malaria-vaccine candidate. *Angew. Chem. Int.* 42, 2368–2371.)

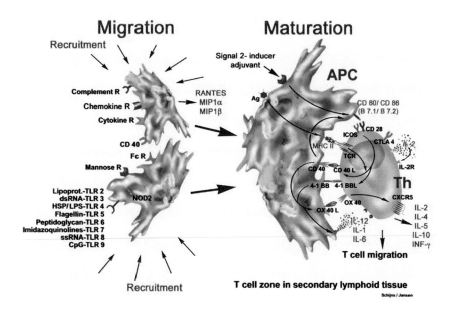

Figure 12.4 ISCOMATRIX™ adjuvant activity is a potent immunomodulator, which has effects on both the innate and adaptive immune systems as indicated in red text (see color plate section). The effects of ISCOMATRIX™ vaccines on the APC include the induction of proinflammatory cytokines (IL-1, IL-6, IL-12), CD80/86, and chemokines (RANTES, MIPI α, MIPI β). ISCOMATRIX™ vaccines also stimulate the expression of T cell cytokines (IL-2, IL-4, IL-5, IL-10, IFN-γ) indicative of a mixed Th1/Th2 response. (Adapted from Figure 1.2, Chapter 1.)

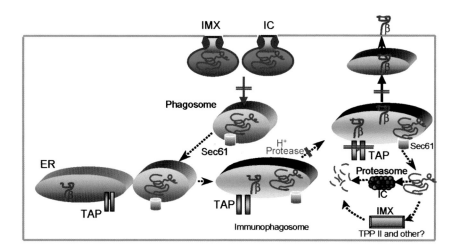

Figure 12.6 Schematic representation of APC uptake and processing of antigen either formulated as an ISCOMATRIX™ vaccine (IMX) or an immune complex (IC). ICs are generally regarded as an efficient means to load APCs for MHC I antigen processing. Using inhibitors of specific cellular processes Schnurr et al. (2005) have shown that the ISCOMATRIX™ adjuvant and IC-mediated cross presentation of antigen requires phagocytosis, acidification, TAP, and the secretory pathway. Double red lines (see color plate section) indicate that inhibition at this point blocks MHC I antigen processing. IC-mediated cross presentation requires proteasome processing whereas ISCOMATRIX™ adjuvant-mediated cross presentation is largely proteasome independent and occurs primarily via Tripeptidyl Peptidase II. The ability to access different antigen processing pathways may increase the range of peptides and hence of the CD8+ T cell response that can be generated in response to ISCOMATRIX™ vaccines.

Cholera Toxin

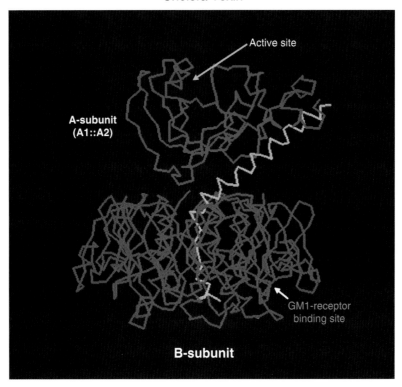

Figure I4.2B Subunit structure and function of cholera toxin.

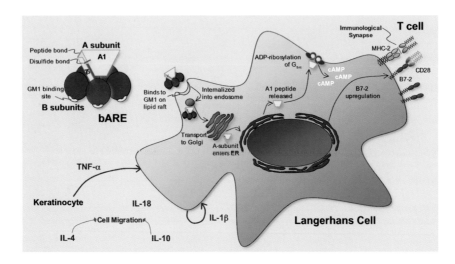

Figure I5.I Effect of bacterial ADP-ribosylating endotoxins (bAREs) in the epidermis. Langerhans cells that are resident in the epidermis can become activated by danger signals from pathogens then travel to the lymph node and initiate an immune response. bAREs can mimic this through pathways that are just now being clarified. See text for details.

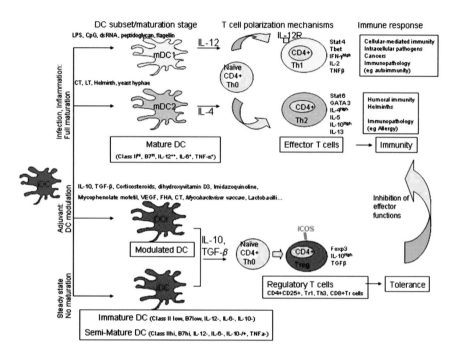

Figure 16.1 The induction of Th1, Th2, or T Reg cells is determined by the type and activation state of dendritic cells (DCs).
In the steady state, immature (iDCs)/semimature DCs capture antigens in the periphery, enter regional lymph nodes, and prime resting T cells to become regulatory T cells. In contrast, microbial product and proinflammatory cytokines produced during infection and inflammation stimulate the terminal maturation of DCs (mDCs) and drive them to prime naive T cells and induce effector Th1 or Th2 responses. Lipopolysaccharides (LPS), polycytosine guanine (CpG) motifs in bacterial DNA, viral double-stranded (ds) RNA, bacterial peptidoglycans, and flagellin stimulate DCs to promote the differentiation of Th1 cells. Cholera toxin (CT), *E. coli* heat-labile enterotoxin (LT), helminths, and yeast hyphae activate DCs to rather support Th2 cell polarization. Tolerogenic/regulatory DCs (DCr) are generated following stimulation with IL-10, TGF-β, immunosuppressive drugs (e.g., corticosteroids, cyclosporin A, rapamycin, mycophenolate mofetil), and pathogen-derived molecules (FHA, CT, PPD from *Mycobacterium tuberculosis*, lactobacilli, *Mycobacterium vaccae*).

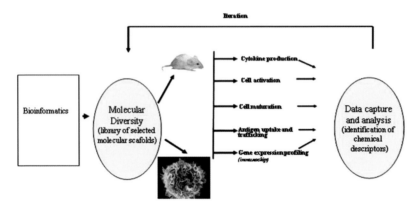

Figure I6.2 A proposed strategy is to screen libraries of natural or synthetic molecules for their activity either in simple animal models or on purified human immune cell subpopulations (dendritic cells in coculture with T cells), using readouts (colorimetric or optical) that can be robotized. Appropriate informatics should be used for both data capture and analysis, thereby allowing identification of molecular descriptors shared by molecules giving positive hits and not present within molecules giving negative hits. Based on such information, biased libraries of chemical entities with selected molecular characteristics can be synthesized, and submitted to a second round of screening.

Development of the IRIV concept

The term "virosome" was originally coined to describe the native virus-like structure of lipid vesicles presenting viral spike proteins from influenza virus when viewed under the electron microscope (Almeida et al., 1975). Virosomes were initially a development of the liposome concept, a concept well recognized for potential in drug, enzyme, and antigen entrapment and delivery. The importance of the work by Almeida et al. was to produce a nonpyrogenic yet immunogenic means of presenting influenza antigen. They also showed that the virosomes were stable structures and that the important fusogenic properties of the hemagglutinin (HA) had been maintained (Almeida et al., 1975). This work was expanded upon by our research and culminated in several patents and the further development of IRIVs and two licensed vaccines containing them (Glück et al., 1992).

Fusogenic properties of IRIVs

Intercalated within a phospholipid bilayer formed predominantly from phosphatidylcholine (PC) and phosphatidylethanolamine (PE), are the influenza virus surface coat proteins HA and neuraminidase (NA). Although influenza NA has been shown to facilitate virus entry into cells (Matrosovich et al., 2004), it is the well-characterized role of HA that forms the basis of the fusogenic properties of IRIVs. HA is a homotrimeric integral membrane protein (M_r 220,000). Each monomer is synthesized as a single polypeptide chain (HA0) that is later cleaved into the fusion-competent form comprised of two polypeptides, HA1 and HA2, linked by a disulfide bond (Wilson et al., 1981).

The initial role of the HA is to facilitate the uptake of IRIVs by APC through endocytosis. HA1 has a high binding affinity towards sialic acid residues that are present in membrane proteins and lipids, and are particularly abundant on APC. Eisenlohr et al. have shown that in the native influenza virus, the binding activity of the HA to sialic acid residues is responsible for focusing the influenza antigen towards the helper T cells (Eisenlohr et al., 1987). In addition, it is thought that the HA1 is responsible for maintaining the membrane-anchored HA2 in a metastable or "spring loaded" state (Bullough et al., 1994).

Once bound the virion presenting the HA is internalized into the endosome via receptor-mediated endocytosis. A fusion reaction involving several stages of membrane rearrangement then occurs, starting with "hemifusion," the merger of only the contacting monolayers, and culminating in a fusion pore and the mixing of the volumes enclosed by the membranes (Leikina et al., 2001). In brief, the acidic environment in the endosome initiates conformational changes in the HA resulting in exposure of the HA2 fusion peptide. This peptide then moves to the tip of the HA where it destabilizes the target membrane and initiates membrane fusion (Durrer et al., 1996). As a result of the merger of the two membranes, the contents of the IRIV are released into the cytosol of the cell.

Immunopotentiation

The adaptive immune system, involving both specificity and memory, is a crucial consideration in the development of vaccines. It is therefore the stimulation of B and T lymphocytes in addition to APC that is of the utmost importance in eliciting an effective immune response.

Studies have shown that B cells recognize the organization of antigens as a marker for foreignness (Bachmann et al., 1995). It has been proposed that highly repetitive antigen organization induces primary B cell responses that are basically T cell independent. This has been associated with B cell receptor crosslinking, as antigens that do not crosslink receptors are ignored by B cells if no linked T help is provided. The structure of the IRIV, with regard to presentation of antigen in a repetitive array, is therefore an important factor in the IRIV immunopotentiating properties.

In addition, the efficient induction of CD8-based cellular immunity occurs through the cytoplasmatic delivery of antigen encapsulated within the IRIV via the stimulation of the endogenous pathway. Following internalization of the IRIV by the APC, maturation signals increase the expression of costimulatory surface molecules, including B7-1, B7-2, and CD40. Interactions between these molecules and CD28 family members expressed on T cells regulate the T cell activation and tolerance (Greenwald et al., 2005). The subsequent activation of specific CD4+ T cells combined with the recognition of antigen presented by the IRIV in the context of the MHC II pathway induces the expression of T helper 1-type cytokines (interferon-γ), tumor necrosis factor α, and granulocyte macrophage colony-stimulating factor (Chapter 1, Figure 1.2). The action of the CD4+ T cells is essential for the generation of long-lasting antibody responses. Furthermore, the feedback signals provided to the APC enhance the presentation of antigen-MHC I complexes that are recognized by antigen-specific CD8+ T cells; these cells then differentiate into cytotoxic CD8+ effector T cells. Comprehensive reviews have summarized the immunological actions of IRIVs in terms of both MHC I presentation, via release of the IRIV contents into the cytoplasm and subsequent processing, and MHC II presentation through the exogenous antigen degradation for antigen which remains in the endolysosome (Moser et al., 2003; Felnerova et al., 2004; Daemen et al., 2005).

Several research groups are currently investigating the potential of IRIVs for use in novel vaccines and therapeutic preparations. It is well established that cytotoxic T lymphocytes (CTLs) play an important role in the control of viral infections and tumors. Recent work on the IRIV concept has therefore concentrated on the induction of CTLs, a development in the vaccine field that has been termed "the fifth [and most recent] revolution" (Plotkin, 2005). To this end, Bungener et al. have also clearly demonstrated that it is the fusion activity of

the IRIV that is key to the induction of a CTL response against IRIV-encapsulated ovalbumin in mice (Bungener et al., 2005). Schumacher et al. have also shown that IRIVs can activate regulatory CD4+ T cells, which in turn enhances and sustains the cellular and humoral immune response (Schumacher et al., 2004).

■ Incorporation of antigens into IRIVs

Directly associated with the immunopotentiating effects of IRIVs is the means by which antigen is included in the IRIV vaccine formulation. Depending on the antigen's properties and the immune response required, antigen could be directly incorporated into the membrane, adsorbed to the IRIV surface, encapsulated within the vesicle, or chemically coupled to a hydrophobic anchor (Figure 11.1). Studies on the biophysical characterization of IRIV vaccine formulations have demonstrated that the best adjuvant properties were found upon a physical association of the antigen with the IRIV, whether this be in terms of chemical, hydrophobic, or alternative means of bonding (Zurbriggen et al., 2000).

Antigens that intrinsically present a hydrophobic domain can be integrated directly into the membrane of the IRIV. However, compounds lacking lipophilic properties have to be modified biochemically in order to enable association, integration, or encapsulation. Although small molecules and synthetic particles may be readily adapted in this fashion, the chemical environment required for such alterations may adversely affect the authentic conformation of large proteins, particularly those of a multimeric nature such as viral nucleocapsids. This in turn may have negative implications on the immunogenicity of the attached antigen and the efficacy of the resulting vaccine.

For some multimeric protein structures, noncovalent adsorption between the antigen and the IRIV may provide for an effective means of coupling, but this is dependent on a sufficiently strong interaction between the

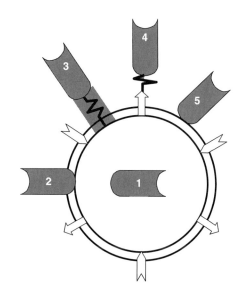

1 encapsulated in the IRIV

2 integrated into lipid bilayer

3 anchored in lipid bilayer

4 crosslinked to HA

5 adsorbed to membrane

Figure II.I **IRIVs present a flexible approach to antigen incorporation.**

IRIV and the antigen. The presentation of hepatitis A antigen on IRIVs has been particularly well elucidated, and remains the only example of a multimeric protein structure having been effectively linked with IRIV without biochemical alterations to its structure (Zurbriggen et al., 2000).

Encapsulation of antigens within IRIVs, essential for strong cellular immune responses and therefore therapeutic vaccine preparations, poses further problems as the current methodology of manufacture means that passive loading of antigen is far from optimal. Improved liposomal packaging methods do exist, but these are of limited use as exposure of the IRIV-bound HA to the low pH or organic solvents frequently used to optimize liposome packaging would result in an irreversible HA conformational change or premature membrane fusion and coagulation of the IRIV particles. However, methods do exist for actively encapsulating peptides and small drugs within IRIVs, such as a proton gradient generated by IRIV-entrapped ammonium sulfate for the loading of cytotoxic drugs, as reported by Waelti et al. (2002).

◼ IRIVs and registered vaccines

The validation of the IRIV concept as a delivery vehicle has been shown through the licensing of IRIV-based vaccines against hepatitis A (Epaxal®, Berna Biotech, Bern, Switzerland) and influenza (Inflexal® V, Berna Biotech, Bern, Switzerland; Invivac is a product of Solvay, Weesp, The Netherlands). The IRIV hepatitis A vaccine was the first to be licensed and has been on the market since 1994; together over 20 million doses of the two IRIV-based vaccines have been applied.

IRIVs can be produced on a large scale, with lot sizes of up to 500,000 doses as standard (Glück et al., 1992). The basic production of the IRIV is similar for both commercial vaccines. Initially monovalent whole influenza virus pools are diluted with a phosphate buffer saline (PBS) solution and ultracentrifuged. The pellet formed is then solubilized with the detergent octaethyleneglycol (OEG) followed by a second ultracentrifugation step and the mixing of the supernatants with lecithin. The preparations are then put through a sterilizing filtration process followed by batch-chromatography and dilution with

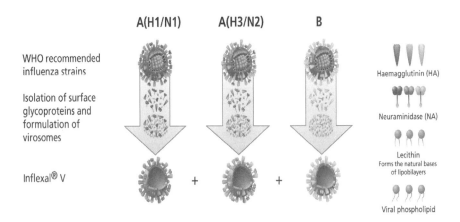

Figure 11.2 The production of Inflexal® V (Berna Biotech, Bern, Switzerland). This is derived from the surface glycoproteins of the three recommended influenza virus strains being isolated and purified prior to reformulation into IRIVs. (See Color Plate Section.)

PBS, the result of which is a pool of mono-valent IRIVs. These are then analyzed for phospholipid content, viral NA and HA content, purity, OEG and endotoxin presence, sterility, and size (Mischler et al., 2002).

In addition, the IRIV hepatitis A vaccine contains formalin-inactivated and highly purified hepatitis A virus particles of strain RG-SB, which are adsorbed to the surface of the IRIV. The trivalent IRIV-based influenza vaccine differs in that it consists of a mixture of three types of monovalent IRIVs (Figure 11.2), each harboring the HA and NA glycoproteins from one of the three strains yearly recommended by the World Health Organization (WHO) (Glück et al., 1997).

The IRIV hepatitis A vaccine has proven to induce a very rapid immune response with 100% seroconversion achieved 10 days after immunization (Wiedermann et al., 1998). The vaccine also demonstrated improved tolerability while being at least as immunogenic as a conventional alum-adjuvanted vaccine (Holzer et al., 1996). The immunogenicity of the IRIV-based influenza vaccine has also been shown by a significant more than four-fold increase in anti-HA antibodies in elderly people (Glück et al., 1994). Comparison trials have also established the superior tolerability of the IRIV-based influenza vaccine when compared

with subunit influenza vaccines (Conne et al., 1997).

IRIVs and malaria prophylaxis

Certain diseases pose a more taxing problem with regard to the development of an efficacious vaccine. Malaria is one of the world's most debilitating diseases with a mortality rate of over one million people per year. The difficulties posed in developing a vaccine against a pathogen such as *Plasmodium falciparium*, the causative agent of malaria, are due to the multiple stages of its life cycle. Although broad antibody responses directed against the parasite are essential for protection, cell-mediated mechanisms are critical for acquired immunity (Breman et al., 2004).

Peptidomimetics have shown promising results in the development of a vaccine against the malaria parasite *Plasmodium falciparium* (Moreno et al., 2002; Pfeiffer et al., 2003; Mueller et al., 2003). The use of synthetic vaccine design technologies has enabled the elicitation of defined antibody responses against conformational epitopes using constrained peptidomimetics (Tsuji et al., 2001). The mimetics function by stimulating the immune system to produce antibodies that

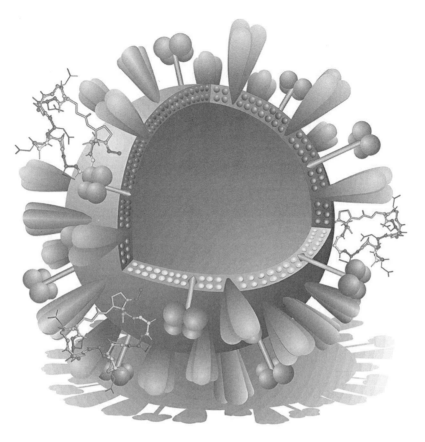

Figure 11.3 Malaria vaccine candidate. This is a peptide epitope of the malaria parasite *Plasmodium falciparum* (mimetic PEV302) attached to an IRIV. (Reproduced with the kind permission of Wiley-VCH, from Pfeiffer, B., Peduzzi, E., Moehle, K., Zurbriggen, R., Gluck, R., Pluschke, G., and Robinson, J.A. (2003). A virosome-mimotope approach to synthetic vaccine design and optimisation: synthesis, conformation and immune recognition of a potential malaria-vaccine candidate. *Angew. Chem. Int.* 42, 2368–2371.) (See Color Plate Section.)

recognize intact pathogens. However, as with many modern, well-defined antigens, poor immunogenicity and low proteolytic stability has limited their use in viable vaccine formulations (Ciba Foundation Symposium, 1986).

Early synthetic malaria vaccine candidates included a linear (NANP)$_3$ peptide conjugated to tetanus toxin in alum. While this vaccine stimulated functional antibodies and was well tolerated, the efficacy was poor (Herrington et al., 1987). In order to improve the immunopotentiating effect of the vaccine, IRIVs have been used in the formulation. By covalently linking multiple copies of a folded conformation of the NANP-repeat

region to IRIVs, they are effectively presented to the immune system in a more native-like state (Figure 11.3) (Moreno et al., 2002; Pfeiffer et al., 2003).

Studies comparing the IRIV-NANP constructs against an alum-adjuvanted mimotope-multiple antigenic peptide (MAP) construct showed noticeable improvements in the pathogen cross-reactive antibody responses when using IRIVs (Moreno et al., 2002). These results are likely to be due to the nature of presentation of the antigen on the IRIV surface in a way that it closely resembles the pathogen. Particularly as alum-adjuvanted formulations, the formation of which may disturb the conformation of the mimetic, preferentially generate antibodies against conformations of the NPNA motif that do not resemble the native CS protein (Moreno et al., 2002).

Following the success of the preclinical testing, a candidate IRIV-based vaccine militating against malaria is currently undergoing clinical trials. In 2004 phase I clinical end points for safety, tolerability, and immunogenicity were achieved in a randomized, placebo-controlled blind study with 46 healthy volunteers. The study is continuing with a third vaccination to evaluate further immunological aspects, the results of which are expected mid-2005 (R. Zurbriggen, personal communication).

■ IRIVs and cancer therapy

Two distinct therapies are currently at the forefront of research in the treatment of cancer: the targeted delivery of cytotoxic drugs, either through delivery vehicles or direct modifications of the drugs, and antibody-directed T cell immunotherapy. The former, more traditional approach, directly uses cytotoxic drugs to induce cell death in the tumor; the latter is based on the manipulation of humoral and cell-mediated immunity. IRIVs can be used for both.

The vast majority of anticancer treatments currently available rely upon cytostatic properties, such as chemotherapy. Generally associated with a lack of selectivity leading to severe adverse events, these treatments have a negative impact on the quality of life of the patients. Several approaches have been investigated in order to reduce the systemic toxicity of chemotherapeutic agents, not least of which is specific targeting of the drug to tumor cells and the use of specifically targeted drug delivery vehicles.

Several pharmacological agents have been developed that can be selectively targeted and may block the action of specific growth factors and their associated receptors. These include bispecific antibodies, monoclonal antibodies (whole molecules, fragments, and conjugated to drugs), antisense oligonucleotides,

small-molecule inhibitors, and liposome-encapsulated drugs (reviewed in Guillemard et al., 2004). Liposome encapsulation is the most intensively studied of these approaches and serves several purposes (reviewed in Felnerova et al., 2004). Initially, the drug has a reduced systemic distribution and is therefore less likely to affect sensitive nontumor organs; particularly if the vehicle used has a low affinity for certain tissues, such as heart, kidney, and gastrointestinal tract. Slow release of the drug is also likely to elicit a lower plasma concentration than an equivalent dose of free drug, potentially reducing toxic adverse events. In addition, the length of time the drugs are present in the blood may be prolonged, potentially increasing their exposure to the targeted sites. A further key stage in the development of the delivery of chemotherapeutic agents has been the selective targeting of tumors by their intrinsic properties, such as their overexpression of particular molecules or the expression of selective molecules.

IRIVs present as a suitable vehicle for the delivery of cytoplasmatic drugs. The retention of pH-dependent HA-mediated membrane fusion by IRIVs coupled with specific targeting of the vehicle provide distinct advantages if an efficient encapsulation of the respective compound can be achieved. Mastrobattista et al. have demonstrated a successful application of the technology in the targeting of ovarian carcinoma cells (Mastrobattista et al., 2001). This was achieved by conjugating antibody Fab′ fragments of monoclonal antibodies (Mabs) to the surface of IRIVs. The use of PEG molecules in the lipid membrane to anchor the antibody Fab′ fragments induced antigen-specific binding to ovarian carcinoma cells while maintaining the fusogenic properties of the IRIVs (Mastrobattista et al., 2001).

Waelti et al. (2002) also demonstrated tumor progression inhibition using similar techniques in a mouse model following treatment with IRIVs that possessed PEG-anchored antibodies for targeting and HA for cytoplasmatic delivery of the encapsulated doxorubicin.

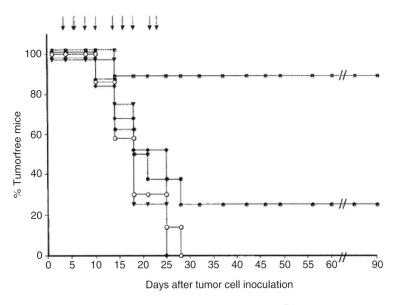

Figure 11.4 Effect of Vir treatment on implanted tumors. rNeu+ tumor cells (2×10^5) were injected subcutaneously, and treatment was started 3 to 5 days later. Intravenous injections of the different Vir formulations, such as Doxo-Vir, Fab'-Doxo-Vir, Fab'-Vir, and free Doxo (all at a concentration of 150 μg/ml doxorubicin), were performed at the indicated time points (arrows) for a period of three weeks (○, control groups; ●, Fab'-Vir; ■, Fab'-Doxo-Vir; ◆, Doxo-Vir; ▼, free Doxo). (Reproduced with the kind permission of AACR from Waelti, E. et al. (2002). Targeting HER-2/neu with antirat Neu virosomes for cancer therapy. *Cancer Res.* 62, 437–444.)

Through the use of an IRIV vector and the conjugation of doxorubicin and Fab′ fragments of an antirat Neu monoclonal antibody, the cytotoxic effect of doxorubicin and the anti-proliferative properties of the monoclonal antibody were effectively combined. Incorporating rNeu-Fab′ fragments to IRIVs in this manner resulted in the selective and efficient *in vivo* inhibition of tumor progression of established rNeu-overexpressing breast tumors. Even at a tumor load representing metastatic spread, this technique was shown to be effective enough to inhibit tumor formation (Figure 11.4) (Waelti et al., 2002).

As an alternative to the use of chemotherapeutic agents, immunotherapy of cancer involving the elicitation of humoral and cell-mediated immune responses has made significant progress, mainly due to a greater understanding of the factors that govern immune tolerance and an increased ability to manipulate specific immune responses.

The identification and targeting of tumor-associated antigen (TAA), combined with a means of generating both cell-mediated anti-tumor immunity (CD8+ CTLs) and B cell antibodies to the respective TAA, may have the potential to eliminate tumors. To this end, the ability to target IRIVs combined with their delivery system properties makes them an effective tool in immunotherapeutic techniques.

The IRIV approach, in the context of a CTL response against parathyroid hormone-related protein (PTH-rP), has been demonstrated by Scardino et al. (2003). Here, the PTH-rP plasmids were purified and encapsulated within the IRIVs and intranasally inoculated into transgenic mice. The resultant PTH-rP-specific CTL response showed antitumor activity. The study also provided evidence that vaccination and subsequent boosting with the same IRIV construct induced a stronger multiepitopic CTL response specific for PTH-rP. The authors proposed that APC engagement by the IRIV via the mucosal vaccination elicited a more effective CD8+ response. This proposition has been elucidated by the same group in further studies (Cusi et al., 2004).

■ References

Almeida, J.D., Edwards, D.C., Brand, C.M., and Heath, T.D. (1975). Formation of virosomes from influenza subunits and liposomes. *Lancet* 2, 899–901.

Bachmann, M.F., Hengartner, H., and Zinkernagel, R.M. (1995). T helper cell-independent neutralizing B cell response against vesicular stomatitis virus: role of antigen patterns in B cell induction? *Eur. J. Immunol.* 25, 3445–3451.

Breman, J.G., Alilio, M.S., and Mills, A. (2004). Conquering the intolerable burden of malaria: what's new, what's needed: a summary. *Am. J. Trop. Med. Hyg.* 71 (2 Suppl.), 1–15.

Bullough, P.A., Hughson, F.M., Skehel, J.J., and Wiley, D.C. (1994). Structure of influenza haemagglutinin at the pH of membrane fusion. *Nature* 371, 37–43.

Bungener, L., Huckriede, A., de Mare, A., de Vries-Idema, J., Wilschut, J., and Daemen, T. (2005). Virosome-mediated delivery of protein antigens in vivo: efficient induction of class I MHC-restricted cytotoxic T lymphocyte activity. *Vaccine* 23, 1232–1241.

Ciba Foundation Symposium 119 (1986). Porter, R. and Whelan, J. (Eds) *Synthetic Peptides as Antigens*. Wiley, Chichester, UK.

Conne, P., Gauthey, L., Vernet, P., Althaus, B., Que, J.U., Finkel, B., Glück, R., and Cryz, S.J., Jr. (1997). Immunogenicity of trivalent subunit versus virosome-formulated influenza vaccines in geriatric patients. *Vaccine* 15, 1675–1679.

Coulter, A., Harris. R., Davis, R., Drane, D., Cox, J., Ryan, D., Sutton, P., Rockman, S., and Pearse, M. (2003). Intranasal vaccination with ISCOMATRIX adjuvanted influenza vaccine. *Vaccine* 21, 946–949.

Cusi, M.G., Terrosi, C., Savellini, G.G., Di Genova, G., Zurbriggen, R., and Correale, P. (2004). Efficient delivery of DNA to dendritic cells mediated by influenza virosomes. *Vaccine* 22, 735–739.

Daemen, T., Mare, A., Bungener, L., Jonge, J., Huckriede, A., and Wilschut, J. (2005). Virosomes for antigen and DNA delivery. *Adv. Drug Del. Rev.* 57, 451–463.

Dietrich, G., Griot-Wenk, M., Metcalfe, I.C., Lang, A.B., and Viret, J.F. (2003). Experience with registered mucosal vaccines. *Vaccine* 21, 678–683.

Durrer, P., Galli, C., Hoenke, S., Corti, C., Gluck, R., Vorherr, T., and Brunner, J. (1996). H+-induced membrane insertion of influenza virus hemagglutinin involves the HA2 amino-terminal fusion peptide but not the coiled coil region. *J. Biol. Chem.* 271, 13417–13421.

Eisenlohr, L.C., Gerhard, W., and Hackett, C.J. (1987). Role of receptor-binding activity of the viral hemagglutinin molecule in the presentation of influenza virus antigens to helper T cells. *J. Virol.* 61, 1375–1383.

Felnerova, D., Moser, C., and Viret, J.F. (2004). Liposomes and virosomes as delivery systems for antigens, nucleic acids and drugs. *Curr. Opin. Biotechnol.* 15, 518–529.

Freund, J., Casals, J., and Hosmer, E.P. (1937). Sensitization and antibody formation after injection of tubercle bacili and parafin oil. *Proc. Soc. Exp. Biol. Med.* 37, 509–513.

Glenny, A.T., Pope, C.G., Waddington, H., and Wallace, V. (1926). The antigenic value of toxoid precipitated by potassium-alum. *J. Path. Bacteriol.* 29, 38–45.

Glück, R. and Cryz, J., Jr. (1997). IRIV vaccine delivery. In Levine, M.M., Woodrow, G.C., Kaper, J.B., and Cobon, G.S. (Eds) *New Generation Vaccines*. Marcel Dekker, New York, pp. 247–252.

Gluck, R., Mischler, R., Brantschen, S., Just, M., Althaus, B., and Cryz, S.J., Jr. (1992). Immunopotentiating reconstituted influenza virus virosome vaccine delivery system for immunization against hepatitis A. *J. Clin. Invest.* 90, 2491–2495.

Glück, R., Mischler, R., Finkel, B., Que, J.U., Scarpa, B., and Cryz, S.J., Jr. (1994). Immunogenicity of new virosome influenza vaccine in elderly people. *Lancet* 344, 160–163.

Glueck, R. (2001). Pre-clinical and clinical investigation of the safety of a novel adjuvant for intranasal immunization. *Vaccine* 20 (Suppl. 1), S42–S44.

Greenwald, R.J., Freeman, G.J., and Sharpe, A.H. (2005). The B7 family revisited. *Annu. Rev. Immunol.* 23, 515–548.

Guillemard, V. and Saragovi, H.U. (2004). Novel approaches for targeted cancer therapy. *Curr. Cancer Drug Targets* 4, 313–326.

Hasegawa, H., Ichinohe, T., Strong, P., Watanabe, I., Ito, S., Tamura, S., Takahashi, H., Sawa, H,. Chiba, J., Kurata, T., and Sata, T. (2005). Protection against influenza virus infection by intranasal administration of hemagglutinin vaccine with chitin microparticles as an adjuvant. *J. Med. Virol.* 75, 130–136.

Herrington, D.A., Clyde, D.F., Losonsky, G. et al. (1987). Safety and immunogenicity in man of a synthetic peptide malaria vaccine against Plasmodium falciparum sporozoites. *Nature* 328, 257–259.

Holzer, B.R., Hatz, C., Schmidt-Sissolak, D., Glück, R., Althaus, B., and Egger, M. (1996). Immunogenicity and adverse effects of inactivated virosome versus alum-adsorbed hepatitis A vaccine: a randomised controlled trial. *Vaccine* 14, 982–986.

MedImmune Vaccines: CAIV-T, influenza virus vaccine live intranasal. (2003). *Drugs Res. Devel.* 4, 312–319.

Leikina, E., LeDuc, D.L., Macosko, J.C., Epand, R., Shin, Y.K., and Chernomordik, L.V. (2001). The 1-127 HA2 construct of influenza virus hemagglutinin induces cell–cell hemifusion. *Biochemistry* 40, 8378–8386.

Levine, M.M. (2003). Can needle-free administration of vaccines become the norm in global immunization? *Nature Med* 9, 99–103.

Mastrobattista, E., Schoen, P., Wilschut, J., Crommelin, D.J., and Storm, G. (2001). Targeting influenza virosomes to ovarian carcinoma cells. *FEBS Lett.* 509, 71–76.

Matrosovich, M.N., Matrosovich, T.Y., Gray, T., Roberts, N.A., and Klenk, H.D. (2004) Neuraminidase is important for the initiation of influenza virus infection in human airway epithelium. *J. Virol.* 78, 12665–12667.

Mischler, R. and Metcalfe, I.C. (2002). Inflexal V a trivalent virosome subunit influenza vaccine: production. *Vaccine* 20 (Suppl. 5), B17–B23.

Moreno, R., Jiang, L., Moehle, K. et al. (2002). Exploiting conformationally constrained peptidomimetics and an efficient human-compatible delivery system in synthetic vaccine design. *Chembiochem.* 2, 838–843. Erratum in *Chembiochem.* 3, 270.

Moser, C., Metcalfe, I.C., and Viret, J.F. (2003). Virosomal adjuvanted antigen delivery systems. *Expert Rev. Vaccines* 2, 189–196.

Mueller, M.S., Renard, A., Boato, F. et al. (2003). Induction of parasite growth-inhibitory antibodies by a virosomal formulation of a peptidomimetic of loop I from domain III of *Plasmodium falciparum* apical membrane antigen 1. *Infect. Immun.* 71, 4749–4758.

Mutsch, M., Zhou, W., Rhodes, P., Bopp, M., Chen, R.T., Linder, T., Spyr, C., and Steffen, R. (2004). Use of the inactivated intranasal influenza vaccine and the risk of Bell's palsy in Switzerland. *N. Engl. J. Med.* 350, 896–903.

Ott, G., Barchfeld, G.L., Chernoff, D., Radhakrishnan, R., van Hoogevest, P., and Van Nest, G. (1995). Design and evaluation of a safe and potent adjuvant for human vaccines. *Pharm. Biotechnol.* 6, 277–296.

Pfeiffer, B., Peduzzi, E., Moehle, K., Zurbriggen, R., Gluck, R., Pluschke, G. et al. (2003). A virosome-mimotope approach to synthetic vaccine design and optimization: synthesis, conformation, and immune recognition of a potential malaria-vaccine candidate. *Angew. Chem. Int. Ed. Engl.* 42, 2368–2371.

Pine, S., Barackman, J., Ott, G., and O'Hagan, D. (2002). Intranasal immunization with influenza vaccine and a detoxified mutant of heat labile enterotoxin from *Escherichia coli* (LTK63). *J. Control. Release* 85, 263–270.

Plotkin, S.A. (2005). Six revolutions in vaccinology. *Pediat. Infect. Dis. J.* 24, 1–9.

Scardino, A., Correale, P., Firat, H., Pellegrini, M., Kosmatopoulos, K., Opolon, P., Alves, P., Zurbriggen, R.,

Gluck, R., Lemonnier, F.A., Francini, G., and Cusi, M.G. (2003). In vivo study of the GC90/IRIV vaccine for immune response and autoimmunity into a novel humanised transgenic mouse. *Br. J. Cancer* 89, 199–205.

Schumacher, R., Adamina, M., Zurbriggen, R., Bolli, M., Padovan, E., Zajac, P., Heberer, M., and Spagnoli, G.C. (2004). Influenza virosomes enhance restricted class I CTL induction through CD4+ T-cell activation. *Vaccine* 22,714–723.

Sesardic, D. and Dobbelaer, R. (2004). European union regulatory developments for new vaccine adjuvants and delivery systems. *Vaccine* 22, 2452–2456.

Tacket, C.O., Losonsky, G., Nataro, J.P., Cryz, S.J., Edelman, R., Kaper, J.B., and Levine, M.M. (1992). Onset and duration of protective immunity in challenged volunteers after vaccination with live oral cholera vaccine CVD 103-HgR. *J. Infect. Dis.* 166, 837–841.

Tsuji, M., Rodrigues, E.G., and Nussenzweig, S. (2001). Progress toward a malaria vaccine: efficient induction of protective anti-malaria immunity. *Biol. Chem.* 382, 553–570.

Van Kampen, K.R., Shi, Z., Gao, P., Zhang, J., Foster, K.W., Chen, D.T., Marks, D., Elmets, C.A., and Tang, D.C. (2005). Safety and immunogenicity of adenovirus-vectored nasal and epicutaneous influenza vaccines in humans. *Vaccine* 23, 1029–1036.

Waelti, E., Wegmann, N., Schwaninger, R., Wetterwald, A., Wingenfeld, C., Rothen-Rutishauser, B., and Gimmi, C.D. (2002). Targeting her-2/neu with antirat Neu virosomes for cancer therapy. *Cancer Res.* 62, 437–444.

Wahdan, M.H., Serie, C., Cerisier, Y., Sallam, S., and Germanier, R. (1982). A controlled field trial of live *Salmonella typhi* strain Ty 21a oral vaccine against typhoid: three-year results. *J. Infect. Dis.* 145, 292–295.

Wiedermann, G., Kundi, M., and Ambrosch, F. (1998). Estimated persistence of anti-HAV antibodies after single dose and booster hepatitis A vaccination (0-6 schedule). *Acta Trop.* 69, 121–125.

Wilson, I.A., Skehel, J.J., and Wiley, D.C. (1981). Structure of the haemagglutinin membrane glycoprotein of influenza virus at 3 A resolution. *Nature* 289, 366–373.

Zurbriggen, R., Novak-Hofer, I., Seelig, A., and Glück, R. (2000). IRIV-adjuvanted hepatitis A vaccine: in vivo absorption and biophysical characterisation. *Prog. Lipid Res.* 39, 3–18.

The ISCOMATRIX™ adjuvant

Debbie Drane and Martin J. Pearse
CSL Limited, Parkville, Australia

■ Introduction

The immunostimulating complex referred to as an "iscom" or ISCOM™ vaccine was first described by Morein et al. in 1984 as a novel structure for antigenic presentation of membrane proteins from enveloped viruses with potent immunomodulatory capability (Morein et al., 1984). Since this discovery many ISCOM™ vaccines have been tested in animal models showing the induction of both humoral and cellular immune responses (Sjolander et al., 1998). ISCOMATRIX™ adjuvant is essentially the same structure as the ISCOM™ vaccine but without the incorporated antigen (Rimmelzwaan and Osterhaus, 1995). Antigens can be formulated with the ISCOMATRIX™ adjuvant to produce ISCOMATRIX™ vaccines which provide the same antigen presentation and immunomodulatory properties as ISCOM™ vaccines but with much broader application. Various ISCOMATRIX™ vaccines have been tested in animal models and more recently in human clinical trials (Kersten et al., 2003). All results to date indicate that ISCOMATRIX™ vaccines are safe and well tolerated in humans with no vaccine-related serious adverse events or clinically significant laboratory abnormalities reported. ISCOMATRIX™ vaccines are capable of inducing strong humoral responses with increases in the magnitude, speed, and longevity of the responses, as well as the capacity for antigen dose reduction when compared to other adjuvants such as aluminum. Additionally, ISCOMATRIX™ vaccines have the ability to induce strong and long lasting CD4+ and CD8+ T cell responses. Furthermore, intranasal delivery of influenza ISCOMATRIX™ vaccine in humans elicited both systemic and mucosal responses, suggesting that the ISCOMATRIX™ adjuvant has significant potential as a mucosal adjuvant. The ability of the ISCOMATRIX™ adjuvant to induce these broad immune responses is due to the fact that it is both an effective antigen delivery vehicle, which can access both the MHC I and MHC II pathways, and a potent immunomodulator of both the innate and adaptive immune systems. The ISCOMATRIX™ adjuvant manufacturing process has been extensively optimized and is simple, reproducible, and well defined as well as being suitable for production at large scale. Overall, the properties of ISCOMATRIX™ vaccines make them viable candidates for the further development and registration of prophylactic and therapeutic human vaccines.

■ Preparation and properties of ISCOMATRIX™ adjuvant

■ Composition

ISCOMATRIX™ adjuvant contains saponin, cholesterol, and phospholipid typically in a phosphate buffered isotonic saline (PBS) at pH 6.2. The saponin used in the ISCOMATRIX™ adjuvant for the development of human vaccines is a multicomponent fraction from the bark extract of the *Quillaia saponaria* tree and is called ISCOPREP™ saponin.

Q. saponaria saponins exhibit potent immuno-modulatory activity and have been used for many years in animal vaccines, although the crude preparations are not suitable for human vaccines due to toxicity and complexity (Dalsgaard, 1970). These problems led to the development of more defined fractions of quillaia, including QS21 (Soltysik et al., 1995) and ISCOPREP^{TM} saponin (Ronnberg et al., 1995). ISCOPREP^{TM} saponin is a well-defined, multicomponent fraction manufactured by CSL using a proprietary process which ensures that the known toxic components of the crude quillaia are not present. It is produced in a liquid formulation and has been extensively characterized to ensure consistency of manufacture. All the reagents used in the fractionation process are chemically defined and none are of animal origin.

During the manufacture of the ISCOMATRIX^{TM} adjuvant cholesterol interacts with saponin to form an extremely strong bond, which is the basis of the unique cage-like structure, and no doubt contributes to the stability of the ISCOMATRIX^{TM} adjuvant (Kersten and Crommelin, 2003). This interaction also substantially reduces the hemolytic activity of the saponin, making it an important component in the formulation of ISCOMATRIX^{TM} adjuvant. The cholesterol used in the manufacturing process at CSL for the ISCOMATRIX^{TM} adjuvant is classified as synthetic, with the starting material for synthesis being plant derived.

The phospholipid component contributes to the morphology and stability of the ISCOMATRIX^{TM} adjuvant (Lovgren and Morein, 1988). The type of phospholipid used is dependent on the formulation properties required, with a wide range of different phospholipids being suitable for the formation of ISCOMATRIX^{TM} adjuvant. Phosphatidylcholine (PC) was traditionally used in the early ISCOM^{TM} vaccines as it was identified as a component of cell membranes that enabled consistent ISCOM^{TM} formation. Although considered safe for use in humans, the PC commonly used was egg derived

and contained a number of different molecules with acyl chains of different lengths making it difficult to produce consistently. Dipalmytoyl-phosphatidylcholine (DPPC) was identified as the optimal phospholipid for the manufacture of ISCOMATRIX^{TM} adjuvant for the development of human vaccines as it is a single chain length, and is manufactured synthetically from plant-derived starting materials.

The nonionic detergent decanoyl-*N*-methylglucanamide (Mega 10) is used to solubilize the cholesterol and phospholipid, but is diluted during manufacture, so that only trace quantities are present in the final product. Mega 10 is chemically defined and synthetically produced.

All the components of the ISCOMATRIX^{TM} adjuvant and the manufacturing process are well defined and either synthetic or derived from plant materials. Substantial effort has been made to ensure that none of the components are of animal origin and that they are sourced from reputable suppliers. These features of the ISCOMATRIX^{TM} adjuvant are important not only for the control and consistency of the raw materials, but also to ensure the acceptability of the adjuvant for use in the clinical development of human vaccines.

■ Physical properties

The physical properties of the ISCOMATRIX^{TM} adjuvant contribute not only to the morphology and stability of the structure, but also to the ability to formulate vaccines with a wide range of antigens. The morphology of the ISCOMATRIX^{TM} adjuvant is generally examined using transmission electron microscopy, where the morphology appears as hollow cage-like spherical structures typically 40 nm in diameter, consisting of subunit rings as shown in Figure 12.1 (Ozel et al., 1989). Other microscopic techniques have also been used to investigate the morphology of ISCOMATRIX^{TM} adjuvant, including cryo-electron microscopy and atomic force microscopy. These techniques have confirmed the spherical nature of the ISCOMATRIX^{TM}

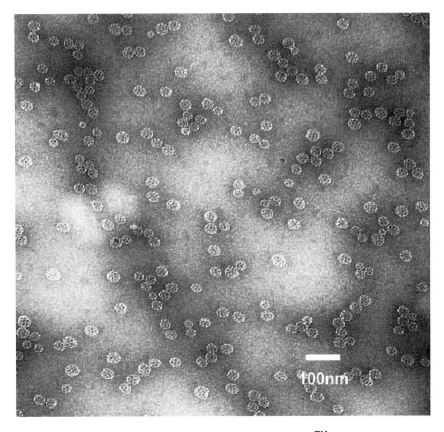

Figure 12.1 Transmission electron micrograph of negatively stained ISCOMATRIX™ adjuvant. The image demonstrates the typical 40 nm cage-like structures.

adjuvant, as well as the typical size and ring-like subunit structure.

A molecular structure proposed by Kersten et al. (1991) described the ISCOMATRIX™ adjuvant as a "soccer ball" arrangement with the multiple micelles held together by hydrophobic interactions, steric factors, and possibly hydrogen bonds. In this model the saponin molecules create pores in cholesterol/DPPC vesicles with only the triterpenoid core of the saponin interacting with the lipid bilayer. Studies using molecular dynamics have supported the general proposal made by Kersten et al. although they also suggest that the saponin molecule is inserted into the bilayer in an extended conformation so that both the triterpenoid core and the acyl side chain interact with the bilayer. The latter structure is more likely as it has been shown that saponin molecules require both the triterpenoid core and acyl side chains to form ISCOMATRIX™ adjuvant (data not shown).

Another important physical property is the surface charge which is approximately −20 mV. This negative charge enables the ISCOMATRIX™ adjuvant to exist in solution as a stable colloid, as well as contributing to formulation capabilities. The typical 40 nm size and particulate nature of the ISCOMATRIX™ adjuvant is also thought to be important for the immunogenicity of ISCOMATRIX™ vaccines, particularly for the delivery of antigens to antigen-presenting cells (APCs), as discussed in more detail in a later section.

As previously described, the interactions of the components and the physical properties contribute to the stability of the ISCOMATRIX™ adjuvant. The cage-like structures form spontaneously and exist in a low-energy state, making them very stable. ISCOMATRIX™ adjuvant is routinely manufactured in PBS pH 6.2 and stored at 2–8°C and is stable for at least 2 years at a range of different concentrations. Studies have also been performed at elevated temperatures and at a range of pH levels. The results of these studies have indicated that ISCOMATRIX™ adjuvant is stable in a wide range of conditions including pH 3 and 45°C. ISCOMATRIX™ adjuvant is not, however, stable for extended periods above pH 8.5, particularly at elevated temperatures. Under these conditions the ISCOPREP™ saponin component undergoes alkaline hydrolysis, which eventually leads to a reduction in the immunomodulatory capability of the ISCOMATRIX™ adjuvant. These studies have enabled the development of stability-indicating assays which can be used to evaluate the ISCOMATRIX™ adjuvant and ISCOMATRIX™ vaccines under various conditions.

Antigens used in the manufacture of vaccines often have specific requirements in terms of buffers, excipients, and storage conditions. ISCOMATRIX™ adjuvant is compatible with a wide range of excipients including solvents, detergents, denaturants, and reducing agents. Additionally, ISCOMATRIX™ adjuvant can be repeatedly freeze thawed, freeze dried, spray dried, or stored frozen for extended periods (Macdonald et al., 1997). This stability enables formulation of ISCOMATRIX™ vaccines with a wide range of antigens under a variety of conditions.

▪ Manufacturing

The ISCOPREP™ saponin used by CSL is fractionated in a dedicated, purpose-built facility using a proprietary process. The process is performed in accordance with good manufacturing practices (GMP) and has been optimized to ensure it is robust and produces a consistent product. A range of in-process testing is performed and the final material is tested according to a predetermined release specification. The crude quillaia used as the starting material for this process undergoes both acceptance and release testing prior to use.

The manufacturing process for ISCOMATRIX™ adjuvant is relatively simple and has been optimized to produce a robust procedure that is well-controlled and suitable for large-scale production. The process is GMP compliant, with in process and release testing performed according to predetermined specifications. A summary of the ISCOMATRIX™ adjuvant manufacturing process is shown in Figure 12.2.

Extensive optimization of the manufacturing process was performed using the principles of design of experiments (DOE). DOE enables a variety of process parameters to be systematically evaluated and analyzed. All aspects of the process were evaluated according to defined product criteria, including key features such as morphology, hemolytic activity, and particle size, as well as process criteria such as filterability and yield. The parameters investigated were extensive and included physical conditions such as time and temperature, as well as process conditions such as the concentration and ratio of starting materials. The data were analyzed using statistical procedures to maximize all the required criteria and resulted in a process that is well controlled, robust, and reproducible.

▪ Formulation methods

The preparation of ISCOM™ vaccines was originally performed using a centrifugation method, which was developed using viral membrane proteins as antigen (Morein et al., 1984). A dialysis procedure was also developed which enabled the use of a broader range of proteins and is now the method most commonly used for laboratory investigations of ISCOM™ vaccines. More recently,

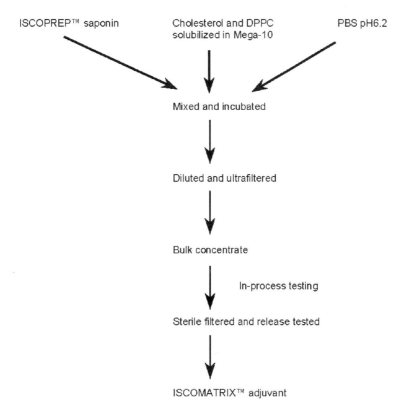

Figure I2.2 Flow chart showing the ISCOMATRIX^{TM} adjuvant manufacturing process. Mega-I0 (decanoyl-*N*-methylglucamide) is a nonionic detergent.

ultrafiltration techniques have been developed which allow the process to be performed at a larger scale. The process for preparing ISCOM^{TM} vaccines to ensure consistency of incorporation of proteins remains quite difficult to control. Additionally, due to the requirement for the protein to contain a hydrophobic region, the range of proteins that can be used is limited. Efforts have been made to develop procedures for introducing hydrophobic regions into proteins using both conjugation and recombinant techniques (Andersson et al., 2000; Morein et al., 1995). Although there has been some success with these methods, they are also difficult to control. Because of these control problems, and limitation on the types of proteins that can be incorporated into ISCOM^{TM} vaccines, recent efforts have focused on the development

of methods to formulate proteins with ISCOMATRIX^{TM} adjuvant.

The method used to formulate ISCOMATRIX^{TM} vaccines is dependent on both the characteristics of the protein and the type of immune response that is required. It is important to ensure that the conditions required for protein conformation and/or solubility are maintained. Additionally, it has been shown experimentally that association between the ISCOMATRIX^{TM} adjuvant and the protein may be required for optimal induction of cellular immune responses (Lenarczyk et al., 2004). Recent studies using the model antigen ovalbumin have shown that CD8+ T cell responses can be induced with an associated formulation using 100-fold less protein than is required for a nonassociated formulation. The capacity to use a lower dose of antigen may be important in situations where manufacture of the protein is difficult and/or expensive, but may be less important for proteins that are relatively inexpensive and easy to manufacture. The mechanisms underlying the efficiency of associated formulations to induce cellular immune responses are described later in this chapter. Interestingly, the induction of antibody responses does not appear to benefit from association, with strong antibody responses induced by both associated and nonassociated formulations (Lenarczyk et al., 2004).

A range of strategies has been developed to associate proteins with preformulated ISCOMATRIX™ adjuvant to produce ISCOMATRIX™ vaccines. These include methods that take advantage of the physical properties of the ISCOMATRIX™ adjuvant such as electrostatic interactions where positively charged proteins will associate with the negatively charged adjuvant. Procedures for modifying either the protein or the adjuvant to maximize this type of association have also been developed (Le et al., 2001).

Other methods for achieving association include modifications to the components of the ISCOMATRIX™ adjuvant to enable coupling of proteins to various exposed chemical groups. One example of this type of modification is called chelating ISCOMATRIX™ adjuvant, in which a metal chelating group is incorporated into the structure, which can then bind proteins containing a metal affinity tag such as hexahistidine (Malliaros et al., 2004). Interestingly, this procedure also allowed association with proteins in denaturants, which could subsequently be removed without affecting association. Activated lipids can also be incorporated into the ISCOMATRIX™ adjuvant to enable coupling using a range of different chemistries (unpublished data).

Nonclinical studies

ISCOM™ and ISCOMATRIX™ vaccines have been shown to elicit strong humoral and cellular immune responses in all species examined to date, including nonhuman primates. The immune responses generated in response to vaccination with ISCOM™ and ISCOMATRIX™ vaccines have recently been reviewed (Pearse and Drane, 2005; Sjolander et al., 2001a).

Humoral immune responses

In mice, ISCOM™ vaccines delivered parenterally induce antibodies of all IgG isotypes, including IgG1 and IgG2a, suggesting a balanced Th1/Th2 response (Sjolander et al., 1997). Consistent with this, both Th1 (e.g., interleukin IL-2, interferon IFN-γ) and Th2 (e.g., IL-4, IL-10) cytokines are also induced. However, ISCOM™ vaccines elicit very weak IgE responses following either intranasal or parenteral delivery (Hu et al., 1998; Sjolander et al., 1997). In contrast, aluminum-based vaccines predominantly elicit IgG1 and IgE antibodies, in concert with the cytokines IL-4 and IL-10, which together are indicative of a Th2 immune response (Kenney et al., 1989; Sjolander et al., 1997). The very low IgE responses elicited in response to ISCOMATRIX™ vaccines reduces the potential for IgE-mediated allergic responses to the vaccine antigen. Induction of hyperallergic responses is a potential problem with aluminum adjuvants, although in practice this rarely occurs (Lindblad, 2004). The induction of both Th1 and Th2 antibodies gives ISCOMATRIX™ vaccines an advantage over aluminum-based vaccines because it results in a broader range of antibody-mediated effector mechanisms being mobilized. Th1 antibodies are particularly important for the clearance of viral infections, because they are potent mediators of complement activation (Coulie and Van Snick, 1985), neutralization, antibody-dependent cell-mediated cellular cytoxicity (ADCC) (Coutelier et al., 1987), opsonization, and phagocytosis (Kipps et al., 1985).

Recent studies in guinea pigs, sheep, and baboons have shown the potential benefit of

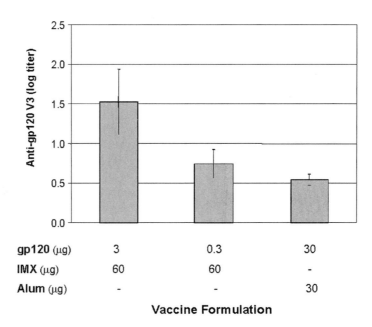

Figure 12.3 Neutralizing antibody responses in guinea pigs. The responses are to HIV gp120 at the antigen dose indicated, following 3 immunizations with ISCOMATRIX™ adjuvant (IMX) or aluminum adjuvant (alum). Antibody responses were determined by EIA on diluted serum (1/25,000).

ISCOMATRIX™ adjuvant in terms of antigen dose reduction for parenterally delivered vaccines. In guinea pigs the human immuno-deficiency virus (HIV) antigen gp120, combined with ISCOMATRIX™ adjuvant, induced neutralizing antibody responses of similar magnitude using 10- to 100-fold less antigen than was required with aluminum hydroxide adjuvant (Figure 12.3). In sheep (Coulter et al., 2003) and baboons (unpublished data) serum hemagglutination inhibition (HAI) titers induced with an influenza ISCOMATRIX™ vaccine were equivalent to or better than unadjuvanted vaccines that contained 10-fold more antigen. Similar antigen dose reduction with influenza ISCOMATRIX™ vaccines has also been observed in humans as shown in a later section.

Antibody responses to ISCOMATRIX™ vaccines have been shown to have increased durability when compared to other adjuvants such as aluminum. In a study in rhesus macaques (antigen not disclosed), antibody responses with an ISCOMATRIX™ vaccine were still maintained at high levels at week 102, whereas antibody responses with the vaccine containing aluminum hydroxide adjuvant had dropped significantly by week 52. Furthermore, the responses at 102 weeks with the ISCOMATRIX™ vaccine were still higher than the peak responses achieved with the aluminum-adjuvanted vaccine (personal communication).

Another important feature of ISCOM™ and ISCOMATRIX™ vaccines is their ability to induce antibody responses in the presence of preexisting antibody. Many pathogens are capable of eliciting antibody responses that do not eliminate the disease, e.g., hepatitis B virus (HBV), hepatitis C virus (HCV), and HIV. A vaccine adjuvant capable of stimulating immune responses in the presence of these antibodies is critical if therapeutic vaccination strategies are to be successful. Furthermore, some vaccines such as the measles vaccine have reduced efficacy in infants, or for boosting in children and adults, because they are inhibited by the presence of low levels of maternally acquired or residual vaccine-induced antibody. Lenarczyk et al., (2004) have recently shown that adoptive transfer of antibodies against the vaccine antigen did not inhibit CD8+ T cell induction by ISCOMATRIX^{TM} vaccines. Additionally, ISCOM^{TM} vaccines have been shown to be immunogenic in the face of passively acquired antibody in neonatal mice, horses, and macaques. In nonhuman primates and horses, active immunity was induced in the presence of maternal antibody against measles virus and equine herpes 2 virus, respectively, with ISCOM^{TM} vaccines, but not conventional killed vaccines (Morein and Lovgren Bengtsson, 1998; Osterhaus et al., 1998).

The ability to function in the presence of preexisting antibodies distinguishes the ISCOMATRIX^{TM} adjuvant from other vaccine delivery modalities, such as live viral vectors, that are "neutralized" by preexisting antibody and therefore cannot be used for repeated dosing.

■ Cellular immune responses

Clearance of viral infection, particularly chronic infection with viruses such as HBV, HCV, HIV and human papilloma virus (HPV) is mainly mediated by MHC I-restricted CD8+ T cells (Hou et al., 1992). It is now also widely accepted that strong CD8+ cytotoxic T lymphocyte (CTL) responses will be vital for successful prophylactic and therapeutic vaccines against these pathogens (Autran et al., 2004) and for cancer immunotherapy (Hariharan et al., 1995).

The induction of MHC I-restricted CD8+ T cells, particularly in humans, has to date proven a significant hurdle for vaccine development. Delivery systems such as DNA and viral vectors have offered some hope, but have potential safety concerns and, in the case of DNA, generally elicit poor cellular responses, in particular CD8+ CTL responses. Additionally, viral vectors as discussed above have the problem of inducing neutralizing antibodies

to the vector, which limits repeated use. Prime-boost combinations of DNA and live viral vector delivery are currently being evaluated and although results have been promising in animal models they are yet to be proven in humans. ISCOM^{TM} and ISCOMATRIX^{TM} vaccines have been shown in numerous studies in animal models to be potent inducers of both T helper (CD4+) and CTL (CD8+) T cell responses to a wide variety of antigens, including naturally occurring immunogens, recombinant proteins, peptides (Sjolander et al., 2001a) and multiple MHC I epitopes arranged in a linear array, referred to as a polytope^{TM} (Le et al., 2001).

Many studies have been performed in nonhuman primates with ISCOM^{TM} vaccines and a few studies with ISCOMATRIX^{TM} vaccines. In most cases strong cellular immune responses have been induced, as reviewed in Sjolander et al., 2001a). In studies which have included comparison with other adjuvants and delivery systems, ISCOM^{TM} vaccines have generally been superior at inducing cellular immune responses, in particular CTL responses (Heeney et al., 1999). We believe this would also apply to ISCOMATRIX^{TM} vaccines due to the similarities between the vaccines. In a study performed with an HCV core ISCOMATRIX^{TM} vaccine in rhesus macaques, strong CD4+ and CD8+ T cell responses against a broad range of epitopes were observed in 100% and 60% of vaccinated animals, respectively. Furthermore, there was evidence to indicate that the animals that did not generate HCV core-specific CD8+ T cell responses to the peptides analyzed were unable to do so because of MHC-restriction (Polakos et al., 2001). The CTL response induced by immunization with the HCV core ISCOMATRIX^{TM} vaccine was extremely long lived, with strong responses still detected almost a year after the final dose. In contrast, the CTL responses generated following vaccination with recombinant vaccinia virus expressing HCV core protein were diminished at week 4 and negligible by week 18 postvaccination. It should be noted, however, that in this study animals only received a single dose of the vaccinia vaccine, as the induction of vaccinia virus-neutralizing antibodies prevents repeat dosing.

Somewhat surprisingly, ISCOM^{TM} vaccines are also able to induce CD8+ T cells in the absence of CD4+ T cell help (Lenarczyk et al., 2004). This may be related to their ability to induce IL-12 (Villacres-Ericsson et al., 1997), thus bypassing the requirement for CD40 ligation (Hu et al., 2002; Smith et al., 1999). The capacity to induce a CD8+ CTL response independently of CD4+ T cell help may have a significant advantage in the development of vaccines where a CD8+ T cell response is required, but where the intended target population has impaired CD4+ T cell function, as is the case for chronic viral infections such as HIV and some cancers.

■ Mucosal immune responses

The majority of licensed vaccines are administered parenterally and predominantly induce systemic immune responses, with limited or no mucosal immune responses. The Sabin oral polio vaccine is an example of a highly effective mucosal vaccine, but like most other successful mucosal vaccines it is dependent on living microorganisms for the induction of a protective immune response. Live vaccines, however, are not the preferred approach for the development of new vaccines, mainly due to safety concerns. For this reason attention has focused on the development of nonliving mucosal vaccines which, although safe, are generally not very immunogenic. Intensive effort has therefore been directed towards the identification of a safe and effective mucosal adjuvant.

Efforts to date have largely focused on cholera toxin (CT) and *Escherichia coli* heat-labile toxin (LT), which have both been shown to have strong mucosal adjuvant activity. The activity of these toxin-based adjuvants is dependent on the presence of the toxic A subunit, which has necessitated the

development of mutant versions of these molecules to improve the safety profile (Peppoloni et al., 2003; Pizza et al., 2001). The recent finding that both CT and CT-B accumulate in the olfactory nerves, epithelial and olfactory bulbs when delivered intranasally (Fujihashi et al., 2002; Van Ginkel et al., 2000), has raised safety concerns regarding the use of toxin-based adjuvants for the development of human vaccines. Additionally, an intranasal LT-adjuvanted virosome-based influenza vaccine was withdrawn from the market due to a possible association between the vaccine and cases of Bell's palsy (Mutsch et al., 2004).

ISCOM^{TM} and ISCOMATRIX^{TM} vaccines have been shown to induce strong immune responses when delivered mucosally. However, in contrast to CT that elicits Th2-biased immune responses (MacDonald, 1999), the responses elicited following mucosal delivery of ISCOM^{TM} vaccines have a more balanced Th1/Th2 profile (Maloy et al., 1995; Sjolander et al., 1997). This appears, as is the case with parenteral delivery, to involve an IL-12-dependent cascade of innate immune responses (Grdic et al., 1999).

Immune responses following intranasal (i.n.) vaccination with ISCOM^{TM} vaccines was recently reviewed by Hu et al. (2001). In mice influenza ISCOM^{TM} vaccines induce CTL as well as strong mucosal (IgG and IgA) and systemic (IgG) antibody responses when delivered by the i.n. route (Sjolander et al., 2001b). Furthermore, the antibody responses generated were equivalent to those obtained with the strong mucosal adjuvant LT.

Studies in mice have demonstrated mucosal antibody responses at distant mucosal sites (genital and intestinal tracts) after i.n. delivery of ISCOM^{TM} vaccines (Hu et al., 1998; Morein et al., 1999). Given the similarities with ISCOMATRIX^{TM} vaccines the same types of responses might also be expected. Systemic and mucosal antibody responses in other species including sheep (Coulter et al., 2003) have also been observed following i.n. delivery of ISCOMATRIX^{TM} vaccines, although they have generally not been as strong as those observed in the mouse. The explanation for this is unclear; however, it is most probably due to inefficient delivery of vaccine to sites of immune induction in these species. In support of this, an influenza ISCOMATRIX[TM] vaccine was shown to be immunogenic following i.n. delivery in humans using a commercially available delivery device optimized for humans. The results of this study are described in more detail in a later section.

ISCOM[TM] vaccines have also been shown to be effective when delivered orally. However, in general the responses have been quite variable, required high and frequent doses, and seem to be restricted to mice (Sjolander and Cox, 1998). Additionally, the nasal passage is the route of infection of a large number of pathogens and the most efficient means of stimulating the common mucosal immune response. Together these observations suggest that i.n. delivery is the preferred option for the development of nonparenteral ISCOMA-TRIX[TM] vaccines. In support of this, i.n. immunization with ISCOM[TM] vaccines has been shown to afford protection against challenge with influenza in mice (Lovgren et al., 1990; Sjolander et al., 2001b) and bovine herpes virus 1 in cattle (Trudel et al., 1988). Intranasal delivery may also be of benefit for vaccination of the elderly as there is evidence to suggest that with aging mucosal immune responses declined more slowly than systemic immune responses (Corrigan and Clancy, 1999).

■ Tumour immunotherapy

As mentioned above, it is generally regarded that a strong tumor antigen-specific CD8+ CTL response will be critical to the success of cancer immunotherapy. In mice ISCOMATRIX[TM] vaccines have been shown to mediate protection in a variety of prophylactic tumor models including EG7 (EL4 thymoma cells expressing ovalbumin, OVA), B16-OVA, Lewis lung-OVA (Lenarczyk et al., 2004), and B16-NY-ESO-1 (Maraskovsky et al., 2004). Although protection in prophylactic mouse models is important, there are many instances where experimental vaccines have succeeded in these models, but the vast majority have failed when more challenging therapeutic models are used. It has been shown that an ISCOMATRIX[TM] vaccine formulated with a recombinant fusion protein consisting of the E6 and E7 proteins from HPV16 has shown some therapeutic effect in mouse tumor model even after a single immunization (Malliaros et al., in preparation). More clinically relevant studies have been performed with an ISCOMATRIX[TM] vaccine containing the NY-ESO-1 protein (Maraskovsky et al., 2004), which is expressed on a variety of human cancers including melanoma, breast, and colon (Scanlan et al., 2002). *In vitro*, the NY-ESO-1 ISCOMATRIX[TM] vaccine was readily taken up by human monocyte-derived dendritic cells (DCs), which on maturation efficiently processed and cross-presented both MHC I and MHC II epitopes to NY-ESO-1-specific CD4+ and CD8+ T cells, respectively. The NY-ESO-1 ISCOMATRIX[TM] vaccine also induced CD8+ T cells in HLA-A2 transgenic mice (Maraskovsky et al., 2004) that were capable of lysing human HLA-A2+ NY-ESO-1+ tumor cells.

■ Clinical experience

■ Clinical overview

In the early to mid-1990s a number of phase I and II studies of various influenza ISCOM[TM] and ISCOMATRIX[TM] vaccines were performed. These studies involved almost 900 participants and showed induction of both antibody and cellular immune responses (Ennis et al., 1999; Rimmelzwaan et al., 2001). The vaccines were moderately reactogenic and at the time not considered to be suitable for further development. Since these studies were performed, the ISCOMATRIX[TM] adjuvant has undergone extensive optimization. Both the prototype and optimized ISCOMATRIX[TM] adjuvant have now been used in a number of clinical studies, which are summarized in

Table 12.1 Summary of completed clinical trials with ISCOMATRIX™ vaccines

Antigen	Number[a]	Number of immunizations	Dose (μg)		Control
			ISCOMATRIX™ adjuvant	Antigen	
NY-ESO-1 (intramuscular)	22	3	12, 36, 120	10, 30, 100	PBS, NY-ESO-1
HPV16 E6E7 (1) (intramuscular)	24	3	120	20, 60, 200	PBS
HPV16 E6E7 (2) (intramuscular)	36	3	60, 120	5, 25, 70, 240	PBS
HCV Core (intramuscular)	24	3	120	5, 20, 50	PBS
Influenza (intramuscular)	55	1	60	15, 45	Influenza
Influenza (intranasal)	24	2	100, 500, 1000	90	PBS

[a]Refers to the number of participants receiving ISCOMATRIX™ vaccines and does not include those who received placebo or antigen control vaccines.

Table 12.1. The NY-ESO-1 and HPV16 E6E7 (1) clinical studies (referred to in Table 12.1) used ISCOMATRIX™ adjuvant manufactured using the prototype process and all the other studies used ISCOMATRIX™ adjuvant from the optimized process. Although not directly compared in a single study, the immune responses to ISCOMATRIX™ vaccines containing the prototype and optimized ISCOMATRIX™ adjuvant are comparable, in terms of both the number of responders and the magnitude of responses, discussed in more detail below. Interestingly, however, the reactogenicity profile of vaccines formulated with optimized ISCOMATRIX™ adjuvant has been improved over that observed with the prototype ISCOMATRIX™ adjuvant. The clinical studies described herein were all phase I, randomized, and placebo and/or antigen controlled, and were designed to assess safety, tolerability, and immunogenicity, with most of the studies including a dose escalation component.

NY-ESO-1 is a cancer testis antigen found on a number of cancer types including melanoma and breast (Chen et al., 1997). The NY-ESO-1 ISCOMATRIX™ vaccine was formulated with E. coli expressed, purified NY-ESO-1 protein (Murphy et al., 2005) and administered to 24 patients aged between 18 and 60 years with resected NY-ESO-1 positive tumors and minimal residual disease. The vaccine was safe, generally well tolerated and induced both humoral and cellular immune responses (Davis et al., 2004).

HPV type 16 infection is associated with a range of cancers including cervical, anal, and vulval (zur Hausen, 2002). The E6 and E7 proteins from HPV are generally regarded as good targets for a therapeutic vaccine as they are expressed on all infected cells and play a role in disease pathogenesis (Munger et al., 1989). The HPV16 E6E7 ISCOMATRIX™ vaccine was formulated with E. coli expressed, purified HPV16 E6E7 fusion protein and evaluated in two studies. The first used the prototype ISCOMATRIX™ adjuvant and was performed in 24 women aged between 18 and 45 years with cervical dysplasia (Frazer et al., 2004). The vaccine was safe, and although generally well tolerated, a small number of women did not complete the treatment schedule due to reactogenicity issues. The vaccine was immunogenic with both humoral and cellular immune responses detected. There was also evidence of reduced viral load in vaccinated subjects; however, the study was too small to reach significance (Frazer et al., 2004). The second HPV16 E6E7 vaccine study included the optimized ISCOMATRIX^{TM} adjuvant formulation and was performed in 36 HLA-A2, healthy male and female volunteers aged between 18 and 45 years. All participants completed the 3 immunization treatment schedule and the vaccine was found to be immunogenic (humoral and cellular responses), safe and well tolerated.

The HCV Core protein is highly conserved among the HCV genotypes and is therefore considered to be a good target for a HCV therapeutic vaccine. The HCV Core ISCOMATRIX^{TM} vaccine was formulated with *E. coli* expressed, purified HCV Core protein and tested in 24 HLA-A2, healthy male volunteers aged between 18 and 45 years. The vaccine was safe and well tolerated and induced humoral immune responses at all doses and cellular immune responses at the highest dose.

The influenza virus vaccine studies were both performed with a trivalent, split virion vaccine. In the first study a single intramuscular immunization of either 5 or 15 μg of hemagglutinin antigen (HA) of each of the 3 strains was tested in 55 healthy male and female volunteers aged between 60 and 65 years. The vaccine was safe and generally well tolerated and induced systemic antibody responses. The second study evaluated two intranasal immunizations of 30 μg of HA of each of the 3 strains with a range of ISCOMATRIX^{TM} adjuvant concentrations in 24 healthy volunteers aged between 18 and 45 years. The vaccine was found to be safe and generally well tolerated and induced both systemic and mucosal antibody responses.

■ Humoral immune responses

Humoral responses were evaluated in all studies using vaccine antigen-specific ELISA, with the exception of antibody to influenza virus where the responses were evaluated by hemagglutination inhibition (HAI). A responder was defined as an individual who

Table 12.2 Humoral immune responses measured by ELISA following 3 immunizations of ISCOMATRIX^{TM} vaccines

Antigen	Dose (μg)		Responders (%)
	ISCOMATRIX^{TM} adjuvant	Antigen	
NY-ESO-1	12	10	100
	36	30	100
	120	100	100
	–	100	25
	–	–	0
HPVl6 E6E7 (1)	120	20	100
	120	60	100
	120	200	100
	–	–	0
HPVl6 E6E7 (2)	120	5	100
	120	25	100
	120	70	100
	120	240	100
	60	70	100
	60	240	100
	–	–	0
HCV Core	120	5	100
	120	20	88
	120	50	100
	–	–	0

experienced a 4-fold rise in antibody titer over preimmunization levels.

In all studies with recombinant proteins over 99% of participants receiving ISCOMATRIX^{TM} vaccines developed humoral immune responses as shown in Table 12.2. Additionally, antibody responses were induced with antigen doses as low as 5 μg as shown in both the HCV Core and HPV16E6E7 (2) studies. There was also a clear benefit for the NY-ESO-1 ISCOMATRIX^{TM} vaccine compared to the NY-ESO-1 alone group with 100% and 25% responders, respectively. No antigen-specific antibody responses were detected in the placebo groups in any of the studies. Although not shown here, the antibody responses generally plateaued following the second immunization, with little evidence of further boosting following the third immunization. The exception to this was with groups that received vaccines containing very low doses of antigen

Table 12.3 Humoral immune respones measured by HAI following a single immunization with influenza ISCOMATRIX™ vaccines

Vaccine	Conversion factor (GMT)			Seroprotection (%) (>40 HAI titer)			Seroconversion (%) (>4-fold increase)		
	HI	H2	B	HI	H2	B	HI	H2	B
Flu 5 µg HA/strain, IMX 60 µg (intramuscular)	5.3	5.2	12.8	100	93	96	50	54	82
Flu 15 µg HA/strain, IMX 60 µg (intramuscular)	7.2	5.9	8.9	96	96	93	59	56	78
Flu 15 µg HA/strain (intramuscular)	6.8	6.7	10.6	93	96	100	67	56	82
Flu 30 µg HA/strain, IMX 100 µg (intranasal)[a]	7.7	4.8	5.4	88	75	75	63	63	50
Flu 30 µg HA/strain, IMX 500 µg (intranasal)[a]	7.3	2.7	5.0	75	100	75	75	25	63
Flu 30 µg HA/strain, IMX 1000 µg (intranasal)[a]	10.4	3.1	10.4	63	100	88	63	25	75

[a] The participants in the intranasal study received two immunizations. There was no difference in the results for any of the above parameters evaluating systemic antibody responses following a second immunization.

where the third immunization was required to reach maximum titer.

The humoral immune responses in the influenza ISCOMATRIX™ vaccine studies are shown in Table 12.3. It should be noted that the two studies were performed at different times, in different populations, and with different formulations, and as such cannot be directly compared. It is interesting to note, however, that the responses by all parameters usually applied to the evaluation of influenza vaccines were relatively similar. Furthermore, the profile of responses induced with the 5 µg of HA per strain ISCOMATRIX™ vaccine delivered intramuscularly (i.m.) were the same as those induced with 15 µg HA per strain either alone or combined with ISCOMATRIX™ adjuvant. This result would indicate ISCOMATRIX™ adjuvant may benefit i.m. influenza vaccines by reducing the dose of antigen required. The humoral immune responses induced following i.n. delivery of the influenza ISCOMATRIX™ vaccine reached maximum titer two weeks after a single immunization with no further boosting observed following the second immunization. This was different to the mucosal immune response, which was boosted following a second immunization as discussed below. These results are of interest because they demonstrate the induction of serum antibody responses to influenza virus following a single i.n. vaccination. Furthermore, the profile of the antibody responses was broadly similar to those observed following i.m. vaccination. Other investigators have found that an influenza ISCOMATRIX™ vaccine induced more rapid antibody responses than the conventional influenza vaccine (Rimmelzwaan et al., 2001). This accelerated induction of antibody responses could be advantageous in epidemic situations when a rapid response to vaccination is required to prevent disease or reduce morbidity and mortality.

■ Cellular immune responses

The cellular immune responses that have been observed in the four clinical trials that have been completed to date with ISCOMATRIX™ vaccines are summarized in

Table 12.4 Cellular immune responses in humans following 3 immunizations with ISCOMATRIX™ vaccines

Antigen	Dose (μg)		T cell responders (%)	
	ISCOMATRIX™ adjuvant	Antigen	CD4+	CD8+
NY-ESO-1	120	100	69[a]	38[e]
	–	100	13[a]	13[e]
	–	–	0[a]	0[e]
HPV16 E6E7 (1)	120	240	80[b]	25[f]
	–	–	0[b]	0[f]
HPV16 E6E7 (2)	120	240	92[c]	27[e]
	–	–	0[c]	0[e]
HCV Core	120	50	88[d]	25[e]
	–	–	0[d]	0[e]

[a] Determined using DTH responses.

[b] Determined using DTH responses and/or IFN-γ expression.

[c] Determined using IFN-γ expression.

[d] Determined using cytokine expression profile (cytokine bead array).

[e] Determined using intracellular staining for IFN-γ with HLA.A2 CD8+ peptides.

[f] Determined using IFN-γ ELISPOT.

Table 12.4. CD4+ T cell responses were detected in the majority of participants receiving ISCOMATRIX™ vaccines. Although the assays used in the studies differed, the response rates were relatively consistent ranging from 69% for the NY-ESO-1 study to 92% for the HPV16 E6E7 (1) study. Additionally, in the NY-ESO-1 study, the comparison with antigen alone showed a clear benefit for the ISCOMATRIX™ vaccine with only 13% responders in the antigen alone group.

CD8+ T cell responses have generally been assessed following stimulation of peripheral blood mononuclear cells (PBMC) with 2–3 HLA-A2 peptide epitopes. Using this type of analysis the CD8+ T cell response to ISCOMATRIX™ vaccines ranged from 25% to 38%. However, there is now compelling evidence that this underestimates the true response rate. When the analyses were repeated for the high dose group from the NY-ESO-1 ISCOMATRIX™ vaccine trial using a pool of overlapping peptides which span the entire protein, a broad range of CD4+ and CD8+ T cell responses were detected in most of the subjects that have been examined to date. Further mapping of these epitopes identified responses against "naturally presented" epitopes as well as previously unidentified epitopes (Davis et al., 2004). Clearly detailed analysis of this kind is preferred; however, at present this requires large blood volumes, which is not always clinically acceptable, and is very labor intensive. As with the CD4+ T cell responses, there was a clear benefit for the NY-ESO-1 ISCOMATRIX™ vaccine over the antigen alone with 38% and 13% responders, in the HLA-A2 peptide assays, respectively.

In general the induction of cellular immune responses required 2–3 immunizations and there has been evidence of an antigen dose response. In most studies the best cellular immune responses, in terms of both magnitude and breadth, were achieved at the highest antigen dose. The ability to give repeated immunizations with the same formulation highlights one of the inherent advantages of ISCOMATRIX™ vaccines over other approaches to induce cellular immune responses, such as DNA/live vector prime boost strategies, or the use of different viral vectors for priming and boosting.

■ Mucosal immune responses

There is now a sizeable body of preclinical and clinical data demonstrating that ISCOMATRIX™ vaccines are highly immunogenic when delivered intranasally, inducing both systemic and mucosal antibody as well as cellular immune responses. Consistent with this, the number of responders with systemic antibody responses was essentially the same following i.n. and i.m. delivery of an influenza ISCOMATRIX™ vaccine, as described above. Mucosal responses, however, were only observed in the participants that received i.n. vaccines. Interestingly, there was no evidence of an adjuvant dose–response with the same number of responders at all doses of ISCOMATRIX™ adjuvant tested. This was surprising as animal studies had

Table 12.5 Influenza-specific mucosal IgA antibody responses detected in the nasal passage following immunization with influenza ISCOMATRIX™ vaccines on days 0 and 21

Dose		Nasal sample	Seroconversion (%) (> 2-fold increase)		
Influenza (µg HA/strain)	ISCOMATRIX™ adjuvant (µg)		HI	H2	B
30	100	Day 21	40	50	38
		Day 42	88	50	50
30	500	Day 21	60	33	50
		Day 42	63	50	75
30	1000	Day 21	80	33	38
		Day 42	88	67	75

indicated that higher doses of ISCOMATRIX™ adjuvant were required for effective i.n. administration. It is possible that this increased efficiency in humans was due to the delivery device, which has been optimized for i.n. delivery. The number of mucosal IgA responders, defined as a greater than 2-fold rise over prevaccination levels, was higher after the second i.n. immunization as shown in Table 12.5. This is perhaps not surprising given that the preimmunization mucosal IgA antibody titers were very low, suggesting that the majority of subjects were "mucosally naive" to influenza.

Whether the capacity to induce broad local (mucosal) and systemic immune response such as this reduces the morbidity and/or mortality of influenza or indeed other respiratory diseases remains to be determined. Furthermore, if i.n. delivery of ISCOMATRIX™ vaccines in humans induces immune responses at distant mucosal sites, as has been observed in mice (Hu et al., 1998; Morein et al., 1999), this route of delivery could be considered for vaccines against sexually transmitted diseases such as chlamydia, HSV-2, HIV, etc.

Safety and tolerability

The issue of reactogenicity of saponin-based adjuvants has been raised as a potential impediment to widespread use in human vaccines. With some saponin-based adjuvants, in particular those based on free saponin such as QS21, this concern has been supported by results in clinical studies. Almost without exception these studies have shown moderate to severe local site reactions which is thought to be associated with the hemolytic activity (Waite et al., 2001). As previously discussed the CSL ISCOMATRIX™ adjuvant has no detectable hemolytic activity when tested *in vitro*, which is proposed to contribute to the improved tolerability profile for ISCOMATRIX™ vaccines. The data discussed below are related to the safety and tolerability of vaccines formulated with the optimized process for ISCOMATRIX™ adjuvant only.

In the clinical trials performed to date using the optimized ISCOMATRIX™ adjuvant there have been no vaccine-related serious adverse events and the vaccines have been generally well tolerated. No medically significant events or clinically significant laboratory abnormalities have been reported nor has there been any adverse event-related withdrawals, or the need for medical intervention following vaccination. The majority of adverse events reported were reactions at the injection site and myalgia. These events are generally mild to moderate in severity, of short duration and self-limiting. The profile of adverse events following i.n. administration of the influenza ISCOMATRIX™ vaccine was broadly similar with transient mild symptoms such as sneezing and sore throat also being reported. Additionally, mild systemic reactions

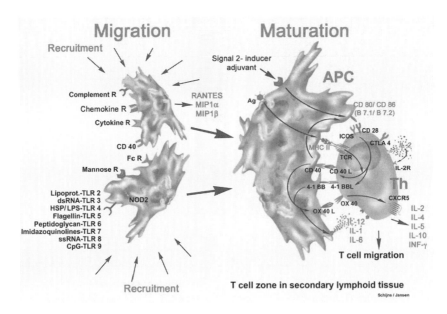

Figure 12.4 ISCOMATRIX™ adjuvant activity is a potent immunomodulator, which has effects on both the innate and adaptive immune systems as indicated in red text (see color plate section). The effects of ISCOMATRIX™ vaccines on the APC include the induction of proinflammatory cytokines (IL-1, IL-6, IL-12), CD80/86, and chemokines (RANTES, MIPI α, MIPI β). ISCOMATRIX™ vaccines also stimulate the expression of T cell cytokines (IL-2, IL-4, IL-5, IL-10, IFN-γ) indicative of a mixed Th1/Th2 response. (Adapted from Figure 1.2, Chapter 1.) (See Color Plate Section.)

including fatigue, headache and myalgia were reported following i.n. administration, although these events were only transient. The profile of systemic reactions (fatigue, headache and myalgia) was similar for the influenza ISCOMATRIX™ and placebo vaccines.

Mechanism of Action

Understanding the mechanism of action of novel adjuvants to be used in human vaccines is important for a number of reasons. Firstly, it will assist in identifying the most appropriate application of the adjuvant in terms of the vaccines in which it is used and how it is used. Secondly, it will provide valuable information that will contribute to the further development of adjuvants with improved immunogenicity profiles and/or adjuvants with properties that better match the requirements of specific indications, e.g., cancer. Thirdly, knowing the mechanism of action of the adjuvant will assist in understanding how the particular vaccine works.

The capacity of ISCOMATRIX™ vaccines to induce both antibody and cellular (CD4+ and CD8+ T cell) responses implies that the adjuvant is functioning via multiple immune mechanisms, involving both innate and adaptive immune mediators. The known effects of ISCOMATRIX™ adjuvant on the immune system are summarized in Figure 12.4. Clearly understanding the full details of this process at the molecular level is beyond the current state of scientific knowledge. However, as the range of immunological tools and reagents expands so does the depth of our understanding of the immunological processes that underpin the potent adjuvant properties of the ISCOMATRIX™ adjuvant. This is particularly relevant with regards the capacity of ISCOMATRIX™ vaccines to induce CD8+ T cell responses.

In a comprehensive recent review, O'Hagan and Valiante (2003) focused on the confusion that has arisen from broad use of the word adjuvant to describe any agent with the "functional ability to enhance *in vivo*

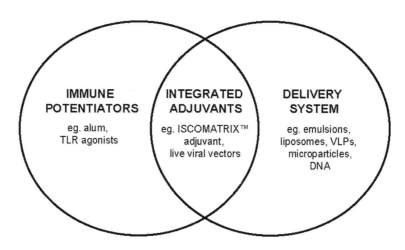

Figure 12.5 O'Hagan and Valiante (2003) proposed classification of adjuvants. They are classified as either immunopotentiators or delivery systems according to their dominant mechanism of action. A modification of this classification to include a third group that has both properties is proposed. This group is referred to as "integrated adjuvants" and includes ISCOMATRIX™ adjuvant and live viral vectors. Because of its particulate nature ISCOMATRIX™ adjuvant is effectively targeted to, and taken up, by APCs. The ISCOMATRIX™ adjuvant also has potent immunomodulatory properties inducing both innate and adaptive immune response mediators (summarized in Figure 12.4).

immunogenicity of the antigens with which they are coadministered." In order to provide greater clarity and rigor to the adjuvant field they proposed separating both traditional and novel adjuvants into either immune potentiators or antigen delivery systems, depending on their dominant mechanism of action. As the name suggests delivery systems mainly function by localizing vaccine components to APCs, which provide a key link between the innate and adaptive immune responses. Immune potentiators, in contrast, activate APCs and other immune regulatory cells. This simple classification will be enormously beneficial; however, like most rules there are always exceptions and the ISCOMATRIX™ adjuvant would appear to be a case in point. There is now a considerable body of data to indicate that the ISCOMATRIX™ adjuvant has both antigen delivery and immune potentiation properties, both of which are likely to be critical to its "adjuvant activity," particularly the capacity to induce CTL responses. A slight modification of the adjuvant classification described by O'Hagan and Valiante to include a third group having both antigen delivery and immunopotentiation properties, referred to as

"integrated adjuvants," would therefore appear justified (Figure 12.5). The properties of the ISCOMATRIX™ adjuvant that justify its inclusion into this group are expanded upon below.

■ Immunomodulation

The ISCOMATRIX™ adjuvant alone, that is in the absence of antigen, has been shown to have potent immunomodulatory effects at the level of the draining lymph node, a phenomena referred to as lymph node priming (Windon et al., 2001). A characteristic of this priming event is that immediately following subcutaneous administration of ISCOMATRIX™ adjuvant, the cellular output from the lymph node draining the injection site transiently (6–12 hours) declines. This is followed 24–48 hours later by a period during which the cellular output from the node increases markedly above the resting levels. This increase in cellular output is associated with increased expression of proinflammatory cytokines such as IL-6, IL-8, and IFN-γ. In the presence of influenza virus antigen (flu Ag) the increase in cellular output from the draining lymph node is significantly greater and persists for longer compared with ISCOMATRIX[TM] adjuvant alone, and is associated with an increase in blast cells and flu Ag-specific antibody in the lymph. Similar observations have also been made when ISCOMATRIX[TM] adjuvant is combined with a purified recombinant protein (unpublished observation). Together these observations demonstrate that ISCOMATRIX[TM] adjuvant is an immune modulator, which maximizes the number of low-frequency antigen-specific cells entering the lymph node, thus increasing the potential for interaction with antigen or APCs, and orchestrates the local immune response via the induction of proinflammatory cytokines. Much of the knowledge of the immunomodulatory capability of the ISCOMATRIX[TM] adjuvant has come from evaluations in animal models with ISCOM[TM] vaccines but it is believed that due to the similarities the information is also likely to be applicable to ISCOMATRIX[TM] vaccines.

Studies in mice using a variety of antigens have shown that ISCOM[TM] vaccines delivered parenterally activate the innate immune system, as reflected by the induction of IL-1, IL-6 and IL-12 expression by APCs (Behboudi et al., 1997; Behboudi et al., 1996; Smith et al., 1999; Villacres-Ericsson et al., 1997). IL-1 and IL-6 cooperate to stimulate naive CD8+ T cells to proliferate and differentiate into CTL effectors (Kovacsovics-Bankowski and Rock, 1995). IL-12, however, shapes the adaptive immune responses (Akira et al., 2001) and plays a key role in the development of CTL, in part due to its role in regulating the expression of IFN-γ (Trinchieri, 1995). Consistent with this, CTL responses are dramatically reduced in IL-12 knockout mice administered ISCOMATRIX[TM] vaccines (Smith et al., 1999). Together these observations suggest that ISCOMATRIX[TM] vaccines directly activate the innate immune system, with IL-12 playing a key role. Activation of the innate immune responses by ISCOMATRIX[TM] adjuvant does not appear to be mediated directly by toll-like receptors (TLRs). However, there is significant overlap in the gene products upregulated by

ISCOM[TM] vaccines and TLR response genes (Guha and Mackman, 2001). The detail of how ISCOM[TM] and ISCOMATRIX[TM] vaccines activate these TLR-independent innate immune responses remains to be elucidated but, as discussed below, may in part be due to the efficiency with which ISCOMATRIX[TM] and ISCOM[TM] vaccines are taken up and processed by APCs. ISCOM[TM] vaccines have also been shown to stimulate the expression of T cell cytokines (IL-2, IL-4, IL-5, IL-10, IFN-γ), indicative of a mixed Th1/Th2 profile (reviewed in Sjolander et al., 1998).

In primates ISCOM[TM] vaccines have also been shown to induce the expression of β chemokines such as RANTES, macrophage inflammatory protein 1α (MIP1α) and MIP1β (Heeney et al., 1998). Chemokines such as these augment Th1 and CTL responses to HIV-1 and HSV-2 (Jameson, 2002). Consistent with this, a correlation was observed between chemokine expression levels and protection in rhesus macaques that were immunized with an HIV-1 ISCOM[TM] vaccine and then challenged with chimeric simian/HIV. The expression of the major costimulatory molecules CD80 and CD86 is also enhanced by ISCOM[TM] vaccines, which may partly explain why they are effective in elderly mice (Morein and Bengtsson, 1999; Sambhara et al., 1997).

Another feature that supports the ISCOMATRIX[TM] adjuvant being regarded as an immune potentiator is the capacity of ISCOM[TM] vaccines to upregulate MHC II expression on APCs (Maraskovsky et al., 2004; Villacres et al., 1998). This may be an important property for the immunotherapy of chronic viral infections such as herpes simplex virus, which downregulates the expression of this molecule.

■ Antigen delivery

To date there is no evidence that cellular uptake of the ISCOMATRIX[TM] adjuvant is mediated by specific membrane-bound receptors. As distinct from a number of adjuvants in development such as CpG and the imidaquinolenes (e.g., R-848), which bind to TLR-9 and TLR-7/8, respectively (O'Neill, 2003), ISCOMATRIX™ adjuvant does not appear to bind to, and subsequently activate, APCs via interaction with TLRs (unpublished observation). TLRs represent a family of cell surface receptors that are specific for pathogen-associated molecular patterns (PAMPs) which are found on a broad range of pathogens (Janeway and Medzhitov, 2002). The role TLR-mediated signaling in the activation of APCs has spawned a growing industry aimed at identifying natural and synthetic ligands for TLRs as novel vaccine adjuvants. However, it is important to keep in mind that APC activation is an important, but clearly not the only adjuvant property required for the induction of cellular responses. This is particularly true for the induction of CD8+ T cells which also requires (as discussed in more detail below) that antigen is delivered in such a way that it gains entry to the cytosol to facilitate access to the MHC I antigen-processing pathway.

The possibility that the ISCOMATRIX™ adjuvant binds to an as yet unidentified receptor cannot be ruled out; however, it appears unlikely. Instead, it is possible that the hydrophobic nature of the ISCOMATRIX™ adjuvant facilitates its interaction with membranes at the cell surface and subcellular organelles such as endosomes (Villacres et al., 1998). In support of this, influenza antigen was detected on cell and organelle membranes, as well as in the cytoplasm when APCs were incubated with influenza ISCOM™ vaccine (Villacres et al., 1998). Furthermore, because of its particulate nature, the ISCOMATRIX™ adjuvant is effectively targeted to, and taken up by, APCs. Being typically 40 nm in diameter, ISCOMATRIX™ adjuvant cage-like structures are similar in size to the viral pathogens that the immune system has evolved to eliminate. Consistent with this, a recent study by Fifis et al. (2004) found the optimal particle size for inducing CTL responses was in the 40–50 nm range, which is very similar to the size of the ISCOMATRIX™ adjuvant, and also to the size of most viruses. Furthermore, ISCOM™ vaccines have been shown to recruit APCs in the form of DCs in vivo (Smith et al., 1999). Once bound to APCs, the antigens in ISCOMATRIX™ vaccines are rapidly taken up and processed for both MHC I and MHC II presentation, as described in more detail in the following section (Schnurr et al., 2005).

■ Antigen processing

There is now a considerable and ever growing body of evidence to demonstrate that ISCOMATRIX™ vaccines efficiently access both the MHC I and MHC II antigen processing pathways, which as discussed above, are critical for the induction of CD4+ and CD8+ T cells, respectively. The ability of ISCOMATRIX™ vaccines to access MHC II antigen processing is perhaps not all that surprising, given that this pathway is primarily fed by cellular uptake of exogenous antigens via the phagocytic pathway (Pfeifer et al., 1993). However, the explanation for why ISCOMATRIX™ vaccines so effectively target the MHC I pathway is not immediately obvious, although recent studies in this area have made considerable progress towards providing an answer to this question.

Most MHC class I-binding peptides are generated in the cytosol as side products of degradation of misfolded proteins which primarily occurs in the proteasome. A subset of the resulting peptides are translocated across the endoplasmic reticulum (ER) membrane by a dedicated peptide transporter, then loaded onto peptide-receptive MHC I molecules in the ER and transported to the cell membrane. Antigenic peptide generation can therefore be regarded as a byproduct of basal protein turnover (Kloetzel, 2004). The requirement for an antigen to be in the cytoplasm to gain access to the MHC I processing pathway has been one of the greatest challenges for the development of subunit vaccines that are capable of inducing CD8+ CTL responses. One of the theoretical benefits

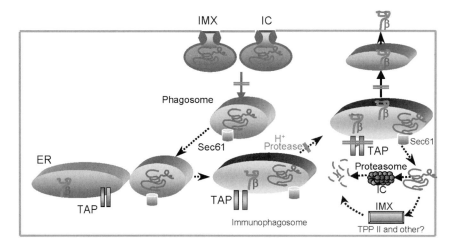

Figure 12.6 Schematic representation of APC uptake and processing of antigen either formulated as an ISCOMATRIX™ vaccine (IMX) or an immune complex (IC). ICs are generally regarded as an efficient means to load APCs for MHC I antigen processing. Using inhibitors of specific cellular processes Schnurr et al. (2005) have shown that the ISCOMATRIX™ adjuvant and IC-mediated cross presentation of antigen requires phagocytosis, acidification, TAP, and the secretory pathway. Double red lines (see color plate section) indicate that inhibition at this point blocks MHC I antigen processing. IC-mediated cross presentation requires proteasome processing whereas ISCOMATRIX™ adjuvant-mediated cross presentation is largely proteosome independent and occurs primarily via Tripeptidyl Peptidase II. The ability to access different antigen processing pathways may increase the range of peptides and hence of the CD8+ T cell response that can be generated in response to ISCOMATRIX™ vaccines. (See Color Plate Section.)

of DNA and live viral vectors as vaccine modalities is that the antigens are expressed in the cytoplasm, and therefore have access to the MHC class I processing pathway. Unfortunately, however, DNA vaccines for reasons unknown have to date worked in mice but not humans and the use of live viral vectors is limited by potential safety concerns and the inability to give repeated doses due to the induction of neutralizing antibodies (Belyakov et al., 1999).

Robson et al. (2003a, 2003b) have shown *in vitro* using mouse cells and an ova ISCOM™ vaccine that bone marrow-derived DCs but not macrophages or naïve B cells prime antigen-specific CD4+ and CD8+ T cells. Furthermore, *in vitro* studies using human cells with an NY-ESO-1 ISCOMATRIX™ vaccine have shown that only CD1c+ blood DCs and monocyte-derived DCs (MoDCs) are capable of presenting epitopes on both MHC I and MHC II, whereas plasmacytoid DCs are limited to MHC II presentation (Schnurr et al., 2005). Detailed examination of antigen

processing of NY-ESO-1 in human MoDCs has shown that ISCOMATRIX™ adjuvant targeted NY-ESO-1 to a fast, proteasome-independent pathway, whereas soluble NY-ESO-1 protein or NY-ESO-1 immune complexes targeted a slow, proteasome-dependent cross-presentation pathway (Schnurr et al., 2005).

As shown in Figure 12.6, both NY-ESO-1 in the form of immune complexes (IC), which are generally regarded as an efficient way to load DCs for MHC I processing (Schuurhuis et al., 2002), and NY-ESO-1 ISCOMATRIX™ vaccine required active phagocytosis, acidification of endosomal compartments, selective use of lysosomal enzymes such as calpains and cysteine proteases, and the transporter TAP (Schnurr et al., 2005). Furthermore, DCs pulsed with NY-ESO-1 ISCOMATRIX™ vaccine resulted in prolonged antigen presentation which efficiently stimulated NY-ESO-1-specific CD4+ and CD8+ T cells for up to 3 days, which was the last time point examined in this study. Prolonged presentation such as this increases the potential for productive DC interaction with rare antigen-specific T cells in draining lymphoid tissues. More detailed *in vitro* analysis of the proteasome-independent antigen processing both in mice using an ovalbumin ISCOM™ vaccine (Robson et al., 2003b) and in humans using an NY-ESO-1 ISCOMATRIX™ vaccine (Schnurr et al., 2005) strongly implicates the enzyme complex Tripeptidyl Peptidase II, a recently identified aminopeptidase with proteolytic activity (Seifert et al., 2003). The ability to access different antigen processing pathways may increase the range of peptides and hence the breadth of the CD8+ T cell responses that can be generated in response to ISCOMATRIX™ vaccines. This would be particularly beneficial in vaccine settings where immune escape is a significant issue, such as RNA viruses (e.g., HIV, HCV) and cancer.

Summary

ISCOMATRIX™ vaccines have now been tested with numerous antigens both in humans and in a variety of experimental animals, and been shown to be safe and highly immunogenic with respect to both humoral and cellular immune responses, including both CD4+ and CD8+ T cells. The ability of the ISCOMATRIX™ adjuvant, in combination with antigen, to induce a broad immune response such as this can be attributed to it having both the properties of an immune modulator and an antigen delivery system. Arguably, live viral vectors are the only other vaccine delivery modality which have similar properties; however, their widespread use is limited by potential safety concerns and the inability to give repeated doses, due to the induction of neutralizing antibodies. ISCOMATRIX™ vaccines, in contrast, have a very good safety profile in humans and, because they do not induce neutralizing antibody responses, can be used for repeat dosing. This obviates the need for different formulations for prime and boost, such as DNA/live vector, or the use of different viruses for priming and boosting, which has

obvious advantages for manufacture, cost, delivery and ease of registration.

The key features of ISCOMATRIX™ vaccines for humoral responses are increases in the magnitude, speed and longevity of the response, as well as the capacity for antigen dose reduction compared to other adjuvants such as aluminum. ISCOMATRIX™ adjuvant therefore is well suited for vaccine applications that require a rapid response, such as epidemic/pandemic situations or travelers vaccines, etc. Longevity of antibody responses would be beneficial in a range of vaccine settings, including vaccines where the primary target population is adolescents such as for sexually transmitted diseases such as chlamydia, HPV and HSV-2. The capacity to induce protective immunity using lower antigen doses is particularly important in situations where the antigen is difficult or expensive to manufacture. ISCOMATRIX™ adjuvant is also well suited for use in combination vaccines or vaccines containing multiple antigens, where there is a strong driver to limit the dose of each vaccine component. Lastly, the addition of the ISCOMATRIX™ adjuvant could also benefit existing vaccines by lowering production costs or improving immunogenicity, particularly in settings where responses are affected by the presence of pre-existing or maternal antibodies.

The key features of ISCOMATRIX™ vaccines for cellular immune responses are the ability to induce strong and long-lasting CD4+ and CD8+ T cell responses. Furthermore, detailed analysis of the cellular responses in recipients of NY-ESO-1 ISCOMATRIX™ vaccine in a recently completed clinical trial demonstrates that CD4+ and CD8+ T cell responses were induced to a wide variety of epitopes in the majority of individuals. The ISCOMATRIX™ adjuvant therefore has significant potential for the development of vaccines where cellular responses are required such HIV, chlamydia and malaria, as well as therapeutic vaccines for chronic infectious disease such as HCV, HBV and cancer. ISCOMATRIX™ adjuvant also demonstrates significant potential as a mucosal adjuvant, particularly for intranasal administration. Manufacture of the ISCOMATRIX™ adjuvant is simple, robust, reproducible, and can be performed at a large scale. The properties and features of the ISCOMATRIX™ adjuvant warrant further clinical investigation for novel human vaccines where cellular and/or humoral immune responses are required, and in vaccines (existing or new) to achieve antigen dose sparing or improved antibody responses.

■ Acknowledgments

The authors acknowledge Gina Kanesoulis for her valuable assistance in preparing the manuscript and to Eugene Maraskovsky, Jeff Boyle, Max Schnurr, Ross Hamilton, and Mary Walker for assistance with preparation of the figures. The authors are also grateful for the valuable contribution of their colleagues at CSL as well as academic and industry partners for their interest and scientific endeavors directed towards better defining our understanding of ISCOMATRIX™ adjuvant, the manufacturing process, and progressing the clinical development of ISCOMATRIX™ vaccines. Thanks also go to Jillian Bennet, John Cox, Jill Haynes, Eugene Maraskovsky, and Kate Noonan for their critical review of the manuscript.

■ References

Akira, S., Takeda, K., and Kaisho, T. (2001). Toll-like receptors: critical proteins linking innate and acquired immunity. *Nature Immunol.* 2, 675–680.

Andersson, C., Sandberg, L., Wernerus, H., Johansson, M., and Lovgren-Bengtsson, K. (2000). Improved systems for hydrophobic tagging of recombinant immunogens for efficient iscom incorporation. *J. Immunol. Methods* 238, 181–193.

Autran, B., Carcelain, G., Combadiere, B., and Debre, P. (2004). Therapeutic vaccines for chronic infections. *Science* 305, 205–208.

Behboudi, S., Morein, B., and Villacres-Eriksson, M. (1996). In vitro activation of antigen-presenting cells (APC) by defined composition of Quillaja saponaria Molina triterpenoids. *Clin. Exp. Immunol.* 105, 26–30.

Behboudi, S., Morein, B., and Villacres-Ericsson, M. (1997). In vivo and in vitro induction of IL-6 by Quillaja saponaria molina triterpenoid formulations. *Cytokine* 9, 682–687.

Belyakov, I.M., Moss, B., Strober, W., and Berzofsky, J.A. (1999). Mucosal vaccination overcomes the barrier to recombinant vaccinia immunization caused by preexisting poxvirus immunity. *Proc. Natl. Acad. Sci. USA* 96, 4512–4517.

Chen, T.-T., Scanlan, M.J., Sahin, U., Tureci, O., Gure, A.O., Tsang, S., Williamson, B., Stockert, E., Pfreundschuh, M., and Old, L.J. (1997). A testicular antigen aberrantly expressed in human cancers detected by autologous antibody screening. *Proc. Natl. Acad. Sci. USA* 94, 1914–1918.

Corrigan, E.M. and Clancy, R.L. (1999). Is there a role for a mucosal influenza vaccine in the elderly? *Drugs Aging* 15, 169–181.

Coulie, P.G. and Van Snick, J. (1985). Enhancement of IgG anti-carrier responses by IgG2 anti-hapten antibodies in mice. *Eur. J. Immunol.* 15, 793–798.

Coulter, A., Harris, R., Davis, R., Drane, D., Cox, J., Ryan, D., Sutton, P., Rockman, S., and Pearse, M. (2003). Intranasal vaccination with ISCOMATRIX((R)) adjuvanted influenza vaccine. *Vaccine* 21, 946–949.

Coutelier, J.P., van der Logt, J.T., Heessen, F.W., Warnier, G., and Van Snick, J. (1987). IgG2a restriction of murine antibodies elicited by viral infections. *J. Exp. Med.* 165, 64–69.

Dalsgaard, K. (1970). Thin-layer chromatographic fingerprinting of commercially available saponins. *Dan. Tidsskr. Farm.* 44, 327–331.

Davis, I.D., Chen, W., Jackson, H., Parente, P., Shackleton, M., Hopkins, W., Chen, Q., Dimopoulos, N. et al. (2004). Recombinant NY-ESO-1 protein with ISCOMATRIX adjuvant induces broad integrated antibody and CD4+ and CD8+ T cell responses in humans. *Proc. Natl. Acad. Sci. USA* 101, 10697–10702.

Ennis, F.A., Cruz, J., Jameson, J., Klein, M., Burt, D., and Thipphawong, J. (1999). Augmentation of human influenza A virus-specific cytotoxic T lymphocyte memory by influenza vaccine and adjuvanted carriers (ISCOMS). *Virology* 259, 256–261.

Fifis, T., Gamvrellis, A., Crimeen-Irwin, B., Pietersz, G.A., Li, J., Mottram, P., McKenzie, I.F., and Plebanski, M. (2004). Size-dependent immunogenicity: therapeutic and protective properties of nano-vaccines against tumors. *J. Immunol.* 173, 148–154.

Frazer, I.H., Quinn, M., Nicklin, J.L., Tan, J., Perrin, L.C., Ng, P., O'Connor, V.M., White, O., Wendt, N., Martin, J., Crowley, J.M., Edwards, S.J., McKenzie, A.W., Mitchell, S.V., Maher, D.W., Pearse, M.J., and Basser, R.L. (2004). Phase 1 study of HPV16-specific immunotherapy with E6E7 fusion protein and ISCOMATRIX™ adjuvant in women with cervical intraepithelial neoplasia. *Vaccine* 23, 172–181.

Fujihashi, K., Koga, T., Van Ginkel, F.W., Hagiwara, Y., and McGhee, J.R. (2002). A dilemma for mucosal vaccination: efficacy versus toxicity using enterotoxin-based adjuvants. *Vaccine* 20, 2431–2438.

Grdic, D., Smith, R., Donachie, A., Kjerrulf, M., Hornquist, E., Mowat, A., and Lycke, N. (1999). The mucosal adjuvant effects of cholera toxin and immune-stimulating complexes differ in their requirement for IL-12, indicating different pathways of action. *Eur. J. Immunol.* 29, 1774–1784.

Guha, M. and Mackman, N. (2001). LPS induction of gene expression in human monocytes. *Cell Signal* 13, 85–94.

Hariharan, K., Braslawsky, G., Black, A., Raychaudhuri, S., and Hanna, N. (1995). The induction of cytotoxic T cells and tumor regression by soluble antigen formulation. *Cancer Res.* 55, 3486–3489.

Heeney, J., Akerblom, L., Barnett, S., Bogers, W., Davis, D., Fuller, D., Koopman, G., Lehner, T., Mooij, P., Morein, B., de Giuli, M.C., Rosenwirth, B., Verschoor, E., Wagner, R., and Wolf, H. (1999). HIV-1 vaccine-induced immune responses which correlate with protection from SHIV infection: compiled preclinical efficacy data from trials with ten different HIV-1 vaccine candidates. *Immunol. Lett.* 66, 189–195.

Heeney, J.L., Teeuwsen, V.J.P., van Gils, M. et al. (1998). β-chemokines and neutralizing antibody titers correlate with sterilizing immunity generated in HIV-1 vaccinated macaques. *Proc. Natl. Acad. Sci. USA* 95, 10803–10808.

Hou, S., Doherty, P.C., Zijlstra, M., Jaenisch, R., and Katz, J.M. (1992). Delayed clearance of Sendai virus in mice lacking class I MHC-restricted CD8+ T cells. *J. Immunol.* 149, 1319–1325.

Hu, H.-M. et al. (2002). CD28, TNF receptor, and IL-12 are critical for CD4-independent cross-priming of therapeutic antitumor CD8+ T cells. *J. Immunol.* 169, 4897–4904.

Hu, K.F., Elvander, M., Merza, M., Akerblom, L., Brandenburg, A., and Morein, B. (1998). The immunostimulating complex (ISCOM) is an efficient mucosal delivery system for respiratory syncytial virus (RSV) envelope antigens inducing high local and systemic antibody responses. *Clin. Exp. Immunol.* 113, 235–243.

Hu, K.F., Lovgren-Bengtsson, K., and Morein, B. (2001). Immunostimulating complexes (ISCOMs) for nasal vaccination. *Adv. Drug Deliv. Rev.* 51, 149–159.

Jameson, S.C. (2002). Maintaining the norm: T-cell homeostasis. *Nature Rev. Immunol.* 2, 547–556.

Janeway, C.A. and Medzhitov, R. (2002). Innate immune recognition. *Annu. Rev. Immunol.* 20, 197–216.

Kenney, J.S., Hughes, B.W., Masada, M.P., and Allison, A.C. (1989). Influence of adjuvants on the quantity, affinity, isotype and epitope specificity of murine antibodies. *J. Immunol. Methods* 121, 157–166.

Kersten, G., Drane, D., Pearse, M., Jiskoot, W., and Coulter, A. (2003). Liposomes and ISCOMs. In Kaufmann, S.H.E. (Ed) *Novel Vaccination Strategies*, Wiley-VCH, Weinheim, pp. 173–196.

Kersten, G.F. and Crommelin, D.J. (2003). Liposomes and ISCOMs. *Vaccine* 21, 915–920.

Kersten, G.F.A., Spiekstra, A., Beuvery, E.C., and Crommelin, D.J.A. (1991). On the structure of immune-stimulating saponin-lipid complexes (iscoms). *Biochim. Biophys. Acta* 1062, 165–171.

Kipps, T.J., Parham, P., Punt, J., and Herzenberg, L.A. (1985). Importance of immunoglobulin isotype in human antibody-dependent, cell-mediated cytotoxicity directed by murine monoclonal antibodies. *J. Exp. Med.* 161, 1–17.

Kloetzel, P.M. (2004). The proteasome and MHC class I antigen processing. *Biochim. Biophys, Acta* 1695, 225–233.

Kovacsovics-Bankowski, M. and Rock, K.L. (1995). A phagosome-to cytosol pathway for exogenous antigens presented on MHC class I molecules. *Science* 267, 243–246.

Le, T.T., Drane, D., Malliaros, J., Cox, J.C., Rothel, L., Pearse, M., Woodberry, T., Gardner, J., and Suhrbier, A. (2001). Cytotoxic T cell polyepitope vaccines delivered by ISCOMs. *Vaccine* 19, 4669–4675.

Lenarczyk, A., Le, T.T.T., Drane, D., Malliaros, J., Pearse, M., Hamilton, R., Cox, J., Luft, T., Garnder, J., and Suhrbier, A. (2004). ISCOM® based vaccines for cancer immunotherapy. *Vaccine* 22, 963–974.

Lindblad, E.B. (2004). Aluminium adjuvants: in retrospect and prospect. *Vaccine* 22, 3658–3668.

Lovgren, K. and Morein, B. (1988). The requirement of lipids for the formation of immunostimulating complexes (iscoms). *Biotechnol. Appl. Biochem.* 10, 161–172.

Lovgren, K., Kaberg, H., and Morein, B. (1990). An experimental influenza subunit vaccine (iscom): induction of protective immunity to challenge infection in mice after intranasal or subcutaneous administration. *Clin. Exp. Immunol. 82*, 435–439.

Macdonald, L., Kleinig, M., and Cox, J. (1997). A single dose (two component) experimental influenza vaccine. *Proc. Intl. Symp. Control. Rel. Bioact. Mater.* 24, 231–232.

MacDonald, T.T. (1999). Effector and regulatory lymphoid cells and cytokines in mucosal sites. *Curr. Top. Microbiol. Immunol.* 236, 113–135.

Malliaros, J., Quinn, C., Arnold, F.H., Pearse, M.J., Drane, D.P., Stewart, T.J., and Macfarlan, R.I. (2004). Association of antigens to ISCOMATRIX adjuvant using metal chelation leads to improved CTL responses. *Vaccine* 22, 3968–3975.

Maloy, K.J., Donachie, A.M., and Mowat, A.M. (1995). Induction of Th1 and Th2 CD4+ T cell responses by oral or parenteral immunization with ISCOMS. *Eur. J. Immunol.* 25, 2835–2841.

Maraskovsky, E., Sjolander, S., Drane, D., Le, T.T.T., Mateo, L., Luft, T., Masterman, K.-A., Tai, T.-Y., Chen, Q., Green, S., Sjolander, A., Pearse, M., Lemonnier, F.A., Chen, W., Cebon, J., and Suhrbier, A. (2004). NY-ESO-1 protein formulated in ISCOMATRIX® adjuvant is a potent anti-cancer vaccine inducing both humoral and CD8+ T cell-mediated immunity and protection against NY-ESO-1+ tumours. *Clin. Cancer Res.* 10, 2879–2890.

Morein, B. and Bengtsson, K.L. (1999). Immunomodulation by iscoms, immune stimulating complexes. *Methods* 19, 94–102.

Morein, B. and Lovgren Bengtsson, K. (1998). Functional aspects of iscoms (review article). *Immunol. Cell Biol.* 76, 295–299.

Morein, B., Sundquist, B., Hoglund, S., Dalsgaard, K., and Osterhaus, A. (1984). Iscom, a novel structure for antigenic presentation of membrane proteins from enveloped viruses. *Nature* 308, 457–460.

Morein, B., Lövgren, K., Rönnberg, B., Sjölander, A., and Villacrés-Eriksson, M. (1995). Immunostimulating complexes. Clinical potential in vaccine development. *Clin. Immunother.* 3, 461–475.

Morein, B., Villacres-Ericsson, M., Ekstrom, J., Hu, K., Behboudi, S., and Lovgren-Bengtsson, K. (1999). ISCOM: a delivery system for neonates and for mucosal administration. *Adv. Vet. Med.* 41, 405–413.

Munger, K., Phelps, W.C., Bubb, V., Howley, P.M., and Schlegel, R. (1989). The E6 and E7 genes of the human papillomavirus type 16 together are necessary and sufficient for transformation of primary human keratinocytes. *J. Virol.* 63, 4417–4421.

Murphy, R. et al. (2005). Recombinant NY-ESO-1 cancer antigen: production and purification of a tumour specific antigen under cGMP conditions. *Prep. Biochem. Biotechnol.* 35, 119–134.

Mutsch, M., Zhou, W., Rhodes, P., Bopp, M. et al. (2004). Use of the inactivated intranasal influenza vaccine and the risk of Bell's Palsy in Switzerland. *N. Engl. J. Med.* 350, 896–904.

O'Hagan, D.T. and Valiante, N.M. (2003). Recent advances in the discovery and delivery of vaccine adjuvants. *Nature Rev. Drug Discov.* 2, 727–735.

O'Neill, L.A. (2003). Therapeutic targeting of Toll-like receptors for inflammatory and infectious diseases. *Curr. Opin. Pharmacol.* 3, 396–403.

Osterhaus, A., van Amerongen, G., and Van Binnendijk, R. (1998). Vaccine strategies to overcome maternal antibody mediated inhibition of measles vaccine. *Vaccine* 16, 1479–1481.

Ozel, M., Hoglund, S., Gelderblom, H.R., and Morein, B. (1989). Quaternary structure of the immunostimulating complex (Iscom). *J. Ultrastr. Molec. Str. Res.* 102, 240–248.

Pearse, M.J. and Drane, D. (2005). ISCOMATRIX adjuvant for antigen delivery. *Adv. Drug Deliv. Rev.* 57, 465–474.

Peppoloni, S., Ruggiero, P., Contorni, M., Morandi, M., Pizza, M., Rappuoli, R., Podda, A., and Del Giudice, G. (2003). Mutants of the Escherichia coli heat-labile enterotoxin as safe and strong adjuvants for intranasal delivery of vaccines. *Expert Rev. Vaccines.* 2, 285–293.

Pfeifer, J.D., Wick, M.J., Roberts, R.L., Findlay, K., Normark, S.J., and Harding, C.V. (1993). Phagocytic processing of bacterial antigens for class I MHC presentation to T cells. *Nature* 361, 359–362.

Pizza, M., Giuliani, M.M., Fontana, M.R., Monaci, E., Douce, G., Dougan, G., Mills, K.H.G., Rappuoli, R., and Del Giudice, G. (2001). Mucosal vaccines: non toxic derivatives of LT and CT as mucosal adjuvants. *Vaccine* 19, 2534–2541.

Polakos, N.K., Drane, D., Cox, J., Ng, P., Selby, M.J., Chien, D., O'Hagan, D.T., Houghton, M., and Paliard, X. (2001). Characterization of hepatitis C virus core-specific immune responses primed in rhesus macaques by a nonclassical ISCOM vaccine. *J. Immunol.* 166, 3589–3598.

Rimmelzwaan, G.F. and Osterhaus, A.D.M.E. (1995). A novel generation of viral vaccines based on ISCOM matrix. In Powell, M.F. and Newman, M.J. (Eds) *Vaccine Design, the Subunit and Adjuvant Approach.* Plenum, New York, pp. 543–558.

Rimmelzwaan, G.F., Nieuwkoop, N., Brandenburg, A., Sutter, G., Beyer, W.E.P., Maher, D., and Bates, J. (2001). A randomized, double blind study in young healthy adults comparing cell mediated and humoral immune responses induced by influenza ISCOM vaccines and conventional vaccines. *Vaccine* 19, 1180–1187.

Robson, N.C., Beacock-Sharp, H., Donachie, A.M., and Mowat, A.M. (2003a). Dendritic cell maturation enhances CD8+ T–cell responses to exogenous antigen via a proteasome–independent mechanism of major histocompatibility complex class I loading. *Immunology* 109, 374–383.

Robson, N.C., Beacock-Sharp, H., Donachie, A.M., and Mowat, A.M. (2003b). The role of antigen-presenting cells and interleukin-12 in the priming of antigen-specific cd4+ T cells by immune stimulating complexes. *Immunology* 110, 95–104.

Ronnberg, B., Fekadu, M., and Morein, B. (1995). Adjuvant activity of non-toxic Quillaja saponaria Molina components for use in ISCOM matrix. *Vaccine* 13, 1375–1382.

Sambhara, S., Woods, S., Arpino, R., Kurichh, A., Tamane, A., Bengtsson, K.L., Morein, B., Underdown, B., Klein, M., and Burt, D. (1997). Influenza (H1N1)-ISCOMs enhance immune responses and protection in aged mice. *Mech. Ageing Dev.* 96, 157–169.

Scanlan, M.J., Gure, A.O., Jungbluth, A.A., Old, L.J., and Chen, Y.T. (2002). Cancer/testis antigens: an expanding family of targets for cancer immunotherapy. *Immunol. Rev.* 188, 22–32.

Schnurr, M., Chen, Q., Shin, A., Chen, W., Toy, T., Jenderek, C., Green, S., Miloradovic, L., Drane, D., Davis, I.D., Villadangos, J., Shortman, K., Maraskovsky, E., and Cebon, J. (2005). Tumor antigen processing and presentation depend critically on dendritic cell type and the mode of antigen delivery. *Blood* 105, 2465–2472.

Schuurhuis, D.H., Ioan-Facsinay, A., Nagelkerken, B., van Schip, J.J., Sedlik, C., Melief, C.J., Verbeek, J.S., and Ossendorp, F. (2002). Antigen–antibody immune complexes empower dendritic cells to efficiently prime specific CD8+ CTL responses in vivo. *J. Immunol.* 168, 2240–2246.

Seifert, U., Maranon, C., Shmueli, A., Desoutter, J.-F., Wesoloski, L., Janek, K., Hendlein, P., Siescher, S., Andrieu, M., de la Salle, H., Weinschenk, T., Schild, H., Laderach, D., Galy, A., Haas, G., Kloetzel, P.-M., Reiss, Y., and Hosmalin, A. (2003). An essential role for tripeptidyl peptidase in the generation of an MHC class I epitope. *Nature Immunol.* 4, 375–379.

Sjolander, A. and Cox, J.C. (1998). Uptake and adjuvant activity of orally delivered saponin and ISCOM vaccines. *Adv. Drug Deliv. Rev.* 34, 321–338.

Sjolander, A., Van't Land, B., and Lovgren, B.K. (1997). Iscoms containing purified Quillaja saponins upregulate both Th1-like and Th2-like immune responses. *Cell Immunol.* 177, 69–76.

Sjolander, A., Cox, J.C., and Barr, I.G. (1998). ISCOMs: an adjuvant with multiple functions. *J. Leukoc. Biol.* 64, 713–723.

Sjolander, A., Drane, D., Maraskovsky, E., Scheerlinck, J.P., Suhrbier, A., Tennent, J., and Pearse, M. (2001a). Immune responses to ISCOM formulations in animal and primate models. *Vaccine* 19, 2661–2665.

Sjolander, S., Drane, D., Davis, R., Beezum, L., Pearse, M., and Cox, J. (2001b). Intranasal immunisation with influenza-ISCOM induces strong mucosal as well as systemic antibody and cytotoxic T-lymphocyte responses. *Vaccine* 19, 4072–4080.

Smith, R.E., Donachie, A.M., Grdic, D., Lycke, N., and Mowat, A.Mc. (1999). Immune-stimulating complexes induce an IL-12-dependent cascade of innate immune responses. *J. Immunol.* 162, 5536–5546.

Soltysik, S., Wu, J.-Y., Recchia, J., Wheeler, D.A., Newman, M.J., Coughlin, R.T., and Kensil, C.R. (1995). Structure/function studies of QS-21 adjuvant: assessment of triterpene aldehyde and glucuronic acid roles in adjuvant function. *Vaccine* 13, 1403–1410.

Trinchieri, G. (1995). Interleukin-12: a proinflammatory cytokine with immunoregulatory functions that bridge innate resistance and antigen-specific adaptive immunity. *Annu. Rev. Immunol.* 13, 251–276.

Trudel, M., Boulay, G., Seguin, C., Nadon, F., and Lussier, G. (1988). Control of infectious bovine rhinotracheitis in calves with a BHV-1 subunit-ISCOM vaccine. *Vaccine* 6, 525–529.

Van Ginkel, F.W., Jackson, R.J., Yuki, Y., and McGhee, J.R. (2000). The mucosal adjuvant cholera toxin redirects vaccine proteins into olfactory tissues. *J. Immunol.* 165, 4778–4782.

Villacres, M.C., Behboudi, S., Nikkila, T., Lovgren-Bengtsson, K., and Morein, B. (1998). Internalization of iscom-borne antigens and presentation under MHC class I or class II restriction. *Cell Immunol.* 185, 30–38.

Villacres-Ericsson, M., Behboudi, S., Morgan, A.J., Trinchieri, G., and Morein, B. (1997). Immunomodulation by Quillaja saponaria adjuvant formulations: in vivo stimulation of interleukin 12 and its effects on the antibody response. *Cytokine* 9, 73–82.

Waite, D.C., Jacobson, E.W., Ennis, F.A., Edelman, R., White, B., Kammer, R., Anderson, C., and Kensil, C.R. (2001). Three double-blind, randomized trials evaluating the safety and tolerance of different formulations of the saponin adjuvant QS-21. *Vaccine* 19, 3957–3967.

Windon, R.G., Chaplin, P.J., Beezum, L., Coulter, A., Cahill, R., Kimpton, W., Drane, D., Pearse, M., Sjolander, A., Tennent, J.M., and Scheerlinck, J.-P.Y. (2001). Induction of lymphocyte recruitment in the absence of a detectable immune response. *Vaccine* 19, 572–578.

Zur Hausen, H. (2002). Papillomaviruses and cancer: from basic studies to clinical application. *Nature Rev. Cancer* 2, 342–350.

Mineral adjuvants

Erik B. Lindblad

Brenntag Biosector, Frederikssund, Denmark

Introduction

Two categories of inorganic mineral compounds have been applied as immunological adjuvants in vaccine formulation, aluminum compounds and calcium phosphate. Of the two the aluminum compounds have the longest history and by far the most comprehensive record of use.

Both adjuvants are generally regarded as safe to use in human vaccines when used in accordance with current vaccination schedules (World Health Organization, 1976; Edelman, 1980).

A.T. Glenny and co-workers were the first to demonstrate the adjuvant effect of aluminum compounds in 1926. Glenny prepared a variety of diphtheria toxoid precipitates and investigated their immunogenicity. Among these were toxoids precipitated by addition of potassium alum ($KAl(SO_4)_2 \cdot 12H_2O$). Glenny observed that injecting the diphtheria toxoid as an alum precipitate led to a significant increase in the immune response against the toxoid (Glenny et al., 1926, 1931). Vaccines prepared in accordance with this principle have been used in practical vaccination and are referred to as *alum-precipitated vaccines.* This approach, however, has a number of drawbacks. It was found (Holt, 1950) that such preparations could be highly heterogeneous, depending upon which anions, such as bicarbonate, sulfate or phosphate, were present at the time of precipitation, e.g., as buffer constituents or growth media residues in the antigen solution. In contrast, preformed aluminum hydroxide, in the form of hydrated colloid "gels," has the ability to adsorb protein antigens from an aqueous solution and such gels can be preformed in a well-defined and standardized way (Maschmann et al., 1931). Vaccine preparations based on adsorption of the antigen onto a preformed aluminum hydroxide adjuvant are referred to as *aluminum-adsorbed vaccines* in contrast to the alum-precipitated vaccines mentioned earlier. Data on the use of alum-precipitated vaccines can be found in older literature (Volk and Bunney, 1942), but in practical vaccination the adsorption onto preformed aluminum hydroxide and aluminum phosphate gels has now almost completely substituted alum precipitation in vaccine formulation. Aluminum phosphate was introduced as an alternative adjuvant two decades after Glenny's work. Ericsson (1946) devised a method in which diphtheria toxoid was coprecipitated into a matrix of aluminum phosphate, corresponding to the alum-precipitation method described earlier. Holt (1947) demonstrated the following year that preformed aluminum phosphate (prepared from aluminum chloride and trisodium phosphate), acted as an adsorbant and was adjuvant active with diphtheria toxoid.

Occasionally the word "alum" is seen in the adjuvant literature to describe both aluminum hydroxide and aluminum phosphate gels, but that is incorrect use of terminology. Potassium alum, $KAl(SO_4)_2 \cdot 12H_2O$, is in accordance with the chemical definition of an alum, whereas neither aluminum hydroxide nor aluminum phosphate is.

Calcium phosphate was introduced as an adjuvant by Edgar Relyveld in 1958 (E.H. Relyveld, personal communication). Also in the case of calcium phosphate the adjuvant can be coprecipitated in the presence of the antigen, or it can be preformed in a carefully controlled chemical environment and subsequently used for adsorption of the antigen in question.

■ Preparation and crystalline structure of mineral adjuvants

Aluminum hydroxide and aluminum phosphate adjuvants are generally prepared by exposing aqueous solutions of aluminum ions, typically as sulfates or chlorides, to alkaline conditions in a well-defined and controlled chemical environment. Various soluble aluminum salts can be used for the production of aluminum hydroxide, but the experimental conditions – temperature, concentration, and even the rate of addition of reagents – strongly influence the results (Willstätter and Kraut, 1923, 1924). Anions present at time of preparation may coprecipitate and change the characteristics away from those of "pure" aluminum hydroxide. Aluminum phosphate gel can be seen as an example of such a preparation where the soluble aluminum salts are exposed to alkaline conditions in the presence of sufficient amounts of phosphate ions. X-ray microanalysis (Figure 13.1) is a way to obtain a ground element "fingerprinting" of mineral adjuvant preparations giving an indication of which salts were used as starting material in the preparation.

Stanley Hem's group at Purdue University has intensively studied for approximately 25 years the physicochemical nature of inorganic mineral gel preparations commonly used as vaccine adjuvants. Using X-ray crystallography and IR spectroscopy they demonstrated a boehmite-like (aluminum oxyhydroxide, AlOOH) pattern in preparations traditionally known as aluminum hydroxide, whereas commercialized aluminum phosphate gel adjuvant was identified as amorphous aluminum hydroxyphosphate (Shirodkar et al., 1990). It was possible to calculate an average primary crystallite size of $4.5 \times 2.2 \times 10 \, nm$ for the boehmite preparations (Johnston et al., 2002). Recently also commercially available calcium phosphate was studied by X-ray

diffraction, Fourier transform infrared (FTIR) spectroscopy, and thermal analysis of an American product. This indicated that calcium phosphate adjuvant with the suggested formula of $Ca_3(PO_4)_2$ could be described as nonstoichiometric hydroxyapatite, $Ca_{10-x}(HPO_4)_x(PO_4)_{6-x}(OH)_{2-x}$, where x varies from 0 to 2 (Jiang et al., 2004). In the original work Relyveld described the calcium phosphate adjuvant, prepared at Institut Pasteur, as nonhydroxyapatite with a stoichiometric formula of $PO_4CaH_2(PO_4)_2Ca_3$ with a Ca/P ratio of approx 1:8 (E.H. Relyveld, personal communication).

Upon injection mineral adjuvant particles are to be phagocytized by the antigen-presenting cells. This is reflected in the particle size distribution of the mineral adjuvant preparations (Figure 13.2). Morphological studies using scanning electron microscopy (SEM) are possible (Figure 13.3). It should be remembered, however, that dehydration of the adjuvant particles in the preparation for SEM may lead to structures not completely identical to those presented to the immune system.

■ Application of mineral adjuvants

In human vaccination aluminum adjuvants have been primarily used in tetanus, diphtheria, pertussis, and poliomyelitis vaccines as part of standard child vaccination programs for approximately 50 years in many countries. Later aluminum adjuvants were also introduced in hepatitis A and hepatitis B virus vaccines. Other aluminum-adsorbed vaccines, against, for example, anthrax, are available for special risk groups. In veterinary medicine aluminum adjuvants have been used in a large number of vaccine formulations against viral (McDougall, 1969; Wilson et al., 1977; Sellers and Herniman, 1974; St. Hyslop and Morrow, 1969; Pini et al., 1965) and bacterial (Thorley and Egerton, 1981; McCandlish et al., 1978; Nagy and Penn, 1974; Ris and Hamel, 1979) diseases, as well as in attempts to make antiparasite vaccines (Leland et al., 1988; Monroy et al., 1989; Carlow and Bianco, 1987;

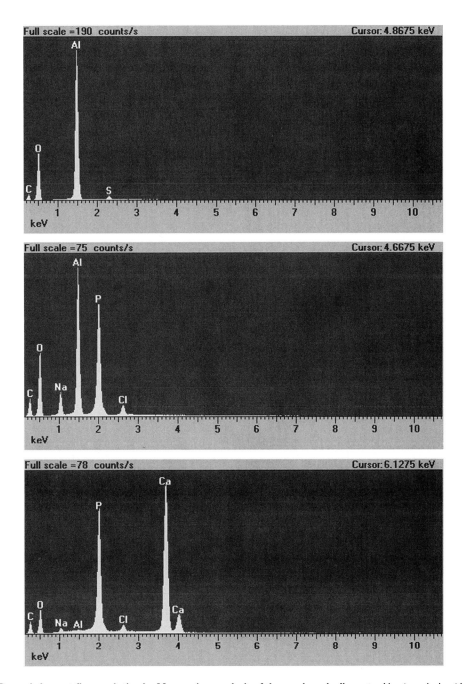

Figure 13.1 Ground element fingerprinting by X-ray microanalysis of three mineral adjuvants. Aluminum hydroxide (top), aluminum phosphate (middle), and calcium phosphate (bottom).

Gamble et al., 1986). Calcium phosphate was used as an adjuvant in vaccines against diphtheria, tetanus, *Bordetella pertussis*, and poliomyelitis (Relyveld, 1986; Coursaget et al., 1986), commercialized by Institut Pasteur. Calcium phosphate was used as an adjuvant in the IPAD series of vaccines by Institut Pasteur for approx. 25 years. Further, calcium

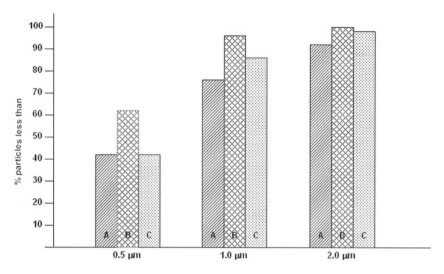

Figure 13.2 Example of particle size distributions of three mineral adjuvants analyzed by ACCUSIZER Model 770A.
Aluminum hydroxide, *Alhydrogel batch 2413* (A), aluminum phosphate, *Adju-Phos batch 8867* (B), and calcium phosphate adjuvant, *batch 034* (C), (Dr. Lisa MacDonald, personal communication.)

phosphate has been tested as an adjuvant in experimental vaccines with the gp160 antigen from HIV (Relyveld and Chermann, 1994). Calcium phosphate has so far not been used as an adjuvant in commercial veterinary vaccines.

Both aluminum hydroxide and calcium phosphate have been used as adjuvant in commercialized adsorbed allergen preparations for hyposensitization of allergic patients (Relyveld et al., 1985).

■ Dosing mineral adjuvants

There are limitations for the content of aluminum and calcium allowed in vaccines for humans, when administered as adjuvants. These limits are 1.25 mg aluminum per dose in Europe (European Pharmacopoeia, 1997), and in the USA 0.85 mg aluminum per dose if determined by assay, 1.14 mg if determined by calculation, and 1.25 mg if safety and efficacy data justify it (Code of Federal Regulations, 2003). In Europe the maximum allowed amount of calcium delivered by calcium phosphate-adjuvanted vaccines is 1.3 mg calcium. There is, however, no obvious toxicological rationale behind limiting the amount of calcium in vaccines to 1.3 mg/dose. Calcium phosphate is a natural constituent of the mammalian organism and it has been a component of bone replacement transplants in much higher amounts with no problems (Tanzer et al., 2004). The optimum dose of adjuvant is normally determined empirically in a pilot trial, but helpful guidelines are available in the literature. In veterinary vaccines there is no defined maximum limit for the allowed content of aluminum adjuvants. Here the dose is normally set from a balance between efficacy and local reactogenicity.

For dose–response relations of both types of mineral adjuvants in combination with bacterial antigens the immunomodulation observed may reflect a composite effect between the mineral adjuvant itself and immunomodulatory and adjuvant-active bacterial substances, such as muramyl peptides from peptidoglycans, lipopolysaccharide (LPS), trehalose dimycolate ("cord factor"), or CpG motifs from bacterial DNA (Krieg, 2002).

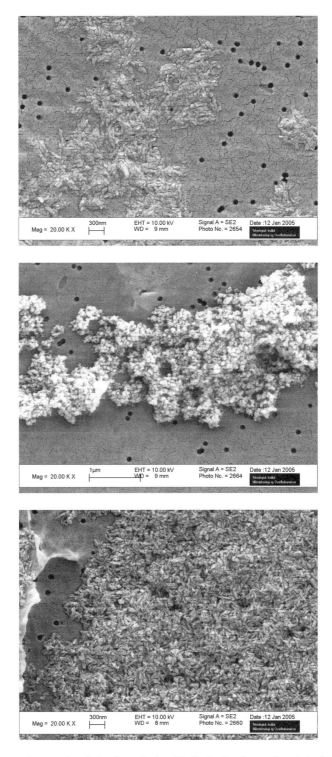

Figure 13.3 Scanning electron micrographs of aluminum hydroxide (top), aluminum phosphate (middle), and calcium phosphate (bottom). Gold coated; ×20,000 magnification. (Photo: Pia Wahlberg, DTI.)

■ Mechanisms of adjuvant activity

The immunostimulating effect of the traditional aluminum adjuvants is highly complex and must be attributed to several different mechanisms. In the older literature (Glenny et al., 1931), the function of a repository adjuvant was originally described as to delay clearing from the injection site and sustain a gradual release of adsorbed antigen from the inoculated depot. Although gradual release and delayed clearing may indeed play a role, it quickly became obvious that a gradual release was insufficient in explaining the mechanisms of adjuvant activity. However, the physical adsorption of antigen onto the adjuvant is still considered to be a very important mechanism for the function of mineral adjuvants. Over the last two decades the role of T cells and cytokine profiles following the application of aluminum adjuvants have also been described. A possible mechanism involving danger signals, heat shock proteins, and Toll-like receptors is discussed at the end of the chapter.

■ Antigen adsorption

The literature contains examples of publications where injection of adjuvant and unadsorbed antigen at distant sites led to immunostimulation towards the antigen (Flebbe and Braley-Mullen, 1986); however, this is not the consistent picture (Gupta et al., 1995), and the nature of the antigen chosen for the work may provide part of the explanation for the deviating conclusions. As a general rule the antigen should be adsorbed onto the adjuvant prior to immunization and the adsorption should be carefully monitored.

A consequence of the physical attachment of the antigen onto the adjuvant is that a soluble antigen upon adsorption may be presented to the immunocompetent cells in a "particulate" manner which could facilitate antigen targeting, i.e., favor uptake by antigen-presenting cells (APCs). A likely explanation is that APCs may be more efficient in antigen uptake by phagocytosis than by pinocytosis. Mannhalter and co-workers demonstrated enhanced uptake of aluminum-adsorbed tetanus toxoid, as compared to the soluble toxoid, by APCs (Mannhalter et al., 1985).

The physicochemical mechanisms behind the antigen adsorption itself are complex and depending upon the nature of the individual antigen some mechanisms may predominate over others.

As a general guideline for many protein antigens adsorption is best accomplished in the pH interval between the isoelectric point (IEP) of the protein antigen and the point of zero charge (PZC) of the adjuvant, which is the equivalent of the IEP, but for the adjuvant. This applies for both aluminum hydroxide and aluminum phosphate adjuvants. In this interval the adjuvant and the antigen will have opposite electrical charges, facilitating electrostatic attraction and adsorption (Figure 13.4).

The surface charge (SCh) in mV of the adjuvant particle was described by Hem (S.L. Hem, personal communication; Wu et al., 1986) by the formula

$$SCh = 59\,mV \times (PZC - pH)$$

In this formula, which is derived from the Nernst equation, "PZC" is the pH value where the net charge of the adjuvant is zero and "pH" is the actual pH value of the chemical environment.

Seeber et al. (1991) concluded that aluminum hydroxide should be superior to aluminum phosphate in adsorbing proteins with an acidic IEP and vice versa for proteins with an alkaline IEP. However, if the antigen contains phosphorylated groups ligand exchange between the antigen-associated phosphate and hydroxyl groups of the adjuvant may account for a high-affinity binding to the adjuvant. This is the case, for example, with HBsAg particles (Iyer et al., 2004), and has been shown in experiments using phosphorylated alpha-casein as model antigen (Iyer et al., 2003).

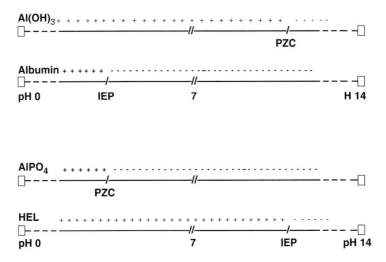

Figure 13.4 In the pH range between the isoelectric point (IEP) of the antigen and the point of zero charge (PZC) of the mineral adjuvant there is basis for electrostatic attraction, due to opposite charge. The alkaline PZC for $Al(OH)_3$ makes it suitable for adsorption of acidic IEP proteins as examplified by albumin, whereas the acidic PZC of $AlPO_4$ makes it suitable for adsorption of alkaline IEP proteins, as examplified by hen egg lysozyme (HEL).

The primary mechanisms responsible for the adsorption have been explained partly by electrostatic attraction and partly by anionic ligand exchange (Hem and White, 1984). In addition other intermolecular binding forces, like hydrophilic–hydrophobic interaction, may play a role in protein adsorption (Al-Shakhshir et al., 1995) and each binding force may play a role in a given antigen–adjuvant combination, depending upon the nature of the antigen and the chemical environment: pH, ionic strength, presence of surfactants, etc. (Rinella et al., 1995, 1998a, 1998b). To complicate the picture even further, antigens with a distinct polarity in terms of one part of the molecule having a clearly acidic IEP and a distant part of the same molecule having a clearly alkaline IEP may bind well to both $Al(OH)_3$ and $AlPO_4$. However, in such cases there may be a difference in the orientation of the adsorbed molecule (Dagoussat et al., 2001).

For testing of adsorptive power of mineral adjuvants when used in diphtheria and tetanus vaccines the established Ramon flocculation test is used. In this test the results are given as Lf (limits of flocculation). The antigen adsorption capacity of calcium phosphate is quantitatively inferior to that of the aluminum compounds, but it is still sufficient to adsorb the required amounts of Lf in conventional diphtheria/tetanus vaccines.

Determination of the protein adsorption capacity of the adjuvant is highly recommended and can be measured by a variety of analytical methods. It is normally done by comparing the protein content in the aqueous phase of the antigen solution before and after adsorption onto the adjuvant. If an antibody specific for the antigen one wishes to adsorb is available, adsorption can be measured by immunoprecipitation techniques. This can be done by quantitative immunoelectrophoresis (Weeke et al., 1975) or by single radial immunodiffusion (Lindblad, 1995). Without the use of an antibody it can be tested spectrophotometrically, e.g., by the BCA method (Smith et al., 1985). However, it should be remembered that contamination with the fine fraction of mineral gel particles can disturb the spectrophotometric readings by light-scatter effects. ELISA methods have been designed (Thiele et al., 1990) in which aluminum-adsorbed antigens could be used directly as antigens in ELISA assays. ELISA methods were also applied for *in vitro* assessment of various viral antigens, i.e., pseudo-rabies, porcine parvovirus, and infectious bovine rhinotracheitis vaccines adsorbed onto aluminum hydroxide adjuvant (Katz et al., 1989).

Differential adsorption of complex mixtures of antigens can be measured by either immunoelectrophoresis or by HPLC. If an antiserum raised against the complex antigen mixture is available, a crossed, two-dimensional immunoelectrophoresis may reveal if single components from the complex solution of proteins remain unadsorbed. To use this approach, the precipitation band pattern from an electrophoresis run on the complex antigen mixture prior to adsorption is compared with the bands of an electrophoresis run on the supernatant of the same mixture after adsorption. Unadsorbed components will retain their immuno-precipitation band pattern, whereas missing bands or reduced height of bands are indicative of complete or partial protein adsorption (Weeke et al., 1975). An HPLC chromatogram of the antigen mixture liquid phase before and after adsorption may provide similar information.

■ T cell reactivity, antibody subclasses, and stimulation of cytokines

In the older literature aluminum adjuvants are often claimed not to be "T cell adjuvants." However, this is mostly based on work from a period where a "T cell adjuvant" was primarily an adjuvant capable of inducing a delayed-type hypersensitivity (DTH) response. It is the case that aluminum adjuvants are not efficient DTH inducers in rodents, as pointed out by Bomford (1980). There is also very little evidence that aluminum adjuvants should be able to generate MHC class I restricted cytotoxic T cells; so far there is only a single report from Dillon et al. (1992) who tested a recombinant influenza vaccine in mice. However, as early as the late 1970s the ability of aluminum adjuvants to induce eosinophilia was shown to require the presence of T cells

(Walls, 1977) and the reaction profile of aluminum adjuvants is now known to comprise stimulation of CD4+ T cells (Grun and Maurer, 1989).

Studies of the impact of interleukins (ILs) in model systems were initiated almost 20 years ago and have more recently been intensified because of the introduction of gene-disrupted mice in research. Among the early observations in classic animal models was the demonstration of Mannhalter that aluminum-adsorbed tetanus toxoid led to an increase in antigen-induced T cell proliferation, apparently due to increased release of IL-1 (Mannhalter et al., 1985). In contrast, there was a lack of importance of IL-1 in the augmentation of the primary antibody response in rabbits immunized with aluminum adjuvant (Sagara et al., 1990).

Grun and Maurer (1989) demonstrated that anti-IL-1α or anti-IL-4 was able to inhibit an antigen-specific T cell proliferative response after immunization with aluminum adjuvant. This was not the case if the mice were immunized with Freund's complete adjuvant (FCA). However, as the proliferative responses were inhibited by anti-CD4 antibody, regardless of the adjuvant used, it indicated that the proliferating CD4+ T cells from mice immunized with aluminum adjuvant were of the Th2 subset. Lindblad et al. (1997) found a corresponding profile in C57BL/6J mice looking at IgG2a and IgG1 subclass assays and RT-PCR for IL-4- and IL-10-specific mRNA in the regional draining lymph nodes at day 7 following vaccination with aluminum-adjuvanted vaccine.

Although it is now generally accepted that aluminum adjuvants are Th2 stimulators, it is interesting that a complex between $Al(OH)_3$ and IL-12 ($Al(OH)_3$/IL-12) induced a Th1 response, rather than a Th2 response, when used as an adjuvant (Jankovic et al., 1999) and the Th1-promoting effect of the $Al(OH)_3$/IL-12 complex was greatly augmented by the coadministration of exogenous IL-18 (Pollock et al., 2003). There are at the moment no corresponding data for calcium phosphate.

A new line of research was initiated with the introduction of gene-disrupted mice, which has facilitated the study of the significance of ILs.

IL-4 gene-disrupted mice immunized with ovalbumin (OVA) + Al(OH)$_3$ elicited IgG2a titers of a similar magnitude to when OVA was injected together with FCA (Brewer et al., 1996). However, interestingly, the group immunized with OVA + Al(OH)$_3$ continued to produce IL-5 (a cytokine normally associated with the Th2 profile). In contrast, when the IL-4–/– mice had been immunized using FCA a similar stimulation of IL-5 was not seen. This supports the idea that the major role of aluminum-induced IL-4 in Th-subset stimulation is to downregulate the Th1 response.

The role of IL-18 in the adjuvant activity of aluminum hydroxide and its effect on Th2 induction has been demonstrated by Pollock et al. (2003). They demonstrated that IL-18-deficient mice immunized with OVA + Al(OH)$_3$ had reduced IL-4 production in lymph node cells compared to wild-type mice. However, if they added exogenous IL-18 it did not further enhance the aluminum-induced Th2 response. Although the aluminum adjuvant led to reduced IL-4 production in IL-18–/– mice, this was not accompanied by a reduced level of serum IgG1. Apparently, there is poor correlation between this particular antibody subclass and IL-4 production.

With calcium phosphate no cytokine data are found in the literature, and the question as to whether calcium phosphate shares the clear Th2 profile of aluminum adjuvants is not fully clarified.

It is not yet possible to investigate surface marker differentiation over time of cell populations *in vivo* due to the biological complexity of the living organism. However, *in vitro* models may lead to observations the

validity of which may later be challenged – with all due care taken – by *in vivo* control experiments.

Rimaniol et al. (2004) recently cultivated human monocytes (PBMC) in medium alone or medium containing aluminum hydroxide adjuvant and observed phenotypic macrophage changes. The changes encountered comprised significant upregulation of HLA-DR, as well as CD86 and CD71. Some 80% of the macrophages obtained were positive for the scavenger receptor CD163. However, incubation with aluminum hydroxide downregulated both Fc$_\gamma$R and CD163. Macrophages, as they expressed a dendritic cell-like phenotype after incubation with aluminum hydroxide (HLA-DR^{high}, CD86^{high}, and CD14−), were further investigated for the expression of dendritic cell-specific markers.

The expression of CD83 increased after 15 hours of incubation with aluminum hydroxide, compared to non-Al(OH)$_3$-stimulated cells. It turned out that adjuvant-stimulated macrophages were also superior in antigen presentation. Based on these findings Rimaniol et al. concluded that stimulation with aluminum adjuvant led to differentiation of the macrophages into a form resembling, but still distinctly different from, dendritic cells.

No similar data are at the moment available for the calcium phosphate adjuvant.

■ Mineral adjuvants and stimulation of IgE

A study of the literature suggests a distinct difference in the profile related to stimulation of IgE between the aluminum- and calcium-based adjuvants.

The ability of aluminum adjuvants to stimulate the production of IgE as part of the overall Th2 profile is well established (Kenney et al., 1989; Hamaoka et al., 1973). Although this has often been mentioned as a disadvantage, it has been difficult to demonstrate cases where vaccination with aluminum adjuvants has led to IgE-mediated allergy towards the vaccine antigen in practical vaccination. In contrast, aluminum adjuvants have been used to hypo-sensitize allergic patients for many years with good results, e.g., with the ALUTARD^{TM} series of vaccines.

A very useful model for studying the IgE/Th2 stimulation in rodent models is to immunize groups of animals using aluminum adjuvant vs. FCA, and assess antibody and cytokine profiles in comparison. Uede and co-workers in Japan (Uede at al., 1982; Uede and Ishizaka, 1982) pioneered this line of research two decades ago using keyhole limpet hemocyanin (KLH) as antigen and demonstrated the involvement glycosylation-enhancing factors and Fc$_\gamma$R+ T cells in a dichotomous regulatory pathway where aluminum adjuvant stimulated the synthesis of IgE whereas FCA suppressed it.

Brewer et al. (1996) used the same approach of comparing the adjuvant profiles of aluminum hydroxide vs. FCA using gene-disrupted mice. They found that there was no IgE production in IL-4 gene-disrupted mice (IL-4–/–) regardless of whether aluminum adjuvant or FCA was used as adjuvant. This suggests that IL-4 is an essential pre-requisite for the induction of IgE by aluminum adjuvants.

With the calcium phosphate adjuvant the literature data suggest that this adjuvant does not lead to significant stimulation of IgE antibodies. Vassilev (1978) compared the reaction in terms of passive cutaneous anaphylaxia (PCA) in guinea pigs after two immunizations with either aluminum or calcium phosphate adjuvant using tetanus toxoid as antigen. He found that calcium phosphate-treated guinea pigs only had insignificant IgE titers compared to the group that had received aluminum-adjuvanted vaccines. In general, the research in this field is sparse and there are at present no data on the IL profile after immunization with calcium phosphate to illustrate possible underlying differences in the mechanisms behind such a distinction.

There are some interesting similarities between the immune response (e.g., stimulation of IgE and eosinophilia) elicited by some helminthic parasites and the immune response following immunization with aluminum adjuvants that make these adjuvants interesting candidates for antiparasitic vaccines. Experimental data suggest a protective superiority of specific IgE after aluminum-adjuvanted vaccination in animal models against schistosomiasis infections (Knopf et al., 1988; Horowitz et al., 1982).

■ Limitations to the applicability of mineral adjuvants

One obvious limitation for the application of aluminum adjuvants lies in the clear Th2 profile of these adjuvants. A Th2-biased immune response is not likely to protect against diseases for which Th1 immunity and MHC class I restricted cytotoxic T lymphocytes (CTLs) are essential for protection, such as with, for example, intracellular parasites or tuberculosis (Lindblad et al., 1997). Another limitation lies in the fact that traditional aluminum- and calcium-adsorbed vaccines are frost sensitive and therefore not lyophilizable.

Aluminum adjuvants failed to provide satisfactory augmentation of the immune response against a number of infectious diseases, such as with influenza and typhoid fever vaccines (Davenport et al., 1968; Cvjetanovic and Uemura, 1965). In some approaches to vaccine preparation, aluminum adjuvants have shown limitations in their applicability in vaccines based on small-size peptides (Francis et al., 1987). In some cases, e.g., with FMD virus peptides, the problem could be overcome by conjugating the peptide to a larger carrier molecule (Francis et al., 1985). In others it could not (Lew et al., 1988; Geerligs et al., 1989). Aluminum adjuvants have been tested in a few DNA vaccine formulations. Here it was shown (Ulmer et al., 2000; Kwissa et al., 2003) that aluminum hydroxide had an inhibiting effect, whereas aluminum phosphate adjuvant augmented the immune response against the antigen encoded by the nucleotide. The high content of phosphate in the DNA molecule apparently gives a high binding affinity of the nucleotide to aluminum hydroxide, which in turn prevents the RNA from getting access to and translating the nucleotides into protein (Kwissa et al., 2003).

In vivo clearing of aluminum and calcium adjuvants

A major difference between aluminum- and calcium-based adjuvants lies in the clearing *in vivo* of the adjuvant inoculum and the metabolic fate of the degradation products. Upon degradation of calcium phosphate the two constituents can be reutilized in the normal metabolic pathways for Ca^{2+} and PO_4^{3-}, whereas in contrast to other metallic ions, like Zn^{2+} and Mg^{2+}, aluminum apparently does not act as an essential trace element or coenzyme in normal metabolism. However, previous claims that aluminum adjuvants are not broken down *in situ* and excreted have been shown to be incorrect.

The mammalian organism is fairly constantly being exposed to aluminum compounds from the environment. As a consequence aluminum is normally found in the blood and serum of humans and animals whether or not they have been vaccinated using aluminum adjuvants. The major source of this aluminum is apparently oral intake with food and drinking water. Martyn et al. (1989), based on a study in Britain, reported the average daily intake of aluminum by humans to be 5–10 mg. This aluminum uptake would be excreted with the urine by individuals with normal renal functions.

The clearing *in vivo* of aluminum adjuvants has been investigated in rabbits using adjuvants prepared from the isotope ^{26}Al (Flarend et al., 1997). Blood and urine-excreted ^{26}Al was followed using accelerator mass spectroscopy for a period of 28 days. As early as 1 hour following intramuscular injection radiolabeled aluminum could be detected in the blood and it was found that approximately three times more ^{26}Al was excreted from animals vaccinated with aluminum phosphate than those vaccinated with aluminum hydroxide. Presumably, interstitial fluid containing organic acids with an α-hydroxy carboxylic acid, able to chelate aluminum, reacted more readily with aluminum phosphate than with aluminum hydroxide (Flarend et al., 1997). It is of interest that following injection of adjuvant containing 0.85 mg aluminum the normal plasma concentration of aluminum in rabbits of 30 ng aluminum/ml only rose by approximately 2 ng aluminum/ml during the experiment. According to the calculation of Flarend a similar aluminum dose injected into humans, provided similar clearing kinetics existed, would lead to an estimated increase of serum aluminum of only 0.04 ng aluminum/ml, equaling 0.8% above the normal level of approximately 5 ng aluminum/ml. Based on these figures it seems that the amount of aluminum administered via vaccination does not contribute significantly to the general exposure to aluminum in humans and serum levels of aluminum.

Side effect profile of mineral adjuvants

Aluminum hydroxide and aluminum phosphate adjuvants have been used for more than half a century, and are generally regarded as safe when used according to current immunization schedules (Edelman, 1980). In 1993 the US NCVDG Working Group on Safety Evaluation of Vaccine Adjuvants with the participation of US Food and Drug Administration representatives concluded that "the extensive experience with this class of adjuvant for vaccine use has indicated that it is safe" (Goldenthal et al., 1993).

There is no evidence that aluminum adjuvants themselves should be immunogenic and act as haptens; accordingly they are not likely to cause harmful immune complex reactions and observations of contact hypersensitivity reactions are not commonly seen (Edelman, 1980; Böhler-Sommeregger and Lindemayr, 1986). The aluminum adjuvants are not in themselves pyrogenic and there is no evidence of carcinogenicity or teratogenicity attributed to their use.

Cases of local reactions have occasionally been reported (Gupta et al., 1993). These may comprise swellings, indurations, erythemas, and cutaneous nodules that can persist for up to eight weeks or sometimes longer (Frost et al., 1985). These reports often describe cases of hyposensitization of allergic patients who receive a large number of injections of adsorbed allergenic extracts over a limited period of time. In a vaccination program in Sweden, Bergfors et al. (2003) found itching local reactions in 0.8% out of 76,000 vaccinees. A number of observations of side effects seen after vaccination with adjuvanted vaccines must, however, be attributed to the vaccine preservatives, like thiomersal, betapropriolactone, or formaldehyde, or, as mentioned, to bacterial toxins from the antigen preparation (Chaby and Caroff, 1988).

The inflammatory focus

Aluminum and calcium adjuvants should, along with water-in-oil emulsions, be regarded as depot-forming or repository adjuvants. With these adjuvants the formation of a temporary inflammatory focus attracting immunocompetent cells shortly after injection must more or less be expected (World Health Organization, 1976). Upon injection macrophages are attracted to the site to phagocytize and clear the inoculum. The local reaction may be negligible if the inoculum is rapidly dispersed from the injection site. However, if the inoculum resides for a prolonged period of time at the injection site (as is the case with repository adjuvants like mineral adjuvants or water-in-oil emulsions) then *in situ* accumulation of phagocytic and immunocompetent cells may in some cases manifest as an inflammatory focus accompanied by a transient swelling, local irritation, and redness. Some observations of aluminum-adsorbed vaccines giving more local reactions than unadsorbed vaccines with plain toxoid (Collier et al., 1979) could in part be explained by the plain toxoid

vaccine being dispersed from the injection site before a local reaction was established.

Any visible or palpable reaction at the injection site is in principle unacceptable, as it hinders the obtaining of a hypothetical and nonreactogenic "ideal adjuvant." However, it is important to realize that the mechanisms described are part of a normally functioning immune system. Hence, it may not be achievable to use repository adjuvants without temporarily also inducing an inflammatory focus around the inoculum. There are inconsistent observations as to whether adsorption onto aluminum adjuvants leads to increased or decreased vaccine reactogenicity (Collier et al., 1979; Aprile and Wardlaw, 1966). However, Butler et al. found that adsorption onto aluminum hydroxide (Alhydrogel™) significantly reduced the side effects with combined DTP vaccines (Butler et al., 1969). The binding affinity of LPS to aluminum hydroxide is well established and is much higher than that to aluminum phosphate (Shi et al., 2001), probably due to the phosphate content of LPS. It is conceivable that the acute toxicity is reduced in adsorbed vaccines simply by a delayed release of toxic vaccine constituents, like pertussis toxin, peptidoglycans from Gram-negative cell walls, or LPS from the injection site. Norimatsu et al. (1995) found that adsorption of LPS onto aluminum hydroxide prior to injection inhibited or mitigated systemic effects like trembling, transient leucopenia, and elevated serum tumor necrosis factor (TNF)-α otherwise observed following intramuscular injection of LPS in saline. Also the level of IL-6 after administration of LPS was reduced if the LPS was adsorbed to aluminum hydroxide prior to injection (Shi et al., 2001).

Attempts have been made to link the presence of a local inflammatory focus in the myofascii (macrophage myofasciitis, MMF) after intramuscular injections of aluminum-adjuvanted vaccines to conditions like myalgia and muscle fatigue, but also to neurological disorders with no obvious aetiological relation to the vaccination (Authier et al., 2001). However, such correlations are associated with statistical problems. Due to the very high vaccination coverage in Western countries it is expected statistically that patients suffering from a wide range of diseases would all have been vaccinated with aluminum-containing vaccines at some point in their medical history. Further, adequate statistical control groups of nonvaccinated individuals may be hard to find in the same population. In a recently published, controlled study in primates it was not possible to detect any histological changes besides the local inflammatory focus itself and no abnormal clinical signs were associated with it (Verdier et al., 2005).

Effect of the injection modus

Vaccinations may be given subcutaneously or intramuscularly and the injection modus is not without importance in relation to local reactogenicity. When immunizing by the subcutaneous route the vaccine inoculum is introduced into a compartment with numerous sensory neurons (in contrast to the intramuscular compartment). The introduction of a local inflammatory response here may more easily lead to irritation and itching reactions. Besides, a transient swelling, as a consequence of the inflammatory focus formed, may be more easily palpable through the skin. When immunizing by the intramuscular route even a similar size swelling may be less easily visible and palpable as it is located in deeper-lying tissue.

Mineral adjuvants and Toll-like receptors

Incubation of dendritic cells with aluminum adjuvant failed to activate the dendritic cells as judged by increased expression of MHC class II and costimulatory molecules. This indicates that aluminum adjuvants, in contrast to bacteria-derived adjuvants (e.g., LPS, CpG), are not *directly* addressing Toll-like receptors (TLRs) (Sun et al., 2003).

However, Lindblad (2004) previously suggested that although aluminum adjuvants were concluded not to act through TLRs as

demonstrated *in vitro* by Brewer's group (Sun et al., 2003), this family of receptors may nevertheless be involved in a secondary reaction to the mineral adjuvants *in vivo* through *a cascade mechanism*. This would be a consequence of local tissue disturbance caused by the repository adjuvant at the injection site and elicitation of *danger signals*, including release of heat shock proteins. The hypothesis is supported primarily by two recent observations. One observation considered supportive was by Asea's group at Harvard Medical School. They demonstrated that extracellular HSP70 added to human monocyte cultures elicited a rapid intracellular Ca^{2+} flux, activated nuclear factor (NF)-κB, and upregulated the expression of proinflammatory cytokines, TNF-α, IL-1β, and IL-6 (Asea et al., 2000). In a follow-up study (Asea et al., 2002) they demonstrated that HSP70 utilized both the TLR2 and TLR4 receptors for proinflammatory signal transduction in a CD14-dependant fashion.

This is particularly interesting when viewed in the context of the investigations of Naim et al. (1997) who found a correlation between the magnitude of the antibody response and the local inflammatory response elicited after injection of different plurivalent metal oxides, including aluminum, and tested as adjuvants.

As both aluminum and calcium adjuvants are repository adjuvants and as both adjuvants lead to local disturbance of tissue integrity and a transient inflammatory response (Goto et al., 1997), I suggest that the mechanism described, addressing TLR2 and TLR4 as a secondary reaction involving HSP70 is common to the function of the two adjuvants.

Conclusion

The aluminum adjuvants have beyond doubt proven their efficiency in a large number of applications as vaccine adjuvants in both human and veterinary immunoprophylaxis with very few problems and they are fairly inexpensive. This may be less relevant from a scientific point of view, but it may be of great importance for establishing effective vaccination programs in developing countries, where funding is limited.

When evaluating the profile of an adjuvant for possible new applications very few adjuvants can match the extremely comprehensive cohorts that are available for aluminum adjuvants in terms of records of efficacy and safety profiles, which after more than half a century of use may reach practically over a lifelong timespan in humans.

The aluminum adjuvants have their limitations, due to their profound Th2 reactivity, which means that there are vaccines in which they will have little or no effect. However, in the future modified formulations with a more balanced Th1–Th2 profile may find their way into practical vaccinology along with more potent Th1 stimulators, like monophosphoryl lipid A (MPL). The potential application of the $Al(OH)_3/IL-12$ complex (Jankovic et al., 1999; Pollock et al., 2003) for use in vaccines for Th1 stimulation is yet to be explored in detail. Over the last ten years there has been an increasing interest in calcium phosphate as adjuvant, both for conventional vaccines (Aggerbeck et al., 1995) and in particular for the preparation of adsorbed allergens. More research will be needed to clarify a possible difference in the ability of the calcium and aluminum based adjuvants in the stimulation of IgE, especially with respect to the cytokine profiles. Only then will it be possible to judge whether or not calcium phosphate is to be regarded as a clear-cut Th2 stimulator.

■ References

Aggerbeck, H., Fenger, C., and Heron, I. (1995). Booster vaccination against diphtheria and tetanus in man. Comparison of calcium phosphate and aluminium hydroxide as adjuvants: II. *Vaccine* 13, 1366–1374.

Al-Shakhshir, R.H., Regnier, F.E., White, J.L., and Hem, S.L. (1995). Contribution of electrostatic and hydrophobic interactions to the adsorption of proteins by aluminium-containing adjuvants. *Vaccine* 13, 41–44.

Aprile, M.A. and Wardlaw, A.C. (1966). Aluminium compounds as adjuvants for vaccines and toxoids in man: a review. *Can. J. Public Health* 57, 343–354.

Asea, A., Kraeft, S-K., Kurt-Jones, E.A., Stevenson, M.A., Chen, L.B., Finberg, R.W., Koo, G.C., and Calderwood, S.K. (2000). HSP70 stimulates cytokine production through a CD14-dependant pathway, demonstrating its dual role as a chaperone and a cytokine. *Nature Med.* 6, 435–442.

Asea, A., Rehli, M., Kabingu, E., Boch, J.A., Bare, O., Auron, P.E., Stevenson, M.A., and Calderwood, S.K. (2002). Novel signal transduction pathway utilized by extracellular HSP70. *J. Biol. Chem.* 277, 15028–15034.

Authier, F.J., Cherin, P., Creange, A., Bonnotte, B., Ferrer, X., Abdelmoumni, A., Ranoux, D., Pelletier, J., Figarella-Branger, D., Granel, B., Maisonobe, T., Coquet, M., Degos, J.D., and Gherardi, R.K. (2001). Central nervous system disease in patients with macrophagic myofasciitis. *Brain* 124 (Pt 5), 974–983

Bergfors, E., Trollfors, B., and Inerot, A. (2003). Unexpectedly high incidence of persistent itching nodules and delayed hypersensitivity to aluminium in children after use of adsorbed vaccines from a single manufacturer. *Vaccine* 22, 64–69.

Böhler-Sommeregger, K., and Lindemayr, H. (1986). Contact sensitivity to aluminium. *Contact Dermatitis* 15, 278–281.

Bomford, R. (1980). The comparative selectivity of adjuvants for humoral and cell-mediated immunity: II. Effect on delayed-type hypersensitivity in the mouse and guinea pig, and cell-mediated immunity to tumour antigens in the mouse of Freund's incomplete and complete adjuvants, Alhydrogel, Corynebacterium parvum, Bordetella pertussis, muramyl dipeptide and saponin. *Clin. Exp. Immunol.* 39, 435–441.

Brewer, J.M., Conacher, M., Satoskar, A., Bluethmann, H., and Alexander, J. (1996). In interleukin-4-deficient mice, alum not only generates T helper 1 responses equivalent to Freund's complete adjuvant, but continues to induce T helper 2 cytokine production. *Eur. J. Immunol.* 26, 2062–2066.

Butler, N.R., Voyce, M.A., Burland, W.L., and Hilton, M.L. (1969). Advantages of aluminium hydroxide adsorbed combined diphtheria, tetanus, and pertussis vaccines for the immunization of infants. *Brit. Med. J.* 1, 663–666.

Carlow, C.K.S. and Bianco, A.E. (1987). Resistance of *Onchocerca lienalis* microfilariae in mice conferred by egg antigens of homologous and heterologous onchocerca species. *Parasitology* 94, 485–496.

Chaby, R. and Caroff, M. (1988). Lipopolysaccharides of Bordetella pertussis endotoxin. In Wardlaw, A.C. and Parton, P. (Eds) Pathogenesis and Immunity in Pertussis. John Wiley, New York, pp. 247–271.

Code of Federal Regulations (2003). Code 21, vol. 7: sec. 610.15 (Constituent Materials), revised 1 April 2003.

Collier, L.H., Polakoff, S., and Mortimer, J. (1979). Reactions and antibody responses to reinforcing doses of adsorbed and plain tetanus vaccines. *Lancet* 1364–1367.

Coursaget, P., Yvonnet, B., Relyveld, E.H., Barres, J.L., Diop-Mar, I., and Chiron, J.P. (1986). Simultaneous administration of diphtheria-tetanus-pertussis-polio and hepatitis B vaccines in a simplified immunization program: immune response to diphtheria toxoid, tetanus toxoid, pertussis, and hepatitis B surface antigen. *Infect. Immun.* 51, 784–787.

Cvjetanovic, B. and Uemura, K. (1965). The present status of field and laboratory studies of typhoid and paratyphoid vaccines. *Bull. WHO* 32, 29–36.

Dagoussat, N., Robillard, V., Haeuw, J.F., Plotnicky-Gilquin, H., Power, U., Corvaia, N., Nguyen, T., Bonnefoy, J.Y., and Beck, A. (2001). A novel bipolar mode of attachment to aluminium-containing adjuvants by BBG2Na, a recombinant subunit hRSV vaccine. *Vaccine* 19, 4143–4152.

Davenport, F.M., Hennessy, A.V., and Askin, F.B. (1968). Lack of adjuvant effect of $AlPO_4$ on purified influenza virus hemagglutinins in man. *J. Immunol.* 100, 1139–1140.

Dillon, S.B., Demuth, S.G., Schneider, M.A., Weston, C.B., Jones, C.S., Young, J.F., Scott, M; Bhatnaghar, P.K., LoCastro, S., and Hanna, N. (1992). Induction of protective class I MHC-restricted CTL in mice by a recombinant influenza vaccine in aluminium hydroxide adjuvant. *Vaccine* 10, 309–318.

Edelman, R. (1980). Vaccine adjuvants. *Rev. Infect. Dis.* 2, 370–383.

Ericsson, H. (1946). Purification and adsorption of diphtheria toxoid. *Nature* 158, 350–351.

European Pharmacopoeia (1997). Vaccines for human use. 3rd edn, p. 1697.

Flarend, R.E., Hem, S.L., White, J.L., Elmore, D., Suckow, M.A., Rudy, A.C., and Dandashli, E.A. (1997). *In vivo* absorption of aluminium containing vaccines using ^{26}Al. *Vaccine* 15, 1314–1318.

Flebbe, L.M. and Braley-Mullen, H. (1986). Immunopotentiating effects of the adjuvants SGP and Quil-A: I. Antibody responses to T-dependent and T-independent antigens. *Cell. Immunol.* 99, 119–127.

Francis, M.J., Fry, C.M., Rowlands, D.J., Brown, F., Bittle, J.L., Houghten, R.A., and Lerner, R.A. (1985). Immunological priming with synthetic peptides of foot-and-mouth disease virus. *J. Gen. Virol.* 66, 2347–2354.

Francis, M.J., Fry, C.M., Rowlands, D.J., Bittle, J.L., Houghten, R.A., Lerner, R.A., and Brown, F. (1987). Immune response to uncoupled peptides of foot-and-mouth disease virus. *Immunology* 61, 1–6.

Frost, L., Johansen, P., Pedersen, S., Veien, N., østergaard, P., and Nielsen M. (1985). Persistent subcutaneous nodules in children hyposensitized with aluminium-containing allergen extracts. *Allergy* 40, 368–372.

Gamble, H.R., Murrell, K.D., and Marti, H.P. (1986). Inoculation of pigs against *Trichinella spiralis* using larval excretory-secretory antigens. *Am. J. Vet. Res.* 47, 2396–2399.

Geerligs, H.J., Weijer, W.J., Welling, G.W., and Welling-Wester, S. (1989). The influence of different adjuvants on the immune response to a synthetic peptide comprising amino acid residues 9–21 of herpes simplex virus type 1. *J. Immunol. Meth.* 124, 95–102.

Glenny, A.T., Pope, C.G., Waddington, H., and Wallace, U. (1926). Immunological notes XVII to XXIV. *J. Pathol.* 29, 31–40.

Glenny, A.T., Buttle, G.A.H., and Stevens, M.F. (1931). Rate of disappearance of diphtheria toxoid injected into rabbits and guinea-pigs: toxoid precipitated with alum. *J. Pathol.* 34, 267–275.

Goldenthal, K.L., Cavagnaro, J.A., Alving, C., and Vogel, F.R. (1993). Safety evaluation of vaccine adjuvants. NCVDG Working Groups. *AIDS Res. Hum. Retroviruses* 9 (Suppl. 1), s47–s51.

Goto, N., Kato, H., Maeyama, J.-I., Shibano, M., Saito, T., Yamaguchi, J., and Yoshihara, S. (1997). Local tissue irritating effects and adjuvant activities of calcium phosphate and aluminium hydroxide with different physical properties. *Vaccine* 15 1364–1371.

Grun, J.L. and Maurer, P.H. (1989). Different T helper cell subsets elicited in mice utilizing two different adjuvant vehicles. The role of endogenous interleukin-l in proliferative responses. *Cell. Immunol.* 121, 134–145.

Gupta, R.K., Relyveld, E.H., Lindblad, E.B., Bizzini, B., Ben-Efraim S., and Gupta, C.K. (1993). Adjuvants: a balance between toxicity and adjuvanticity. *Vaccine* 11, 293–306.

Gupta, R.K., Rost, B.E., Relyveld, E., and Siber, G.R. (1995). Adjuvant properties of aluminum and calcium compounds. In: Powell, M.F. and Newman, M.J. (Eds) *Vaccine Design: The Subunit and Adjuvant Approach*. Plenum Press, New York.

Hamaoka, T., Katz, D.H., Bloch, K.J., and Benacerraf, B. (1973). Hapten-specific IgE antibody responses in mice: I. Secondary IgE response in irradiated recipients of syngeneic primed spleen cells. *J. Exp. Med.* 138, 306–311.

Hem, S.L. and White, J.L. (1984). Characterization of aluminium hydroxide for use as an adjuvant in parenteral vaccines. *J. Parent. Sci. Technol.* 38, 2–11.

Holt, L.B. (1947). Purified precipitated diphtheria toxoid of constant composition. *Lancet* i, 282–285.

Holt, L.B. (1950). *Developments in Diphtheria Prophylaxis*, Heinemann, London.

Horowitz, S., Smolarsky, M., and Arnon, R. (1982). Protection against *Schistosoma mansoni* achieved by immunization with sonicated parasite. *Eur. J. Immunol.* 12, 327–332.

Hyslop, N.St.G. and Morrow, A.W. (1969). The influence of aluminium hydroxide content, dose volume and the inclusion of saponin on the efficacy of inactivated foot-and-mouth disease vaccines. *Res. Vet. Sci.* 10, 109–120.

Iyer, S., HogenEsch, H., and Hem, S.L. (2003). Effect of the degree of phosphate substitution in aluminium hydroxide adjuvant on the adsorption of phosphorylated proteins. *Pharm. Dev. Tech.* 8, 81–86.

Iyer, S., Robinett, R.S.R., HogenEsch, H., and Hem, S.L. (2004). Mechanism of adsorption of hepatitis B surface antigen by aluminium hydroxide adjuvant. *Vaccine* 22, 1475–1479.

Jankovic, D., Caspar, P., Zweig, M., Garcia-Moll, M., Showalter, S.D., Vogel, F.R., and Sher, A. (1999). Adsorption to aluminium hydroxide promotes the activity of IL-12 as an adjuvant for antibody as well as type 1 cytokine responses to HIV-1 gp 120. *J. Immunol.* 163, 4481–4488.

Jiang, D., Premachandra, G.S., Johnston, C., and Hem, S.L. (2004). Structure and adsorption properties of commercial calcium phosphate adjuvant. *Vaccine* 23, 693–698.

Johnston, C.F., Wang, S.-L., and Hem, S.L. (2002). Measuring the surface area of aluminium hydroxide adjuvant. *J. Pharm. Sci.* 91, 1702–1706.

Katz, J.B., Hanson, S.K., Patterson, P.A., and Stoll, I.R. (1989). In vitro assessment of viral antigen content in inactivated aluminium hydroxide adjuvanted vaccines. *J. Virol. Methods* 25, 101–108.

Kenney, J.S., Hughes, B.W., Masada, M.P., and Allison, A.C. (1989). Influence of adjuvants on the quantity, affinity, isotype and epitope specificity of murine antibodies. *J. Immunol. Meth.* 121, 157–166.

Knopf, P.M., Goldberg, M., Grossi, C.A., Cappello, M., and Coulter, S.T. (1988). Induction of resistance to *Schistosoma mansoni* by immunization with subfractions of worms. *Am. J. Trop. Med. Hyg.* 38, 515–528.

Krieg, A.M. (2002). CpG motifs in bacterial DNA and their immune effects. *Annu. Rev. Immunol.* 20, 709–760.

Kwissa, M., Lindblad, E.B., Schirmbeck, R., and Reimann, J. (2003). Co-delivery of a DNA vaccine and a protein vaccine with aluminium phosphate stimulates a potent and multivalent immune response. *J. Mol. Med.* 81, 502–510.

Leland, S.E., Sofield, W.L., and Minocha, H.C. (1988). Immunogenic effects of culture-derived exoantigens of *Cooperia punctata* on calves before and after challenge exposure with infective larvae. *Am. J. Vet. Res.* 49, 366–379.

Lew, A.M., Anders, R.F., Edwards, S.J., and Langford, C.J. (1988). Comparison of antibody avidity and titre elicited by peptide as a protein conjugate or as expressed in vaccinia. *Immunology* 65, 311–314.

Lindblad, E.B. (1995). Aluminium adjuvants. In Stewart-Tull (Ed) *The Theory and Practical Application of Adjuvants.* John Wiley, New York, pp. 21–35.

Lindblad, E.B. (2004). Aluminium compounds for use in vaccines. *Immunol. Cell Biol.* 82, 497–505.

Lindblad, E.B., Elhay, M.J., Silva, R., Appelberg, R., and Andersen, P. (1997). Adjuvant modulation of immune responses to tuberculosis subunit vaccines. *Infect. Immun.* 65, 623–629.

Mannhalter, J.W., Neychev, H.O., Zlabinger, G.J., Ahmad, R., and Eibl, M.M. (1985). Modulation of the human immune response by the non-toxic and non-pyrogenic adjuvant aluminium hydroxide: effect on antigen uptake and antigen presentation. *Clin. Exp. Immunol.* 61, 143–151.

Martyn, C.N., Barker, D.J.P., Osmond, C., Harris, E.C., Edwardson, J.A., and Lacey, R.F. (1989). Geographical relation between Alzheimer's disease and aluminium in drinking water. *Lancet* 1, 59–62.

Maschmann, E., Küster, E., and Fischer, W. (1931). Über die Fähigkeit des Tonerde-Präparates B, Diphtherie-Toxin zu adsorbieren. *Ber. Dtsch. Chem. Ges.* 64, 2174–2178.

McCandlish, I.A.P., Thompson, H., and Wright, N.G. (1978). Vaccination against canine bordetellosis using an aluminium hydroxide adjuvant vaccine. *Res. Vet. Sci.* 25, 51–57.

McDougall, J.S. (1969). Avian infectious bronchitis: the protection afforded by an inactivated virus vaccine. *Vet. Rec.* 85, 378–380.

Monroy, F.G., Adams, J.H., Dobson, C., and Bast, I.J. (1989). *Nematospiroides dubius*: influence of adjuvants on immunity in mice vaccinated with antigens isolated by affinity chromatography from adult worms. *Exp. Parasitol.* 68, 67–73.

Nagy, L.K. and Penn, C.W. (1974). Protective antigens in bovine pasteurellosis. *Dev. Biol. Stand.* 26, 65–76.

Naim, J.O., van Oss, C.J., Wu, W., Giese, R.F., and Nickerson, P.A. (1997). Mechanisms of adjuvancy: I. Metal oxides as adjuvants. *Vaccine* 15, 1183–1193.

Norimatsu, M., Ogikubo,Y., Aoki, A., Takahashi,T., Watanabe, G., Taya, K., Sasamoto, S., Tsuchiya, M., and Tamura, Y. (1995). Effects of aluminium adjuvant on systemic reactions of lipopolysaccharides in swine. *Vaccine* 13, 1325–1329.

Pini, A., Danskin, D., and Coackley, W. (1965). Comparative evaluation of the potency of beta-propiolactone inactivated Newcastle disease vaccines prepared from a lentogenic and a velogenic strain. *Vet. Rec.* 77, 127–129.

Pollock, K.G.J., Conacher, M., Wei, X.-Q., Alexander, J., and Brewer, J.M. (2003). Interleukin-18 plays a role in both the alum-induced T helper 2 response and the T helper 1 response induced by alum-adsorbed interleukin-12. *Immunology* 108, 137–143.

Relyveld, E.H. (1986). Preparation and use of calcium phosphate adsorbed vaccines. *Develop. Boil. Stand.* (S. Karger, Basel), 65, 131–136.

Relyveld, E.H. and Chermann, J.C. (1994). Humoral response in rabbits immunized with calcium phosphate adjuvanted HIV-1 gp160 antigen. *Biomed. Pharmacother.* 48, 79–83.

Relyveld, E.H., Ickovic, M.-R., Henocq, E., and Garcelon, M. (1985). Calcium phosphate adjuvanted allergens. *Ann. Allergy* 54, 521–529.

Rimaniol, A.-C., Gras, G., Verdier, F., Capel, F., Grigoriev, V.B., Porcheray, F., Sauzeat, E., Fournier, J.-G., Clayette, P., Siegrist, C.-A., and Dormont, D. (2004). Aluminium hydroxide adjuvant induces macrophage differentiation towards a specialized antigen-presenting cell type. *Vaccine* 22, 3127–3135.

Rinella, J.V., White, J.L., and Hem, S.L. (1995). Effect of anions on model aluminium-adjuvant-containing vaccines. *J. Colloid Interf. Sci.* 172, 121–130.

Rinella, J.V., Workman, R.F., Hermodson, M.A., White, J.L., and Hem, S.L. (1998a). Elutability of proteins from aluminium-containing vaccine adjuvants by treatment with surfactants. *J. Colloid Interf. Sci.*, 197, 48–56.

Rinella, J.V., White, J.L., and Hem, S.L. (1998b). Effect of pH on the elution of model antigens from aluminium-containing adjuvants. *J. Colloid Interf. Sci.* 205, 161–165.

Ris, D.R. and Hamel, K.L. (1979). *Leptospira interrogans* serovar. pomona vaccines with different adjuvants in cattle. *NZ Vet. J.* 27, 169–171.

Sagara, T., Mori, S., Ohkawara, S., Goto, F., Takagi, K., and Yoshinaga, M. (1990). A limited role of IL-1 in immune-enhancement by adjuvants. *Immunology* 71, 251–257.

Seeber, S.J., White, J.L., and Hem, S.L. (1991). Predicting the adsorption of proteins by aluminium-containing adjuvants. *Vaccine* 9, 201–203.

Sellers, R.F. and Herniman, K.A.J. (1974). Early protection of pigs against foot-and-mouth disease. *Br. Vet. J.* 130, 440–445.

Shi, Y., HogenEsch, H., Regnier, F.E., and Hem, S.L. (2001). Detoxification of endotoxin by aluminium hydroxide adjuvant. *Vaccine* 19, 1747–1752.

Shirodkar, S., Hutchinson, R.L., Perry, D.L., White, J.L., and Hem, S.L. (1990). Aluminium compounds used as adjuvants in vaccines. *Pharm. Res.* 7, 1282–1288.

Smith, P.K., Krohn, R.I., Hermanson, G.T., Gartner, F.H., Provenzano, M.D., Fujimoto, E.K., Goeke, N.M., Olson, B.J., and Klenk, D.C. (1985). Measurement of protein using bicinchoninic acid. *Anal. Biochem.* 150, 76–85.

Sun, H., Pollock, K.G.J., and Brewer, J.M. (2003). Analysis of the role of vaccine adjuvants in modulating dendritic cell activation and antigen presentation in vitro. *Vaccine* 21, 849–855.

Tanzer, M., Gollish, J., Leighton, R., Orrell, K., Giacchino, A., Wells, P., Shea, B., and Wells, G. (2004). The effect of adjuvant calcium phosphate coating on a porous-coated femoral stem. *Clin. Orthop.* July, 153–160.

Thiele, G.M., Rogers, J., Collins, M., Yasuda, N., Smith, D., and McDonald, T.L. (1990). An enzyme-linked immunosorbent assay for the detection of antitetanus toxoid antibody using aluminium-adsorbed coating antigen. *J. Clin. Lab. Anal.* 4, 126–129.

Thorley, C.M. and Egerton, J.R. (1981). Comparison of alum-adsorbed or non-alum-adsorbed oil emulsion vaccines containing, either pilate or non-pilate *Bacteroides nodosus* cells in inducing and maintaining resistance of sheep to experimental foot rot. *Res. Vet. Sci.* 30, 32–37.

Uede, T. and Ishizaka, K. (1982). Formation of IgE binding factors by rat T lymphocytes: VI. Cellular mechanisms for the formation of IgE-potentiating factor and IgE-suppressive factor by antigenic stimulation of antigen primed spleen cells. *J. Immunol.* 129, 1391–1397.

Uede, T., Huff, T.F., and Ishizaka, K. (1982). Formation of IgE binding factors by rat T lymphocytes: V. Effect of adjuvant for the priming immunization on the nature of IgE binding factors formed by antigenic stimulation. *J. Immunol.* 129, 1384–1390.

Ulmer, J.B., DeWitt, C.M., Chastain, M., Friedman, A., Donelly, J.J., McClements, W.L., Caulfield, M.J., Bohannon, K.E., Volkin, D.B., and Evans, R.K. (2000). Enhancement of DNA vaccine potency using conventional aluminum adjuvants. *Vaccine* 18, 18–28.

Vassilev, T.L. (1978). Aluminium phosphate but not calcium phosphate stimulates the specific IgE response in guinea pigs to tetanus toxoid. *Allergy* 33, 155–159.

Verdier, F., Burnett, R., Michelet-Habchi, C., Moretto, P., Fievet-Groyne, F., and Sauzeat, E. (2005). Aluminium assay and evaluation of the local reaction at several time points after intramuscular administration of aluminium containing vaccines in the Cynomolgus monkey. *Vaccine* 23, 1359–1367.

Volk, V.K. and Bunney, W.E. (1942). Diphtheria immunization with fluid toxoid and alum-precipitated toxoid. *Am. J. Public Health* 32, 690–699.

Walls, R.S. (1977). Eosinophil response to alum adjuvants: involvement of T cells in non-antigen-dependent mechanisms. *Proc. Soc. Exp. Biol. Med.* 156, 431–435.

Weeke, B., Weeke, E., and Løwenstein, H. (1975). The adsorption of serum proteins to aluminium hydroxide gel examined by means of quantitative immunoelectrophoresis. In Axelsen, N.H. (Ed) *Quantitative Immuno-electrophoresis. New Developments and Applications.* Universitetsforlaget, pp. 149–154.

Wilson, J.H.G., Hermann-Dekkers, W.M., Leemans-Dessy, S., and de Meijer, J.W. (1977). Experiments with an inactivated hepatitis leptospirosis vaccine in vaccination programmes for dogs. *Vet. Rec.* 100, 552–554.

Willstätter, R. and Kraut, H. (1923). Über ein Tonerde-Gel von der Formel Al (OH)$_3$: II. Mitteilung über Hydrate und Hydrogele. *Ber. Dtsch. Chem. Ges.* 56, 1117–1121.

Willstätter, R. and Kraut, H. (1924). Über die Hydroxide und ihre Hydrate in den verschiedenen Tonerde-Gelen: V. Mitteilung über Hydrate und Hydrogele. *Ber. Dtsch. Chem. Ges.* 57, 1082–1091.

World Health Organization (1976). Immunological adjuvants. Technical Report Series 595, Geneva.

Wu, P.P., Feldkamp, J.R., White, J.L., and Hem, S.L. (1986). Effect of surface charge of carbonate-containing aluminium hydroxide on particle interactions in aqueous suspensions. *J. Colloid Interf. Sci.* 110, 601–603.

Mucosal adjuvants based on cholera toxin and *E. coli* heat-labile enterotoxin

Jan Holmgren, Ali M. Harandi, Michael Lebens, Jia-Bin Sun
Göteborg University, Göteborg, Sweden

Fabienne Anjuère and Cecil Czerkinsky
INSERM Unit 720, Nice, France

Introduction

The mucosal immune system consists of an integrated network of lymphoid cells that work in concert with innate host factors to promote host defense. The mucous membranes covering the respiratory, gastrointestinal, and urogenital tracts as well as the eye conjunctiva, the inner ear, and the ducts of all exocrine glands are endowed with powerful mechanical and chemical cleansing mechanisms that degrade and repel most foreign matters. The mucosal organs also contain a number of other cells of the innate immune system, including phagocytic neutrophils and macrophages, dendritic cells, natural killer cells, and mast cells. Through a variety of mechanisms these cells are essential in the immune defense against pathogens and are also pivotal for initiating adaptive mucosal immune responses. In addition, a large and highly specialized innate and adaptive mucosal immune system protects these surfaces and thereby also the body interior against potential insults from the environment. In a healthy human adult, this local immune system contributes almost 80% of all immunocytes.

There is currently a great interest in developing mucosal vaccines against a variety of microbial pathogens. The main protective mechanism then usually is the generation of a local secretory immune response with secretory IgA (SIgA) antibodies as the primary effector molecules, but additional humoral and cell-mediated mucosal protective mechanisms have also been identified (for a recent review see Holmgren and Czerkinsky, 2005).

Less well appreciated, mucosally induced tolerance also appears to be a promising form of immunomodulation for treating certain autoimmune diseases and allergies (Figure 14.1). The aim is then to induce a state of peripheral immunological tolerance against antigens being the targets for these harmful immune reactions by administering the same or related (bystander) antigens through a mucosal,

Possible outcomes of mucosal immunization:
Protective immunity and/or "oral tolerance"

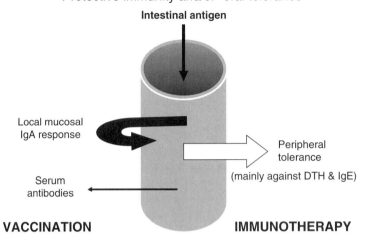

Figure 14.1 Mucosal immunization. This may lead to either or both of a protective mucosal immune response (with secretory IgA as the main protective antibody) and/or to "oral tolerance" resulting in peripheral, mainly regulatory T cell-mediated, suppression of systemic immune responses to the mucosally administered antigen with potential applicability for immunotherapy against allergic and autoimmune diseases and against chronic infection-associated inflammation.

usually oral route (so-called "oral tolerance"). The mechanisms involved in oral tolerance induction and effects are complex and not fully defined, but a main mechanism involves the generation of suppressor-regulatory T cells (Wu and Weiner, 2003; Holmgren and Czerkinsky, 2005).

A few mucosal vaccines have recently become available and shown to work well despite a lack of any specific adjuvants. However, it has become increasingly appreciated that the development of a broader range of mucosal vaccines, whether for prevention of infectious diseases or for oral tolerance immunotherapy, will require access to efficient antigen delivery and adjuvant systems that can help to present the appropriate antigens to the mucosal immune system and stimulate the desired type of response. The most potent and best-studied mucosal adjuvants are cholera toxin (CT) and the closely related *Escherichia coli* heat-labile enterotoxin (LT). However, since these proteins are clearly too toxic to be considered for human use, intense efforts have been made recently to generate partly or wholly detoxified derivatives of these toxins

with retained adjuvant activity. Here we briefly review and discuss these advances, including the potential for using even unattenuated CT or LT as adjuvants for *ex vivo* dendritic cell (DC) vaccination purposes. We also summarize the very promising results achieved when using the nontoxic B subunit components of these toxins (CTB or LTB) as combined carrier and adjuvant systems for inducing "oral tolerance" protection against harmful immune responses to self-antigens and some allergens.

The need for mucosal vaccines and adjuvants

The primary reason for using a mucosal route of vaccination is that most infections affect or start from a mucosal surface, and that in these infections topical application of a vaccine is often required to induce a protective immune response. Examples include (i) gastrointestinal infections such as those caused by *Helicobacter pylori*, *Vibrio cholerae*, enterotoxigenic *Escherichia coli* (ETEC), campylobacter, *Clostridium difficile*, rotaviruses, and calici viruses; (ii) respiratory infections caused, for example, by *Mycoplasma pneumoniae*, influenza virus, and respiratory syncytial virus; and (iii) sexually transmitted genital infections caused by, for example, HIV, chlamydia, *Neisseria gonorrhoeae*, and herpes simplex virus (HSV). Taken together, these infections represent an enormous challenge for development of vaccines targeted to induce immunity that can either prevent the infectious agent from attaching and colonizing at the mucosal epithelium (noninvasive bacteria) or from penetrating and replicating in the mucosa (viruses and invasive bacteria), and/or that can block microbial toxins from binding to and affecting epithelial and other target cells. Compared to parenteral vaccines, mucosal vaccines would also be easier and safer to administer, carry less risk of transmitting infections, and could also simplify vaccine manufacturing, thereby increasing the potential for local vaccine production in developing countries.

As mentioned, although much less well recognized than mucosal vaccination against infection, mucosal immunization could also be used to induce peripheral tolerance. This phenomenon, often referred to as "oral tolerance" because it was initially documented by the effect of oral administration of antigen, is characterized by the fact that an individual who has ingested or inhaled an antigen may become refractory or have diminished capability to develop an immune response when reexposed to the same antigen introduced by a parenteral route. Oral tolerance is an important physiological mechanism to avoid development of T cell-mediated delayed-type hypersensitivity and other allergic reactions to ingested food proteins and other antigens, in case these antigens would reach the body interior in an undegraded form. Oral tolerance, at variance with many other forms of immunotherapy, is specific for the antigen initially ingested or inhaled and does not influence the development of systemic immune responses against other antigens. As a result the induction of oral tolerance has become an attractive strategy for prevention and potential treatment of illnesses that are caused by immunopathological reactions against specific antigens that may be encountered or expressed in preferentially nonmucosal tissues including both foreign antigens and autoantigens (Wu and Weiner, 2003).

However, despite the many attractive features of mucosal immunization it has often proved difficult in practice to stimulate strong mucosal IgA immune responses and protection by oral-mucosal administration of antigens. In general, the results to date of mucosal vaccination efforts using soluble protein antigens have, with a few notable exceptions, been rather disappointing. Indeed, only half a dozen of the vaccines that are currently approved for human use are administered mucosally. These are the oral polio vaccine, two types of oral vaccines against cholera (composed of either killed whole-cell cholera vibrios plus cholera toxin B subunit or of a live-attenuated cholera vaccine strain), an oral live-attenuated typhoid vaccine, an oral live-attenuated rotavirus vaccine, an oral adenovirus vaccine (restricted to military personnel), an oral BCG strain licensed in Brazil for vaccination against tuberculosis, and since a few years ago also an intranasal cold-adapted live-attenuated influenza vaccine. Likewise, in the area of oral tolerance, although promising results were obtained in initial clinical trials that used this principle for immunotherapy of autoimmune diseases, such as multiple sclerosis and rheumatoid arthritis, larger randomized placebo-controlled multicenter trials failed to show any significant therapeutic benefits of these agents over those achieved by the placebo (Wu and Weiner, 2003; Chaillous et al., 2000; Wiendl and Hohlfeld, 2003; Postlethwaite, 2001). More uniformly promising results, however, are at hand when mucosal immunization, mainly by the sublingual-oral route, has been used as a means for inducing "hyposensitization" and thus suppressing allergic responses against specific allergens causing rhinitis and/or asthma (Di Rienzo et al., 2003; Mastrandrea, 2004; Holmgren and Czerkinsky, 2005; Wilson et al., 2005).

To overcome the obstacles to the development of a broader range of mucosal vaccines and mucosal immunotherapies, and being the subject for this chapter, there is a need to find more efficient means of delivering the appropriate antigens to the mucosal immune system, and/or to develop effective, safe mucosal adjuvants or immunoregulatory agents that, depending on the goal and the systems used, will provide protective immunity against infectious agents or induce suppression of peripheral immunopathological disorders. Ideally, such systems should (i) protect the vaccine from physical elimination and enzymatic digestion, (ii) target mucosal inductive sites including M cells, and (iii) at least for vaccines against infections, appropriately stimulate the innate immune system to generate effective adaptive immunity.

Cholera toxin and *E. coli* heat-labile enterotoxin as mucosal immunogens and adjuvants

Some but not all types of *Vibrio cholerae* bacteria produce CT, the enterotoxin that is responsible for the severe, life-threatening diarrhea in cholera disease. CT is mainly produced by *V. cholerae* belonging to serogroup O1, that comprises the Inaba and Ogawa serotypes and the classic and El Tor biotypes. Until recently the O1 serogroup was regarded to be the only of 138 recognized *V. cholerae* O groups that could cause cholera epidemics (for a recent review see Sack et al., 2004). Since 1993, however, a new *V. cholerae* serogroup, O139, which is a mutated variant of an O1 El Tor strain, has also been found to cause outbreaks of cholera and to produce similar amounts of CT as *V. cholerae* O1 bacteria (Sack et al., 2004). CT production has also been demonstrated from a related vibrio species, *V. mimicus* (Dotevall et al., 1986).

The CT molecule was together with diphtheria toxin the first bacterial toxin that was well characterized with regard to its molecular structure and function (Holmgren, 1981). CT is an AB_5 toxin which consists of a monomeric toxic-active A subunit (CTA) and of a B subunit (CTB) composed of five identical subunits (Figure 14.2). Through its CTB component, CT binds specifically and pentavalently to

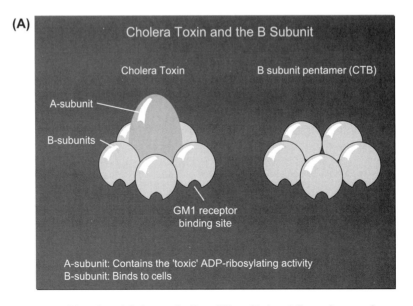

Figure 14.2 Subunit structure and function of cholera toxin (A and B) and industrially used system for recombinant production of the cholera toxin B subunit (C).

(B) Cholera Toxin

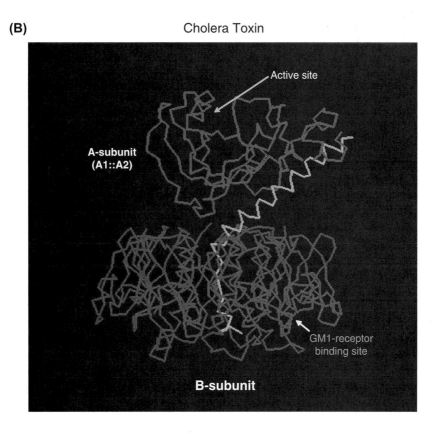

(C) **Large scale recombinant production of cholera B subunit for vaccine use**

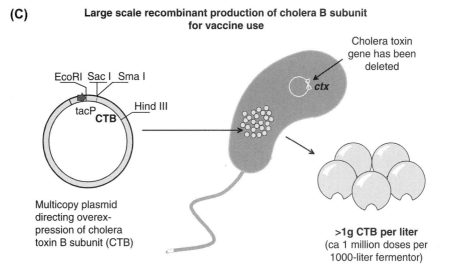

Figure 14.2 Continued. (See Color Plate Section for Figure 14.2B.)

cellular receptors, identified as the GM1 ganglioside, expressed on intestinal epithelial (and most other) cells which enables the entry of the toxin into the cell. Following the internalization and intracellular transport of toxin through a recently well "mapped" pathway through endosomes, the Golgi system, and endoplasmic reticulum (Lencer and Tsai, 2003), the A subunit is activated by proteolytic cleavage of the peptide loop linking the enzymatically active A1 domain from the CTB-associating A2 domain. A1 is then translocated into the cytoplasm where it associates with the Gs protein of adenylate cyclase at the inside of the plasma membrane, binds NAD, and transfers an ADP-ribose group ("ADP-ribosylates") onto Gs leading to increased cyclic AMP production in the affected cells (Holmgren, 1981; Lencer and Tsai, 2003; de Haan and Hirst, 2003).

LT, being produced by different strains of ETEC, has an analogous AB_5 structure and shares about 80% homology with CT (de Haan and Hirst, 2003). LT from human ETEC strains differs in a few residues from LT from porcine ETEC isolates. Both human and porcine LT bind with similar affinity as CT to GM1 gangliodside, but different from CT, LT can also bind to some other structurally related receptors comprising both glycoproteins and complex glycolipids (Holmgren et al., 1982; Bäckström et al., 1997). The immunological and adjuvant properties also appear to be very similar, if not identical, between CT and LT. While most studies to date have been undertaken with CT the findings will be assumed to also hold true for LT, and vice versa, unless there is specific evidence to the contrary, which there is in a few specific regards (to be discussed).

Both CT and LT are exceptionally potent oral-mucosal immunogens. This property can be explained by three characteristic features of the molecules: (i) consistent with their functions as enterotoxins, CT and LT are remarkably stable to proteases, bile salts, and other compounds in the intestine; (ii) as mentioned, both CT and LT bind with high affinity to GM1 ganglioside receptors, which are present not only on the villous and crypt enterocytes but also on Peyer's patch M cells as well as on all known antigen-presenting cells (APCs) present within Peyer's patches, the intestinal mucosa and draining mesentesic lymph nodes; this facilitates efficient uptake and presentation of the toxins to the gut mucosal immune system; and (iii) CT and LT have strong inherent adjuvant and immuno-modulating activities as discussed below.

The toxicity of CT has precluded its use for human vaccination. Instead, nontoxic CTB has been extensively used as a mucosal immunogen in humans without any side effects. Indeed, recombinantly produced CTB (Figure 14.2C) is an important component of an oral cholera vaccine for human use (Dukoral®, SBL Vaccin, Sweden). In addition to CTB, this vaccine also contains inactivated whole-cell cholera vibrios and is now being registered in more than 50 countries worldwide (Holmgren and Bergquist, 2004). This vaccine has proved to be very safe and efficiently immunogenic in both adults and children. Thus, when given in 2 or 3 oral doses, the oral cholera vaccine has been found to stimulate the same levels of intestinal IgA antitoxin and anti-bacterial (mainly anti-lipopolysaccharide) anti-bodies as seen in convalescents from severe clinical cholera disease and also to induce very long-lasting (more than 5 years) immunologic memory in the intestinal mucosa (Svennerholm et al., 1984). A high protective efficacy of the vaccine has also been demonstrated, being 80–90% for the first 6 months after vaccination in both endemic and non-endemic populations, and remaining at or above 60% for at least 2 more years in vaccinated adults and children above an age of 5 years. In children below age 5, the short-term efficacy, which is significantly attributed to antitoxic immunity, is very high (100% for the first 6 months when tested in a field trial in Bangladesh), but wanes more rapidly than in older children and adults (Clemens et al., 1986, 1990). The vaccine has also recently proved to be safe and effective (80–90% protection) when used as a public health intervention tool in Mozambique in a population with a high frequency of HIV-infected individuals (Lucas et al., 2005). Because of the close immunological relationship between the CTB component of the oral cholera vaccine and the B subunit part of the LT that is being produced by many strains of *E. coli* causing cholera-like diarrheal disease (ETEC diarrhea), the CTB whole-cell cholera vaccine also offers 60–80% short-term protection against ETEC diarrhea (Clemens et al., 1988b; Holmgren and Bergquist, 2004), and the cholera vaccine has also been found to reduce substantially overall diarrhea morbidity in areas where cholera and ETEC diarrheas are common (Clemens et al., 1988a).

Based on its excellent safety and immunogenicity in humans when given by the oral route, CTB has also been used for studies of mucosal immune responses in humans after other routes of immunization. Indeed, much of our current knowledge of the localization of the mucosal immune responses after different routes of immunization and of the links between mucosal inductive and expression sites in humans have emerged from studies in volunteers using CTB as immunogen (reviewed in Holmgren and Czerkinsky, 2005).

Besides being strong mucosal immunogens, both CT and LT are powerful mucosal adjuvants. They strongly potentiate the immunogenicity of most other antigens, whether these are linked to or simply admixed with the toxins, provided that the other antigen is given at the same time and at the same mucosal surface as the toxins (Lycke and Holmgren, 1986). CT/LT can affect several steps in the induction of a mucosal immune response, which alone or in combination might explain their strong adjuvant action after oral immunization (Holmgren et al., 1993; Lycke, 1997; Plant and Williams, 2004). Thus, CT/LT has been found to (i) induce increased permeability of the intestinal epithelium leading to enhanced uptake of coadministered antigen; (ii) recruit immature DCs in the intestinal epithelium and promote their emigration and differentiation in draining MLNs; (iii) induce enhanced antigen presentation by various APCs; (iv) promote isotype differentiation in B cells leading to increased IgA formation; and (v) exert complex stimulatory as well as inhibitory effects on T cell proliferation and cytokine production. In addition, both CT and LT have been shown to not only avoid to induce oral tolerance but also to abrogate otherwise efficient regimens for tolerance induction by oral antigen administration (Elson and Ealding, 1984).

Among these many effects, those leading to enhanced antigen presentation by various APCs are probably of the greatest importance for the adjuvant activity. CT/LT markedly increases antigen presentation by dendritic cells, macrophages, and B cells (George-Chandy et al., 2001) and has also been found, at least *in vitro*, to stimulate intestinal epithelial cells to become effective APCs. Consistent with this activity, CT/LT upregulates the expression of MHC/HLA-DR molecules, CD80/B7.1 and CD86/B7.2 costimulatory molecules, as well as chemokine receptors such as CCR7 and CXCR4 on both murine and human dendritic cells and other APCs (George-Chandy et al., 2001; Gagliardi et al., 2002; Eriksson et al., 2003). Importantly, CT/LT also induces the secretion of interleukin (IL)-1β from dendritic cells (Lycke and Holmgren, 1986) thus supporting similar observations made earlier for macrophages. IL-1 not only induces the maturation of dendritic cells, but is also by itself an efficient mucosal adjuvant when coadministered with protein antigens and might mediate a significant part of the adjuvant activity of CT (George–Chandy et al., 2001).

Importantly, in a recent study we could further show that feeding mice with CT induced a rapid and transient mobilization of a new CD11c$^+$CD8$^-$ DC subset near the intestinal epithelium (Anjuère et al., 2004). This recruitment was associated with an increased production of the chemokine CCL20/MIP-3α in the small intestine and was followed by a massive accumulation of a more mature type of DCs (CD8^{int}) in MLN. MLN DCs from CT-treated mice were more potent activators of naive T cells than DCs from control mice and induced mainly a Th2 type response *in vitro*. This increase in immunostimulating properties was accounted for by CD8^{int} and CD8$^-$ DCs, where CD8$^+$ DCs remained insensitive to CT treatment. Adoptive transfer experiments showed that these two DC subsets, unlike CD8$^+$ DCs, were able to present antigens orally coadministered with CT in an immunostimulating manner. Consistently, the CD8^{int} and CD8$^-$ subsets expressed higher levels of costimulatory molecules than CD8$^+$ and corresponding conrol DCs, and more specifically orally administered CT upregulated the expression of costimulatory molecules CD40, CD80 and CD86 on CD8^{int} and CD8$^-$ DCs but only CD40 on CD8$^+$ DCs. The ability of CT to mobilize large numbers of immature DCs in the intestinal epithelium, probably as a result of CT-induced production of the CCL20/MIP-3α chemokine by intestinal epithelial cells, and to promote their emigration, maturation and enhanced antigen-presenting capacity in draining lymph nodes could explain much of the exceptional adjuvant activity of this toxin on mucosal immune responses.

It has been suggested mainly based on *in vitro* studies, that CT primarily induces Th2-type immune responses characterized by CD4+ T cells producing IL-4, IL-5, IL-6, and IL-10 and by the production of IgA, IgG1, and IgE antibodies. LT, in contrast, has been reported to induce a mixed Th1- and Th2-type immune response. However, other studies have shown that CT can also induce mixed Th1- and Th2-type immune responses, in contrast to CTB, which appears to induce a more restricted Th2 type of immune response (Eriksson et al., 2003). Thus dendritic cells, which had been pretreated *in vitro* with a protein antigen (ovalbumin, OVA) linked to or admixed with CT and then injected into mice, induced in an antigen-specific manner both Th1 and CTL responses in addition to a Th2 response. In contrast, dendritic cells pulsed *in vitro* with OVA linked to CTB only gave rise

to a Th2 type of immune response (Eriksson et al., 2003).

■ Development of nontoxic derivatives as mucosal adjuvants

To avoid the toxicity problems with whole CT or LT, the isolated or recombinantly produced CTB and LTB proteins have been explored for their ability to augment immune responses against coadministered antigens. However, their capacity as mucosal adjuvants has proved to be much less than that of the holotoxins. Indeed, both CTB and LTB are poor adjuvants when given to animals together with noncoupled antigens by the oral route, although they display a more significant adjuvant activity when administered via the nasal route. Adjuvanticity of CTB or LTB is much improved when coupled to antigens (Figure 14.3), due to the increased uptake of the coupled antigen across the mucosal barrier as well as to the more efficient uptake and presentation of the coupled antigen not only by dendritic cells and macrophages but also by naive B cells (George-Chandy et al., 2001).

Recently, as illustrated in Figure 14.4A, site-directed mutagenesis has permitted the generation of LT and CT mutants that have reduced toxicity, but which retain significant adjuvanticity when given to animals by the nasal-mucosal route or, even though by that route they perform less well, by the oral-mucosal route, even though less effective (Pizza et al., 2001). Two of these, best characterized, proteins are mutants of LT: LTK63 (in which the serine residue in LTA has been replaced by a lysine residue (Di Tommaso et al., 1996) and LTK72 (in which the alanine residue 72 in LTA has been replaced by an arginine) (Giuliano et al., 1998). LTK63 is practically devoid of enzymatic and toxic activity, whereas LTR72 retains some residue enzymatic activity. Both of these mutant proteins behaved as significant mucosal adjuvants for coadministered antigens given intranasally, inducing strong systemic and mucosal antigen-specific antibody responses. LTR72

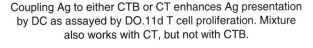

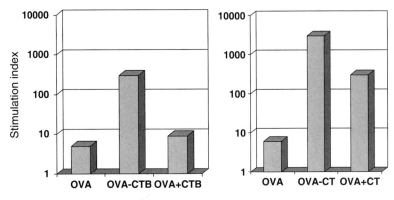

Coupling Ag to either CTB or CT enhances Ag presentation by DC as assayed by DO.11d T cell proliferation. Mixture also works with CT, but not with CTB.

Figure I4.3 Coupling an antigen to cholera toxin B subunit or to cholera toxin enhances uptake and presentation by different antigen-presenting cells including dendritic cells (DC), B cells, and macrophages.

was by far the strongest adjuvant and induced antibody titers to the coadministered antigen, being similar to those induced using the wild-type LT as mutant. Although there has been a report of increased protection against *Helicobacter pylori* infection in mice by intragastric vaccination with *H. pylori* antigens together with LTK63 as adjuvant (Marchetti et al., 1998), it remains to be shown whether a fully nontoxic LT mutant molecule such as LTK63 can serve as a useful adjuvant for increasing the gastrointestinal IgA antibody response to an orally or intragastrically coadministered protein antigen.

Other LT mutants have been generated by substituting amino acid residues in the loop of the A subunit, thus rendering the toxin insensitive to proteases and thereby also not susceptible to the intracellular proteolytic activation which releases the toxic enzymatic A1 subunit to exert its toxic activity (Dickinson and Clements, 1995; Lu et al., 2002). Similar to LTK63 and LTR72 the most extensively studied of this type of mutant proteins (LTR192G) enhances protective humoral and cellular immune responses to intranasally, and reportedly also to orally coadministered antigens. Again, it remains to be established

whether after the oral route there was a significant enhancement in specific gut mucosal IgA responses.

To achieve detoxification of CT, yet another type of mutants was recently described in which peptides are added to the CTA1 amino end (Sanchez et al., 2002). The added peptides seem to reduce both enterotoxicity and ADP-ribosylating activity by sterically blocking the toxic active site within CTA1. In general, in these (like in all other detoxified) constructs, adjuvanticity decreased with decreasing enterotoxicity/ADP-ribosylating activity. However, a mutant (eCT6), with 10- to 20-fold lower enterotoxicity than CT in rabbit intestinal loops, displayed a level of adjuvanticity comparable to that of the wild-type CT. Another mutant with a longer peptide linked to CTA1 (eCT23) and no detectable toxic activity, although being much less potent in adjuvant activity than either CT or eCT6, was superior to CTB as both a mucosal immunogen and as an adjuvant for a coadministered antigen.

A different approach that has been used to circumvent the harmful drawbacks of CT or LT adjuvants is to link the enzymatically active A subunit domain of the toxin to a cell-binding

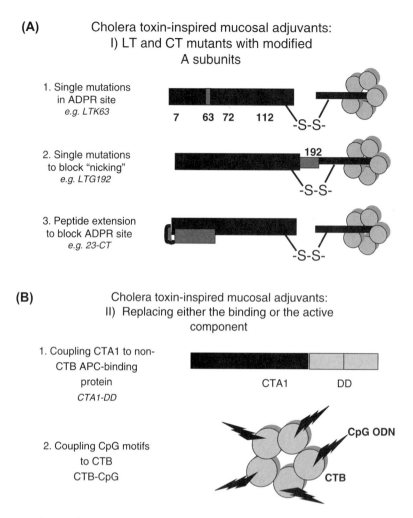

(A)   Cholera toxin-inspired mucosal adjuvants:
                     I) LT and CT mutants with modified
                                A subunits

1. Single mutations
   in ADPR site
   e.g. LTK63

2. Single mutations
   to block "nicking"
   e.g. LTG192

3. Peptide extension
   to block ADPR site
   e.g. 23-CT

(B)   Cholera toxin-inspired mucosal adjuvants:
                     II) Replacing either the binding or the active
                                component

1. Coupling CTA1 to non-
   CTB APC-binding
   protein
   CTA1-DD

2. Coupling CpG motifs
   to CTB
   CTB-CpG

Figure 14.4 Different approaches used to generate mucosal adjuvants by modifications of cholera toxin or *E. coli* heat-labile toxin or their subunits (for further discussion see text).

moiety other than the natural B subunit, such as the cell-binding domain of *Staphylococcus aureus* protein A (CTA1-DD) (Ågren et al., 1999) (Figure 14.4B). CTA1-DD, like most of the above mentioned other toxin derivatives, functions when applied nasally but not when given orally. This limitation has recently been overcome by the incorporation of CTA1-DD fused to a short peptide into immune stimulating complexes (ISCOMS). Oral vaccination with the ISCOM-CTA1-DD complex induced systemic and mucosal responses with both Th1 and Th2 characteristics (Mowat et al., 2001); whether this relatively complicated complex

can be practically produced to also comprise a real vaccine of course remains to be seen.

Recent work from our laboratory has also identified bacterial DNA, or synthetic oligodeoxynucleotides (ODN), containing unmethylated so-called CpG motifs covalently linked to the B subunit of cholera toxin (CTB::CpG) as a particularly promising novel mucosal immunomodulating adjuvant (Figure 14.4B). CpG ODN is known to stimulate cells that express Toll-like receptor 9 thereby initiating an immunomodulating cascade. Although previously mainly considered for systemic use, CpG ODN has been found after different routes of mucosal administration to markedly enhance both innate and adaptive mucosal immunity in animal models (Harandi et al., 2003; Harandi and Holmgren, 2004). Most strikingly, it has recently been shown that the immunostimulatory effect of CpG DNA is significantly enhanced when chemically conjugated to CTB (Harandi and Holmgren, 2004; Adamsson et al., to be published). When the effect on murine splenocytes was compared, the CpG ODN coupled to CTB induced much stronger chemokine responses than achieved with CpG ODN alone, and when tested on human white blood cells even more pronounced differences were found. Thus, while *in vitro* treatment of human peripheral blood mononuclear cells with an optimal human CpG ODN did not give rise to any appreciable levels of CC chemokine responses, CpG ODN coupled to CTB elicited strong CC chemokine responses. The corresponding optimal CTB-CpG conjugate when administered intravaginally elicited stronger CC chemokine responses in the murine female genital tract mucosa compared with those of CpG ODN. The mechanism(s) for the increased immunostimulatory property of CTB::CpG conjugate remains to be defined, but may be due both to an increased CTB-mediated uptake of coupled CpG ODN across the mucosal barrier and by target cells and possibly also by a quantitatively or qualitatively changed CTB/GM1-directed intracellular transport of CpG intracellularly (Adamsson et al., to be published).

Some concerns have recently been raised about the use of CT- or LT-derived adjuvants for use in intranasal vaccines (Fujihashi et al., 2002; Couch, 2004). This was based on reports from studies in mice that intranasally administered CT and LT could be localized by immunohistochemical methods in the olfactory bulb of the brain, apparently as a result of retrograde transport via the olfactory nerve (Fujihashi et al., 2002). This observation may or may not be linked to the increased frequency of facial paresis noted after vaccination of humans with an intranasally administered

subunit influenza virus hemagglutinin vaccine that had been adjuvanted with 2 μg of (fully active) LT per dose, leading to the withdrawal of this vaccine from the market after a short time. Such retrograde transport of proteins binding to nerve endings is a long known phenomenon described for various viruses and viral attachment proteins, such as the influenza virus hemagglutinin and it has also been shown for CTB and LTB. This by itself has not been associated with any demonstrable negative consequences for as long as the antigen is not replicating (live viruses) or causing inflammation or edema swelling (as may be the case for CT or LT with retained ADP ribosylating toxic activity). At a specially organized conference to discuss and advise on the safety evaluation of toxin adjuvants delivered intranasally (NIAID Conference, 2001), it was emphasized that special attention and more animal studies should be undertaken to exclude short-term or long-term adverse reactions following intranasal administration of attenuated LT and CT adjuvants. The intranasal use of highly purified CTB or LTB in humans, however, appears to be completely safe, as supported by several clinical studies undertaken with recombinantly produced, highly purified CTB administered intranasally in different doses to human volunteers (de Fijter et al., 1996; Bergquist et al., 1997; Rudin et al., 1998, 1999; Johansson et al., 2001). In the latter studies, intranasal doses of CTB up to 250 μg appear to not give rise to any significant adverse reactions. Intranasal administration of a higher dose, 1000 μg, however, was associated with disturbing local irritation resulting in sneezing, itching, and a tendency to a running nose lasting for up to a few hours in some vaccinees; however, even at this high dose of CTB there was no evidence of any longer-lasting adverse reactions and no suggestion of any effects on olfactory nerve perceptions (smelling). Recently a clinical trial was also undertaken using the LTK63 protein in different doses for adjuvanting the immunogenicity of a coadministered subunit influenza vaccine (Stephenson et al., 2005); no

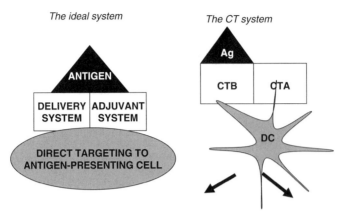

Cholera Toxin and Dendritic Cell Vaccination:
Combining positive elements for maximal immunogenicity

The ideal system

The CT system

Toxicity of CT is avoided by washing DC before reinfusion into host,
which should allow for safe clinical use!

Figure 14.5 Cholera toxin (or *E. coli* LT) to which antigen has been coupled is a powerful and clinically promising vaccine formulation for dendritic cell vaccination aimed at inducing strong B cell, CD4+ T cell, and CD8+ T cell immune responses.

significant adverse reactions were observed and, quite promisingly, there was a significant adjuvanting effect on the IgA antibody responses to the flu vaccine in both serum and nasal secretions after the highest dose (30 µg) of LTK63 adjuvant coadministered.

■ CT and CTB as adjuvants for dendritic cell vaccination

Dendritic cells are professional APCs which act as sentinels throughout the body. Vaccination with autologous monocyte/bone marrow-derived dendritic cells pulsed with an appropriate antigen together with a suitable adjuvant *ex vivo* represents a promising approach to immunotherapeutic vaccination, e.g., in patients with cancer or severe infections. The *ex vivo*-pulsed dendritic cells are autologous and can be washed free of any unprocessed antigen and adjuvant before they are re-infused to the patient. This also makes it a promising prospective to be able to use even such strong (but toxic) adjuvants as unmodified CT or LT for stimulating the dendritic cells to become maximally

immunogenic without risks of causing toxic side effects *in vivo* (Figure 14.5).

Conjugation of antigen to either CT or CTB greatly facilitated MHC class II-restricted antigen presentation by dendritic cells (George–Chandy et al., 2001; Eriksson et al., 2003). This was associated with both an upregulated secretion of IL-1β by the pulsed dendritic cells and increased expression of CD80 and CD86 on the dendritic cell surface. Dendritic cells pulsed with CT- or CTB-conjugated antigen were found to be superior to dendritic cells pulsed with free antigen at inducing CD4+ T cell and B cell responses *in vivo* (Eriksson et al., 2003). However, while CTB-antigen conjugates almost exclusively stimulated immune responses with a Th2-type profile, conjugates based on CT were shown to drive the *in vivo* responses towards a mixed Th1 and Th2 phenotype (Eriksson et al., 2003). Vaccination with dendritic cells pulsed with antigen and CT, but not vaccination with dendritic cells pulsed with the same antigen coupled to CTB or antigen alone, also induced antigen-specific CD8+ T cells that produced interferon (IFN)-β, were cytotoxic for tumor antigen-expressing (E.G7) tumor cells *in vitro*, and were able to infiltrate and eliminate an already established E.G7 tumor *in vivo* (Eriksson et al., 2004; Sun et al., 2004). We propose that the use of CT as a combined carrier/delivery system and adjuvant for dendritic cell vaccination represents a novel attractive strategy for therapeutic antitumor vaccination, at least for tumors that express sufficient amounts of tumor-specific peptide antigens linked to their MHC class I antigens.

■ Mucosal immunotherapy based on cholera toxin B subunit

As mentioned, mucosal tolerance is a mechanism whereby the immune system refrains from responding in a deleterious manner to harmless antigens that are contacted through mucosal surfaces. This permits mammals to coexist with their normal flora and to eat large amounts of foreign food proteins without inducing harmful systemic immune responses. Since induction of mucosal tolerance is antigen specific but can be expressed in a nonspecific manner ("bystander suppression") via the production of suppressive cytokines by regulatory T cells in the inflamed microenvironment of the target organ, this approach has been utilized to suppress immune responses against self antigens. It has been possible to prevent or to delay onset of experimental autoimmune diseases in a variety of animal systems by feeding selected autoantigens or peptide derivatives (reviewed by Wu and Weiner, 2003). In addition to the oral route, virtually all other routes of mucosal administration (nasal, buccal, rectal, genital) are also effective to induce tolerance although to a different degree. The dosage, the route, and frequency of autoantigen administration have proven to be critical for the outcome and to engage different regulatory mechanisms. Thus, whereas low doses of nasally administered antigens favor expansion of regulatory T cells producing IL-10, low doses of orally administered antigen promote activation of CD8+ and/or CD4+ regulatory T cells

producing TGF-β. Large doses of antigens appear to induce anergy of effector CD4+ T cells while massive doses can induce their apoptosis (Wu and Weiner, 2003). While mucosal tolerance is usually effective in animal models for preventing inducible autoimmune diseases, its efficacy has been more variable and limited when utilized as an intervention strategy in animals in which the disease had already been induced or had spontaneously developed. This may explain in part the disappointing results of recent phase III clinical trials of oral tolerance in patients with type I diabetes (Chaillous et al., 2000), multiple sclerosis (Wiendl, 2002), and rheumatoid arthritis (Postlethwaite, 2001), diseases in which there may be multiple target autoantigens that remain largely unknown.

A significant improvement has been achieved by coadministering CTB as an immunomodulating agent to enhance the tolerogenic activity of autoantigens as well as allergens given orally or nasally. The use of antigen coupled to CTB has been found to minimize by several hundred-fold the amount of antigen/tolerogen needed and also to reduce the number of doses that would otherwise be required by reported protocols of orally induced tolerization (Sun et al., 2004). Further, and most important, at divergence from the use of free antigen, CTB-linked antigens have been shown to work also in an already sensitized individual. In experimental systems this has resulted in effective suppression of various pathological immune responses associated with experimental autoimmune diseases (Sun et al., 1996; Bergerot et al., 1997; Arakawa et al., 1998; Tarkowski et al., 1999), type I allergies (Tamura et al., 1997; Rask et al., 2000), and allograft rejection (Ma et al., 1998; Sun et al., 2000) also when the CTB-antigen conjugate was administered as therapy rather than for prevention (Figure 14.6).

The physical coupling of antigen to CTB or LTB appears to be of great importance for tolerance induction by the oral route. This is probably because this facilitates the parallel transport of antigen and adjuvant across the

Cholera toxin B subunit for mucosal immunotherapy:
Use of antigens coupled to CTB has resulted in increased
efficacy compared with use of antigen alone in many
experimental disease systems

- ■ Autoimmune diseases
  - ➤ Type I diabetes;
  - ➤ Multiple sclerosis;
  - ➤ Rheumatoid arthritis
  - ➤ Uveitis (e.g. Behcet´s disease) etc.
- ■ Graft rejections
- ■ Allergies
- ■ Immunopathology in chronic infections

In one case (Bechet´s disease) there is now also clinical proof of
principle!

Figure l4.6 Coupling relevant self antigens or allergens to CTB markedly enhances their ability to induce oral tolerance and suppress disease in animal models, and in the first clinical application tested also in patients with Behcet's disease.

intestinal epithelium and also ensures the coordinated uptake of both the antigen and the immunomodulating agent (CTB or LTB) by the same APCs, which would otherwise be difficult at a large mucosa such as that in the intestine. However, when given intranasally also a mixture of antigen and CTB or LTB can lead to efficient induction of tolerance, probably due to the much smaller size and greater permeability of the nasal mucosa allowing for easier transport and co-localization to the same APCs (Bregenholt et al., 2003; Luross et al., 2002).

While there are many studies documenting the efficacy of mainly CTB but also LTB in inducing peripheral tolerance to coadministered cell antigens or allergens in animal systems, it was only recently that initial proof of principle could be demonstrated in humans. Thus, based on previous encouraging results in a rat model of heat-shock protein-induced uveitis (Phipps et al., 2003), a small phase I/II trial in patients with Behcet's disease (BD) was undertaken with very encouraging results (Stanford et al., 2004). BD is an autoimmune eye disease often associated with extraocular manifestations and abnormal T cell reactivity to a specific peptide ("BD peptide") within

the human 60 kD heat shock protein. Oral administration of CTB-BD peptide conjugate, three times weekly, had no adverse effects and enabled gradual withdrawal, without any relapse of uveitis, of existing treatment with immunosuppressive drugs in 5 out of 8 unselected patients with BD. Indeed, relapse of uveitis was prevented after complete withdrawal of existing treatment in 4 of 5 patients, in whom the preexisting immunosuppressive treatment had maintained the patient in clinical remission prior to initiating the tolerizing regime. Most strikingly, remission was maintained up to 1 year following withdrawal of the peptide-CTB treatment, without a need of any systemic immunosuppression. Associated with the control of uveitis in the BD patients was a lack of peptide-specific CD4+ T cell proliferation and various other immunological parameters. This study is the first instance where mucosal tolerization with a CTB-specific antigen conjugate has been tested in humans. The promising results of this study clearly need to be confirmed by a placebo-controlled phase III trial. However, if the efficacy of the BD peptide-CTB oral tolerance treatment observed here were to be confirmed, this novel treatment strategy may be applicable generally to autoimmune diseases in which oral tolerization with specific antigen alone has not been effective.

The specific actions in the strong enhancement of oral tolerance by CTB-antigen conjugates are probably complex and may include: (i) increased uptake of tolerizing antigen across the mucosal surface; (ii) increased high-affinity delivery of both specific antigen and CTB to the relevant mucosal APCs; and (iii) a direct immunomodulatory effect of bound CTB on these APCs. Effective treatment with different CTB-antigen conjugates or fusion proteins are associated with the development of actively tolerogenic APCs as well as of different types, both CD25+ and CD25–, suppressive-regulatory T cells in mucosal tissues and draining lymph nodes (Sun et al., 2000; Li et al., 2001; Boirivant et al., 2001; Anjouere et al., to be published; Sun et al., to be published). Depending on the nature of the conjugated antigen, the route of administration (oral, nasal) of the conjugate, and the animal species used in the different study models, treatment with CTB-antigen conjugates has variably affected the capacity of lymph node T cells to produce Th1 or Th2 cytokines. A striking observation in all models of autoimmune diseases tested was the finding that treatment with CTB-antigen complexes suppressed leukocyte infiltration into the target organ. This suggests that the mechanisms governing induction of tolerance by feeding or inhaling CTB-linked antigens may involve modifications of the migratory behavior of inflammatory cells.

Furthermore, tolerization also results in a local downregulation in the target tissue of certain chemokines, such as MCP-1 and RANTES, known selectively to promote both the attraction and differentiation of inflammatory-pathogenic Th1 cells (Sun et al., 2000). CTB has also been shown to be antiinflammatory *per se*. Oral feeding of CTB both prevents and cures Th1-driven experimental colitis in mice, through an unidentified mechanism involving a reduced production of IL-12 within the large bowel (Boirivant et al., 2001).

Conclusions

The last decade has brought much progress in the development of especially CTB as an oral-mucosal vaccine immunogen protecting against cholera and/or ETEC diarrhea as well as serving as a model immunogen in humans for studying the immune responses in different mucosal tissues after oral, nasal, vaginal, or rectal immunizations. Together with findings showing that CTB or LTB also can serve as efficient mucosal carriers for inducing mucosal immune responses to various immunogenic antigens or peptides chemically linked to or genetically fused to CTB/LTB, it seems likely that mucosal vaccines against various microbial pathogens may be developed based on CTB or LTB as vectors.

Significant progress has also been made in developing detoxified CT and LT molecules that display adjuvant activity with little or no toxicity. Although so far only one study in humans has been undertaken, it seems likely based on the rapid pace of investigation in the field that the future holds much promise for detoxified CT and LT derivatives as mucosal adjuvants also for human use.

Further, even without attenuation CT and LT have shown promising properties as adjuvants for *ex vivo* dendritic cell vaccination leading to dramatically increased antibody as well as cellular immune responses after reinfusion of the *ex vivo*-pulse vaccinated dendritic cells in mice. It remains to be determined whether these promising features would also hold true for dendritic cell vaccination in humans using, for example, various tumor vaccine antigens in combination with or linked to CT or LT.

Finally, the prospects for using CTB (or LTB) for inducing so-called oral tolerance to various chemically linked or genetically fused organ-specific antigens or selected allergens for immunotherapeutic purposes has taken a big step forward with the demonstration in a first clinical trial of very promising effects using this principle in patients with Behcet's disease. If the promising results of this study can be confirmed in future clinical studies, this novel strategy may be applicable to a variety of autoimmune diseases and potentially also allergic diseases in which oral tolerization with specific antigen alone has not been effective.

■ References

Agren, L.C., Ekman, L., Lowenadler, B., and Nedrud, J.H. (1999). Adjuvanticity of the cholera toxin A1-based gene fusion protein, CTA1-DD, is critically dependent on the ADP-ribosyltransferase and Ig-binding activity. *J. Immunol.* 162, 2432–2440.

Anjuère, F., Luci, C., Lebens, M., Rousseau, D., Hervouet, C., Milon, G., Holmgren, J., Ardavin, C., and Czerkinsky, C. (2004). In vivo adjuvant-induced mobilization and maturation of gut dendritic cells after oral administration of cholera toxin. *J Immunol.* 173, 5103–5111.

Arakawa, T., Yu, J., Chong, D.K., Hough, J., Engen, P.C., and Langridge, W.H. (1998). A plant-based cholera toxin B subunit-insulin fusion protein protects against the development of autoimmune diabetes. *Nature Biotechnol.* 16, 934–938.

Bäckström, M., Shahabi, V., Johansson, S., Teneberg, S., Kjellberg, A., Miller-Podraza, H., Holmgren, J. and Lebens, M. (1997). Structural basis for differential receptor binding of cholera and *Escherichia coli* heat-labile toxins: influence of heterologous amino acid substitutions in the cholera B-subunit. *Mol. Microbiol.* 24, 489–497.

Bergerot, I., Ploix, C., Petersen, J., Moulin, V., Rask, C., Fabien, N., Lindblad, M., Mayer, A., Czerkinsky, C., Holmgren, J., and Thivolet, C. (1997). A cholera toxoid-insulin conjugate as an oral vaccine against spontaneous autoimmune diabetes. *Proc. Natl. Acad. Sci. USA* 94, 4610–4614.

Bergquist, C., Johansson, E-L., Lagergård, T., Holmgren, J., and Rudin, A. (1997). Intranasal vaccination of humans with recombinant cholera toxin B subunit induces systemic and local antibody responses in the upper respiratory tract and the vagina. *Infect. Immun.* 65, 2676–2684.

Boirivant, M., Fuss, I., Ferroni, L., De Pascale. M., and Strober, W. (2001). Oral administration of recombinant cholera toxin subunit B inhibits IL-12-mediated murine experimental (trinitrobenzene sulfonic acid) colitis. *J. Immunol.* 166, 3522–3532.

Bregenholt, S., Wang, M., Wolfe, T., Hughes, A., Baerentzen, L., Dyrberg, T., von Herrath, M.G., and Petersen, J.S. (2003). The cholera toxin B subunit is a mucosal adjuvant for oral tolerance induction in type 1 diabetes. *Scand. J. Immunol.* 57, 432–438.

Chaillous, L., Lefevre, H., Thivolet, C., Boitard, C., Lahlou, N., Atlan, G., Bouhanick, B., Mogenet, A., Nicolino, M., Carel, J.C., Lecomte, P., Marecha, R., Bougneres, P., Charbonnel, B., and Sai, P. (2000). Oral insulin administration and residual beta-cell function in recent-onset

type 1 diabetes: a multicentre randomised controlled trial. *Lancet* 12, 545–549.

Clemens, J., Sack, D.A., Harris, J.R., Atkinson, W., Chakraborty, J., Khan, M.R., Stanton, B.F., Kay, B.A., Khan, M.U., Yunus, M.D., Svennerholm, A.-M., and Holmgren, J. (1986). Field trial of oral cholera vaccines in Bangladesh. *Lancet* I, 124–127.

Clemens, J.D., Sack, D.A., Harris, J.R., Chakraborty, J., Khan, M.R., Stanton, B.F., Ali, M., Ahmed, F., Yunus, M., Kay, B.A., Khan, M.U., Rao, M.R., Svennerholm, A.-M., and Holmgren, J. (1988a). Impact of B subunit killed whole-cell and killed whole-cell-only oral vaccines against cholera upon treated diarrhoeal illness and mortality in an area endemic for cholera. *Lancet* I, 1375–1379.

Clemens, J.D., Sack, D.A., Harris, J.R., Chakraborty, J., Neogy, P.K., Stanton, B., Huda, N., Khan, M.U., Kay, B.A., Khan, M.R., Ansaruzzaman, M., Yunus, M., Rao, M.R., Svennerholm, A.-M., and Holmgren, J. (1988b). Cross-protection by B subunit-whole cell cholera vaccine against diarrhea associated with heat-labile toxin-producing enterotoxigenic *Escherichia coli*: results of a large-scale field trial. *J. Infect. Dis.* 158, 372–377.

Clemens, J.D., Sack, D.A., Harris, J.R., Van Loon, F., Chakraborty, J., Ahmed, F., Rao, M.R., Khan, M.R., Yunus, M.D., Huda, N., Stanton, B.F., Kay, B.A., Walter, S., Eeckels, R., Svennerholm, A.-M., and Holmgren, J. (1990). Field trial of oral cholera vaccines in Bangladesh: results from three-year follow-up. *Lancet* i, 270–273.

Couch, R.B. (2004). Nasal vaccination, Escherichia coli enterotoxin, and Bell's palsy. *N. Engl. J. Med.* 350, 860–861.

De Fijter, J.W., Eijgenraam, J.W., Braam, C.A., Holmgren, J., Daha, M.R., van Es, L.A., and van den Wall Blake, A.W.L. (1996). Deficient IgA1 immune response to nasal cholera toxin subunit B in primary IgA nephropathy. *Kidney Int.* 50, 952–961.

De Haan, L. and Hirst, T.R. (2003). Cholera toxin and related enterotoxins: a cell biological and immunological perspective. *J. Nat. Toxins* 9, 281–297.

Di Rienzo, V., Marcucci, F., Puccinelli, P., Parmiani, S., Frati, F., Sensi, L., Canonica, G.W., and Passalacqua, G. (2003). Long-lasting effect of sublingual immunotherapy in children with asthma due to house dust mite: a 10-year prospective study. *Clin. Exp. Allergy* 33, 206–210.

Di Tommaso, A., Saletti, G., Pizza, M., Rappuoli, R., Dougan, G., Abrignani, S., Douce, G., and de Magistris, M.T. (1996). Induction of antigen specific antibodies in vaginal secretions by using a nontoxic mutant of heat-labile enterotoxin as a mucosal adjuvant. *Infect. Immun.* 64, 974–979.

Dickinson, B.L. and Clements, J.H. (1995). Dissociation of *Escherichia coli* heat-labile enterotoxin adjuvanticity from ADP-ribosyltransferase activity. *Infect. Immun.* 63, 1617–1623.

Dotevall, H., Jonson-Strömberg, G., Sanyal, S., and Holmgren, J. (1985). Characterization of enterotoxin and soluble hemagglutinin from *Vibrio mimicus*: identity with *V. cholerae* O1 toxin and hemagglutinin. *FEMS Microbiol. Lett.* 27, 17–22.

Elson, C.O. and Ealding, W. (1984). Cholera toxin feeding did not induce oral tolerance in mice and abrogated oral tolerance to an unrelated protein antigen. *J. Immunol.* 133, 2892–2897.

Eriksson, K., Fredriksson, M., Nordström, I., and Holmgren, J. (2003). Cholera toxin and its B subunit promote dendritic cell vaccination with different influence on Th1/Th2 development. *Infect. Immun.* 71, 1740–1747.

Eriksson, K., Sun, J.B., Nordström, I., Fredriksson, M., Lindblad, M., Li, B.L., and Holmgren, J. (2004). Coupling of antigen to cholera toxin for dendritic cell vaccination promotes the induction of MHC class I-restricted cytotoxic T cells and the rejection of a cognate antigen-expressing model tumour. *Eur. J. Immunol.* 34, 1272–1281.

Fujihashi, K., Koga, T., van Ginkel, F.W., Hagiwara, Y., and McGhee, J.R. (2002). A dilemma for mucosal vaccination: efficacy versus toxicity using enterotoxin-based adjuvants. *Vaccine* 20, 2431–2438.

Gagliardi, M., Sallusto, F., Marinaro, M., Vendetti, S., Riccomi, A., and De Magistris, M. (2002). Effects of the adjuvant cholera toxin on dendritic cells: stimulatory and inhibitory signals that result in the amplification of immune responses. *Ing. J. Med. Microbiol.* 291, 571–575.

George-Chandy, A., Eriksson, K., Lebens, M., Nordstrom, I., Schön, E., and Holmgren, J. (2001). Cholera toxin B subunit as a carrier molecule promotes antigen presentation and increases CD40 and CD86 expression on antigen-presenting cells. *Infect. Immun.* 69, 5716–5725.

Guiliano, M.M., Del Giudice, G., Giannelli, V., Dougan, G., Douce, G., Rappuoli, R., and Pizza, M. (1998). Mucosal adjuvanticity and immunogenicity of LTR72, a novel mutant of *Escherichia coli* heat-labile enterotoxin with partial knockout of ADP-ribosyltransferase activity. *J. Exp. Med.* 187, 1123–32.

Harandi, A.M. and Holmgren, J. (2004). CpG DNA as a potent inducer of mucosal immunity: implications for immuno-prophylaxis and immunotherapy of mucosal infections. *Curr. Opin. Invest. Drugs* 5, 141–145.

Harandi, A.M., Eriksson, K., and Holmgren, J. (2003). A protective role of locally administered immunostimulatory CpG oligodeoxynucleotide in a mouse model of genital herpes infection. *J. Virol.* 77, 953–962.

Holmgren, J. (1981). Actions of cholera toxin and the prevention and treatment of cholera. *Nature* 292, 413–417.

Holmgren, J. and Bergquist, C. (2004). Oral B subunit killed whole-cell cholera vaccines. In Levine M.M. et al. (Eds) *New Generation Vaccines*, 3rd edn. Marcel Decker, New York, pp. 499–510.

Holmgren, J. and Czerkinsky, C. (2005). Mucosal immunity and vaccines. *Nature Med.*, 11 (Suppl. 4), S45–S53.

Holmgren, J., Fredman, P., Lindblad, M., Svennerholm, A.-M., and Svennerholm, L. (1982). Rabbit intestinal glycoprotein receptor for *Escherichia coli* heat-labile enterotoxin lacking affinity for cholera toxin. *Infect. Immun.* 38, 424–433.

Holmgren, J., Lycke, N., and Czerkinsky, C. (1993). Cholera toxin and cholera B subunit as oral-mucosal adjuvant and antigen vector system. *Vaccine* 11, 1179–1184.

Johansson, E.-L., Wassén, L., Holmgren, J., Jertborn, M., and Rudin, A. (2001). Nasal and vaginal vaccinations have differential effects on antibody responses in vaginal and cervical secretions in humans. *Infect. Immun.* 69, 7481–7486.

Lencer, W.I. and Tsai, B. (2003). The intracellular voyage of cholera toxin: going retro. *Trends Biochem. Sci.* 12, 639–645.

Li, B.-L., Sun, J.-B., and Holmgren, J. (2001). Adoptive transfer of mucosal T cells or dendritic cells from animals fed with cholera toxin B subunit alloantigen conjugate induces allogeneic T cell tolerance. *Adv. Exp. Med. Biol.* 495, 271–275.

Lu, X., Clements, J.D., and Katz, J.M. (2002). Mutant *Escherichia coli* heat-labile enterotoxin [LT(R192G)] enhances protective humoral and cellular immune responses to orally administered inactivated influenza vaccine. *Vaccine* 20, 1019–1029.

Lucas, M. et al. (2005). High-level effectiveness of a mass oral cholera vaccination in Beira, Mozambique. *N. Engl. J. Med.* 352, 757–767.

Luross, J.A., Heaton, T., Hirst, T.R., Day, M.J., and Williams, N.A. (2002). *Escherichia coli* heat-labile enterotoxin B subunit prevents autoimmune arthritis through induction of regulatory CD4+ T cells. *Arthritis Rheum.* 46, 1671–1682.

Lycke, N. (1997). The mechanism of cholera toxin adjuvanticity. *Res. Immunol.* 148, 504–520.

Lycke, N. and Holmgren, J. (1986). Strong adjuvant properties of cholera toxin on gut mucosal immune responses to orally presented antigens. *Immunology* 59, 301–308.

Ma, D., Mellon, J., and Niederkorn, J. (1998). Conditions affecting enhanced corneal allograft survival by oral immunization. *Invest. Ophthalmol. Vis. Sci.* 39, 1835–1846.

Marchetti, M., Rossi, M., Giannelli, V., Giuliani, M.M., Pizza, M., Censini, S., Covacci, A., Massari, P., Pagliaccia, C., Manetti, R., Telford, J.L., Douce, G., Dougan, G., Rappuoli, R., and Ghiara, P. (1998). Protection against *Helicobacter pylori* infection in mice by intragastric vaccination with *H. pylori* antigens is achieved using a non-toxic mutant of *E. coli* heat-labile enterotoxin (LT) as adjuvant. *Vaccine* 16, 33–37.

Mastrandrea, F. (2004). The potential role of allergen-specific sublingual immunotherapy in atopic dermatitis. *Am. J. Clin. Dermatol.* 5, 281–294.

Mowat, A.M., Donachie, A.M., Jagewall, S., Schön, K., Lowenadler, B., Dalström, K., Kaastrup, P., and Lycke, N. (2001). CTA1-DD-immune stimulating complexes: a novel, rationally designed combined mucosal vaccine adjuvant effective with nanogram doses of antigen. *J. Immunol.* 167, 3398–3405.

NIAID Conference (2001). Safety evaluation of toxin adjuvants delivered intranasally. www.niaid.nih.gov/dmid/enteric/intranasal.htm.

Phipps, P.A., Stanford, M.R., Sun, J.-B., Xiao, B.G., Holmgren, J., Shinnic, T., Hasa, A., Mizushima, Y., and Lehner, T. (2003). Prevention of mucosally induced uveitis with a HSP60-derived peptide linked to cholera toxin B subunit. *Eur. J. Immunol.* 33, 224–232.

Pizza, M., Giuliani, M., Fontana, M., Monaci, E., Douce, G., Dougan, G., Mills, K.H., Rappuoli, R., and Del Giudice, G. (2001). Mucosal vaccines: non toxic derivatives of LT and CT as mucosal adjuvants. *Vaccine* 19, 2534–2541.

Plant, A. and Williams, N.A. (2004). Modulation of the immune response by the cholera-like enterotoxins. *Curr. Top. Med. Chem.* 4, 509–519.

Postlethwaite, A.E. (2001). Can we induce tolerance in rheumatoid arthritis? *Curr. Rheumatol. Rep.* 3, 64–69.

Rask, C., Holmgren, J., Fredriksson, M., Lindblad, M., Nordström, I., Sun, J.-B., and Czerkinsky, C. (2000). Prolonged oral treatment with low doses of allergen conjugated to cholera toxin B subunit suppresses immunoglobulin E antibody responses in sensitized mice. *Clin. Exp. Allergy* 30, 1024–1032.

Rudin, A., Johansson, E.-L., Bergquist, C., and Holmgren, J. (1998). Differential kinetics and distribution of antibodies in serum and nasal and vaginal secretions after nasal and oral vaccination in humans. *Infect. Immun.* 66, 3390–3396.

Rudin, A., Riise, G.C.. and Holmgren, J. (1999). Antibody responses in the lower respiratory tract and male urogenital tract in humans after nasal and oral vaccination with cholera toxin B subunit. *Infect. Immun.* 67, 2884–2890.

Sack, D.A., Sack, B.R., Nair, G.B., and Siddique, A.K. (2004). Cholera. *Lancet* 363, 223–233.

Sanchez, J., Wallerstrom, G., Fredriksson, M., Angstrom, J., and Holmgren, J. (2002). Detoxification of cholera toxin without removal of its immunoadjuvanticity by the addition of (STa-related) peptides to the catalytic subunit. A potential new strategy to generate immunostimulants for vaccination. *J. Biol. Chem.* 277, 33369–33377.

Staats, H.F. and Ennis, F.A. Jr. (1999). IL-1 is an effective adjuvant for mucosal and systemic immune responses when co-administered with protein immunogens. *J. Immunol.* 162, 6141–6147.

Stanford, M., Whittall, T., Bergmeier, L.A., Lindblad, M., Lundin, S., Shinnick, T., Mizushima, Y., Holmgren, J., and Lehner, T. (2004). Oral tolerization with peptide 336–351 linked to cholera toxin B subunit in preventing relapses of uveitis in Behcet's disease. *Clin. Exp. Immunol.* 137, 201–208.

Stephenson, I., Nicholson, K.G., Rudin, A., Colegate, A., Podda, A., Bugarini, R., del Giudice, G., Minutello, A., Bonnington, S., Holmgren, J., Mills, K.H.G., and Zambon, M.C. (2005). Trivalent nasal inactivated influenza vaccine with non-toxigenic Escherichia coli enterotoxin and novel biovector as mucosal adjuvants: a randomised phase I trial. *Vaccine*, in press.

Sun, J.-B., Holmgren, J., and Czerkinsky, C. (1994). Cholera toxin B subunit: an efficient transmucosal carrier-delivery

system for induction of peripheral immunological tolerance. *Proc. Natl. Acad. Sci. USA* 91, 10795–10799.

Sun, J.-B., Rask, C., Olsson, T., Holmgren, J., and Czerkinsky, C. (1996). Treatment of experimental autoimmune encephalomyelitis by feeding myelin basic protein conjugated to cholera toxin B subunit. *Proc. Natl. Acad. Sci. USA* 93, 7196–7201.

Sun, J.-B., Li, B-L., Czerkinsky, C., and Holmgren, J. (2000). Enhanced immunological tolerance against allograft rejection by oral administration of allogeneic antigen linked to cholera toxin B subunit. *J. Clin. Immunol.* 97, 130–139.

Sun, J.-B., Xiao, B.-G., Lindblad, M., Li, B.-L., Link, H., Czerkinsky, C., and Holmgren, J. (2000). Oral administration of cholera toxin B subunit conjugated to myelin basic protein protects against experimental autoimmune encephalomyelitis by inducing transforming growth factor-b-secreting cells and suppressing chemokine expression. *Int. Immunol.* 12, 1449–1457.

Sun, J.-B., Eriksson, K., Li, B.-L., Lindblad, M., Azem, J., and Holmgren, J. (2004). Vaccination with dendritic cells pulsed *in vitro* with tumor antigen conjugated to cholera toxin efficiently induces specific tumoricidal CD8+ cytotoxic lymphocytes dependant on cyclic AMP activation of dendritic cells. *Clin. Immunol.* 112, 35–44.

Svennerholm, A.-M., Jertborn, M., Gothefors, L., Karim, A.M.M.M., Sack, D.A, and Holmgren, J. (1984). Mucosal antitoxic and antibacterial immunity after cholera disease and after immunization with a combined B subunit-whole cell vaccine. *J. Infect. Dis.* 149, 884–893.

Tamura, S., Hatori, E., Tsuruhara, T., Aizawa, C., and Kurata, T. (1997). Suppression of delayed-type hypersensitivity and IgE antibody responses to ovalbumin by intranasal administration of *Escherichia coli* heat-labile enterotoxin B subunit-conjugated ovalbumin. *Vaccine* 15, 225–229.

Tarkowski, A., Sun, J.-B., Holmdahl, R., Holmgren, J., and Czerkinsky, C. (1999). Treatment of experimental autoimmune arthritis by nasal administration of a type II collagen-cholera toxoid conjugate vaccine. *Arthritis Rheum.* 42, 1628–1634.

Wiendl, H. and Hohlfeld, R. (2002). Therapeutic approaches in multiple sclerosis: lessons from failed and interrupted treatment trials. *BioDrugs* 16, 183–200.

Wilson, D.R., Torres Lima, M., and Dirham, S.R. (2005). Sublingual immunotherapy for allergic rhinitis: systematic review and meta-analysis. *Allergy* 60, 4–12.

Wu, H.Y. and Weiner, H.L. (2003). Oral tolerance. *Immunol. Res.* 28, 265–284.

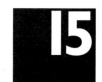

Transcutaneous immunization using the heat-labile enterotoxin of *E. coli* as an adjuvant

Richard T. Kenney and Gregory M. Glenn
Iomai Corporation, Gaithersburg, Maryland

Introduction

The skin represents the first line of host defense against many pathogens and has a sophisticated structure to achieve this purpose. Immune cells trafficking through the area sample the epidermal space to detect invading microorganisms that might penetrate the specialized physical barrier on the surface. When danger is perceived, these cells become activated and carry the signal to the draining lymph node to orchestrate a systemic immune response. Application of vaccine antigens and adjuvants to the skin, also known as transcutaneous immunization (TCI), can mimic these events to stimulate protective responses to the organisms they represent. This review discusses the nature of the anatomical barrier of the skin and some of the known mechanisms for activation and augmentation of the immune response to antigens applied to the skin.

We have focused on the development of products that allow delivery of vaccine antigens into the skin using a patch or similar means. Along the way we have discovered the utility of disrupting the most superficial layers of the skin before applying the antigens, as well as the importance of adjuvants in

activating the responding cells. All of the clinical work with TCI has been done using the heat-labile enterotoxin of *E. coli* (LT) or a mutant of this toxin as the adjuvant. Stimulation of the skin immune system in this manner leads to strong and effective responses in preclinical models and in our human trials, and this immune responsiveness, in combination with a high safety margin, has fostered a great deal of interest in targeting the skin with vaccines. We discuss some of the preclinical and clinical findings that support the utility of TCI, as well as some of the regulatory implications of developing a new antigen/adjuvant delivery system. We then compare TCI with several other approaches that are moving out of the laboratory and into the clinic.

Background

Mammalian skin is divided at the basal lamina between the dermis, which has direct vascular, lymphatic, and nervous connection to the subcutaneous tissues and the rest of the body, and the overlying epidermis, which is composed of four layers of cells at different stages of differentiation that migrate away from the deeper tissues and are eventually sloughed off the surface (Morganti et al., 2001).

The stratum basale (SB), or the layer of cells separating the dermis and epidermis, is composed of large columnar cells that form intercellular attachments with adjacent cells through desmosomes and with the basal lamina through hemidesmosomes, laminin, and integrins (Marchisio et al., 1991). An extensive keratin network, primarily made up of keratins K5 and K14 in this layer, serves to prevent both water loss and the absorption of foreign substances (Moll et al., 1982). As these cells divide and migrate upward from the basal layer, they gradually acquire the characteristics of a fully differentiated corneocyte and are eventually sloughed at the skin surface. Cells in the stratum spinosum (SP), the next layer up, lose the capacity to divide, enlarge and flatten, and their water content diminishes. Production of the earlier keratins gives way to favor K1 and K10, which aggregate to form filaments. A specialized protein envelope begins to form, composed of involucrin and the transglutaminase that is responsible for eventually crosslinking these substrates into the insoluble cornified envelope (Thacher and Rice, 1985). The keratin filaments are packed further together in the stratum granulosum (SG) with filaggrin, resulting in the formation of macrofibrils. Granular lamellar bodies composed of profilaggrin or loricrin form in this layer and generate ceramides, cholesterol, and free fatty acids that replace some of the membrane amphiphilic phospholipids and contribute to the permeability barrier of the skin (Elias et al., 1988). The cells reach their final state of differentiation in the stratum corneum (SC) as flat horny cells filled with keratin bundles. The lamellar contents are released to form a lipid-enriched intercellular matrix surrounding the corneocytes, generating a bricks-and-mortar structure with the cells essentially embedded within the lipid matrix. The lipids in the SC block microbes and the inward diffusion of aqueous material through the epidermis and help retain water within the body.

The epidermis is a dynamic immune environment as well, with constant trafficking of immune cells in and out. Bone marrow-derived Langerhans cells (LCs) are a type of dendritic cell that reside in the epidermis and act as sentinels, transmitting danger signals by capturing antigens and presenting them to T cells in the draining lymph node (Olszewski et al., 1995; Banchereau and Steinman, 1998). They form a monolayer network of cells, being evenly distributed throughout the suprabasal regions of the epidermis (Berman et al., 1983; Yu et al., 1994). While they account for only 1–3% of the epidermal cells, confocal microscopy has shown that LCs cover 25% of the total human skin surface area to efficiently trap antigens. Following sensitization, up to 30% of resident LCs leave the skin and migrate via afferent lymphatics to the draining node (Cumberbatch et al., 2001). Epidermal keratinocytes are likely to play a role in initiating the immune response, since they provide the tumor necrosis factor (TNF)-α that is necessary to stimulate LC migration (Cumberbatch et al., 1999). In addition to TNF-α, LC-derived interleukin (IL)-1β has been shown to be required for migration, at least in mice (Cumberbatch et al., 1997). The number of LCs and their responsiveness to TNF-α decreases with age, which may account for some of the immune senescence associated with the elderly (Bhushan et al., 2002). More recently, IL-18 has been shown to act upstream from both TNF-α and IL-1β and may be necessary to sustain their expression (Cumberbatch et al., 2001, 2003), whereas IL-4 and IL-10 antagonize trafficking (Wang et al., 1999). The chemokine receptor CCR7 appears to be essential for mobilization of LCs from the epidermis to the dermis and for entry of these cells into the dermal lymphatic vessels (Ohl et al., 2004). Injection of a vaccine into the muscle completely bypasses this rich immune milieu, while in TCI antigens and adjuvant are applied directly to the skin where LCs take them up, become activated, and migrate to the draining lymph node to present the resultant peptides and initiate the systemic immune response.

Molecular structure

LT and cholera toxin (CT) act as potent immune stimulators in the context of the skin and share closely related structure and function, with over 80% sequence identity in both of the A and B subunits and very similar tertiary structure (O'Neal et al., 2004). The peptide chains in both LT and CT are encoded on a single cistron containing two genes that overlap by four bases. Once synthesized in the cytosol, the subunits are translocated across the inner membrane into the periplasm, where one A subunit and five B subunits are assembled into a single heterohexameric holo-toxin protein (Fan et al., 2004). Active secretion of the toxins across the outer membrane by the type II bacterial protein secretion system occurs by the general secretion pathway (Gsp) and the extracellular protein secretion (Eps) export machinery for enterotoxigenic *E. coli* (ETEC) and *Vibrio cholerae*, respectively (Sandkvist et al., 2000; Tauschek et al., 2002).

The crystal structure of LT was first solved in 1991 (Sixma et al., 1991) and has been substantially refined since then (reviewed in Fan et al., 2004). The A subunit contains two functional parts: the wedge-shaped A1 domain that carries the enzyme site is tethered in place by the A2 domain that consists of an elongated alpha-helix, ending in a tail that extends through the pore formed by the B pentamer (Spangler, 1992). The B subunit of LT binds via the ubiquitous GM1-ganglioside receptor, a glycosphingolipid found ubiquitously on the cell surface of mammalian cells (Holmgren, 1973; Sixma et al., 1992), as does the closely related CT. Binding affinities of the toxins to GM1 is extremely high, with dissociation constants of 5.7×10^{-10} and 4.6×10^{-12} for LT and CT, respectively (Kuziemko et al., 1996; MacKenzie et al., 1997). Crystallization of LT bound to lactose revealed that the GM1-binding sites are located at the base of the B pentamer and form a firm platform for docking (Sixma et al., 1992). LTD33, a B-subunit receptor-binding mutant, was able to serve as an equipotent adjuvant for an intranasal influenza vaccine (de Haan et al., 1998), but it was unable to serve as an effective oral adjuvant for ovalbumin (OVA) (Guidry et al., 1997). Intranasal LTB was only able to adjuvant the influenza response when binding was intact, since the LTB-D33 mutant had no effect on the response. Thus, binding to the GM1 receptor is required for antigenicity and seems important, although not completely required, for adjuvanticity (reviewed in de Haan and Hirst, 2004).

Trafficking within the cell

Molecular trafficking is complex and still incompletely understood, but the details that are known from studies in various cell types may provide insights into the mechanisms of immunopotentiation (Figure 15.1). CT-coated gold particles were shown in early electron microscopy studies to bind to the GM1 receptors localized in uncoated plasma membrane invaginations (Montesano et al., 1982) that were later shown to be caveolae (Parton, 1994). These structures can bud off into the cytosol to form transendocytic carriers and may serve as the usual mechanism for the initiation of CT toxicity (Parton and Richards, 2003). Internalization and the ability to elicit a cAMP-dependent Cl^- secretory response requires localization in lipid rafts, which are detergent-insoluble cell surface islands of highly ordered saturated lipids and choles-terol. Construction of a series of chimeric toxins with the more distantly related *E. coli* heat-labile type II enterotoxin (LTIIb), which preferentially binds the ganglioside GD1a, showed a loss of the toxin secretory response when CTA was bound to this receptor through the LTIIb-B subunit and a competent response with the reciprocal chimera bound to GM1, which was also shown to be raft-associated (Wolf et al., 1998). Thus, toxin-binding localization at these specialized cell membrane microdomains may provide a distinct trafficking pathway that can lead to toxicity (Orlandi and Fishman, 1998; Fishman and Orlandi, 2003).

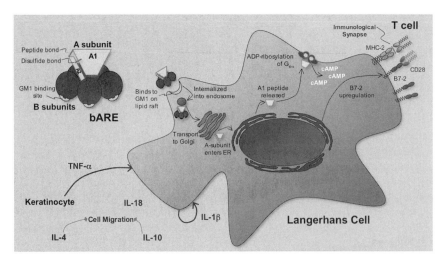

Figure 15.1 Effect of bacterial ADP-ribosylating endotoxins (bAREs) in the epidermis. Langerhans cells that are resident in the epidermis can become activated by danger signals from pathogens, then travel to the lymph node and initiate an immune response. bAREs can mimic this through pathways that are just now being clarified. See text for details. (See Color Plate Section.)

Once internalized, CT-coated gold particles can be found in endosomes that are also positive for EEA1, a marker for early sorting endosomes (Wilson et al., 2000). The toxin is then delivered to the Golgi complex by retrograde vesicular transport where the A and B subunits dissociate (Majoul et al., 1996). The A subunit traffics to the endoplasmic reticulum (ER) by a coatomer (COP) I-mediated retrograde pathway (Girod et al., 1999). Delivery of CTA and LTA to the ER is facilitated by a KDEL retrieval motif on the carboxy terminus of the A2 subunit (Lencer et al., 1995; Majoul et al., 1998). The recent crystallization of active CT highlights the importance of this A2 tail structure and its interaction with B_5 (O'Neal et al., 2004) in comparison with LT (Sixma et al., 1993). Release of the catalytic A1 polypeptide (residues 1–192 or –194 for CT and LT, respectively) from the A2 portion (residues 193– or 195–240), which attaches the A chain to the receptor-binding pentamer of B subunits (B_5), requires proteolysis of the peptide bond as well as reduction of the disulfide bond between Cys_{187} and Cys_{199} to allow full enzymatic activity (Mekalanos et al., 1979). This appears to be under the control of the ER-associated degradation (ERAD) system, which is active in the folding of nascent proteins and recognizes misassembled proteins (Teter et al., 2003). The A1 peptide is then translocated into the cytosol via the sec61 protein translocation complex (Schmitz et al., 2000), where it has its enzymatic activity.

Cell biology

After being liberated into the cytoplasm, the active toxin ADP-ribosylates Arg 201 of the α -subunit of the heterotrimeric G-signaling protein ($G_{s\alpha}$) at the cell surface, which locks the protein in its GTP-bound form resulting in the persistent activation of adenylate cyclase and elevated production of cAMP within the cell (Sharp and Hynie, 1971; Moss et al., 1977). In intoxicated intestinal epithelial cells, the increased cAMP causes a marked efflux of chloride ions and inhibition of sodium ion absorption, causing an osmotic gradient that pulls water molecules into the lumen of the gut, leading to watery diarrhea. On the skin, CT and LT cause enhanced presentation of antigens, migration away from the site, and activation of LCs. Their adjuvanticity appears to correlate with the level of ribosyl-transferase activity, just as it does in oral and most nasal immunization studies (Lycke et al., 1992; Scharton-Kersten et al., 2000). The LTG192 mutant is an interesting exception to the rule, in that it has no modification to the enzymatic site and no ribosyl-transferase activity due to the mutation in the A1–A2 cleavage site, yet it retains its adjuvanticity (Dickinson and Clements, 1995; Kotloff et al., 2001). The double mutant LTK112/D33 was also found to retain adjuvant properties with intranasal vaccination, although anti-LT antibodies were not induced due to lack of GM1 binding (de Haan et al., 1999).

Activation actually starts with inhibition of processing of new antigens, although pre-existing peptide-MHC-II complexes can still be presented (Matousek et al., 1998; Watts and Amigorena, 2000; Petrovska et al., 2003), and it is strictly dependent on the presence of cAMP (Bagley et al., 2002). The final stages of LC activation relate to the ability of native LT preferentially to cause upregulation of the costimulatory molecule B7-2. The B7-1 (CD80) and B7-2 (CD86) antigen-presenting cell (APC) ligands differentially bind to T cell receptors CTLA-4 and CD28 in the immunological synapse, respectively (Hammond et al., 2001a; Pentcheva-Hoang et al., 2004). Upon binding to its ligand, CD28 can increase T cell proliferation by enhancing the transcription and mRNA stability of IL-2. In contrast, when ligand is bound to CTLA-4, T cell activation is restricted by inhibiting IL-2 production, IL-2 receptor expression, and cell cycle progression. Before stimulation, CD28 is uniformly distributed around the T cell plasma membrane and CTLA-4 is in intracellular vesicles. Binding of the APC B7-2 causes CD28 to concentrate in the synapse, while B7-1 ligand binding mediates CTLA-4 localization on the surface (Pentcheva-Hoang et al., 2004). Thus, the amount of B7-2 on the surface of LCs reflects their ability to present antigen that had been collected at the skin surface and activate T cells in the draining node. Although the link to ADP-ribosylation has not been fully characterized, there is a strong correlation between the enhancement of B7-2 expression and enzymatic activity of the toxin. The effect of native LT was compared with a nonenzymatic mutant LTK112 on several types of APCs: B cells, macrophages, and bone marrow-derived dendritic cells (DCs) (Martin et al., 2002). LTK112 substantially upregulates B7-1 in DCs, whereas native LT strongly upregulates surface expression of B7-2 in all three cell types compared to LTK112. Another group found similar correlation between enzymatic activity and B7-2 expression based on exposure to native LT, the partially active LTR72 mutant, and the nontoxic mutant LTK63 (Ryan et al., 2000), although the latter retains some adjuvant activity (Beignon et al., 2002).

Purified cholera toxin B subunit (pCTB) and mutant toxins that retain at least some ribosyl-transferase activity can also act as adjuvants (Matousek et al., 1998; Simmons et al., 2001), as opposed to recombinant CTB (rCTB) that has no associated enzymatic subunit and little to no activity (Hammond et al., 2001b; Simmons et al., 2001). The recombinant LTB subunit retains some adjuvant activity, however, following intranasal delivery (Richards et al., 2001), although the reasons for the difference with CTB are not completely clear. It may do this by changing the trafficking pattern of coadministered antigen into nonacidic endosomal compartments (Millar and Hirst, 2001). While the holotoxin is known to break mucosal tolerance (Clements et al., 1988), this effect requires receptor binding, at least for LTB, since the receptor-binding mutant LTD33 was unable to prevent the induction of collagen-induced arthritis (Williams et al., 1997). LTB also causes a shift from a Th1-dominated response to a Th2-associated one with increased IL-10 production and inhibition of IL-12 (Braun et al., 1999; Richards et al., 2001; Turcanu et al., 2002).

■ Safety and efficacy of bAREs

Even though skin delivery of some antigens can stimulate detectable antibody development, robust humoral and cellular responses consistently require the presence of an adjuvant

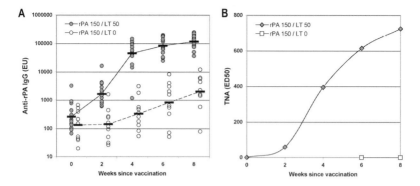

Figure I5.2 Immune response to TCI. Sixteen New Zealand white rabbits were vaccinated by TCI with a dry adhesive patch containing rPA I50 μg/LT 50 μg after skin pretreatment with a nonwoven abrasive pad to disrupt the stratum corneum on weeks 0, 2, 4, and 6 along with ten rabbits in the rPA I50 μg alone control group (Kenney et al., 2004). (A) The kinetic rPA IgG ELISA responses are shown individually and the geometric mean for each, with $p < 0.000I$ at all periods after the first dose. (B) TNA titers of pooled sera from the same group of rabbits treated with rPA/LT. No toxin-neutralizing activity was found in rabbits treated with rPA alone.

(Glenn et al., 1998a; Glenn and Alving, 1999a, 1999b; Baca-Estrada et al., 2000; Chen et al., 2001a; Güereña-Burgueño et al., 2002; Kenney et al., 2004). A large variety of adjuvants are under development or in use in licensed vaccines (Singh and O'Hagan, 1999; Kenney and Edelman, 2004). The most potent ones in the context of the skin appear to be the bacterial ADP-ribosylating exotoxins (bAREs), including LT, CT, and their mutants and subunits, as well as pseudomonas exotoxins A and diphtheria toxin. Millions of humans are exposed annually to the native toxins by way of natural infection with ETEC or cholera, suggesting that topical use would not induce long-term side effects. While there are dose limitations with mucosal delivery, bAREs have been extensively studied as mucosal adjuvants via intranasal and oral routes (Dickinson and Clements, 1995; Snider, 1995; Freytag and Clements, 1999; Michetti et al., 1999; Gluck et al., 2000; Holmgren et al., 2003; Zurbriggen et al., 2003). The skin, however, appears to be a protected site for adjuvant delivery, perhaps because proteins have difficulty penetrating the epidermis to reach the systemic circulation and any LT molecules that might get through would quickly become bound to the GM1 receptors on the first cell surface they encounter. Doses that are

many times the oral toxic dose have been given safely by TCI in clinical settings (Glenn et al., 2000; Güereña-Burgueño et al., 2002).

Our studies have primarily focused on CT, LT, and their derivatives, given their potency and the breadth of information available on these adjuvants (Lycke, 1997; Freytag and Clements, 1999; Michetti et al., 1999). Early studies of TCI clearly showed the critical need for an adjuvant for successful induction of high-level antibodies to a coadministered antigen (Glenn et al., 1998a). We and others have shown the utility of an adjuvant in developing a robust immune response to TCI using animal models as well as in clinical studies (Baca-Estrada et al., 2000; Scharton-Kersten et al., 2000; Chen et al., 2001a; Güereña-Burgueño et al., 2002; Kenney et al., 2004). As an example, Figure 15.2 shows the effect of immunizing rabbits transcutaneously using recombinant anthrax protective antigen (rPA) without and with LT. The skin is quite efficient, and some antibody response to antigen alone is often seen compared to the baseline titers. However, when a relatively low dose of adjuvant is combined with the antigen on the skin, a dramatic increase in response is seen, which can be as great or greater than the response to the same antigen given parenterally. Adjuvant is required for

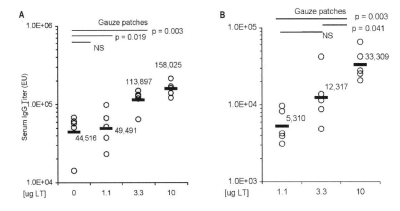

Figure I5.3 Immunostimulation of an intradermal vaccination with an LT patch. C57BL/6 mice were immunized by ID injection of 0.5Lf tetanus toxoid at the base of the tail and the indicated amounts of LT (0, 1.1, 3.3, or 10 μg) were applied to a gauze patch over the injection site after emery paper pretreatment. Patches were applied for 24 hours, removed, and the skin rinsed. The "no LT" group was shaved but was not pretreated and did not receive a patch. All groups were immunized on study day 1 and serum collected on day 15. Sera were evaluated for IgG titers to tetanus (panel A) and LT (panel B) by ELISA. The geometric mean titer and p-value for a t-test of the logs is indicated.

the development of robust neutralizing antibodies in this rPA system in rabbits, as well as in mice in an influenza system (Guebre-Xabier et al., 2003).

The use of adjuvant on the skin results in both primary and secondary serum antibody responses to the coadministered antigens (Glenn et al., 1999). TCI appears to induce boostable, long-lasting immune responses. In addition, prior immunization does not appear to inhibit responses to different antigens, suggesting the action of the adjuvant is initiated in a protected space such as in the epidermis, away from neutralizing antibodies (Tierney et al., 2003). Memory responses seen after boosting immunizations using TCI suggest that T cell responses are induced (Hammond et al., 2001b). T cell proliferative responses in spleen and lymph node preparations from mice revealed the induction of antigen-specific immunity, as well as mixed but predominantly Th2 cytokine profiles. In addition, intramuscularly primed animals responded vigorously to topical boosting. Other adjuvants, including bacterial DNA, cytokines, lipopolysaccharide (LPS), and LPS analogs have been shown to have activity in the context of the skin, but their comparative potency needs to be further

evaluated (Scharton-Kersten et al., 2000). Taken together, the results suggest the responses to TCI are systemic and are at least qualitatively similar to the humoral and cellular responses associated with classic immunization mechanisms.

A related approach is the augmentation of the response to an injected antigen by topical application of LT, which then serves as an immunostimulant (IS^{TM}). In preclinical models, these responses are strongest when the antigen is given intradermally and the adjuvant is placed directly over the injection site (Guebre-Xabier et al., 2003). Typical S-shaped dose-response curves can be generated for both antigen and adjuvant depending on the dose of adjuvant, as shown with a tetanus model in Figure 15.3A and B, respectively. Intradermal tetanus toxoid given to mice with or without increasing doses of LT induced a significant antibody response, but only with 3.3 μg LT or more in the patch. The dramatic increase in antibody response with an IS^{TM} patch can also be seen with an aging immune system (Guebre-Xabier et al., 2004), raising the possibility that the typical immunosenescence found in the elderly can be overcome. LT can act as an antigen as well and generates a strong dose-related serological response, with or without a coadministered antigen (Figure 15.3B), which is convenient for assessing delivery from the patch.

The immunity that develops to antigens and adjuvant on the skin is functionally relevant as well. Protective responses have been demonstrated in several models. Tetanus toxoid (TTx) delivered with increasing doses of LT resulted in a robust antibody response that was clearly dependent on the adjuvant dose (Scharton-Kersten et al., 2000). Only the animals that received adjuvant were fully protected on a subsequent challenge with systemic tetanus toxin. Studies of TCI in many antigen systems support the importance of the adjuvant for the development of protective antibodies. Adjuvant was required for the development of neutralizing antibodies following TCI with diphtheria toxin (Hammond et al., 2001a). The adjuvant was shown to play a crucial role in the protective responses for both live respiratory syncytial virus (RSV) (Godefroy et al., 2003) and chlamydia (Berry et al., 2004) challenges. While adjuvant was not required for protection in an aerosolized spore anthrax challenge, since all animals that received recombinant protective antigen (rPA) were protected, it was needed for the development of detectable levels of toxin neutralizing antibodies, which is more predictive for protection across species (Kenney et al., 2004). More recent studies have shown that TCI with a helper peptide derived for HIV IIIB and the immunodominant cytotoxic T lymphocyte (CTL) epitope from the V3 loop of the HIV IIIB strain of HIV can induce CTLs located in the intestinal Peyers patches (Belyakov et al., 2004). The CTL response correlated with protection against intrarectal challenge with gp160-expressing vaccinia virus. Interestingly, whereas the majority of LCs clearly migrated from the skin to the draining lymph nodes, some LCs containing fluorescently labeled LT appeared in the Peyers patches. LCs isolated after immunization could still present antigen, suggesting that a population of DCs

may present antigen directly to the mucosal immune system.

The passive transfer of immunity by injection of serum or cells into an immune animal is a key indicator of a mechanistic relationship between an immunization strategy and functional success in protection. Demonstration of a human disease correlate in an animal model can provide insights into the development of vaccines. ETEC, the most commonly identified pathogen causing diarrheal disease in travelers, is one of the main causes of foodborne disease in developing countries (Todd, 1997) and is an important cause of waterborne outbreaks (Daniels et al., 2000; Huerta et al., 2000). It is estimated that ETEC causes more than 600 million cases of diarrhea per year and more than 400,000 deaths, yet a fully predictive animal model has been difficult to substantiate. We investigated the potential that immunity to LT has for inducing relevant immune responses to ETEC infection, as suggested by recent epidemiological findings that LT is the sole correlate of disease (Steinsland et al., 2003). Using a model originally developed to study cholera toxin (Richardson et al., 1984), mice immunized by TCI with LT and a recombinant ETEC surface protein (rCS6) were orally challenged with LT in a sodium bicarbonate ($NaHCO_3$) buffer (Yu et al., 2002). High levels of anti-LT IgG were detected in the sera of the immunized mice (geometric mean for BALB/c mice, 36,249 ELISA units (EU); geometric mean for C57BL/6 mice, 54,792 EU). Mice immunized by TCI also developed detectable anti-LT IgG, IgA, and secretory IgA in the feces and vaginal secretions. For the oral toxin challenge experiments, two strains of mice with different sensitivities to challenge were used. C57BL/6 mice are much more sensitive to the effects of LT challenge than BALB/c mice, and protection in both strains suggests that the protective effect might be observed in more genetically diverse settings. As shown in Figure 15.4A and B, significant protection against LT challenge was observed in both strains ($p < 0.05$). The host-protective role of antitoxin antibody in the

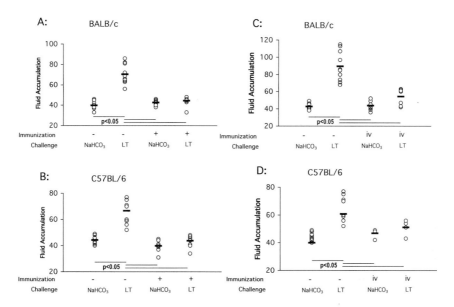

Figure 15.4 Serum from topically immunized mice passively protects naive mice from oral toxin challenge. BALB/c and C57BL/6 mice were vaccinated on the skin with LT for 1 hour on days 1 and 24 (A and B) or passively immunized by transfer of serum from topically immunized mice (C and D). Naive and immunized (active and passive) animals were subdivided into two groups and challenged by giving either 10% $NaHCO_3$ ($N = 10$) alone or LT in 10% $NaHCO_3$ orally. Actively immunized mice (A and B) were challenged 14 days after the second immunization. Passively vaccinated animals were challenged within either 12 hours of intravenous injection of the immune serum (C57BL/6) or 1 hour after intravenous injection (BALB/c). Fluid accumulation was assessed 6 hours after the challenge. (From Yu, J. et al. (2002). *Infect. Immun.* **70**, 1056–1068. Reprinted courtesy of American Society for Microbiology.)

serum was then evaluated by quantifying the amount of intestinal swelling elicited by oral LT challenge of naive and passively immunized mice that had received serum from animals immunized by TCI. The effect of passive immunization was evaluated in both BALB/c and C57BL/6 mice. Oral administration of LT to naive mice consistently induced fluid accumulation. In contrast, passively immunized mice accumulated negligible fluid, and the amount was comparable to that observed in the groups fed buffer alone (Figure 15.4C and D). Thus, the passively immunized mice given antibody from topically immunized mice were protected from the sequelae of oral toxin challenge.

While influenza vaccination has been shown to be effective in all age groups (Hak et al., 2005), immunosenescence in the elderly puts them at higher risk and makes them more vulnerable to disease (Murasko et al., 2002). We sought to augment the immune response

to vaccination in this age group with the addition of an IS[TM] patch (Frech et al., 2005). Hemagglutination inhibition is generally recognized as a correlate for protection in influenza and serves as the basis for annual relicensure in Europe (EMEA, 1997). Groups of healthy young adults or healthy elderly volunteers (≥ 60 years old) were vaccinated with a commercial influenza vaccine intramuscularly and compared with a group of elderly similarly vaccinated, but also treated with an IS[TM] patch containing $45\,\mu g$ LT (Figure 15.5). As expected, the elderly had a decreased response in comparison with the young. Young adults had 69, 56, and 61% seroconversion rates for A/New Caledonia, A/Panama, and B/Shandong, respectively. These rates were significantly higher or showed a trend compared to corresponding seroconversion rates in the elderly without a patch (40% ($p = 0.005$), 36% ($p = 0.06$), and 38% ($p = 0.03$), respectively). The addition of an IS[TM] patch to

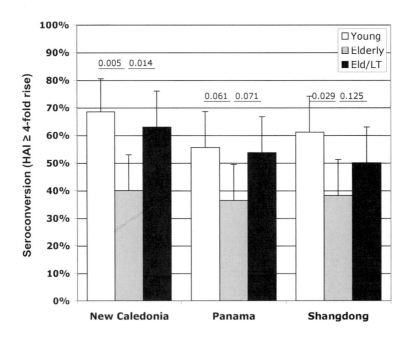

Figure I5.5 Seroconversion rates for A/New Caledonia, A/Panama, and B/Shandong following LT immunostimulation of intramuscular influenza vaccination in the elderly. Healthy young or elderly (≥ 60 years old) subjects were dosed at day 0 with influenza vaccine intramuscularly and their serum was assessed for HAI titers at day 2I. A third group of elderly subjects was dosed intramuscularly and an LT patch was applied near the vaccination site. The rates of seroconversion, or a four-fold rise in serum antibody, are shown for each strain in the vaccine, along with the significance of comparisons between groups. (Reprinted from Frech, S.A., Kenney, R.T., Spyr, C.A., Lazar, H., Viret, J.F., Herzog, C., Gluck, R., and Glenn, G.M. (2005). Improved immune responses to influenza vaccination in the elderly using an immunostimulant patch. *Vaccine* 23, 946–950. Copyright 2005, with permission from Elsevier.)

the elderly improved these seroconversion rates to 63, 54, and 50%, respectively. The seroconversion rates in elderly volunteers receiving the patch were not significantly different from those in healthy adults, and represent a substantial absolute improvement in seroconversion of the elderly over those not receiving the patch. Seroprotection, the percentage of subjects achieving an HAI titer ≥ 1 : 40 postvaccination, was achieved in most subjects for the A/New Caledonia and A/Panama strains, and lower levels were seen for the B/Shandong, reflecting the relative naivety of subjects to this strain. The percent change in seroprotection rates following vaccination was highest for the healthy adults, followed by the group receiving an IS^{TM} patch. Overall, the IS^{TM} patch group improved the elderly seroprotection rates by 26, 20, and 16% compared to influenza vaccination alone for the A/New Caledonia, A/Panama, and B/Shandong

strains, respectively. The IS^{TM} patch appears to be a practical intervention that takes advantage of the highly competent skin immune system to enhance immune responses to influenza vaccination.

Systemic and mucosal responses

Despite the novel approach, the development of immune responses to TCI is similar to those induced by classic immunization by other routes. Serum antibodies can be induced by antigen delivered to the skin and are greatly augmented by the simple admixture with LT. Priming and boosting responses are readily identified. The use of bAREs by TCI can induce strong cell-mediated immunity to the coadministered antigens, resulting in increased cellular memory with a balanced T-helper cytokine profile and the development of antigen-specific CTLs (Hammond et al.,

2001b; Kahlon et al., 2003; Seo et al., 2003). Tracking antigen after delivery to the LCs may be difficult because of the extremely small amount of material that is required to elicit immune responses. However, cells from draining lymph nodes can be readily assayed for the presence of FITC after application to the skin. The addition of LT or CT to the solution applied to the skin caused the upregulation of surface-expressed CD86 as well as a simultaneous increase in the number of FITC-positive LCs in the draining node (Hammond et al., 2001a). There is a clear association between the site of skin application and the regional location of the node, suggesting that activated LCs migrate only to the draining lymph node where they can initiate a typical immune response and coordinate the development of T cell memory (Glenn et al., 2003).

The skin and mucosa share similar immune elements, including LCs, secretory organs, and the presence of secretory IgA, particularly in the sweat glands (Okada et al., 1988). Early studies showed that both IgG and IgA are stimulated in TCI with LT and CT as adjuvants (Glenn et al., 1998b). Topical application of bAREs and coadministered antigens, such as rCS6, tetanus, and herpes, induces mucosal antibodies (El-Ghorr et al., 2000; Glenn et al., 2000; Scharton-Kersten et al., 2000) as well as mucosal cellular responses (Gockel et al., 2000; Kenney et al., 2004). Mice immunized transcutaneously with CT produce anti-CT neutralizing IgG and IgA antibodies in the stool and in pulmonary secretions (Glenn et al., 1998b). Antigen-specific ASCs can be detected in the vaginal mucosa of mice immunized topically using CT and TTx (Gockel et al., 2000) and in the serum of humans vaccinated with LTG192 and rCS6 (Güereña-Burgueño et al., 2002). TCI can also augment the mucosal immune response to oral vaccination with *Vibrio cholerae* expressing CTB (John et al., 2002). In addition, mucosal anti-LT IgG and IgA antibodies were detected in humans immunized topically with LT, consistent with the repeated observations in mice

(Glenn et al., 2000). Antibodies detected in TCI studies may represent transudates into the mucosa, yet recent data have shown that anti-LT antibodies detected in the stool and lung wash contain the secretory component of IgA, indicating that local mucosal antibody production occurs (Yu et al., 2002). Taken together, these data suggest that antibody-secreting cells and possibly memory T cells have homed to the mucosa to generate functional immune responses in the gut.

■ Delivery optimization

The SC functions as a barrier for the penetration of fluids, large molecules, particles, and microbes. Transdermal delivery of drugs to the systemic circulation is generally limited to a maximum of 500 kDa, even with strategies to enhance penetration. On the other hand, the target for protein delivery in TCI is the LCs that reside in the epidermis, so the larger molecules have a much shorter distance to travel to have their effect. Hydration alone results in swelling of the keratinocytes and creation of aqueous channels in intercellular spaces (Roberts and Walker, 1993) that can allow antigens into the skin to initiate an immune response (Glenn et al., 1998a). Preclinical studies of relatively simple techniques to physically disrupt the SC, such as with abrasives used clinically to improve conductivity for electrocardiograms, have shown marked improvements in antibody generation (Glenn and Alving, 1999b; Glenn et al., 2003). The same materials used in conjunction with hydrating solution improve antigen delivery, creating a single simple pretreatment swab for use prior to patch placement. Studies in our laboratory have explored this concept and demonstrated its feasibility and effect on the delivery of both an antigen and adjuvant. In preclinical studies, the optimized application of a simple, wet patch compares well with the efficiency of adjuvanted, injected antigen (Figure 15.2). Other groups have developed microenhancer array devices (Mikszta et al.,

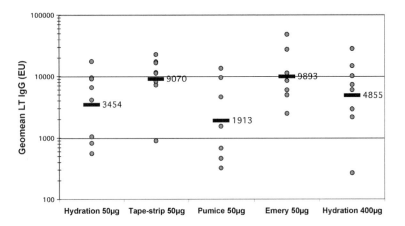

Figure 15.6 Response to various skin pretreatments. Disruption of the stratum corneum can augment delivery of proteins to the Langerhans cells to provide substantial improvements in antibody titers. Eight subjects per group were dosed at days 0 and 21 with 50 μg or 400 μg LT following pretreatment with hydration alone, tape stripping, pumice pads, or emery paper. Serum LT-specific IgG measured by ELISA is shown after the second dose at day 42 and the geometric mean is calculated.

2002) to disrupt the SC or epidermal powder jet injectors to penetrate the space with similar effect (Partidos, 2003; Chen et al., 2004; Dean and Chen, 2004).

Quantitation of the antibody response has been the most useful measure of patch delivery, since the proteins are unable to traverse into the dermis and functional activation of APCs is the target for this approach; however, interspecies differences in the skin have made the development of animal models difficult. Hairless guinea pigs have similar SC and epidermal thickness, so they can be used to study the histology of mild abrasives or devices to disrupt the SC, but the high lipid content of their skin inhibits the delivery of proteins and makes them unsuitable for vaccination studies. Human SC is relatively easy to disrupt and, despite the differences in the thickness of the epidermal layers, murine studies show similar responsiveness so mice have been useful for screening pretreatment methods for immune responses (Scharton-Kersten et al., 2000; Yu et al., 2002; Guebre-Xabier et al., 2003). Hairy guinea pigs are somewhat more difficult to work with, although their larger size and SC thickness can make them useful for modeling certain types of pretreatment strategies and the study

of the immunogenicity of later stage vaccine products. Hair follicles have been suggested to play an important role in topical administration, but this hypothesis would not explain the consistent enhancement seen with SC disruption. The likelihood that follicles are not significant antigen transit pathways is supported by the observation that out-bred CD1 mice with normal hair follicle development, and hairless SKH mice (same genetic background) with sparse, vestigial follicles respond equally well to topical immunization and disruption of the SC (Glenn et al., 2003).

Clinical studies have been conducted to evaluate skin pretreatment methods for optimization of the response. In early studies with no pretreatment, up to 500 μg LT was needed to show immunogenicity (Glenn et al., 2000). Figure 15.6 shows the effect of simple hydration or mild disruption of the SC on the delivery of LT after two doses using commercially available medical products. Following pretreatment, all groups were vaccinated twice, at days 0 and 21, with a TCI patch composed of gauze containing 50 μg LT (groups 1–4) or 400 μg LT (group 5) that was then covered with an adhesive. No significant adverse events were observed after either vaccination, apart from a mild self-limited maculopapular rash that occasionally developed with or without associated pruritis at the site of vaccination. Baseline geometric mean LT IgG values ranged from 280 to 430 EU. All subjects seroconverted with at least a two-fold rise in LT IgG titer, apart from one subject each in groups 1, 3, and 5. Hydration with glycerol/IPA alone produced a moderate response at the lower dose of 50 μg LT (group 1), but there was little added dose response with 400 μg LT (group 5). Pretreatment of the skin with tape stripping followed by hydration with glycerol/IPA (group 2) or with hydration followed by ten strokes of emery paper (group 4) led to nearly a three-fold improvement in immunogenicity compared to the same dose with hydration alone, suggesting improved LT delivery. Interestingly, treatment with a pumice pad seemed to decrease the efficiency of LT delivery, perhaps as a result of particles filling the spaces in the SC that did get disrupted. The data indicate that at least an eight-fold reduction in the dose of LT is possible with mild emery abrasion or tape stripping. More recent trials have demonstrated similar immunogenicity with as little as 45 μg LT with the use of a nonwoven abrasive pad and a weaker, but measurable, response with 15 μg LT. In general, we have seen geometric mean LT IgG titers of 5,000–10,000 EU or more and seroconversion in over 90% of subjects with 45–50 μg LT dosed twice by TCI using various pretreatment methodologies (R.T. Kenney et al., unpublished observations).

◼ Regulatory considerations

Worldwide regulatory guidance on the development and testing of vaccines has expanded significantly in the past decade. In general, vaccines are held to the same standards as other drugs and biologics, in that the purity, safety, potency, and effectiveness of the products must be demonstrated before licensure. Advice with respect to adjuvants has been relatively sparse, although a European guidance document on this topic was recently finalized (EMEA, 2005). Adjuvants are not licensed separately, but since they are active they essentially define the products they complement as combinations. They require the same level of detail in characterization and description of the quality in manufacture as any other drug substance. The mechanism of association with the antigen needs to be studied and described in detail, as well as the dose and necessity for each component. Nonclinical toxicity and clinical testing may need to be done with the adjuvant alone as well as in combination with the antigen. Dose-finding studies should be performed in the target population if possible, although studies in healthy adults may suffice. Confirmatory studies defining safety and efficacy may need to be done in several populations, depending on the scope of intended use. The regulatory requirements in the USA are similar, although there are no guidance documents available specifically addressing the situation with adjuvants. In addition to the regulations found in 21 CFR 312 and 610, products are generally dealt with on a case-by-case basis.

The use of bAREs as adjuvants, whether by TCI or some other route of administration, would thus be expected to be regulated in the same fashion. As new vaccines, the route to licensure depends on the specific circumstances for the indication and the feasibility of conducting an efficacy study, as outlined in a recent European guidance (EMEA, 1999). In some situations, such as the development of a vaccine for almost any biowarfare agent, the conduct of an efficacy trial would not be possible. The "animal rule" has been established to help demonstrate the utility of this type of vaccine for humans (Horne et al., 2004). While adjuvants typically enhance the immunogenicity and presumably efficacy of a new moiety, safety is the primary concern for new adjuvants. LT was the adjuvant in an intranasal influenza vaccine licensed in Switzerland and Germany, but this was withdrawn when an association with Bell's palsy was found (Mutsch et al., 2004). Extensive efforts were made to study the safety in animal models;

however, a causal relationship could not be demonstrated (Zurbriggen et al., 2003). However, application of LT to the skin in TCI appears to be safe, even in high doses, as demonstrated in multiple clinical trials (reviewed in Glenn et al., 2003). As with any other vaccine, regulatory approval of patch vaccination will depend on the demonstration of the safety of the final product in a representative population and its effectiveness through the use of a surrogate marker or efficacy studies.

■ Comparison with other skin delivery technologies

Several groups have noted the potential for robust responses with delivery of vaccines to the skin. PowderJect (now part of Powdermed) has developed an epidermal powder immunization (EPI) technology that delivers vaccine antigens or DNA plasmids on microscopic beads or with sugar excipients formulated as particles, and recently reported the results of the first clinical trial (Dean and Chen, 2004). Theoretically, any vaccine that is stable as a dried powder or in a particulate form can be delivered using EPI, and PowderJect has successfully induced significant immune responses with a number of plasmids that contain genes of interest (Fynan et al., 1993; Schirmbeck et al., 1995; Chen et al., 2000; Yoshida et al., 2000) as well as recombinant proteins (Chen et al., 2001b, 2002; Osorio et al., 2003) and inactivated viruses (Chen et al., 2001b, 2003; Dean and Chen, 2004). Both humoral and cellular immunity can be induced in responses that are protective against experimental challenge (Chen et al., 2000, 2003, 2004) and the addition of adjuvants such as QS-21 (Chen et al., 2003), CpG DNA (Chen et al., 2001b; Osorio et al., 2003), CT and LT (Arrington et al., 2002; Osorio et al., 2003), or LTR72 (Chen et al., 2004) to these formulated antigen vaccines significantly enhances the immune responses.

Progress in moving epidermal DNA vaccination into the clinic has been slow, although the potential to enhance CTL responses is appealing. Two reports from PowderJect tested the safety and immunogenicity of hepatitis B DNA vaccination using their needle-free system to deliver gold particles coated with DNA. In the first study, a dozen healthy volunteers showed mild to moderate local reactions to $1–4\,\mu g$ DNA given three times (Roy et al., 2000). While all volunteers developed seroprotective responses ($\geq 10\,mIU/ml$), the level of peak antibody production was 4- to 10-fold lower than what is reported for the licensed recombinant vaccine (Van Damme et al., 1989; West, 1989); however, the eight subjects that received a subsequent vaccination with recombinant HBsAg developed elevated antibody responses suggesting they had been fully primed. All volunteers had detectable IFN-γ-secreting cells by ELISPOT and HLA-A2 positive volunteers also had antigen-specific CD8+ T cells as assessed by peptide tetramers that secreted IFN-γ and a functional antigen-specific CTL response. The second study was conducted in eleven hepatitis B vaccine nonresponders and five poor responders using $4\,\mu g$ of the plasmid DNA encoding the HBsAg dried onto gold particles given epidermally by a jet injector in one or three doses (Rottinghaus et al., 2003). Local reactions to the vaccine were mild and well tolerated. Three subjects had no response, but the rest had at least a peak titer $\geq 10\,mIU/ml$ and three had titers >1000.

Electroporation (EP) in the context of vaccination involves the application of a high-voltage electric current across the SC, leading to a reversible breakdown of the membrane and the formation of pores that can allow macromolecules to pass into the deeper epidermis (Prausnitz et al., 1993). Pulse electric fields in the range 50–1000 V for micro- or millisecond periods have been shown to enhance the permeation of a broad range of compounds including small drugs (Vanbever et al., 1994), oligonucleotides (Zewert et al., 1995), proteins (Zewert et al., 1999), and drug-loaded microparticles (Prausnitz et al., 1996). While the concept seems amenable to use with vaccines, little preclinical and no clinical data have been published. EP can enhance the gene expression of intradermally injected DNA in both mice and human skin xenografts on nude mice (Zhang et al., 2002). EP was used to enhance delivery of topically applied diphtheria toxoid and a myristylated hepatitis B peptide (Misra et al., 1999). The EP route elicited higher responses to the peptide than intradermal immunization, but lower responses to diphtheria toxoid.

Other technologies are emerging as potential means for delivery of antigens and adjuvants or disruption of the SC. Sonophoresis uses ultrasound waves to perturb the SC and facilitate the permeation of small molecules (Mitragotri et al., 1995; Weimann and Wu, 2002); however, the applicability to vaccination needs to be further investigated. Microporation by means of heated probes to vaporize the SC has been shown to enhance immune responses to adenoviral-based vaccines 10- to 100-fold in mice (Bramson et al., 2003). Microneedles can be used as skin pretreatment followed by topical application of plasmid to enhance gene activity (Mikszta et al., 2002) or application of recombinant proteins to give protective responses against anthrax (Mikszta et al., 2005). A coated microneedle technology called macroflux may allow rapid delivery of antigen and adjuvant to the epidermis. A study in hairless guinea pigs found that with an average penetration of $100\,\mu m$ up to $20\,\mu g$ ovalbumin could be delivered in as little as 5 seconds (Matriano et al., 2002). These and other technologies being developed to enhance skin delivery of macromolecules have the potential greatly to facilitate the response to vaccines delivered topically.

■ Summary

The skin is an active site of complex interactions with the environment involving stimulation of the resident keratinocytes as well as the transient populations of immune cells. The body has physical permeation barriers to retain hydration and exclude macromolecules and microorganisms. Permeation of these barriers through physical or chemical means allows the safe delivery of antigens and adjuvants with TCI that mimic pathogens to induce typical vaccine responses without the use of needles that would bypass this rich immune setting. New insights into the mechanism of action of the most potent adjuvants, the bAREs, may lead to refinement of the approach and the development of novel mutants that could minimize toxicity yet retain adjuvanticity. Progress on SC disruption techniques can enhance the efficiency of delivery, theoretically allowing reduced cost and lower risk of adverse effects. Optimization of delivery and product development are challenges that remain to be accomplished before licensure, yet the basic biological principles of protein macromolecule delivery resulting in immune responses have been clearly established.

■ Acknowledgments

The authors thank David Flyer, Jianmei Yu, Mimi Guebre-Xabier, and Guoling Xi for research support, Wanda Hardy for administrative assistance, and Jeff Cogen for review and comments on the manuscript.

■ References

Arrington, J., Braun, R.P., Dong, L., Fuller, D.H., Macklin, M.D., Umlauf, S.W., Wagner, S.J., Wu, M.S., Payne, L.G., and Haynes, J.R. (2002). Plasmid vectors encoding cholera toxin or the heat-labile enterotoxin from *Escherichia coli* are strong adjuvants for DNA vaccines. *J. Virol.* 76, 4536–4546.

Baca-Estrada, M.E., Foldvari, M., Ewen, C., Badea, I., and Babiuk, L.A. (2000). Effects of IL-12 on immune responses induced by transcutaneous immunization with antigens formulated in a novel lipid-based biphasic delivery system. *Vaccine* 18, 1847–1854.

Bagley, K.C., Abdelwahab, S.F., Tuskan, R.G., Fouts, T.R., and Lewis, G.K. (2002). Cholera toxin and heat-labile enterotoxin activate human monocyte-derived dendritic cells and dominantly inhibit cytokine production through a cyclic AMP-dependent pathway. *Infect. Immun.* 70, 5533–5539.

Bancherau, J. and Steinman, R.M. (1998). Dendritic cells and the control of immunity. *Nature* 392, 245–252.

Beignon, A.S., Briand, J.P., Rappuoli, R., Muller, S., and Partidos, C.D. (2002). The LTR72 mutant of heat-labile enterotoxin of *Escherichia coli* enhances the ability of peptide antigens to elicit CD4(+) T cells and secrete gamma interferon after coapplication onto bare skin. *Infect. Immun.* 70, 3012–3019.

Belyakov, I.M., Hammond, S.A., Ahlers, J.D., Glenn, G.M., and Berzofsky, J.A. (2004). Transcutaneous immunization induces mucosal CTLs and protective immunity by migration of primed skin dendritic cells. *J. Clin. Invest.* 113, 998–1007.

Berman, B., Chen, V.L., France, D.S., Dotz, W.I., and Petroni, G. (1983). Anatomical mapping of epidermal Langerhans cell densities in adults. *Br. J. Dermatol.* 109, 553–558.

Berry, L.J., Hickey, D.K., Skelding, K.A., Bao, S., Rendina, A.M., Hansbro, P.M., Gockel, C.M., and Beagley, K.W. (2004). Transcutaneous immunization with combined cholera toxin and CpG adjuvant protects against *Chlamydia muridarum* genital tract infection. *Infect. Immun.* 72, 1019–1028.

Bhushan, M., Cumberbatch, M., Dearman, R.J., Andrew, S.M., Kimber, I., and Griffiths, C.E. (2002). Tumour necrosis factor-alpha-induced migration of human Langerhans cells: the influence of ageing. *Br. J. Dermatol.* 146, 32–40.

Bramson, J., Dayball, K., Evelegh, C., Wan, Y.H., Page, D., and Smith, A. (2003). Enabling topical immunization via microporation: a novel method for pain-free and needle-free delivery of adenovirus-based vaccines. *Gene Ther.* 10, 251–260.

Braun, M.C., He, J., Wu, C.Y., and Kelsall, B.L. (1999). Cholera toxin suppresses interleukin (IL)-12 production and IL-12 receptor beta1 and beta2 chain expression. *J. Exp. Med.* 189, 541–552.

Chen, D., Endres, R.L., Erickson, C.A., Weis, K.F., McGregor, M.W., Kawaoka, Y., and Payne, L.G. (2000). Epidermal immunization by a needle-free powder delivery technology: immunogenicity of influenza vaccine and protection in mice. *Nature Med.* 6, 1187–1190.

Chen, D., Erickson, C.A., Endres, R.L., Periwal, S.B., Chu, Q., Shu, C., Maa, Y.F., and Payne, L.G. (2001a). Adjuvantation of epidermal powder immunization. *Vaccine* 19, 2908–2917.

Chen, D., Weis, K.F., Chu, Q., Erickson, C., Endres, R., Lively, C.R., Osorio, J., and Payne, L.G. (2001b). Epidermal powder immunization induces both cytotoxic T-lymphocyte and antibody responses to protein antigens of influenza and hepatitis B viruses. *J. Virol.* 75, 11630–11640.

Chen, D., Zuleger, C., Chu, Q., Maa, Y.F., Osorio, J., and Payne, L.G. (2002). Epidermal powder immunization with a recombinant HIV gp120 targets Langerhans cells and induces enhanced immune responses. *AIDS Res. Hum. Retroviruses* 18, 715–722.

Chen, D., Endres, R., Maa, Y.F., Kensil, C.R., Whitaker-Dowling, P., Trichel, A., Youngner, J.S., and Payne, L.G. (2003). Epidermal powder immunization of mice and monkeys with an influenza vaccine. *Vaccine* 21, 2830–2836.

Chen, D., Burger, M., Chu, Q., Endres, R., Zuleger, C., Dean, H., and Payne, L.G. (2004). Epidermal powder

immunization: cellular and molecular mechanisms for enhancing vaccine immunogenicity. *Virus Res.* 103, 147–153.

Clements, J.D., Hartzog, N.M., and Lyon, F.L. (1988). Adjuvant activity of *Escherichia coli* heat-labile enterotoxin and effect on the induction of oral tolerance in mice to unrelated protein antigens. *Vaccine* 6, 269–277.

Cumberbatch, M., Dearman, R.J., and Kimber, I. (1997). Langerhans cells require signals from both tumour necrosis factor-alpha and interleukin-1 beta for migration. *Immunology* 92, 388–395.

Cumberbatch, M., Griffiths, C.E., Tucker, S.C., Dearman, R.J., and Kimber, I. (1999). Tumour necrosis factor-alpha induces Langerhans cell migration in humans. *Br. J. Dermatol.* 141, 192–200.

Cumberbatch, M., Dearman, R.J., Antonopoulos, C., Groves, R.W., and Kimber, I. (2001). Interleukin (IL)-18 induces Langerhans cell migration by a tumour necrosis factor-alpha- and IL-1beta-dependent mechanism. *Immunology* 102, 323–330.

Cumberbatch, M., Dearman, R.J., Griffiths, C.E., and Kimber, I. (2003). Epidermal Langerhans cell migration and sensitisation to chemical allergens. *Apmis* 111, 797–804.

Daniels, N.A., Neimann, J., Karpati, A., Parashar, U.D., Greene, K.D., Wells, J.G., Srivastava, A., Tauxe, R.V., Mintz, E.D., and Quick, R. (2000). Traveler's diarrhea at sea: three outbreaks of waterborne enterotoxigenic *Escherichia coli* on cruise ships. *J. Infect. Dis.* 181, 1491–1495.

De Haan, L. and Hirst, T.R. (2004). Cholera toxin: a paradigm for multi-functional engagement of cellular mechanisms. *Mol. Memb. Bio.* 21, 77–92.

De Haan, L., Verweij, W.R., Feil, I.K., Holtrop, M., Hol, W.G., Agsteribbe, E., and Wilschut, J. (1998). Role of GM1 binding in the mucosal immunogenicity and adjuvant activity of the *Escherichia coli* heat-labile enterotoxin and its B subunit. *Immunology* 94, 424–430.

De Haan, L., Holtrop, M., Verweij, W.R., Agsteribbe, E., and Wilschut, J. (1999). Mucosal immunogenicity and adjuvant activity of the recombinant A subunit of the *Escherichia coli* heat-labile enterotoxin. *Immunology* 97, 706–713.

Dean, H.J. and Chen, D. (2004). Epidermal powder immunization against influenza. *Vaccine* 23, 681–686.

Dickinson, B.L. and Clements, J.D. (1995). Dissociation of *Escherichia coli* heat-labile enterotoxin adjuvanticity from ADP-ribosyltransferase activity. *Infect. Immun.* 63, 1617–1623.

El-Ghorr, A.A., Williams, R.M., Heap, C., and Norval, M. (2000). Transcutaneous immunisation with herpes simplex virus stimulates immunity in mice. *FEMS Immunol. Med. Microbiol.* 29, 255–261.

Elias, P.M., Menon, G.K., Grayson, S., and Brown, B.E. (1988). Membrane structural alterations in murine stratum corneum: relationship to the localization of polar lipids and phospholipases. *J. Invest. Dermatol.* 91, 3–10.

EMEA (1997). CPMP Note for Guidance on Harmonisation of Requirements for Influenza Vaccines, CPMP/BWP/

214/96. European Agency for the Evaluation of Medicinal Products, Human Medicines Evaluation Unit, London.

EMEA (1999). CPMP Note for Guidance on Clinical Evaluation of New Vaccines, CPMP/EWP/463/97. European Agency for the Evaluation of Medicinal Products, Human Medicines Evaluation Unit, London.

EMEA (2005). CPMP Guideline on Adjuvants in Vaccines for Human Use, CHMP/VEG/134716/2004. European Medicines Agency Evaluation of Medicines for Human Use, London.

Fan, E., O'Neal, C.J., Mitchell, D.D., Robien, M.A., Zhang, Z., Pickens, J.C., Tan, X.J., Korotkov, K., Roach, C., Krumm, B., Verlinde, C.L., Merritt, E.A., and Hol, W.G. (2004). Structural biology and structure-based inhibitor design of cholera toxin and heat-labile enterotoxin. *Int. J. Med. Microbiol.* 294, 217–223.

Fishman, P.H. and Orlandi, P.A. (2003). Cholera toxin internalization and intoxication. *J. Cell Sci.* 116, 431–432; author reply 432–433.

Frech, S.A., Kenney, R.T., Spyr, C.A., Lazar, H., Viret, J.F., Herzog, C., Gluck, R., and Glenn, G.M. (2005). Improved immune responses to influenza vaccination in the elderly using an immunostimulant patch. *Vaccine* 23, 946–950.

Freytag, L.C. and Clements, J.D. (1999). Bacterial toxins as mucosal adjuvants. *Curr. Top. Microbiol. Immunol.* 236, 215–236.

Fynan, E.F., Webster, R.G., Fuller, D.H., Haynes, J.R., Santoro, J.C., and Robinson, H.L. (1993). DNA vaccines: protective immunizations by parenteral, mucosal, and gene-gun inoculations. *Proc. Natl. Acad. Sci. USA* 90, 11478–11482.

Girod, A., Storrie, B., Simpson, J.C., Johannes, L., Goud, B., Roberts, L.M., Lord, J.M., Nilsson, T., and Pepperkok, R. (1999). Evidence for a COP-I-independent transport route from the Golgi complex to the endoplasmic reticulum. *Nature Cell Biol.* 1, 423–430.

Glenn, G.M. and Alving, C.R. (1999a) Adjuvant for transcutaneous immunization. US Patent No. 5,980,898. United States of America as represented by the US Army Medical Research & Material Command, Washington, DC.

Glenn, G.M. and Alving, C.R. (1999b) Use of penetration enhancers and barrier disruption agents to enhance the transcutaneous immune response induced by ADP-ribosylating exotoxin. European Patent No. 1061951.

Glenn, G.M., Rao, M., Matyas, G.R., and Alving, C.R. (1998a). Skin immunization made possible by cholera toxin. *Nature* 391, 851.

Glenn, G.M., Scharton-Kersten, T., Vassell, R., Mallett, C.P., Hale, T.L., and Alving, C.R. (1998b). Transcutaneous immunization with cholera toxin protects mice against lethal mucosal toxin challenge. *J. Immunol.* 161, 3211–3214.

Glenn, G.M., Scharton-Kersten, T., Vassell, R., Matyas, G.R., and Alving, C.R. (1999). Transcutaneous immunization with bacterial ADP-ribosylating exotoxins as antigens and adjuvants. *Infect. Immun.* 67, 1100–1106.

Glenn, G.M., Taylor, D.N., Li, X., Frankel, S., Montemarano, A., and Alving, C.R. (2000). Transcutaneous immunization: a human vaccine delivery strategy using a patch. *Nature Med.* 6, 1403–1406.

Glenn, G.M., Kenney, R.T., Ellingsworth, L.R., Frech, S.A., Hammond, S.A., and Zoeteweij, J.P. (2003). Transcutaneous immunization and immunostimulant strategies: capitalizing on the immunocompetence of the skin. *Expert Rev. Vaccines* 2, 253–267.

Glenn, G.M., Flyer, D.C., Al-Khalili, M., and Ellingsworth, L.R. (2005). In Moingeon, P. (Ed) *Vaccines: Frontiers in Design and Development.* Horizon Scientific Press, Wymondham, UK, pp. 81–104.

Gluck, R., Mischler, R., Durrer, P., Furer, E., Lang, A.B., Herzog, C., and Cryz, S.J., Jr. (2000). Safety and immunogenicity of intranasally administered inactivated trivalent virosome-formulated influenza vaccine containing *Escherichia coli* heat-labile toxin as a mucosal adjuvant. *J. Infect. Dis.* 181, 1129–1132.

Gockel, C.M., Bao, S., and Beagley, K.W. (2000). Transcutaneous immunization induces mucosal and systemic immunity: a potent method for targeting immunity to the female reproductive tract. *Mol. Immunol.* 37, 537–544.

Godefroy, S., Goestch, L., Plotnicky-Gilquin, H., Nguyen, T.N., Schmitt, D., Staquet, M.J., and Corvaia, N. (2003). Immunization onto shaved skin with a bacterial enterotoxin adjuvant protects mice against respiratory syncytial virus (RSV). *Vaccine* 21, 1665–1671.

Guebre-Xabier, M., Hammond, S.A., Epperson, D.E., Yu, J., Ellingsworth, L., and Glenn, G.M. (2003). Immunostimulant patch containing heat-labile enterotoxin from *Escherichia coli* enhances immune responses to injected influenza virus vaccine through activation of skin dendritic cells. *J. Virol.* 77, 5218–5225.

Guebre-Xabier, M., Hammond, S.A., Ellingsworth, L.R., and Glenn, G.M. (2004). Immunostimulant patch enhances immune responses to influenza virus vaccine in aged mice. *J. Virol.* 78, 7610–7618.

Guidry, J.J., Cardenas, L., Cheng, E., and Clements, J.D. (1997). Role of receptor binding in toxicity, immunogenicity, and adjuvanticity of *Escherichia coli* heat-labile enterotoxin. *Infect. Immun.* 65, 4943–4950.

Güereña-Burgueño, F., Hall, E.R., Taylor, D.N., Cassels, F.J., Scott, D.A., Wolf, M.K., Roberts, Z.J., Nesterova, G.V., Alving, C.R., and Glenn, G.M. (2002). Safety and immunogenicity of a prototype enterotoxigenic *Escherichia coli* vaccine administered transcutaneously. *Infect. Immun.* 70, 1874–1880.

Hak, E., Buskens, E., van Essen, G.A., de Bakker, D.H., Grobbee, D.E., Tacken, M.A., van Hout, B.A., and Verheij, T.J. (2005). Clinical effectiveness of influenza vaccination in persons younger than 65 years with high-risk medical conditions: the PRISMA study. *Arch. Intern. Med.* 165, 274–280.

Hammond, S.A., Guebre-Xabier, M., Yu, J., and Glenn, G.M. (2001a). Transcutaneous immunization: an emerging route of immunization and potent immunostimulation strategy. *Crit. Rev. Ther. Drug Carrier Syst.* 18, 503–526.

Hammond, S.A., Walwender, D., Alving, C.R., and Glenn, G.M. (2001b). Transcutaneous immunization: T cell responses and boosting of existing immunity. *Vaccine* 19, 2701–2707.

Holmgren, J. (1973). Comparison of the tissue receptors for *Vibrio cholerae* and *Escherichia coli* enterotoxins by means of gangliosides and natural cholera toxoid. *Infect. Immun.* 8, 851–859.

Holmgren, J., Czerkinsky, C., Eriksson, K., and Mharandi, A. (2003). Mucosal immunisation and adjuvants: a brief overview of recent advances and challenges. *Vaccine* 21 (Suppl. 2), S89–S95.

Horne, A.D., Clifford, J., Goldenthal, K.L., Kleppinger, C., and Lachenbruch, P.A. (2004). Preventive vaccines against bioterrorism: evaluation of efficacy and safety. *Vaccine* 23, 84–90.

Huerta, M., Grotto, I., Gdalevich, M., Mimouni, D., Gavrieli, B., Yavzori, M., Cohen, D., and Shpilberg, O. (2000). A waterborne outbreak of gastroenteritis in the Golan Heights due to enterotoxigenic *Escherichia coli*. *Infection* 28, 267–271.

John, M., Bridges, E.A., Miller, A.O., Calderwood, S.B., and Ryan, E.T. (2002). Comparison of mucosal and systemic humoral immune responses after transcutaneous and oral immunization strategies. *Vaccine* 20, 2720–2726.

Kahlon, R., Hu, Y., Orteu, C.H., Kifayet, A., Trudeau, J.D., Tan, R., and Dutz, J.P. (2003). Optimization of epicutaneous immunization for the induction of CTL. *Vaccine* 21, 2890–2899.

Kenney, R., Yu, J., Guebre-Xabier, M., Lambert, A., Heller, B., Ellingsworth, L., Eyles, J., Williamson, E.D., and Glenn, G. (2004). Induction of protective immunity against lethal anthrax challenge with a patch. *J. Infect. Dis.* 190, 774–782.

Kenney, R.T., and Edelman, R. (2004). In Levine, M.M. (Ed) *New Generation Vaccines*, 3rd edn. Marcel Dekker, New York, pp. 213–223.

Kotloff, K.L., Sztein, M.B., Wasserman, S.S., Losonsky, G.A., DiLorenzo, S.C., and Walker, R.I. (2001). Safety and immunogenicity of oral inactivated whole-cell *Helicobacter pylori* vaccine with adjuvant among volunteers with or without subclinical infection. *Infect. Immun.* 69, 3581–3590.

Kuziemko, G.M., Stroh, M., and Stevens, R.C. (1996). Cholera toxin binding affinity and specificity for gangliosides determined by surface plasmon resonance. *Biochemistry* 35, 6375–6384.

Lencer, W.I., Constable, C., Moe, S., Jobling, M.G., Webb, H.M., Ruston, S., Madara, J.L., Hirst, T.R., and Holmes, R.K. (1995). Targeting of cholera toxin and *Escherichia coli* heat labile toxin in polarized epithelia: role of COOH-terminal KDEL. *J. Cell Biol.* 131, 951–962.

Lycke, N. (1997). The mechanism of cholera toxin adjuvanticity. *Res. Immunol.* 148, 504–520.

Lycke, N., Tsuji, T., and Holmgren, J. (1992). The adjuvant effect of *Vibrio cholerae* and *Escherichia coli* heat-labile enterotoxins is linked to their ADP-ribosyltransferase activity. *Eur. J. Immunol.* 22, 2277–2281.

MacKenzie, C.R., Hirama, T., Lee, K.K., Altman, E., and Young, N.M. (1997). Quantitative analysis of bacterial toxin affinity and specificity for glycolipid receptors by surface plasmon resonance. *J. Biol. Chem.* 272, 5533–5538.

Majoul, I., Sohn, K., Wieland, F.T., Pepperkok, R., Pizza, M., Hillemann, J., and Soling, H.D. (1998). KDEL receptor (Erd2p)-mediated retrograde transport of the cholera toxin A subunit from the Golgi involves COPI, p23, and the COOH terminus of Erd2p. *J. Cell Biol.* 143, 601–612.

Majoul, I.V., Bastiaens, P.I., and Soling, H.D. (1996). Transport of an external Lys-Asp-Glu-Leu (KDEL) protein from the plasma membrane to the endoplasmic reticulum: studies with cholera toxin in Vero cells. *J. Cell Biol.* 133, 777–789.

Marchisio, P.C., Bondanza, S., Cremona, O., Cancedda, R., and De Luca, M. (1991). Polarized expression of integrin receptors (alpha 6 beta 4, alpha 2 beta 1, alpha 3 beta 1, and alpha v beta 5) and their relationship with the cytoskeleton and basement membrane matrix in cultured human keratinocytes. *J. Cell Biol.* 112, 761–773.

Martin, M., Sharpe, A., Clements, J.D., and Michalek, S.M. (2002). Role of B7 costimulatory molecules in the adjuvant activity of the heat-labile enterotoxin of *Escherichia coli*. *J. Immunol.* 169, 1744–1752.

Matousek, M.P., Nedrud, J.G., Cieplak, W., Jr., and Harding, C.V. (1998). Inhibition of class II major histocompatibility complex antigen processing by *Escherichia coli* heat-labile enterotoxin requires an enzymatically active A subunit. *Infect. Immun.* 66, 3480–3484.

Matriano, J.A., Cormier, M., Johnson, J., Young, W.A., Buttery, M., Nyam, K., and Daddona, P.E. (2002). Macroflux microprojection array patch technology: a new and efficient approach for intracutaneous immunization. *Pharm. Res.* 19, 63–70.

Mekalanos, J.J., Collier, R.J., and Romig, W.R. (1979). Enzymic activity of cholera toxin: II. Relationships to proteolytic processing, disulfide bond reduction, and subunit composition. *J. Biol. Chem.* 254, 5855–5861.

Michetti, P., Kreiss, C., Kotloff, K.L., Porta, N., Blanco, J.L., Bachmann, D., Herranz, M., Saldinger, P.F., Corthesy-Theulaz, I., Losonsky, G., Nichols, R., Simon, J., Stolte, M., Ackerman, S., Monath, T.P., and Blum, A.L. (1999). Oral immunization with urease and *Escherichia coli* heat-labile enterotoxin is safe and immunogenic in *Helicobacter pylori*-infected adults. *Gastroenterology* 116, 804–812.

Mikszta, J.A., Alarcon, J.B., Brittingham, J.M., Sutter, D.E., Pettis, R.J., and Harvey, N.G. (2002). Improved genetic immunization via micromechanical disruption of skin-barrier function and targeted epidermal delivery. *Nature Med.* 8, 415–419.

Mikszta, J.A., Sullivan, V.J., Dean, C., Waterston, A.M., Alarcon, J.B., Dekker, J.P., 3rd, Brittingham, J.M., Huang, J., Hwang, C.R., Ferriter, M., Jiang, G., Mar, K., Saikh, K.U., Stiles, B.G., Roy, C.J., Ulrich, R.G., and Harvey, N.G. (2005). Protective immunization against inhalational anthrax: a comparison of minimally invasive delivery platforms. *J. Infect. Dis.* 191, 278–288.

Millar, D.G. and Hirst, T.R. (2001). Cholera toxin and *Escherichia coli* enterotoxin B-subunits inhibit macrophage-mediated antigen processing and presentation: evidence for antigen persistence in non-acidic recycling endosomal compartments. *Cell Microbiol.* 3, 311–329.

Misra, A., Ganga, S., and Upadhyay, P. (1999). Needle-free, non-adjuvanted skin immunization by electroporation-enhanced transdermal delivery of diphtheria toxoid and a candidate peptide vaccine against hepatitis B virus. *Vaccine* 18, 517–523.

Mitragotri, S., Blankschtein, D., and Langer, R. (1995). Ultrasound-mediated transdermal protein delivery. *Science* 269, 850–853.

Moll, R., Franke, W.W., Schiller, D.L., Geiger, B., and Krepler, R. (1982). The catalog of human cytokeratins: patterns of expression in normal epithelia, tumors and cultured cells. *Cell* 31, 11–24.

Montesano, R., Roth, J., Robert, A., and Orci, L. (1982). Non-coated membrane invaginations are involved in binding and internalization of cholera and tetanus toxins. *Nature* 296, 651–653.

Morganti, P., Ruocco, E., Wolf, R., and Ruocco, V. (2001). Percutaneous absorption and delivery systems. *Clin. Dermatol.* 19, 489–501.

Moss, J., Osborne, J.C., Jr., Fishman, P.H., Brewer, H.B., Jr., Vaughan, M., and Brady, R.O. (1977). Effect of gangliosides and substrate analogues on the hydrolysis of nicotinamide adenine dinucleotide by choleragen. *Proc. Natl. Acad. Sci. USA* 74, 74–78.

Murasko, D.M., Bernstein, E.D., Gardner, E.M., Gross, P., Munk, G., Dran, S., and Abrutyn, E. (2002). Role of humoral and cell-mediated immunity in protection from influenza disease after immunization of healthy elderly. *Exp. Gerontol.* 37, 427–439.

Mutsch, M., Zhou, W., Rhodes, P., Bopp, M., Chen, R.T., Linder, T., Spyr, C., and Steffen, R. (2004). Use of the inactivated intranasal influenza vaccine and the risk of Bell's palsy in Switzerland. *N. Engl. J. Med.* 350, 896–903.

O'Neal, C.J., Amaya, E.I., Jobling, M.G., Holmes, R.K., and Hol, W.G. (2004). Crystal structures of an intrinsically active cholera toxin mutant yield insight into the toxin activation mechanism. *Biochemistry* 43, 3772–3782.

Ohl, L., Mohaupt, M., Czeloth, N., Hintzen, G., Kiafard, Z., Zwirner, J., Blankenstein, T., Henning, G., and Forster, R. (2004). CCR7 governs skin dendritic cell migration under inflammatory and steady-state conditions. *Immunity* 21, 279–288.

Okada, T., Konishi, H., Ito, M., Nagura, H., and Asai, J. (1988). Identification of secretory immunoglobulin A in human sweat and sweat glands. *J. Invest. Dermatol.* 90, 648–651.

Olszewski, W.L., Grzelak, I., Ziolkowska, A., and Engeset, A. (1995). Immune cell traffic from blood through the normal human skin to lymphatics. *Clin. Dermatol.* 13, 473–483.

Orlandi, P.A. and Fishman, P.H. (1998). Filipin-dependent inhibition of cholera toxin: evidence for toxin internalization and activation through caveolae-like domains. *J. Cell Biol.* 141, 905–915.

Osorio, J.E., Zuleger, C.L., Burger, M., Chu, Q., Payne, L.G., and Chen, D. (2003). Immune responses to hepatitis B surface antigen following epidermal powder immunization. *Immunol. Cell Biol.* 81, 52–58.

Partidos, C.D. (2003). Delivering vaccines into the skin without needles and syringes. *Expert Rev. Vaccines* 2, 753–761.

Parton, R.G. (1994). Ultrastructural localization of gangliosides; GM1 is concentrated in caveolae. *J. Histochem. Cytochem.* 42, 155–166.

Parton, R.G. and Richards, A.A. (2003). Lipid rafts and caveolae as portals for endocytosis: new insights and common mechanisms. *Traffic* 4, 724–738.

Pentcheva-Hoang, T., Egen, J.G., Wojnoonski, K., and Allison, J.P. (2004). B7-1 and B7-2 selectively recruit CTLA-4 and CD28 to the immunological synapse. *Immunity* 21, 401–413.

Petrovska, L., Lopes, L., Simmons, C.P., Pizza, M., Dougan, G., and Chain, B.M. (2003). Modulation of dendritic cell endocytosis and antigen processing pathways by *Escherichia coli* heat-labile enterotoxin and mutant derivatives. *Vaccine* 21, 1445–1454.

Prausnitz, M.R., Bose, V.G., Langer, R., and Weaver, J.C. (1993). Electroporation of mammalian skin: a mechanism to enhance transdermal drug delivery. *Proc. Natl. Acad. Sci. USA* 90, 10504–10508.

Prausnitz, M.R., Gimm, J.A., Guy, R.H., Langer, R., Weaver, J.C., and Cullander, C. (1996). Imaging regions of transport across human stratum corneum during high-voltage and low-voltage exposures. *J. Pharm. Sci.* 85, 1363–1370.

Richards, C.M., Aman, A.T., Hirst, T.R., Hill, T.J., and Williams, N.A. (2001). Protective mucosal immunity to ocular herpes simplex virus type 1 infection in mice by using *Escherichia coli* heat-labile enterotoxin B subunit as an adjuvant. *J. Virol.* 75, 1664–1671.

Richardson, S.H., Giles, J.C., and Kruger, K.S. (1984). Sealed adult mice: new model for enterotoxin evaluation. *Infect. Immun.* 43, 482–486.

Roberts, M.S. and Walker, M. (1993) *Water, the Most Natural Penetration Enhancer*. Marcel Dekker, New York.

Rottinghaus, S.T., Poland, G.A., Jacobson, R.M., Barr, L.J., and Roy, M.J. (2003). Hepatitis B DNA vaccine induces protective antibody responses in human non-responders to conventional vaccination. *Vaccine* 21, 4604–4608.

Roy, M.J., Wu, M.S., Barr, L.J., Fuller, J.T., Tussey, L.G., Speller, S., Culp, J., Burkholder, J.K., Swain, W.F., Dixon, R.M., Widera, G., Vessey, R., King, A., Ogg, G., Gallimore, A., Haynes, J.R., and Heydenburg Fuller, D. (2000). Induction of antigen-specific CD8+ T cells, T helper cells, and protective levels of antibody in humans by particle-mediated administration of a hepatitis B virus DNA vaccine. *Vaccine* 19, 764–778.

Ryan, E.J., McNeela, E., Pizza, M., Rappuoli, R., O'Neill, L., and Mills, K.H. (2000). Modulation of innate and acquired immune responses by *Escherichia coli* heat-labile toxin: distinct pro- and anti-inflammatory effects of the nontoxic

AB complex and the enzyme activity. *J. Immunol.* 165, 5750–5759.

Sandkvist, M., Bagdasarian, M., and Howard, S.P. (2000). Characterization of the multimeric Eps complex required for cholera toxin secretion. *Int. J. Med. Microbiol.* 290, 345–350.

Scharton-Kersten, T., Yu, J., Vassell, R., O'Hagan, D., Alving, C.R., and Glenn, G.M. (2000). Transcutaneous immunization with bacterial ADP-ribosylating exotoxins, subunits, and unrelated adjuvants. *Infect. Immun.* 68, 5306–5313.

Schirmbeck, R., Bohm, W., Ando, K., Chisari, F.V., and Reimann, J. (1995). Nucleic acid vaccination primes hepatitis B virus surface antigen-specific cytotoxic T lymphocytes in nonresponder mice. *J. Virol.* 69, 5929–5934.

Schmitz, A., Herrgen, H., Winkeler, A., and Herzog, V. (2000). Cholera toxin is exported from microsomes by the Sec61p complex. *J. Cell Biol.* 148, 1203–1212.

Seo, N., Furukawa, F., Tokura, Y., and Takigawa, M. (2003). Vaccine therapy for cutaneous T-cell lymphoma. *Hematol. Oncol. Clin. North Am.* 17, 1467–1474.

Sharp, G.W. and Hynie, S. (1971). Stimulation of intestinal adenyl cyclase by cholera toxin. *Nature* 229, 266–269.

Simmons, C.P., Ghaem-Magami, M., Petrovska, L., Lopes, L., Chain, B.M., Williams, N.A., and Dougan, G. (2001). Immunomodulation using bacterial enterotoxins. *Scand. J. Immunol.* 53, 218–226.

Singh, M. and O'Hagan, D. (1999). Advances in vaccine adjuvants. *Nature Biotechnol.* 17, 1075–1081.

Sixma, T.K., Pronk, S.E., Kalk, K.H., Wartna, E.S., van Zanten, B.A., Witholt, B., and Hol, W.G. (1991). Crystal structure of a cholera toxin-related heat-labile enterotoxin from *E. coli*. *Nature* 351, 371–377.

Sixma, T.K., Pronk, S.E., Kalk, K.H., van Zanten, B.A., Berghuis, A.M., and Hol, W.G. (1992). Lactose binding to heat-labile enterotoxin revealed by X-ray crystallography. *Nature* 355, 561–564.

Sixma, T.K., Kalk, K.H., van Zanten, B.A., Dauter, Z., Kingma, J., Witholt, B., and Hol, W.G. (1993). Refined structure of *Escherichia coli* heat-labile enterotoxin, a close relative of cholera toxin. *J. Mol. Biol.* 230, 890–918.

Snider, D.P. (1995). The mucosal adjuvant activities of ADP-ribosylating bacterial enterotoxins. *Crit. Rev. Immunol.* 15, 317–348.

Spangler, B.D. (1992). Structure and function of cholera toxin and the related *Escherichia coli* heat-labile enterotoxin. *Microbiol. Rev.* 56, 622–647.

Steinsland, H., Valentiner-Branth, P., Gjessing, H.K., Aaby, P., Molbak, K., and Sommerfelt, H. (2003). Protection from natural infections with enterotoxigenic *Escherichia coli*: longitudinal study. *Lancet* 362, 286–291.

Tauschek, M., Gorrell, R.J., Strugnell, R.A., and Robins-Browne, R.M. (2002). Identification of a protein secretory pathway for the secretion of heat-labile enterotoxin by an enterotoxigenic strain of *Escherichia coli*. *Proc. Natl. Acad. Sci. USA* 99, 7066–7071.

Teter, K., Jobling, M.G., and Holmes, R.K. (2003). A class of mutant CHO cells resistant to cholera toxin rapidly degrades the catalytic polypeptide of cholera toxin and exhibits increased endoplasmic reticulum-associated degradation. *Traffic* 4, 232–242.

Thacher, S.M. and Rice, R.H. (1985). Keratinocyte-specific transglutaminase of cultured human epidermal cells: relation to cross-linked envelope formation and terminal differentiation. *Cell* 40, 685–695.

Tierney, R., Beignon, A.S., Rappuoli, R., Muller, S., Sesardic, D., and Partidos, C.D. (2003). Transcutaneous immunization with tetanus toxoid and mutants of *Escherichia coli* heat-labile enterotoxin as adjuvants elicits strong protective antibody responses. *J. Infect. Dis.* 188, 753–758.

Todd, E.C. (1997). Epidemiology of foodborne diseases: a worldwide review. *World Health Stat. Q.* 50, 30–50.

Turcanu, V., Hirst, T.R., and Williams, N.A. (2002). Modulation of human monocytes by *Escherichia coli* heat-labile enterotoxin B-subunit; altered cytokine production and its functional consequences. *Immunology* 106, 316–325.

Van Damme, P., Vranckx, R., Safary, A., Andre, F.E., and Meheus, A. (1989). Protective efficacy of a recombinant deoxyribonucleic acid hepatitis B vaccine in institutionalized mentally handicapped clients. *Am. J. Med.* 87, 26S–29S.

Vanbever, R., Lecouturier, N., and Preat, V. (1994). Transdermal delivery of metoprolol by electroporation. *Pharm. Res.* 11, 1657–1662.

Wang, B., Zhuang, L., Fujisawa, H., Shinder, G.A., Feliciani, C., Shivji, G.M., Suzuki, H., Amerio, P., Toto, P., and Sauder, D.N. (1999). Enhanced epidermal Langerhans cell migration in IL-10 knockout mice. *J. Immunol.* 162, 277–283.

Watts, C. and Amigorena, S. (2000). Antigen traffic pathways in dendritic cells. *Traffic* 1, 312–317.

Weimann, L.J. and Wu, J. (2002). Transdermal delivery of poly-l-lysine by sonomacroporation. *Ultrasound Med. Biol.* 28, 1173–1180.

West, D.J. (1989). Clinical experience with hepatitis B vaccines. *Am. J. Infect. Control* 17, 172–180.

Williams, N.A., Stasiuk, L.M., Nashar, T.O., Richards, C.M., Lang, A.K., Day, M.J., and Hirst, T.R. (1997). Prevention of autoimmune disease due to lymphocyte modulation by the B-subunit of *Escherichia coli* heat-labile enterotoxin. *Proc. Natl. Acad. Sci. USA* 94, 5290–5295.

Wilson, J.M., de Hoop, M., Zorzi, N., Toh, B.H., Dotti, C.G., and Parton, R.G. (2000). EEA1, a tethering protein of the early sorting endosome, shows a polarized distribution in hippocampal neurons, epithelial cells, and fibroblasts. *Mol. Biol. Cell* 11, 2657–2671.

Wolf, A.A., Jobling, M.G., Wimer-Mackin, S., Ferguson-Maltzman, M., Madara, J.L., Holmes, R.K., and Lencer, W.I. (1998). Ganglioside structure dictates signal transduction by cholera toxin and association with caveolae-like membrane domains in polarized epithelia. *J. Cell Biol.* 141, 917–927.

Yoshida, A., Nagata, T., Uchijima, M., Higashi, T., and Koide, Y. (2000). Advantage of gene gun-mediated over intramuscular inoculation of plasmid DNA vaccine in reproducible induction of specific immune responses. *Vaccine* 18, 1725–1729.

Yu, J., Cassels, F., Scharton-Kersten, T., Hammond, S.A., Hartman, A., Angov, E., Corthesy, B., Alving, C., and Glenn, G. (2002). Transcutaneous immunization using colonization factor and heat-labile enterotoxin induces correlates of protective immunity for enterotoxigenic *Escherichia coli*. *Infect. Immun.* 70, 1056–1068.

Yu, R.C., Abrams, D.C., Alaibac, M., and Chu, A.C. (1994). Morphological and quantitative analyses of normal epidermal Langerhans cells using confocal scanning laser microscopy. *Br. J. Dermatol.* 131, 843–848.

Zewert, T.E., Pliquett, U.F., Langer, R., and Weaver, J.C. (1995). Transdermal transport of DNA antisense oligonucleotides by electroporation. *Biochem. Biophys. Res. Commun.* 212, 286–292.

Zewert, T.E., Pliquett, U.F., Vanbever, R., Langer, R., and Weaver, J.C. (1999). Creation of transdermal pathways for macromolecule transport by skin electroporation and a low toxicity, pathway-enlarging molecule. *Bioelectrochem. Bioenerg.* 49, 11–20.

Zhang, L., Nolan, E., Kreitschitz, S., and Rabussay, D.P. (2002). Enhanced delivery of naked DNA to the skin by non-invasive in vivo electroporation. *Biochim. Biophys. Acta* 1572, 1–9.

Zurbriggen, R., Metcalfe, I.C., Gluck, R., Viret, J.F., and Moser, C. (2003). Nonclinical safety evaluation of *Escherichia coli* heat-labile toxin mucosal adjuvant as a component of a nasal influenza vaccine. *Expert Rev. Vaccines* 2, 295–304.

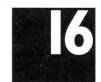

T cell adjuvants and novel strategies for their identification

Laurence Van Overvelt and Philippe Moingeon
Stallergenes, Antony, France

■ Abstract

A better understanding of T lymphocyte biology paves the ground for the design of adjuvants activating specific subsets of T lymphocytes. For vaccination purposes, distinct CD4$^+$ T cell types should be targeted, depending on the final aim: (i) Th1 cells producing IL2, TNFα and IFNγ, in order to stimulate cytotoxic T cell responses against cancers or chronic infectious pathogens (ii) Th2 cells producing IL4 and IL5, to induce sustained antibody responses against infectious pathogens, most particularly in the elderly and young infants (iii) Regulatory T cells producing IL10 and/or TGFβ to control inappropriate antigen-specific immune responses in patients with autoimmune diseases or allergies.

This review covers the current status of T cell adjuvant development and testing in humans, as well as the emerging immunological foundations for the design of new T cell adjuvants. The latter include detailed information on the biology of toll-like receptors, dendritic cell maturation, T lymphocyte polarization and memory. This scientific basis allows moving from conventional empirical approaches to rational design and high throughput screening approaches applied to both biological and synthetic chemical entities. This should yield in the future well-characterized, safe and efficient adjuvants up or down regulating T cell effector and regulatory functions as appropriate in a broad range of clinical indications.

Keywords: adjuvant, rational design, T lymphocyte polarization

■ Status of T cell adjuvant testing in humans

In the context of growing regulatory pressure, a challenge faced by vaccine developers is to rely upon better-defined molecular immunogens, expressed in the form of recombinant proteins, peptides, lipopeptides, plasmid DNA, or recombinant viruses, as opposed to whole attenuated or inactivated pathogens (Bonnet et al., 2000; Moingeon et al., 2001; O'Hagan and Valiante, 2003; Levine and Sztein, 2004). However, such "molecular vaccines" are in general poorly immunogenic, and selective signals for activation of innate and acquired immune systems need to be reintroduced using an appropriate adjuvant. Until recently, vaccines have been designed essentially to stimulate antibody responses against molecules expressed at the surface of bacteria or viruses, and thus conventional vaccine formulations have been poorly efficient at inducing strong T cell responses in humans. It is now broadly admitted that involvement of a T helper component is important to sustain an efficient and long-lived antibody response, as for example is intended with conjugate vaccines associating bacterial capsular carbohydrates with carrier proteins. Also Th1 immune responses and strong class I-restricted cytotoxic T lymphocyte (CTL) responses are needed to control chronic infectious diseases associated with viruses (e.g., HIV1, herpes simplex virus 1 (HSV1), human oncogenic papillomaviruses (HPV) 16 or 18) or intracellular pathogens (e.g., *Plasmodium falciparum*, *Mycobacterium tuberculosis*) (Hunter, 2002). Similarly, a working assumption is that therapeutic cancer vaccines should elicit both humoral and Th1 cellular immune responses against target antigen(s) (Offringa et al., 2000; Moingeon et al., 2001; Klein, 2001). Beyond infectious diseases, selected autoimmune diseases and allergies are currently considered as targets for vaccines directed against well-characterized antigens. Interestingly, in such diseases, symptoms are often linked to the existence of inappropriate Th1 or Th2 responses, against autoantigens or allergens, respectively. Thus, redirecting the immune response in an antigen-specific manner by stimulating regulatory T lymphocytes (T Regs) capable of establishing long-term tolerance is likely to be beneficial in those pathologies (Akbari et al., 2003; Sakaguchi, 2004; Taylor et al., 2004). Altogether, stimulation of specific T lymphocyte subpopulations is a well-identified goal for most modern vaccines, with the type of T cell to be targeted varying depending upon the indication.

A series of adjuvants that have been tested in humans for their capacity to increase or modulate cellular immune responses against antigens are listed in Table 16.1. Some of these adjuvants facilitate long-term persistence of the antigen at the administration site (the so-called "depot" effect seen with some emulsions). Others, such as particulate delivery systems (e.g., virosomes, liposomes, nonionic block copolymers, alginate microspheres, ISCOMS, virus-like particles), enhance antigen capture by professional antigen-presenting cells (APCs) (Eldridge et al., 1991; Katz et al., 2003). Other adjuvants (e.g., natural/synthetic bacterial products) act as immune potentiators that specifically elicit the production of cytokines by APCs relevant to the induction of either a Th1 or Th2 response (O'Hagan and Valiante, 2003; Levine and Sztein, 2004). Cytokines such as IL-2, GM-CSF, IL-12, and Flt3L have also been used directly as adjuvants

in humans, mostly in cancer patients but in the absence of a long-lasting biological activity and in the context of significant safety issues, their impact in vaccinology has been limited (Table 16.1). An efficient stimulation of Th2 responses (helper T cell stimulation supporting strong antibody responses) against numerous antigens has been successfully achieved in humans with aluminum salts (Vogel, 2000). By contrast, significant enhancement, both in terms of magnitude and duration, of Th1 immune responses is yet to be obtained, even if some lymphoproliferative and, to a much less extent, cytotoxic T cell responses or antigen-specific production of IFN-γ have been observed with selected antigen–adjuvant combinations, involving for example monophosphoryl lipid A (MPL), ISCOMs, emulsions, or oligonucleotide CpGs (see Table 16.1) (Aguado et al., 1999; Saul et al., 1999; Moingeon et al., 2002; Edelman, 2002; Engers et al., 2003; Burdin et al., 2004). At present we lack adjuvants capable of stimulating regulatory T cells, although the field is raising considerable interest (see below). Although the development of adjuvants has been largely empirical, our current understanding of the physiology of immune responses allows consideration of a "rational" approach to the design and development of molecularly characterized T cell adjuvants (Schijns et al., 2000; Berzofsky et al., 2001; Moingeon et al., 2001). In this review, we discuss a number of such new findings, as they relate to the induction of effector or regulatory responses mediated by distinct T cell subsets.

■ T lymphocyte polarization

■ Th1/Th2 balance

The concept of polarization of immune responses following antigen stimulation was initially proposed based on the identification of Th1 and Th2 subsets within CD4+ helper T cells, both in mice and subsequently in humans (Abbas et al., 1996; Carter and Dutton, 1996; Mosmann and Sad, 1996).

Table 16.1 Main categories of T cell adjuvants for human vaccines (Aguado et al., 1999; Moingeon et al., 2001; Edelman, 2002; Engers et al., 2003; Burdin et al., 2004)

Adjuvant/formulation	Comments
Th2 adjuvants	
Mineral salts	Calcium phosphate. Potential alternative to aluminum salts. Used in commercial allergy vaccines against grass pollen or house dust mites.
	Aluminum salts (hydroxide, phosphate) are licensed for human use with numerous vaccines. Well tolerated. Induction of strong antibody responses.
	SBAS-4/ASO4 (alum + MPL). Antibody titers, seroconversion rates, and lymphoproliferative responses were significantly stronger than with alum when tested in combination with recombinant proteins (e.g., hepatitis B S antigen or gD glycoprotein from HSV).
Carrier proteins	DT, TT, CRM, *Pseudomonas aeruginosa* exoprotein A. Proteins bearing T helper epitopes, and conjugated with capsular carbohydrates from infectious pathogens in a number of commercial (*Streptococcus pneumoniae*, *Haemophilus influenza*, meningococci type A and C) and exploratory (*Staphylococcus aureus*, *Pseudomonas aeruginosa*) vaccines. Such vaccines elicit stronger and more sustained antibody responses, most particularly in young infants and in the elderly.
Th1 adjuvants	
Emulsions	QS21 (purified saponin from *Quillaja saponaria*). Local reactogenicity. Enhanced antibody responses when tested with malaria vaccine (SPf66), HIV (gp120), or melanoma antigens as well as conjugate polysaccharidic vaccine against *Neisseria pneumoniae*. Limited induction of Th1 responses in humans, despite good results obtained in animal models.
	SBAS-2/ASO2 (squalene/water + MPL +QS21). Stimulation of antibody responses (using HIV-1 rgp120 as an antigen) and some level of cell-mediated immunity (T cell proliferation) but no CTLs. When tested with a candidate malaria vaccine, induction of high antiplasmodium CSP lymphoproliferative and antibody responses but no induction of CD8+ CTLs, leading to short-lived protection (less than 6 months) against challenge of naive individuals by infected mosquitoes.
	MF59 (stabilized squalene/water). Well tolerated (part of a licensed influenza vaccine). Improved immunogenicity over alum, when tested with an hepatitis B vaccine, or with HIV1 (gp120), CMV(rgB) subunits.
	Montanide ISA51 (stabilized water/Drakeol) and ISA720 (stabilized water/squalene). Both are well tolerated. In combination with an HIV candidate vaccine, ISA51 induced strong anti-Tat antibody and lymphoproliferative responses. Together with a malaria subunit vaccine (MSP1, MSP2, Resa AMA1), ISA720 elicited antibody responses equivalent to alum and strong T cell lymphoproliferative response.
	Incomplete Freund adjuvant: enhanced antibody (anti p24) and DTH responses when used with gp120-depleted inactivated HIV1. Stimulation of β-chemokine (Rantes, MIP-1α MIP-1β) production following p24 stimulation.
	Induction of T cell responses (IFN-γ production) against gp100 tumor antigen peptides in melanoma patients.
Natural/synthetic bacterial products	Monophosphoryl lipid A (MPL): Well tolerated. Limited increase of cellular responses in humans against bacterial or tumor-associated antigens. In combination with a pneumococcal conjugate vaccine, induced Th1 responses to the carrier protein, without enhancement of antibody responses to polysaccharide.
	RC-529 (synthetic MPL-like acylated monosaccharide). In combination with alum, enhances antibody responses against HBs antigen in humans. Th1 and mucosal adjuvant in mice.
	OM-174 (lipid A derivative from *E. coli*) and synthetic analogs based on a common triacyl motif, induce maturation of human dendritic cells *in vitro*. Well tolerated in humans.
	Detox (stabilized squalene/water + MPL +CWS). A Detox-containing melanoma vaccine (Melacine) has been registered in Canada. Detox enhances both cellular and humoral responses against melanoma-associated antigens.

(Continued)

Table 16.1 Continued

Adjuvant/formulation	Comments
	Toxins (CT, PT, LT): prototypic mucosal adjuvants, efficient in numerous animal models. In humans, detoxified bacterial toxins (i.e., mutated toxins or B subunits) lacking ADP-ribosylase activity are considered. Enhancement of seric and mucosal IgA production. CT or LT as adjuvants in patch-based transcutaneous immunization elicit balanced Th1/Th2 responses. In humans modest adjuvant effect of LT by oral route. A flu vaccine formulated with LT has faced safety issues.
	CpG oligonucleotides: at least three classes of oligonucleotides are now defined, based on the motif and chemical backbone, with respect to their distinct capacity to activate human B, NK, or dendritic cells *in vitro*. Immunostimulatory CpGs act as potent Th1 adjuvants in mice and monkeys, but such an activity remains to be documented in humans (enhanced antibody responses against the HBs antigen or flu antigens, but no reported effect on CTL activity). Currently being tested in association with the Amb a1 peanut allergen in humans.
Immunoadjuvants	Cytokines: when used as recombinant proteins in cancer patients, some T cell stimulation has been documented, as well as some toxicity (vascular leak syndrome for IL-2 and hepatotoxicity for IL-12). Enhancement of antibody responses against recombinant proteins with GM-CSF. More recently, utilization of poxviruses expressing locally (intratumorally) immunostimulatory cytokines (e.g., IL-2, IL-12). Administration of Flt3L with HBS Ag increases number of immature DCs in peripheral blood, but has no impact on antibody response against the antigen.
	Accessory molecules: the accessory molecule (B7.1), expressed with the CEA antigen within the canarypox vector ALVAC, enhances cellular responses in colorectal cancer patients. An anti-CTLA4 antibody administered to cancer patients previously vaccinated enhances immune responses to the vaccine. The LAG-3 molecule is a good Th1 adjuvant in murine and induces DC maturation *in vitro*. Being tested in humans in a phase I study.
Particulate formulations	Liposomes (DMPC/Chol). Well tolerated and slight enhancement of CD8+ CTL response to flu antigens. DC Chol: stimulates balanced Th2/Th1 responses in humans, when tested with *H. pylori* urease. Virosomes: well tolerated. Stimulation of antibody responses to hepatitis A or flu viruses. Licensed in those two indications in Switzerland. ISCOMS (cage-shaped complex of saponins and lipids). Local reactogenicity. Increase of influenza-specific CD8+ CTL response. Second generation (ISCOMATRIX) based on purified saponins, currently being tested with HPV16 (E6/E7) fusion protein. PLGA: particles eliciting Th1 and Th2 responses in murine. Ongoing trial with tetanus toxoid in humans.
T Reg adjuvants	
Bacterial/parasitic/ viral products	Regulatory/IL10-producing T cells appear to be induced by the FHA from *Bordetella pertussis*, lactobacilli, *Mycobacterium vaccae*, LPS, nonstructural protein 4 from hepatitis C virus, CT, PPD from *Mycobacterium tuberculosis*, and helminths.
Synthetic molecules	In murine models, imidazoquinolines (ligands for TLR 7), corticosteroids, cyclosporin A, rapamycin, mycophenolate mofetil, aspirin, dihydroxyvitamin D3, prostaglandins, N-acetyl-L-cysteine, anti-DEC-205 antibodies enhance T Reg responses.

CSP: *P. falciparum* circumsporozoite; CTL: cytotoxic T lymphocyte; CWS: cell wall skeleton from *Mycobacterium phlei*; DT: diphtheria toxoid; FHA: filamentous hemaglutinin; HB: hepatitis B; HPV: human papilloma virus; MTP-PE: muramyl tripeptide dipalmitoyl phosphatidyl ethanolamine; PLGA: poly(D,L)lactide-co-glycolic acid; PPD: protein purified derivative; TAAs: tumor-associated antigens; TLR: Toll-like receptor; TT: tetanus toxoid.

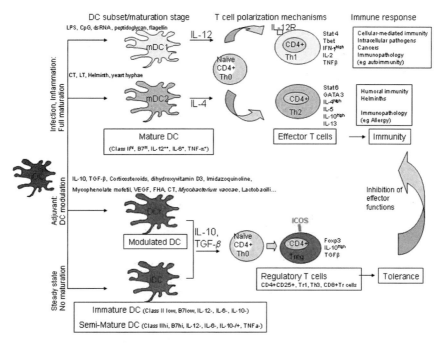

Figure 16.1 The induction of Th1, Th2, or T Reg cells is determined by the type and activation state of dendritic cells (DCs).
In the steady state, immature (iDCs)/semimature DCs capture antigens in the periphery, enter regional lymph nodes, and prime resting T cells to become regulatory T cells. In contrast, microbial product and proinflammatory cytokines produced during infection and inflammation stimulate the terminal maturation of DCs (mDCs) and drive them to prime naive T cells and induce effector Th1 or Th2 responses. Lipopolysaccharides (LPS), polycytosine guanine (CpG) motifs in bacterial DNA, viral double-stranded (ds) RNA, bacterial peptidoglycans, and flagellin stimulate DCs to promote the differentiation of Th1 cells. Cholera toxin (CT), *E. coli* heat-labile enterotoxin (LT), helminths, and yeast hyphae activate DCs to rather support Th2 cell polarization. Tolerogenic/regulatory DCs (DCr) are generated following stimulation with IL-10, TGF-β, immunosuppressive drugs (e.g., corticosteroids, cyclosporin A, rapamycin, mycophenolate mofetil), and pathogen-derived molecules (FHA, CT, PPD from *Mycobacterium tuberculosis*, lactobacilli, *Mycobacterium vaccae*). (See Color Plate Section.)

These subsets are characterized by the pattern of cytokines they produce and the immune responses they induce both physiologically as well as under pathological conditions. Th1 cells produce IL-2 and IFN-γ, and are important for the clearance of intracellular pathogens. They also are involved in autoimmune diseases (O'Garra and Robinson, 2004). In mice, Th1 responses are associated with the production of IgG2a/2b antibodies. Th2 cells produce IL-4, IL-5, and IL-13 supporting antibody responses (e.g., IgG1, and IgE in murine) which play a role in the clearance of extracellular pathogens. Inappropriate activation of Th2 cells results in allergic inflammatory reactions and type I hypersensitivity. The molecular mechanisms leading to Th1 or Th2 polarization following antigen stimulation of

Th0 naive T cells are partially known (Pulendran, 2004b). The dose of antigen, the strength of signals transduced through the T cell receptor (Rengarajan et al., 2000; Mullen et al., 2001; Pulendran, 2004a), as well as costimulation signals provided by various subsets of dendritic cells appear to be involved (Figure 16.1). The cytokine milieu surrounding newly activated T cells is one of the most important factors (Rengarajan et al., 2000; Mullen et al., 2001). In the presence of IL-12 secreted by macrophages or dendritic cells (DCs), Th1 differentiation occurs through the activation of Stat4 (signal transducer and activator of transcription 4) and T-Bet transcription factors which upregulate IFN-γ production while repressing Th2 cytokines such as IL-4 and IL-5. Conversely, IL-4 stimulation of Th0 cells activates Stat6 and initiates Th2 differentiation. The latter involves the zinc finger protein GATA3, which upregulates the expression of IL-5 and IL-13, and inhibits the production of IFN-γ. DC functions, including the production of cytokines affecting T cell polarization, are modulated during natural exposure to pathogens (Figure 16.1) (Pulendran, 2004a). DCs express conserved pathogen-recognition receptors (PRRs) (scavenger receptors, C-type lectins, or Toll-like receptors, TLRs) which enable these cells to recognize bioactive molecules (pathogen-associated molecular patterns, PAMPs) presented by pathogens (Janeway and Medzhitov, 2002; Takeda et al., 2003; Iwasaki and Medzhitov, 2004; Cook et al., 2004). T cell adjuvants mimicking danger signals by targeting specific TLRs can influence the interface between DCs and T cells in the presence of the antigen, both in terms of differentiation and activation signals, thereby having an impact on the Th1/Th2 balance. Some TLR ligands are being considered as Th1 adjuvant candidates, including, for example, TLR9 agonists containing CpG motifs (Krieg, 2002), TLR4 agonists such as MPL and synthetic analogs (Persing et al., 2002), or TLR7 agonists such as imidazoquinolines (Hemmi et al., 2002). In contrast, helminths express sugar moieties that trigger a set of unidentified cell-bound PRRs that prime DCs for promoting rather the development of Th2 cells (de Jong et al., 2002). Importantly, distinct subsets of human DCs express different TLRs (e.g., monocyte-derived DCs express predominantly TLR4, whereas plasmacytoid DCs express TLR9) (Kadowaki et al., 2001). Thus, the analysis of patterns of TLR expression on immune cells may be useful to select the most appropriate TLR agonists to be used as adjuvants, depending on the foreseen route of immunization, and the responses desired.

■ Regulatory T cells

Recently, different subsets of T cells with immunomodulatory and suppressive properties have been identified, including naturally occurring (CD4+ CD25+) and peripherally induced regulatory T cells following exposure to antigen (Tr1, Th3, CD8+ Tr) (Jonuleit and Schmitt, 2003; Thompson and Powrie, 2004). Collectively, regulatory T cells represent 5 to 10% of peripheral CD4+ T cells in mice and humans. They are usually present as anergic cells (with a low spontaneous proliferation rate) and are highly dependent on exogenous IL-2. Such T cells regulate T and B lymphocyte activation directly by cell–cell contact or through the production of immunosuppressive cytokines such as TGF-β and IL-10, or both (O'Garra and Vieira, 2004). Regulatory T cells can modulate immune responses against viruses, bacteria, and parasites, and control the establishment of chronic infection (Mills and McGuirk, 2004; Stassen et al., 2004a). They also inhibit both Th1 and Th2 responses (Stassen et al., 2004b; O'Garra and Barrat, 2003), and the development of T cell memory following infection or vaccination (Lundgren et al., 2003). Given their role in the regulation of peripheral and mucosal tolerance to self and foreign antigens, regulatory T cells could be targeted by vaccines to prevent the onset of autoimmune diseases (Hori et al., 2003; von Herrath and Homann, 2003; Horwitz et al., 2004), to achieve transplantation tolerance (Wood and Sakaguchi, 2003; Jonuleit et al., 2003), and to treat allergy (Akbari et al., 2003; Taylor et al., 2004; Romagnani, 2004; Stock et al., 2004). Whereas in those indications, antigen-specific activation of T Regs is needed, it might be useful to rather attenuate their function in order to enhance immune responses, for example to a tumor vaccine (Jonuleit and Schmitt, 2005; Belardelli et al., 2004).

TGF-β and IL-10 are important for the generation of CD4+CD25+ (Chen et al., 2003; Yamagiwa et al., 2001; Rao et al., 2005), Tr1 (Groux et al., 1997; Levings et al., 2001), and Th3 T Regs. Regulatory T cells can also be activated through the stimulation of TLR4 (e.g., with LPS), thereby increasing their capacity to downregulate inflammation and T cell activation (Caramalho et al., 2003; Sakaguchi, 2003). In vitro, IL-10-producing

T Regs can be induced by stimulation of naive T cells with vitamin D3 and dexamethasone (Barrat et al., 2002) or anti-CD46 and anti-CD3 antibodies (Kemper et al., 2003). Bacterial proteins such as filamentous hemagglutinin (FHA) from *Bordetella pertussis* or purified protein derivative (PPD) from *Mycobacterium tuberculosis* can induce Tr1 cells *in vivo* in mice (McGuirk et al., 2002) and IL-10-producing T cells in humans (Boussiotis et al., 2000), respectively. In this context, adjuvants triggering the production of IL-10 and TGF-β, or stimulating ICOS (Akbari et al., 2002) or TLR4, are likely to upregulate regulatory T cell activity. It has also been suggested that the type and activation state of DCs control the differentiation of naive T cells into T Regs (Groux et al., 2004; Jonuleit et al., 2001; Jonuleit et al., 2003; Morelli and Thomson, 2003; Rutella and Lemoli, 2004). Altogether, induction of DC maturation by inflammatory stimuli is key in directing naive T cells to differentiate into effector Th1 or Th2 cells (Figure 16.1). In contrast, immature DCs are rather tolerogenic and favor the development of T Regs, possibly as a physiological mechanism for the maintenance of peripheral T cell tolerance. Several protocols have been developed to enhance the tolerogenic potential of DCs, relying upon (i) specific cytokines, (ii) biological or synthetic reagents, and (iii) genetic engineering of DCs. Such functionally blocked DCs can induce T Regs that suppress a broad range of effector T cell responses (Morelli and Thomson, 2003; Rutella and Lemoli, 2004).

■ Nonconventional natural T lymphocytes

Synthetic activators of nonconventional T cells can represent powerful adjuvants due to their capacity to reveal interesting immune effector functions (e.g., cytotoxicity, cytokine production) associated with such cells. For example, NKT cells express an invariant TCR (Vα24/Vβ 11 in humans) and are specific for a restricted set of conserved ligands (distinct from peptides) (Bendelac et al., 2001; Kronenberg and Gapin, 2002). NKT cells are cytolytic, secrete high levels of cytokines, and thus exhibit potent antitumor as well as antiinfectious properties (Kronenberg and Gapin, 2002). These cells can be activated by the synthetic glycolipid α-galactosylceramide (α-GalCer) (Burdin and Kronenberg, 1999), to further stimulate CD4+ or CD8+ memory T cells as well as Th1 responses (Hayakawa et al., 2001). Gamma/delta T lymphocytes (γδ T cells), which constitute less than 5% of circulating lymphocytes, are mainly present in the skin, gut, as well as reproductive tract mucosae. These γδ T cells likely play a role of immune surveillance against cancer and infectious pathogens (Carding and Egan, 2002). They can be specifically activated by small antigens, such as organic phosphoesters, alkylamines, or nucleotide-conjugates, to exhibit cytolytic activity or to produce cytokines (Espinosa et al., 2001; Sireci et al., 2001).

■ Memory T cells

Since a major objective of T cell vaccines is to elicit long-term immune protection, an ideal T cell adjuvant should activate memory T cell mechanisms. Three stages have been delineated in the development of memory T cells following antigen stimulation: an expansion phase, a contraction phase, and a memory phase associated with long-term persistence of antigen-specific T cells which recirculate and are homeostatically regulated in an antigen-independent manner (Sallusto et al., 2004). Memory T cells express a phenotype distinct from naive T lymphocytes. Two major memory T cell subsets, namely central memory (CD45RA, CD62L^{high}CCR7$^+$) and effector memory cells (CD45RO, CD62L^{low}CCR7), have been described, which exhibit different homing properties to peripheral lymph nodes and nonlymphoid tissues, respectively (Wherry et al., 2003). In order to enhance memory T cell generation, adjuvants should increase the initial burst size, limit the contraction phase, and favor homeostatic survival of established memory T cells. Adjuvants enhancing the initial antigen load and persistence positively impact the expansion phase. To this end, prime-boost strategies using heterologous vectors may improve the antigen load available to the immune system (Haglund et al., 2002; Moingeon, 2002) by minimizing the impact of antivector immunity on antigen capture by APCs. Candidate adjuvants to limit the contraction phase are those that can induce *in vivo* the release of IL-7, IL-2 (Schluns and Lefrancois, 2003), or other T cell growth factors, or which can provide anti-apoptotic signals. In this regard, LPS appears to mediate part of its adjuvant activity by ensuring T cell survival following the induction of the IKB family member Bcl-3 molecule (Mitchell et al., 2001).

■ Implications for vaccine design

■ Designing immunogenic T cell antigens

Class I- and/or class II-restricted T cell epitopes can be identified within target antigen(s) based on the presence of known anchor residues conferring binding to a given MHC haplotype (Rammensee et al., 1997; Offringa et al., 2000). Such peptides can subsequently be tested for direct binding to MHC molecules to confirm the affinity and the stability of the interaction. Also, it is possible to "enhance" such T cell epitopes to make them more immunogenic, either by introducing random mutations, or modifications based on structural information regarding the interaction between MHC class I (or class II) molecules, peptides, and T cell receptor complexes (Ding et al., 1999; Reinherz et al., 1999). T cell epitope improvement can be undertaken at the level of residues involved in the interaction either with the MHC groove or with the T cell receptor complex, with the aim of enhancing the affinity of such interactions. Such approaches have been used successfully to enhance the immunogenicity of T cell epitopes within tumor-associated antigens (Parkhurst et al., 1996; Zaremba et al., 1997), and to reveal the immunogenicity of cryptic epitopes when presented together

with immunodominant T cell epitopes (Tine et al., 2005).

■ Targeting and conditioning antigen-presenting cells

Given that DCs play an important role in Th1, Th2, or T Reg polarization, most T cell adjuvants will act at this level. Candidate adjuvants can, for example, attract DCs and/or facilitate antigen entry to have it expressed in a precise subcellular compartment (e.g., cytosol or endosome) to promote subsequent association with MHC class I or class II receptors and presentation of MHC-peptide complexes at the cell surface. Several receptors expressed on APCs can be targeted to allow cross-priming or receptor-mediated endocytosis. This includes receptors for apopotic bodies or dying cells (such as CD14, $\alpha v\beta 5$, CD36), scavenger receptors, receptors for heat-shock proteins, mannose/fucose receptors, and chemokine receptors (Moingeon et al., 2001). Also, vectors such as live attenuated pathogens, lipopeptides, recombinant viruses (based for example on pox viruses, adenoviruses, or alphaviruses), or virus-like particles share in common the property to express the antigen inside DCs (Bonnet et al., 2000; Klein, 2001; Moingeon et al., 2002). Importantly, with the exception of T Reg adjuvants, a T cell adjuvant should also provide signals leading to both DC maturation and T cell costimulation. Maturation or "conditioning" of APCs can be achieved by crosslinking CD40 molecules (e.g., with CD40L or anti-CD40 antibodies), by cytokines such as TNF-α, or by engaging PAMPs such as TLR4. Thus, adjuvants designed specifically to elicit strong Th1 cellular immune responses should consist in a molecule – or combination thereof – capable of facilitating antigen entry in the cytosol or in the lysosomal compartment of professional APCs and to control the maturation of such APCs so that they can optimally prime naive T lymphocytes to differentiate along the appropriate pathway (Moingeon et al., 2001).

■ New schemes and routes of immunization

In order to elicit T cell responses, a common practice today is to associate multiple vectors, as part of heterologous prime-boost vaccination schemes. In such an approach, the antigen is presented to the immune system using first a priming vector, and subsequently a distinct vector as an antigen presentation platform (Tartaglia et al., 1998; Haglund et al., 2002). Associations between DNA and poxviruses, or vaccinia and canarypox, for example, are capable of inducing broad immune responses in animals, but also in humans (Moingeon, 2002).

In parallel, new routes of immunization beyond intramuscular or subcutaneous routes are being tested in humans in order to enhance T cell responses. For example, recombinant canarypox viruses expressing tumor-associated antigens are being administered to cancer patients through the intravenous route (Van der Burg et al., 2002) or directly into lymph nodes under radioguidance (Tartaglia et al., 2001). Another approach, termed transcutaneous immunization, relies on the application to hydrated skin of a mixture of antigen and adjuvant (e.g., the CT or LT holotoxins) with the aim of targeting the antigen to skin Langherans cells (Sun et al., 1994; Hammond et al., 2001). This latter approach when used in humans appears to elicit a mixed Th1/Th2 immune response. Lastly, the sublingual, nasal, and oral routes of immunization are being tested in humans with a number of candidate allergy vaccines to induce immune tolerance, likely through the induction of allergen-specific regulatory T cells (McSorley et al., 1998; Taylor et al., 2004).

■ New strategies to screen synthetic T cell adjuvants

One difficulty in the development of T cell vaccines or adjuvants is the limited predictability of animal models. Thus preclinical selection of candidate adjuvants should be made in parallel using simple animal models, as well as *in vitro* human culture systems. In this context, a strategy is rather to assess adjuvants in exploratory studies in humans, obviously after firmly establishing the safety of such candidate adjuvants in preclinical studies. Since immunogenicity is used as a readout of adjuvant efficacy, this requires that T cell responses should be monitored in detail, both on a qualitative and quantitative standpoint (Offringa et al. 2000; Moingeon et al., 2001). In this regard the utilization of soluble HLA tetramers in combination with appropriate peptides allows the detection of antigen-specific T cells (both class I and class II restricted), even with low precursor frequencies (Coulie et al., 2001). Also real-time PCR analysis of mRNA for transcription factors such as T Bet, GATA-3, or Fox p3 allows the early detection of T cell polarization events. Functional assays to further dissect T cell responses include conventional lymphoproliferation as well as the measurement of cytokine or chemokine production following antigen stimulation (using elispot, or intracellular cytokine staining). Biological molecules, mostly of bacterial origin, can be used as a source of candidate adjuvants in that such molecules can be recognized as "danger" signals by the immune system. While the natural origin of such molecules makes them rather acceptable by regulatory authorities, the number and diversity of such molecules is limited. Also, biological adjuvants of nonhuman origin are immunogenic by themselves, thereby eliciting antibody responses that will likely limit their efficacy in immunization schemes relying upon multiple administration. Thus, a strategy is to capitalize on the power of medicinal chemistry to synthesize small molecular analogs to such biological immunostimulants. Also, a "pharmaceutical" approach to adjuvant screening can focus on biased libraries of synthetic molecules representing modified versions of a model molecule (e.g., a known synthetic agonist of a TLR), looking for improved efficacy and safety as part of a "lead optimization" strategy.

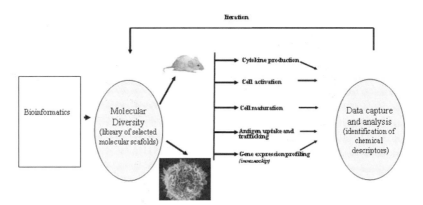

Figure 16.2 A proposed strategy is to screen libraries of natural or synthetic molecules for their activity either in simple animal models or on purified human immune cell subpopulations (dendritic cells in coculture with T cells), using readouts (colorimetric or optical) that can be robotized. Appropriate informatics should be used for both data capture and analysis, thereby allowing identification of molecular descriptors shared by molecules giving positive hits and not present within molecules giving negative hits. Based on such information, biased libraries of chemical entities with selected molecular characteristics can be synthesized, and submitted to a second round of screening. (See Color Plate Section.)

A high-efficiency screening strategy for synthetic adjuvants, allowing evaluation of up to several hundred molecules a day, is shown schematically in Figure 16.2. It includes:

- A bioinformatics step to define molecular characteristics (e.g., charge, hydrophobicity) of biological molecules with interesting properties, to be mimicked by the adjuvant.
- Synthesis of biased chemical scaffolds, providing access to a variety of molecules with characteristics similar to model biological molecules.
- Development at microscale level of simple readout assays using human *in vitro* systems (based on colorimetric/fluorescence/optical readouts to facilitate automation). It is likely that most T cell adjuvants will act on APCs, and also possibly directly on T cells.
- Data capture and analysis, leading to the identification of physicochemical characteristics (molecular descriptors) associated with molecules giving positive hits in screening assays. Both positive (hit) and negative (no hit) information can be used in an iterative process as a basis to design secondary biased libraries of molecules sharing such molecular descriptors, which can then be submitted to a second round of screening.

- Selected candidate adjuvants should subsequently be fully characterized using gene profiling techniques with respect to the genes they induce or downregulate, when incubated with various subsets of human immune cells. Such a detailed molecular characterization of future adjuvants is necessary to understand both their mechanism of action, but also their potential toxicity profile, thereby easing subsequent acceptance by regulatory authorities of a "new chemical entity."

■ Conclusions

Adjuvants for human vaccines capable of stimulating strong T cell responses are desperately needed, and are yet to be developed. Vaccines comprising such active components would help to control chronic infectious diseases, and are likely mandatory for successful therapeutic vaccination approaches, e.g., against cancer or autoimmune diseases. Recent insights into proinflammatory signals have opened the way to a more rational design of immunoadjuvants. Improved knowledge on the interface between innate and adoptive immunity provides clues for designing new formulations eliciting selective T cell responses.

While adjuvants inducing Th2 responses are available, there is a strong residual need to design and develop adjuvants eliciting Th1 or T Reg responses. Adjuvants can in this regard attract professional APCs, express the antigen intracellularly in order to facilitate cross-priming, and provide appropriate maturation and activation signals for both APCs and T lymphocytes. A suggested strategy to identify new T cell adjuvants is to move from an empirical to a rational approach and from biological to synthetic molecules, to harness the power of medicinal chemistry and access molecular diversity. The development of a new candidate adjuvant will be facilitated by such a strategy, which integrates within the screening process a detailed characterization at a cellular and molecular level of its mode of action.

■ References

Abbas, A.K., Murphy, K.M., and Sher, A. (1996). Functional diversity of helper T lymphocytes. *Nature* 383, 787–793.

Aguado, T., Engers, H., Pang, T., and Pink, R. (1999). Novel adjuvants currently in clinical testing: November 2–4, 1998, Fondation Mérieux, Annecy, France. A meeting sponsored by the World Health Organization. *Vaccine* 17, 2321–2328.

Akbari, O., Freeman, G.J., Meyer, E.H., Greenfield, E.A., Chang, T.T., Sharpe, A.H., Berry, G., DeKruyff, R.H., and Umetsu, D.T. (2002). Antigen-specific regulatory T cells develop via the ICOS-ICOS-ligand pathway and inhibit allergen-induced airway hyperreactivity. *Nature Med.* 8, 1024–1032.

Akbari, O., Stock, P., DeKruyff, R.H., and Umetsu, D.T. (2003). Role of regulatory T cells in allergy and asthma. *Curr. Opin. Immunol.* 15, 627–633.

Barrat, F.J., Cua, D.J., Boonstra, A., Richards, D.F., Crain, C., Savelkoul, H.F., de Waal-Malefyt, R., Coffman, R.L., Hawrylowicz, C.M., and O'Garra, A. (2002). *In vitro* generation of interleukin 10-producing regulatory CD4(+) T cells is induced by immunosuppressive drugs and inhibited by T helper type 1 (Th1)- and Th2-inducing cytokines. *J. Exp. Med.* 195, 603–616.

Belardelli, F., Ferrantini, M., Parmiani, G., Schlom, J., and Garaci, E. (2004). International meeting on cancer vaccines: how can we enhance efficacy of therapeutic vaccines? *Cancer Res.* 64, 6827–6830.

Bendelac, A., Bonneville, M. and Kearney, J.F. (2001). Autoreactivity by design: innate B and T lymphocytes. *Nature Rev. Immunol.* 1, 177–186.

Berzofsky, J.A., Ahlers, J.D., and Belyakov, I.M. (2001). Strategies for designing and optimizing new generation vaccines. *Nature Rev. Immunol.* 1, 209–219.

Bonnet, M.C., Tartaglia, J., Verdier, F., Kourilsky, P., Lindberg, A., Klein, M., and Moingeon, P. (2000). Recombinant viruses as a tool for therapeutic vaccination against human cancers. *Immunol. Lett.* 74, 11–25.

Boussiotis, V.A., Tsai, E.Y., Yunis, E.J., Thim, S., Delgado, J.C., Dascher, C.C., Berezovskaya, A., Rousset, D., Reynes, J.M., and Goldfeld, A.E. (2000). IL-10-producing T cells suppress immune responses in anergic tuberculosis patients. *J. Clin. Invest.* 105, 1317–1325.

Burdin, N. and Kronenberg, M. (1999). CD1-mediated immune responses to glycolipids. *Curr. Opin. Immunol.* 11, 326–331.

Burdin, N., Guy, B., and Moingeon, P. (2004). Immunological foundations to the quest for new vaccine adjuvants. *Biodrugs* 18, 79–93.

Caramalho, I., Lopes-Carvalho, T., Ostler, D., Zelenay, S., Haury, M., and Demengeot, J. (2003). Regulatory T cells selectively express toll-like receptors and are activated by lipopolysaccharide. *J. Exp. Med.* 197, 403–411.

Carding, S.R. and Egan, P.J. (2002). Gamma delta T cells: functional plasticity and heterogeneity. *Nature Rev. Immunol.* 2, 336–345.

Carter, L.L. and Dutton, R.W. (1996). Type 1 and type 2: a fundamental dichotomy for all T cell subsets. *Curr. Opin. Immunol.* 8, 336–342.

Chen, W., Jin, W., Hardegen, N., Lei, K.J., Li, L., Marinos, N., McGrady, G., and Wahl, S.M. (2003). Conversion of peripheral CD4+CD25– naive T cells to CD4+CD25+ regulatory T cells by TGF-beta induction of transcription factor Foxp3. *J. Exp. Med.* 198, 1875–1886.

Cook, D.N., Pisetsky, D.S., and Schwartz, D.A. (2004). Toll-like receptors in the pathogenesis of human disease. *Nature Immunol.* 5, 975–979.

Coulie, P.G., Karanikas, V., Colau, D., Lurquin, C., Landry, C., Marchand, M., Dorval, T., Brichard, V., and Boon, T. (2001). A monoclonal cytolytic T-lymphocyte response observed in a melanoma patient vaccinated with a tumor-specific antigenic peptide encoded by gene MAGE-3. *Proc. Natl. Acad. Sci. USA* 98, 10290–10295.

De Jong, E.C., Vieira, P.L., Kalinski, P., Schuitemaker, J.H., Tanaka, Y., Wierenga, E.A., Yazdanbakhsh, M., and Kapsenberg, M.L. (2002). Microbial compounds selectively induce Th1 cell-promoting or Th2 cell-promoting dendritic cells in vitro with diverse the cell-polarizing signals. *J. Immunol.* 168, 1704–1709.

Ding, Y.-H., Baker, B.M., Garboczi, D.N., Biddison, W.E., and Wiley, D.C. (1999). Four A6-TCR/peptide/HLA-A2 structures that generate very different T cell signals are nearly identical. *Immunity* 11, 45–56.

Edelman, R. (2002). The development and use of vaccine adjuvants. *Mol. Biotechnol.* 21, 129–148.

Eldridge, J.H., Staas, J.K., Meulbroek et al. (1991). Biodegradable microspheres as a vaccine delivery system. *Mol. Immunol.* 28, 287–294.

Engers, H., Kieny, M.P., Malhotra, P. et al. (2003). Third meeting on novel adjuvants currently in or close to clinical testing. *Vaccine* 21, 3503–3524.

Espinosa, E., Belmant, C., Pont, F. et al. (2001). Chemical synthesis and biological activity of bromohydrin pyrophosphate, a potent stimulator of human gamma delta T cells. *J. Biol. Chem.* 276, 18337–18344.

Groux, H., O'Garra, A., Bigler, M., Rouleau, M., Antonenko, S., de Vries, J.E., and Roncarolo, M.G. (1997). A CD4+ T-cell subset inhibits antigen-specific T-cell responses and prevents colitis. *Nature* 389, 737–742.

Groux, H., Fournier, N., and Cottrez, F. (2004). Role of dendritic cells in the generation of regulatory T cells. *Semin. Immunol.* 16, 99–106.

Haglund, K., Leiner, I., Kerksiek, K. et al. (2002). Robust recall and long-term memory T-cell responses induced by prime-boost regimens with heterologous live viral vectors expressing human immunodeficiency virus type 1 Gag and Env proteins. *J. Virol.* 76, 7506–7517.

Hammond, S.A., Walwender, D., Alving, C.R., and Glenn, G. (2001). Transcutaneous immunization: T cell responses and boosting of existing immunity. *Vaccine* 19, 2701–2707.

Hayakawa, Y., Takeda, K., Yagita, H. et al. (2001). Differential regulation of Th1 and Th2 functions of NKT cells by CD28 and CD40 costimulatory pathways. *J. Immunol.* 166, 6012–6018.

Hemmi, H., Kaisho, T., Takeuchi, O. et al. (2002). Small anti-viral compounds activate immune cells via the TLR7 MyD88-dependent signaling pathway. *Nature Immunol.* 3, 196–200.

Hori, S., Takahashi, T., and Sakaguchi, S. (2003). Control of autoimmunity by naturally arising regulatory CD4+ T cells. *Adv. Immunol.* 81, 331–371.

Horwitz, D.A., Zheng, S.G., Gray, J.D., Wang, J.H., Ohtsuka, K., and Yamagiwa, S. (2004). Regulatory T cells generated ex vivo as an approach for the therapy of autoimmune disease. *Semin. Immunol.* 16, 135–143.

Hunter, R.L. (2002). Overview of vaccine adjuvants: present and future. *Vaccine* 20, S7–S12.

Iwasaki, A. and Medzhitov, R. (2004). Toll-like receptor control of the adaptive immune responses. *Nature Immunol.* 5, 987–995.

Janeway, C.A., Jr. and Medzhitov, R. (2002). Innate immune recognition. *Annu. Rev. Immunol.* 20, 197–216.

Jonuleit, H. and Schmitt, E. (2003). The regulatory T cell family: distinct subsets and their interrelations. *J. Immunol.* 171, 6323–6327.

Jonuleit, H. and Schmitt, E. (2005). Regulatory T-cells in antitumor therapy: isolation and functional testing of CD4+CD25+ regulatory T-cells. *Methods Mol. Med.* 109, 285–296.

Jonuleit, H., Schmitt, E., Steinbrink, K., and Enk, A.H. (2001). Dendritic cells as a tool to induce anergic and regulatory T cells. *Trends Immunol.* 22, 394–400.

Jonuleit, H., Adema, G., and Schmitt, E. (2003). Immune regulation by regulatory T cells: implications for transplantation. *Transpl. Immunol.* 11, 267–276.

Kadowaki, N., Ho, S., Antonenko, S. et al. (2001). Subsets of human dendritic cell precursors express different Toll-like receptors and respond to different microbial antigens. *J. Exp. Med.* 194, 863–869.

Katz, D.E., DeLorimier, A.J., Wolf, M.K. et al. (2003). Oral immunization of adult volunteers with microencapsulated enterotoxigenic *Escherichia coli* (ETEC) CS6 antigen. *Vaccine* 21, 341–346.

Kemper, C., Chan, A.C., Green, J.M., Brett, K.A., Murphy, K.M., and Atkinson, J.P. (2003). Activation of human CD4+ cells with CD3 and CD46 induces a T-regulatory cell 1 phenotype. *Nature* 421, 388–392.

Klein, M. (2001). Current progress in the development of human immunodeficiency virus vaccines: research and clinical trials. *Vaccine* 19, 2210–2215.

Krieg, A.M. (2002). CpG motifs in bacterial DNA and their immune effects. *Annu. Rev. Immunol.* 20, 709–30.

Kronenberg, M. and Gapin, L. (2002). The unconventional lifestyle of NKT cells. *Nature Rev. Immunol.* 2, 557–568.

Levine, M.M. and Sztein, M.B. (2004). Vaccine development strategies for improving immunization: the role of modern immunology. *Nature Immunol.* 5, 460–464.

Levings, M.K., Sangregorio, R., Galbiati, F., Squadrone, S., de Waal, M.R., and Roncarolo, M.G. (2001). IFN-alpha and IL-10 induce the differentiation of human type 1 T regulatory cells. *J. Immunol.* 166, 5530–5539.

Lundgren, A., Suri-Payer, E., Enarsson, K. et al. (2003). Helicobacter pylori-specific CD4(+) CD25(high) regulatory T cells suppress memory T-cell responses to H. pylori in infected individuals. *Infect. Immun.* 71, 1755–1762.

McGuirk, P., McCann, C., and Mills, K.H. (2002). Pathogen-specific T regulatory 1 cells induced in the respiratory tract by a bacterial molecule that stimulates interleukin 10 production by dendritic cells: a novel strategy for evasion of protective T helper type 1 responses by Bordetella pertussis. *J. Exp. Med.* 195, 221–231.

McSorley, S., Rask, C., Pichot, R. et al. (1998). Selective tolerization of Th1 like cells after nasal administration of a cholera toxoid-LACK antigen. *Eur. J. Immunol.* 28, 424–430.

Mills, K.H. and McGuirk, P. (2004). Antigen-specific regulatory T cells: their induction and role in infection. *Semin. Immunol.* 16, 107–117.

Mitchell, T., Hildeman, D., Keoll, R. et al. (2001). Immunological adjuvants promote activated T cell survival via induction of Bcl-3. *Nature Immunol.* 2, 397–402.

Moingeon, P. (2002). Strategies for designing vaccines eliciting Th1 responses in humans, *J. Biotech.* 98, 189–198.

Moingeon, P., Haensler, J., and Lindberg, A. (2001). Towards the rational design of Th1 adjuvants. *Vaccine* 19, 4363–4372.

Moingeon, P., De Taisne, C., and Almond, J. (2002). Delivery technologies for human vaccines. *Br. Med. Bull.* 62, 29–44.

Morelli, A.E. and Thomson, A.W. (2003). Dendritic cells: regulators of alloimmunity and opportunities for tolerance induction. *Immunol. Rev.* 196, 125–146.

Mosmann, T.R. and Sad, S. (1996). The expanding universe of T cell subsets: Th1, Th2 and more. *Immunol. Today* 17, 138–146.

Mullen, A.C., High, F.A., Hutchins, A.S., Lee, H.W., Villarino, A.V., Livingston, D.M., King, A.L., Cereb, N., Yao, T-P, Yang, S.Y., and Reiner, S.L. (2001). Role of T-bet in commitment of T_H1 cells before IL-12-dependent selection. *Science* 292, 195–199.

Offringa, R., van der burg, S., ossendorp, F., Toes, R., and Melief, C. (2000). Design and evaluation of antigen-specific vaccination strategies against cancer. *Curr. Opin. Immunol.* 12, 576–582.

O'Garra, A. and Barrat, F.J. (2003). In vitro generation of IL-10-producing regulatory CD4+ T cells is induced by immunosuppressive drugs and inhibit by Th1- and Th2-inducing cytokines. *Immunol. Lett.* 85, 135–139.

O'Garra, A. and Robinson D. (2004). Development and function of T helper 1 cells. *Adv. Immunol.* 83, 133–162.

O'Garra, A. and Vieira, P. (2004). Regulatory T cells and mechanisms of immune system control. *Nature Med.* 10, 801–805.

O'Hagan, D.T. and Valiante, N.M. (2003). Recent advances in the discovery and delivery of vaccine adjuvants. *Nature Rev. Drug Discov.* 2, 727–735.

Parkhurst, M.R., Salgaller, M.L., Southwood, S., Robbins, P.F., Sette, A., Rosenberg, S.A., and Kawakami Y. (1996). Improved induction of melanoma-reactive CTL with peptides from the melanoma antigen gp100 modified at HLA-A*0201-binding residues. *J. Immunol.* 157, 2539–2548.

Persing, D.H., Coler, R.N., Lacy, M.J. et al. (2002). Taking toll: lipid A mimetics as adjuvants and immunomodulators. *Trends Microbiol.* 10, S32–S37.

Pulendran, B. (2004a). Modulating vaccine responses with dendritic cells and Toll-like receptors. *Immunol. Rev.* 199, 227–250.

Pulendran, B. (2004b). Modulating TH1/TH2 responses with microbes, dendritic cells, and pathogen recognition receptors. *Immunol. Res.* 29, 187–196.

Rammensee, H.G., Bachman, J., and Stevanovic, S. (1997). *MHC Ligands and Peptide Motifs.* Springer Verlag, Heidelberg.

Rao, P.E., Petrone, A.L., and Ponath, P.D. (2005). Differentiation and expansion of T cells with regulatory function from human peripheral lymphocytes by stimulation in the presence of TGF-β. *J. Immunol.* 174, 1446–1455.

Reinherz, E.L., Tan, K., Tang, L., Kern, P., Liu, J-H, Xiong, Y, Hussey, R.E., Smolyar, A., Hare, B., Zhang, R., Joachimiak, A., Chang, H-C, Wagner, G., and Wang, J.-H. (1999). The crystal structure of a T cell receptor in complex with peptide and MHC class II. *Science* 286, 1913–1917.

Rengarajan, J., Szabo, S.J., and Glimcher, L.H. 2000. Transcriptional regulation of Th1/Th2 polarization. *Immunol. Today* 21, 478–486.

Romagnani, S. (2004). The increased prevalence of allergy and the hygiene hypothesis: missing immune deviation, reduced immune suppression, or both? *Immunology.* 112, 352–363.

Rutella, S. and Lemoli, R.M. (2004). Regulatory T cells and tolerogenic dendritic cells: from basic biology to clinical applications. *Immunol. Lett.* 94, 11–26.

Sakaguchi, S. (2003). Control of immune responses by naturally arising CD4+ regulatory T cells that express toll-like receptors. *J. Exp. Med.* 197, 397–401.

Sakaguchi, S. (2004). Naturally arising CD4+ regulatory t cells for immunologic self-tolerance and negative control of immune responses. *Annu. Rev. Immunol.* 22, 531–562.

Saul, A., Lawrence, G., Smillie, A. et al. (1999). Human phase I vaccine trials of 3 recombinant asexual stage malaria antigens with Montanide ISA720 adjuvant. *Vaccine* 17, 3145–3159.

Sallusto, F., Geginat, J., and Lanzavecchia, A. (2004). Central memory and effector memory T cell subsets: function, generation, and maintenance. *Annu Rev Immunol.* 22, 745–63.

Schijns, V. (2000). Immunological concepts of vaccine adjuvant activity. *Curr. Opin. Immunol.* 12, 456–463.

Schluns, K.S. and Lefrancois, L. (2003). Cytokine control of memory T-cell development and survival. *Nature Rev. Immunol.* 3, 269–279.

Sireci, G., Espinosa, E., Di Sano, C. et al. (2001). Differential activation of human gamma delta cells by nonpeptide phosphoantigens. *Eur. J. Immunol.* 31, 1628–1635.

Stassen, M., Schmitt, E., and Jonuleit, H. (2004a). Human CD(4+)CD(25+) regulatory T cells and infectious tolerance. *Transplantation* 77, S23–S25.

Stassen, M., Jonuleit, H., Muller, C., Klein, M., Richter, C., Bopp, T., Schmitt, S., and Schmitt, E. (2004b). Differential regulatory capacity of CD25+ T regulatory cells and preactivated CD25+ T regulatory cells on development, functional activation, and proliferation of Th2 cells. *J. Immunol.* 173, 267–274.

Stock, P., Akbari, O., Berry, G., Freeman, G.J., DeKruyff, R.H., and Umetsu, D.T. (2004). Induction of T helper type 1-like regulatory cells that express Foxp3 and protect against airway hyper-reactivity. *Nature Immunol.* 5, 1149–1156.

Sun, J.B., Holmgren, J., and Czerkinsky, C. (1994). Cholera toxin B subunit: an efficient transmucosal delivery system for induction of peripheral immunological tolerance. *Proc. Natl. Acad. Sci. USA* 91, 10795–10800.

Takeda, K., Kaisho, T., and Akira, S. (2003). Toll-like receptors. *Annu. Rev. Immunol.* 21, 335–376.

Tartaglia, J., Excler, J.L., ElHabib, R., Limbach, K., Meignier, B., Plotkin, S., and Klein, M. (1998). Canary pox virus-based vaccines: prime-boost strategies to induce cell-mediated and humoral immunity against HIV. *AIDS Res. Hum. Retroviruses* 14, S291–S298.

Taylor, A., Verhagen, J., Akdis, C.A., and Akdis, M. (2004). T regulatory cells in allergy and health: a question of allergen specificity and balance. *Int. Arch. Allergy Immunol.* 135, 73–82.

Thompson, C. and Powrie, F. (2004). Regulatory T cells. *Curr. Opin. Pharmacol.* 4, 408–414.

Tine, J., Firat, H., Payne, A., Russo, G., Davis, S.W., Tartaglia, J., Lemonnier, F., Langlade-Demoyen, P., and Moingeon, P. (2005). Enhanced multiepitope vaccines elicit CD8+ cytoxic T cells against both immunodominant and crytic epitopes. *Vaccine* 23, 1085–1091.

Vogel, F.R. (2000). Improving vaccine performance with adjuvants. *Clin. Infect. Dis.* 30 (Suppl. 3), S266–S270.

Van der Burg, S.H., Visseren, M.J., Brandt, R.M., Kast, W.M., and Melief, C.J. (1996). Immunogenicity of peptides bound to MHC class I molecules depends on the MHC-peptide complex stability. *J. Immunol.* 156, 3308–3314.

Von Herrath, M. and Homann, D. (2003). Introducing baselines for therapeutic use of regulatory T cells and cytokines in autoimmunity. *Trends Immunol.* 24, 540–545.

Wherry, E.J., Teichgraber, V., Becker, T.C. et al. (2003). Lineage relationship and protective immunity of memory CD8 T cell subsets. *Nature Immunol.* 4, 225–234.

Wood, K.J. and Sakaguchi, S. (2003). Regulatory T cells in transplantation tolerance. *Nature Rev. Immunol.* 3, 199–210.

Yamagiwa, S., Gray, J.D., Hashimoto, S., and Horwitz, D.A. (2001). A role for TGF-beta in the generation and expansion of CD4+CD25+ regulatory T cells from human peripheral blood. *J. Immunol.* 166, 7282–7289.

Zaremba, S., Barzaga, E., Zhu, M., Soares, N., Tsang, K.-Y., and Schlom, J. (1997). Identification of an enhancer agonist cytotoxic T lymphocyte peptide from human carcinoembryonic antigen. *Cancer Res.* 57, 4570–4577.

Vaccination to treat noninfectious diseases: surveying the opportunities

Stephen W. Martin and Martin F. Bachmann
Cytos Biotechnology AG, Zürich-Schlieren, Switzerland

■ Introduction

Vaccination for the treatment and prevention of infectious diseases has been the most successful medical intervention from a public health perspective. The application of vaccination for treating noninfectious diseases is becoming more common and there are many recent examples of applying vaccine technology to a diverse range of noninfectious diseases (Bachmann and Dyer, 2004). In this review we attempt to separate the immunological requirements of different classes of noninfectious diseases to show the underlying immunological mechanisms that have to be considered in the design of appropriate vaccines. Broadly this encompasses treatments requiring the strong induction of immune responses, both humoral and cell mediated, or the downmodulation of an existing pathological immune response, either through immune deviation or suppression (Figure 17.1). We highlight the desired adjuvant qualities required for each approach and look at some of the potential dangers that may result from using vaccine formulations that push the immune system too far in one particular direction.

■ The immune system

The immune system is a complicated interconnected network of cells and molecules designed to protect the host from infection. It is clear that there is cross-talk between the various arms of the immune system, with recent advances focusing on the way "innate" immune components are required for initiating and directing the quality (and quantity) of the later "adaptive" immune response (Iwasaki and Medzhitov, 2004).

In the case of infectious diseases mediated by viruses, bacteria, or parasites there are numerous layers of immunological defense. The innate immune response is alerted rapidly to infection by events such as tissue damage, the binding of natural antibody, complement fixation, and the induction of inflammatory mediators (cytokines, vasoactive compounds), as well as granulocyte and phagocyte recruitment and activation (Carroll, 2004; Iwasaki and Medzhitov, 2004). The induction of the adaptive immune response is critically dependent on the interactions between T cells and antigen-presenting cells (APCs), of which the major player is the dendritic cell (DC) (Guermonprez et al., 2002). Immature DCs

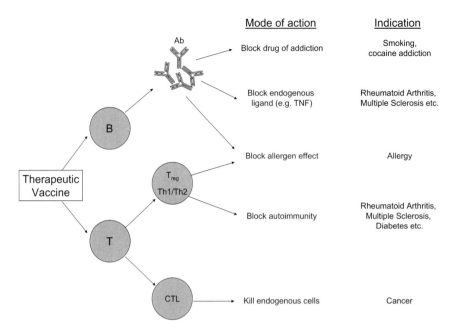

Figure 17.1 Mechanism of action of different therapeutic vaccines. Depending on the required vaccine effect, the mechanism of action of different therapeutic vaccines will rely on the type of immune response induced, whether antibody- or cell-mediated immunity (CTLs, Th1/Th2, and T_{reg}). Examples of relevant disease indications for each approach are indicated.

resident in peripheral tissues sample antigen from the environment and, if activated via pattern recognition receptors by pathogen-associated molecular patterns, are induced to migrate to secondary lymphoid tissues where they mature, present pathogen-derived peptides on MHC molecules in the context of costimulatory molecules, and become capable of efficiently priming naive CD4+ and CD8+ T cells.

T cell priming requires cell contact between the T cell and APC, leading to stimulation of the T cell receptor (TCR) by antigen presented by MHC molecules as well as the reception of costimulatory signals. This induces T cell proliferation and, under appropriate conditions, differentiation into effector cells. Effector T cells then downregulate lymphoid tissue homing receptors and migrate to sites of inflammation where effector CD8+ T cells are able to lyse infected target cells. The class of T cell help induced in CD4+ antigen-specific T cells at this stage is critical for fine-tuning the type of response that is mounted, a process

known as T cell polarization. The impact of polarization also feeds back into the innate system, for example Th1 T cell help is required for optimal macrophage activation and host protection in response to intracellular pathogens (Yamamura et al., 1991).

CD4+ T cell help is also required in the humoral response for inducing isotype switching in B cells, as well as supporting germinal center formation, the production of high-affinity long-lived plasma cells, and the formation of memory B cells. Furthermore, CD4+ T helper cells are known to be important for the normal development of memory CD8+ T cells (Janssen et al., 2003; Shedlock and Shen, 2003). Thus, T helper cells are key coordinators of the immune response required for the optimal development of antibody and cytotoxic T lymphocyte (CTL) responses.

The processes described above governing the induction of immune responses are relatively well defined. This contrasts with a lack of detailed understanding of how immune responses are downregulated. The most important mechanism of downmodulating immune responses is probably the successful clearance of the pathogen (essentially the removal of antigen), directly leading to a decline in the response. In contrast, under conditions of persistent infection, when the pathogen cannot be eliminated, additional mechanisms act to minimize damage inflicted onto the host by the immune system. T cell responses may be exhausted and specific T cells are either deleted or become nonfunctional (Moskophidis et al., 1993; Wherry et al., 2003; Zhou et al., 2004). In addition, high levels of persisting antigen may favor the production of antiinflammatory cytokines further reducing immune responses. It is this balance between the induction of effector responses vs. the exhaustion of T cell responses and the production of anti-inflammatory cytokines that immunologists try to influence in order to induce protective immunity vs. the amelioration of autoimmune diseases.

■ Induction of an immune response by vaccination: general considerations

Vaccination is a highly successful intervention whereby the immune system is primed by prior antigen exposure to provide protective immunity upon encounter with the specific pathogen and reencounter with its antigens. A key parameter for the success of a vaccine is therefore its immunogenicity. The most immunogenic form of vaccines against pathogens are live but attenuated strains, with killed forms of the pathogen and recombinant pathogen subunit vaccines showing reduced immunogenicity. In essence, this reduced immunogenicity is due to an inability of these vaccines to stimulate appropriately the immune system. These vaccines have lost the "flavor" of a pathogen. Current vaccine strategies for inducing an immune response therefore aim at combining safe, but poorly immunogenic vaccines with additional stimuli that drive an efficient immune response. Essentially three strategies are followed to trick the immune system into viewing a

recombinant vaccine as a pathogen. (i) Pathogens usually replicate in the host and pathogen-derived antigens are presented for extended time periods. This is mimicked by giving vaccines in a depot-forming adjuvant, a typical example of which is alum. (ii) Pathogens potently activate the innate immune system often through pattern recognition receptors, such as Toll-like receptors (TLRs). This is mimicked by adding TLR ligand to the vaccine, for example monophosphoryl lipid A (MPL) or CpGs, triggering TLR 4 and 9, respectively. (iii) Pathogens are macromolecular structures that are efficiently phagocytozed. In addition, many pathogens exhibit highly repetitive surfaces that efficiently crosslink B cell receptors, leading to potent antibody responses. This is mimicked by increasing the size and organization of the antigen by using virus-like particles, virosomes, or nanoparticles for vaccination (Gamvrellis et al., 2004). Currently the development of safe and effective vaccine formulations is a high priority (Petrovsky and Aguilar, 2004). This is especially true if vaccine technology is to be broadened and applied to noninfectious diseases (Table 17.1). Several challenges exist for this approach that will require good adjuvants, as it will be especially difficult to manipulate successfully aberrant immune responses (allergy and autoimmunity), ineffective immune responses (cancer immunotherapy), or immune responses against self antigens.

Adjuvants in antibody-based immunotherapy

■ Overview

The ability of antibodies to bind and neutralize pathogens is critical for the maintenance of vaccine-induced protective immunity against many life-threatening viral and bacterial infections (Zinkernagel, 2003). In the field of treatments for chronic noninfectious diseases, such as rheumatoid arthritis or multiple sclerosis (MS), the use of monoclonal antibodies is well established for targeting cells or blocking

Table 17.1 An overview of possible vaccination strategies, including some of the potential advantages and disadvantages of each approach

Aim	Vaccination strategy	Advantages	Disadvantages
Induction of humoral immunity	Passive administration of monoclonal antibodies	Effective; reversible	Cost; side effects; large and frequent dosing required
	Active vaccination targeting self antigens	Cost effective; long lasting; with VLP technology humoral immunity is induced without needing adjuvants	Reversibility? Possibility of ADCC/CDC; T cell-driven inflammation possible if strong adjuvants are used
Induction of T cell immunity in cancer immunotherapy	Transfer of *ex vivo* expanded T cells	Cells guaranteed to be specific	Cost; labor intensive; low persistence after transfer
	Improvement of antigen immunogenicity	Coadministered adjuvants boost antitumor and antipeptide responses (depot effects, costimulatory and pathogen-like signals, antigen in particulate form); DCs matured *ex vivo* provide extra adjuvant effects	Therapy requiring *ex vivo* expansion of T cells or DCs is expensive and labor intensive; responses to antigens in cancer immunotherapy are often observed with little associated clinical benefit
	Removal of tolerance mechanisms	Improves effectiveness of vaccination	May increase the risk of autoimmunity
Deviation or suppression of existing responses	SIT for allergy	Effective	Time consuming; risk of anaphylaxis; limited to certain allergens
	Provide Th1 stimuli with the allergen, either mixed or directly linked	Decreases time required for desensitization; successful in animal models of autoimmunity	Risk of side effects for some adjuvants (CpG); toxicity associated with direct application of cytokines. Risk of inducing autoimmunity?
	Provide Th2 stimuli to treat auto immunity	Successful in animal models of autoimmunity	Risk of inducing allergy?
	Enhance T_{reg} suppression to treat autoimmunity	Successful in animal models of autoimmunity	Risk of compromising tumor immunosurveillance?

specific molecular interactions (Reichert, 2001). Monoclonal antibodies are very specific and are often effective; however, there are several potential problems with their passive administration as a treatment, including unfavorable pharmacokinetics and expense.

An alternative for such passive vaccination with monoclonal antibodies would be some form of active vaccination to induce the production of neutralizing antibodies in the host. This approach is envisaged to be more cost effective and longer lasting; however, the challenge in active vaccination is to find immunogenic formulations of antigen which are sufficient to induce strong antibody responses but are controllable and free from

adverse effects such as T cell-driven inflammation. Given that many active vaccination therapies for chronic noninfectious diseases would target self antigens, the balance between the breaking of self tolerance and the avoidance of immunopathology becomes critical. The key criterion of safety may in fact prevent the use of strong adjuvants in active vaccination strategies aimed at inducing antibodies against self antigens (Table 17.1).

■ Passive vaccination

Passive vaccination using chimeric, humanized, or fully human monoclonal antibodies has become a major success story of modern biotechnology, representing over 30% of biopharmaceuticals in clinical trials (Hudson and Souriau, 2003). We will not provide extensive coverage here and suggest the reader consult one of several recent reviews on the subject (Hudson and Souriau, 2003; Waldmann, 2003). We wish only to compare and contrast passive immunotherapy with the active induction of antibodies using therapeutic vaccination for the treatment of noninfectious diseases.

Passive immunotherapy using monoclonal antibodies has several attractive features. Monoclonals exhibit generally high target selectivity. For example, Eculizumab™ (Kaplan, 2002), a monoclonal specific for complement C5, has a picomolar affinity for its target and blocks complement activation at close to the theoretical 1:2 molar ratio (Thomas et al., 1996). Monoclonal antibodies can also be used as carriers of other bioactive molecules such as toxins or radionuclides, a recent example being Zevalin™, the first radionuclide-containing monoclonal treatment to be approved by the US Food and Drug Administration (FDA). Monoclonal antibodies are metabolized with distinct pharmacokinetics, giving potentially full reversibility of their effects. In addition, the engineering of smaller antibody fragments (e.g., single chain Fv) or design of new antibody-based molecules (e.g., "diabodies") may increase the bioavailability of the drug (Hudson and Souriau, 2003), although the half-life of such molecules is usually very short.

Despite these qualities there are several limitations to passive antibody immunotherapy. It is expensive and, due to unfavorable pharmacokinetics, often requires repeated administration at high doses. This can lead to serious side effects such as infusion sickness and risks the induction of inactivating anti-antibodies (antiallotypic and antiidiotypic) as well as being inconvenient for patients. In addition the targeting of cell surface molecules may induce antibody-dependent cytotoxicity (ADCC), a desirable effect in

some cases (e.g., Rituxan® for the treatment of non-Hodgkin's lymphoma) but not appropriate if the target molecule is to be blocked without inducing tissue damage.

■ Active vaccination

The alternative to passive antibody immunotherapy is to vaccinate individuals against a variety of foreign and self antigens to generate neutralizing antibodies. This approach has proven safe and effective in a number of animal models and clinical trial settings in humans. It has the potential advantages that well-established existing vaccine technology and delivery mechanisms can be used to induce long-lived polyclonal neutralizing immune responses against the target of interest, resulting in convenience for the patient and reduced cost of goods.

The induction of neutralizing antibodies against a given antigen requires that specific B cells and T cells of the right specificity are present and able to be activated. For therapeutic vaccines targeting self antigens the mechanisms of tolerance may interfere with the induction of an appropriate response. Autoreactive B lymphocytes are in fact present in the periphery yet are held in check primarily by a lack of T cell help, as well as mechanisms of anergy (Goodnow, 1992). However, self-reactive B cells can be activated under appropriate circumstances allowing the therapeutic induction of antiself antibodies by vaccination.

Most therapeutic vaccination strategies for noninfectious diseases target self antigens. However, there is one notable recent example of the use of foreign antigens to treat drugs of addiction, including nicotine (Nabi, Xenova, Cytos) and cocaine (Xenova). The use of these small drug molecules as antigens provides less of a safety concern as it does not require the breaking of self tolerance. Some positive phase II clinical trial results were recently reported by Nabi and Cytos for their nicotine vaccines and by Xenova for its cocaine vaccine.

A number of strategies have been proposed for inducing neutralizing antibodies against self antigens, including linking self antigens to foreign carrier proteins, incorporating foreign T helper epitopes into self antigens, using DNA vaccination to enhance antiself responses, and using virus-like particles (VLPs) to display self antigens in a highly immunogenic form.

In foreign carrier protein strategies, vaccination by linking small hormone self molecules such as human chorionic gonadotropin (GC) (Talwar et al., 1976), gonadotropin-releasing hormone (GnRH) (Mettens and Monteyne, 2002), gastrin (Watson et al., 1999; Watson et al., 2000; Smith et al., 2001), and angiotensin (Gardiner et al., 2000) to diphtheria toxoid or tetanus toxoid has proven successful in inducing neutralizing antibodies. Several of these vaccines have been tested in human clinical trials, CG and GnRH vaccines showed promise as both immunocontraceptives (Talwar et al., 1994; Mettens and Monteyne, 2002) and cancer immunotherapeutics (Simms et al., 2000; Moulton et al., 2002); and a gastrin vaccine showed efficacy for the treatment of advanced pancreatic cancer (Brett et al., 2002).

Perhaps the most striking recent use of active vaccination targeting a small self molecule has been in the development of a treatment for Alzheimer's disease. Human amyloid beta (Aβ) peptides derived from the amyloid precursor protein (APP) accumulate as plaques in the brain of Alzheimer's patients. Transgenic mice expressing a plaque-forming variant of human APP can be vaccinated with Aβ peptides in strong adjuvant, generating a humoral response that reduces plaque burden (Schenk et al., 1999) and improves mental performance in the mice (Morgan et al., 2000). In a phase IIa clinical trial of the vaccine in Alzheimer's patients, antibody responses against Aβ peptides were associated with a delay of cognitive decline (Hock et al., 2003). Despite these promising results, the clinical trial was halted after a subset of patients developed meningoencephalitis (Orgogozo et al., 2003). This side effect of the vaccine formulation highlights the potential problems of active vaccination in the presence of strong

adjuvants and is discussed later with other potential risks.

One problem with using large foreign carrier proteins is the potential for strong anticarrier T cell responses and the masking of B cell epitopes on the self protein. This may be overcome by linking peptides to the self antigen that contain strong foreign T helper cell epitopes (Sad et al., 1992), although this approach is restricted to individuals carrying the requisite MHC haplotype for peptide presentation. Along similar lines is a recent approach to break self tolerance by genetically engineering strong foreign T helper epitopes directly into self antigens without disturbing the antigen structure (Dalum et al., 1996). The resulting response appears effective in animals carrying mismatched MHC molecules, suggesting novel T helper epitopes are being formed by the genetic insertion into the self antigen (Dalum et al., 1999). This approach has been effective in treating disease in several animal models, including arthritis (Dalum et al., 1999) and asthma (Hertz et al., 2001), although success in these models requires the coadministration of highly inflammatory adjuvants.

DNA vaccination with immunostimulatory DNA encoding self antigens has been reported recently as a method to induce autoantibodies. The production of autoantibodies after DNA vaccination specific for a variety of cytokines and chemokines, including macrophage inhibitory factor-1, tumor necrosis factor (TNF)-α, and FasL provided beneficial results in experimentally induced autoimmune diseases such as experimental autoimmune encephalomyelitis (EAE) and adjuvant induced arthritis (Youssef et al., 1998; Wildbaum and Karin, 1999; Youssef et al., 1999; Wildbaum et al., 2000; Youssef et al., 2000). Interestingly the DNA vaccination strategy did not induce autoantibodies in the absence of disease, but rather augmented the production of autoantibodies that would normally be produced at low level during the autoimmune disease. This approach may hold promise in autoimmune diseases where an existing autoimmune reaction against a self antigen simply needs to be enhanced to have a therapeutic benefit.

The use of VLPs to make antigens more immunogenic by presentation to the immune system as a highly ordered array holds promise as a vaccine delivery system, especially as high neutralizing antibody titers can be obtained even in the absence of adjuvants. The rationale for this vaccine carrier system comes from observations that antibody responses against the glycoprotein of vesicular stomatitis virus (VSV) could only be elicited in transgenic mice expressing this antigen if the glycoprotein was presented to the immune system as a highly ordered array on the surface of virions, but not in a disorganized soluble or membrane-bound form (Bachmann et al., 1993). It may be that only highly repetitive antigens able to efficiently crosslink surface antigen receptors on B cells are able to "rescue" autoreactive B cells from peripheral tolerance mechanisms (Bachmann et al., 1993). VLP vectors in current use are usually single coat proteins of viruses which are recombinantly expressed and self assemble into particles that resemble the live virus but lack viral genetic material and hence infectivity. Antigens are then displayed by these particles either as genetic fusions (Chackerian et al., 1999), by streptavidin-biotin conjugation (Chackerian et al., 2001), or by chemical crosslinking (Jegerlehner et al., 2002b), with the density of self antigen on the surface of the particle playing a critical role in the induction of strong neutralizing IgG antibody responses (Chackerian et al., 2002; Jegerlehner et al., 2002a). VLP-based vaccines have been tested in clinical trials to induce immune responses against human papillomavirus (Evans et al., 2001; Harro et al., 2001; Pastrana et al., 2001; Ault et al., 2004; Brown et al., 2004; Fife et al., 2004), Norwalk virus (Ball et al., 1999), HIV (Weber et al., 1995; Benson et al., 1999), and a model peptide coupled to bacteriophage-derived VLPs (Spohn and Bachmann, 2003). In all cases the vaccines proved to be safe, well tolerated, and immunogenic. A major advantage of VLPs over other carrier technologies for inducing antibody responses against self antigens is that adjuvants are not required to produce strong neutralizing IgG responses, a point we will return to when we highlight some of the potential problems associated with active vaccination.

■ *Potential and actual problems with active vaccination*

Toxic effects from autoantibodies. There are several important safety concerns surrounding active vaccination against self antigens, especially with respect to the possible presence of continual high titer autoantibodies in the serum. Firstly, autoantibodies binding to cell surface antigens would have the potential to induce antibody-dependent cytotoxicity and complement-dependent cytotoxicity. This effect is harnessed, for example, in the action of anti-CD20 monoclonal antibodies for treating non-Hodgkin's lymphoma (Reff et al., 1994; Kennedy et al., 2004). Current active vaccination strategies have avoided this issue by immunizing against soluble secreted self antigens such as growth factors, hormones, and cytokines. This brings another potential danger, however, in the form of immune complex formation, which may lead to nephritis if complexes are deposited in the kidney. A polyclonal antibody response against an abundant soluble self antigen would need to be carefully monitored to ensure safety. Monoclonal antibodies, despite their single specificity, also have this safety concern, particularly if polymeric proteins such as TNF or IgE are targeted.

Reversibility. Unlike passive immunotherapy with monoclonal antibodies, in which the drug is metabolized with distinct kinetics, active immunotherapy by vaccination relies on the cessation of an immune response for reversibility. This is potentially problematic, as vaccination of patients that already have immune defects, in particular autoimmunity, may provoke a continuous autoantibody response against the self antigen. Available reversibility data in animals for self antigens linked to carrier proteins, genetically fused to foreign T helper epitopes or presented on the surface of VLPs show that most responses decline over several months. In human trials of CG conjugated to tetanus toxoid and diphtheria toxoid, antibody titers declined rapidly after each vaccination and this decline was not affected by repeated vaccination (Talwar et al., 1994). Similarly autoantibodies to TNF-α and ubiquitin induced in mice after immunization with recombinant self proteins incorporating foreign T helper epitopes showed a ~90% reduction 5–6 months after the last immunization (Dalum et al., 1996; Dalum et al., 1999). In contrast, mice immunized with a chemical conjugate of interleukin (IL)-9 and ovalbumin showed sustained high inhibitory autoantibody titers over one year after the final vaccination (Richard et al., 2000). In papilloma VLP-based immunizations, autoantibody titers against CCR5 declined by 2- to 8-fold within 6 months of the last immunization (Chackerian et al., 1999). Vaccination against TNF-α using the same VLP system led to a reversible autoantibody response with a 60-fold reduction in titers one year after the last boost (Chackerian et al., 2001). In general current information suggests autoantibody titers induced by active vaccination of antigens linked with foreign T help components are reversible; however, this may depend on the vaccine target and formulation and will have to be carefully investigated for each new vaccine candidate. By contrast, DNA vaccination to enhance autoantibody production against a particular target may not always show such reversibility, as autoantibody production closely followed disease course in experimental animals, for example in an acute EAE model autoantibody titers declined (Youssef et al., 1998), while in a chronic adjuvant arthritis model autoantibody titers were maintained (Youssef et al., 2000).

T cell-mediated side effects. The potential dangers of active vaccination were highlighted in a recent phase IIa clinical trial for the treatment of Alzheimer's disease (Gelinas et al., 2004;

Robinson et al., 2004). Treatment by active vaccination against Aβ was halted after some of the patients developed meningoencephalitis. Interestingly autopsy data from a patient who developed meningoencephalitis showed evidence of T cell infiltration and an immune response against Aβ (Nicoll et al., 2003). Vaccine efficacy was observed in a sub-cohort of patients by the observation that the production of high anti-Aβ antibody titers was associated with delayed cognitive decline (Hock et al., 2003), but clearly the immunization induced unwanted T cell-driven inflammatory side effects. This may have been due to immunization with a form of Aβ-containing T cell epitopes in conjunction with the Th1 polarizing adjuvant QS-21. At the very least this experience must serve as a cautionary tale for active vaccination strategies and highlight the need for inducing strong antibody responses without inflammatory T cells. This may be possible by removing known T cell epitopes from antigens (Gelinas et al., 2004) or using vaccine technologies such as VLPs that induce strong antibody responses without requiring inflammatory adjuvants.

Adjuvants to stimulate T cell immunity

Outlook

The other major arm of the adaptive immune system besides the antibody response is T cell-mediated immunity. In the field of noninfectious diseases, the boosting of T cell immunity, particularly CD8+ CTLs, is especially important in the search for an immunotherapy for cancer. Adjuvants will play an important role in the development of any successful cancer vaccine, as methods are clearly required to increase the immunogenicity of tumor antigens, stimulate innate tumor immunity, remove immunosuppressive pathways, and deal with the challenge of vaccination in immunocompromised and elderly patients (Table 17.1).

Is there hope for the successful treatment of cancer by vaccination? Prophylactic vaccination to prevent infection with the limited number of viral infections directly associated with the development of cancer is clearly feasible (Finn, 2003); however, therapeutic vaccination to treat existing cancers is proving more difficult. Current evidence suggests the immune system is able to respond to tumors, as tumor-specific T cell and antibody responses can be detected in patients (Houghton et al., 2001) and both immunocompromised humans and mice with defined immunological defects show greater susceptibility to spontaneous and induced tumors (Shankaran et al., 2001). Despite this, the poorly immunogenic form in which tumor antigens are usually presented to the immune system means robust antitumor T cell responses are not easily induced. Ideally for vaccination, a tumor antigen should be tumor-specific, or abundantly expressed by the tumor and essential for the tumor phenotype.

The low immunogenicity of tumor antigens can be the result of tumor-derived factors, which can form an immunosuppressive environment by, for example, downmodulating or secreting MHC class I homologs (Groh et al., 2002) or secreting immunosuppressive cytokines such as IL-10 and VEGF (Gabrilovich et al., 1996a). In addition, any given cancer immunotherapeutic is initially a "second line" treatment. To show efficacy in this situation requires eliciting an immune response in elderly or immunocompromised patients who may have had several previous therapies (Finn, 2003). Many proposed cancer treatments, for example those involving the *ex vivo* culture of DCs, tumor cells, or tumor-reactive T cells, are also very labor intensive and expensive, suggesting that their widespread use may be difficult to achieve (Berzofsky et al., 2004).

■ Adjuvants and vaccines to enhance innate immunity

Tumor surveillance by innate immune cells capable of producing interferon (IFN)-γ, such as NK, NKT, and $\gamma\delta$ T cells is important at least in animal models of tumor immunity (Street et al., 2004). Attempts to boost the

antitumor activity of this arm of the immune system in humans, however, are in their infancy. For example, while systemic IL-12 administration was shown to be effective in enhancing tumor rejection in experimental animals (Nastala et al., 1994), it resulted in liver toxicity in humans.

NKT cells are immune cells expressing $\alpha\beta$ TCRs that recognize glycolipids presented by the nonclassic MHC molecule CD1d (Godfrey and Kronenberg, 2004). These cells produce large amounts of cytokines (IFN-γ, IL-13, IL-4) rapidly upon activation in part due to pre-stored cytokine mRNA. There is some debate about whether NKT cells mediate or hinder antitumor immune reactions. It has been shown that NKT cells are a major source of IL-13, which acts via a myeloid intermediate to generate transforming growth factor (TGF)-β, an immunosuppressive cytokine able to inhibit antitumor activity by CD8+ CTLs in murine cancer models (Terabe et al., 2000; Terabe et al., 2003). From this finding it may be a useful strategy to target IL-13 produced by NKT cells and downstream TGF-β to boost antitumor immunity (Ahlers et al., 2002). Alternatively, in cancer patients the NKT cell cytokine secretion repertoire is reportedly skewed towards Th2 (IL-4), producing NKT cells that some have termed "regulatory" (Terabe and Berzofsky, 2004). The capacity to re-secrete IFN-γ can be restored by immunization with DCs pulsed with the CD1d ligand α-Gal-Cer (Nieda et al., 2004) and this is actively being pursued as a cancer therapy to boost innate immunity.

■ Adjuvants and vaccines based on humoral immunity

Passive monoclonal antibody therapy is used for some tumors, although it is not generally applicable to solid tumors for reasons of bioavailability (Hudson and Souriau, 2003). Active vaccination to induce a humoral antitumor immune response has been described by using the unique variable regions of heavy and light chain immunoglobulin genes as a tumor-specific antigen. A recent report used

DCs pulsed with peptides from specific B cell lymphoma idiotypes followed by idiotype-KLH vaccination to induce both cell-mediated and humoral immunity in B cell lymphoma patients (Timmerman et al., 2002).

Adjuvants and vaccine strategies to enhance the immunogenicity of tumor antigens

Vaccination with modified tumor cells

The advantage of using tumor cells for vaccination (either autologous cells or cancer cell lines) is that the formulations contain tumor-specific antigens. The major disadvantage is that the production of autologous tumor-derived cell lines is expensive and labor intensive. The use of cancer cell lines could circumvent this limitation; for example, Melacine® and Canvaxin™ are vaccines derived from melanoma cell lines that have been trialled for the treatment of malignant melanoma. However, clinical trial data from these products are not impressive (Sondak et al., 2002; Sosman et al., 2002).

The immunogenicity of killed tumor cells can be improved by transduction with cytokine genes, for example GM–CSF, which acts to recruit more DCs to the site of vaccine administration, presumably increasing tumor antigen presentation to the immune system (Dranoff et al., 1993). Several clinical trials of cytokine-secreting tumor cell vaccines have been completed or are ongoing (Soiffer et al., 1998; Simons et al., 1999; Jaffee et al., 2001; Salgia et al., 2003).

Vaccination with peptides

Vaccination with peptides derived from tumor-specific antigens allows the immune response to be focused to the parts of tumor antigens that are different from normal tissue antigens. This may be desirable from a safety point of view, as the risk of inducing autoimmunity is presumably reduced. In addition, peptide antigens are relatively stable, safe, and cost effective. The biggest hurdles for this approach include making the peptide formulation sufficiently immunogenic, defining appropriate peptides, and the limited patient range of a given peptide due to MHC restriction.

In order to increase immunogenicity, peptides are often administered with adjuvants, including coadministered cytokines, e.g., GM-CSF, CD40L, IL-12, and IL-15 (Ahlers et al., 2002). In addition CpG oligonucleotides can be used as an adjuvant to activate numerous immune cells (Klinman et al., 1996). Peptides can also be delivered on the surface of mature autologous DCs, an approach that is discussed in more detail below. The problem of identifying "unique" patient-specific tumor antigens may be circumvented by using tumor-derived heat shock proteins as a source of tumor peptides (Lewis, 2004).

Is peptide-based vaccination successful? In clinical trials of peptide-based cancer vaccines it is often possible to detect immune responses against the peptide in a subset of patients, but this does not necessarily correlate with tumor regression (Rosenberg et al., 1998; Lee et al., 2001; Phan et al., 2003).

Viral vectors expressing tumor antigens

Viral vectors, including adenoviruses, vaccinia, and avipox vectors, have been used to express tumor antigens and immunostimulatory cytokines (Marshall et al., 2000; Zhu et al., 2000). However, these viral vectors are immunogenic themselves, so two major concerns for this approach are the effect of preexisting neutralizing humoral immunity, as well as the problem of the immunodominance of responses against the vector compared to those against the tumor antigen (Berzofsky et al., 2004).

Dendritic cell-based vaccines

Dendritic cells have been used as a kind of vaccine adjuvant for the delivery of tumor antigens to the immune system in an immunogenic form. While approaches such as direct antigen delivery by targeting DCs with antibodies (Bonifaz et al., 2002) or the use of particulate vaccine formulations (Gamvrellis et al., 2004) are being pursued, evidence of impaired DC function in animal models of cancer (Gabrilovich et al., 1996a, 1996b) and cancer patients has led to the *ex vivo* expansion and maturation of autologous DCs becoming a major focus of cancer immunotherapy (Berzofsky et al., 2004; Blattman and Greenberg, 2004). DCs cultured *ex vivo* can be either loaded with tumor peptides or tumor lysates (Gabrilovich et al., 1996b; Paglia et al., 1996; Zitvogel et al., 1996; Ashley et al., 1997; Nair et al., 1997), fused with irradiated tumor cells (Siders et al., 2003) or transformed with genes encoding tumor antigens by plasmid and viral vectors (Wan et al., 1997; Akiyama et al., 2000; Esslinger et al., 2002; Chen et al., 2003a). The major advantage of this method for antigen delivery is that activated DCs are the key APCs involved in priming CTL responses. Increasing the number and quality of these cells that carry tumor-specific antigens should therefore increase the number and quality of tumor-specific CTLs.

As well as transferring mature DCs loaded with tumor antigens, additional signals can be provided by transducing DCs with costimulatory and cytokine genes (Zitvogel et al., 1996), or by the coadministration of adjuvants such as cytokines, DC maturation signals, and CTLA-4 blockade to increase and sustain T cell activation (Gamvrellis et al., 2004).

In clinical trials with cancer patients there have been encouraging but variable results with DC vaccination to date, which probably reflects the variety of protocols, tumor antigens, and formulations being trialled. For example, Banchereau et al. (2001) showed clinical responses in 7 out of 17 melanoma patients after DC immunization with peptides from four defined melanoma antigens. In another study, however, while DC immunization with undefined tumor antigens from solid tumor lysates elicited DTH responses in several patients, no partial or complete clinical responders were observed (Stift et al., 2003). One important issue in the field of DC vaccination is the need to ensure that DCs used for clinical trials in humans are reproducibly matured (Schuler et al., 2003).

■ Approaches to downmodulate immunosuppressive pathways

In contrast to the methods outlined above, which aim to boost antitumor T cell immunity, an alternative possibility is to turn off immunosuppressive pathways which act to limit the T cell response. Interruption of CTLA-4 signaling, for example, acts to enhance T cell-mediated rejection of tumors in experimental animals (Leach et al., 1996; Hurwitz et al., 1998; van Elsas et al., 2001). This approach has been trialled in humans, with anti-CTLA-4 blocking antibodies provoking clear antitumor responses when administered either after (Hodi et al., 2003) or concurrently with (Phan et al., 2003) therapeutic vaccines. CTLA-4 knockout mice exhibit a strong progressive lymphoproliferative disease, reflecting the role of this inhibitory pathway in the maintenance of self tolerance (Waterhouse et al., 1995). In a similar way, interference with the CTLA-4 pathway in experimental models (van Elsas et al., 2001) and in human clinical trials (Phan et al., 2003) is associated with autoimmune symptoms.

Immune suppression mediated by CD4+ CD25+ regulatory T cells (T_{regs}) can also play a role in antitumor immunity. Recent studies have shown enhanced tumor immunity in mice upon depletion of the T_{reg} subset using antibodies against CD25 (Sutmuller et al., 2001; Golgher et al., 2002; Turk et al., 2004; Prasad et al., 2005). However, the importance of T_{reg} in the management of peripheral tolerance (Sakaguchi et al., 1995) suggests that such treatments in cancer patients may lead to autoimmune symptoms. Additionally, activated effector T cells also express CD25, so a reliance on this marker for T_{reg} depletion may not be advisable (Blattman and Greenberg, 2004).

Adjuvants inducing immune deviation or immunosuppression

■ Overview

Immune deviation and immunosuppression involve downmodulating an existing immune response for therapeutic benefit. This may involve switching the type of immune response from one sort to another, for example deviation of Th2 to Th1, or involve suppression of an immune response, for example through the induction of T_{regs}.

Two noninfectious disease classes to which strategies of immune deviation and immunosuppression are currently being applied are allergy and autoimmunity. These are characterized by aberrant immune responses to innocuous environmental allergens or to host tissue antigens, respectively, and are increasing in incidence, especially in industrialized countries (Yazdanbakhsh et al., 2002).

Allergy and autoimmunity have been described as being at opposite ends of a regulatory axis, with allergic diseases showing a strong Th2 bias in cytokine production (Robinson et al., 1992) and antibody isotypes such as IgE, while autoimmunity (at least for organ-specific disease) shows a strong Th1 bias (Ando et al., 1989; Campbell et al., 1991). This provides a clear therapeutic rationale: in order to treat one or the other disease the immune system should be "deviated" back toward some sort of balance point. In addition, both allergy and autoimmunity can be viewed as chronic immune responses to which specific immunosuppression could be applied, especially through the manipulation of peripheral tolerance mechanisms such as T_{regs} (Wills-Karp et al., 2001; Yazdanbakhsh et al., 2002).

The following sections discuss the biology of Th1/Th2 cells as well as the characteristics of T_{regs} and will subsequently show possible ways to tip the balance of these responses towards protection from allergy or autoimmune diseases (Table 17.1).

◾ The Th1/Th2 paradigm

The subdivision of effector CD4+ "helper" T cells into Th1 and Th2 subsets grew out of work demonstrating an inverse relationship between "humoral" and "cell-mediated" immunity (Parish, 1971; Parish and Liew, 1972). It was subsequently shown that murine and human CD4+ T cells could be subdivided on

the basis of their cytokine production profile (Mosmann et al., 1986; Wierenga et al., 1990; Parronchi et al., 1991), with the Th1 subset producing predominantly IFN-γ and IL-2, while the Th2 subset produces predominantly IL-4, IL-5, and IL-13. Under this scheme it was proposed that Th1-driven immunity, particularly through the activation of macrophages, is crucial for protection against intracellular pathogens (Scott et al., 1988; Heinzel et al., 1989; Yamamura et al., 1991); by contrast Th2-driven immunity (in particular IL-4 production) is crucial for protection against helminth infection (Urban et al., 1991; Kopf et al., 1993). It was shown that Th1 or Th2 cytokines also lead to distinct antibody isotype profiles, Th1 giving predominantly IgG2a and Th2 promoting switching to IgG1 and IgE (Snapper and Paul, 1987; Stevens et al., 1988).

The control of Th1 vs. Th2 polarization is complicated and controversial (Kapsenberg, 2003), with many factors playing a role, including the nature of the pathogen and the pattern recognition receptor signals induced, the subsequent cytokine and costimulatory environment derived from innate immune cells and DCs (Hsieh et al., 1993; Macatonia et al., 1995), the maturation and activation state of APCs, the nature of T cell antigen receptor (TCR) signals, MHC haplotypes, and antigen dose (Parish and Liew, 1972; Bretscher et al., 1992; Hosken et al., 1995). In general, strong signals drive Th1 responses while weak signals favor the development of Th2 responses. Consequently, a commonly followed path to vaccinate against allergies is the induction of allergen-specific Th1 responses by adding TLR ligands to the vaccine formulation. Intriguingly, although many parasites and in particular helminths induce Th2 responses, little is known about parasite-derived ligands driving the responses in this direction.

Recently T-bet and GATA-3 have been described as master transcription factors required for the development of Th1 or Th2 phenotypes, respectively (Murphy and Reiner, 2002). These transcription factors lie downstream of TCR, costimulatory, and cytokine signals and are involved in reinforcing both Th1 (IFN-γ secretion, IL-12 sensitivity) and Th2 (IL-4, IL-5, and IL-13 secretion) phenotypes. Interestingly, GATA-3 induces its own transcription, offering an explanation of the stable phenotype of at least Th2 cells.

Regulatory T cells

The recent revival of interest in T cell subsets having regulatory functions has important implications for the treatment of noninfectious diseases, especially where aberrant T cell responses need to be suppressed or where weak T cell responses need to be enhanced.

The renewed significance of thymus-produced "natural" T_{regs} derived from the finding that CD4+CD25+ T cells were present in naive animals and involved in the suppression of organ-specific CD4+ T cell-mediated autoimmunity (Sakaguchi et al., 1995). Since then cells with a similar phenotype (CD4+ cells expressing CD25, GITR, CTLA-4, and CD62L) have been shown to suppress pathogen and antigen-specific immune responses, as well as the activation and proliferation of CD8+ T cells. These cells have also been described in humans. CD25+ regulatory cells are a minor population (<10%) of CD4+ T cells and are thought to be produced either in the thymus (natural T_{regs}) or in responses to suboptimal antigen encounter in the periphery (induced T_{regs}, including IL-10 producing "Tr1" and TGF-β producing "Th3" subsets). There is also considerable variation in the phenotypes of T cells exhibiting regulator (i.e., suppressive) effects, with CD25+, CD62L+, and CD45RB^{lo} cells all providing protection from different autoimmune syndromes (Alyanakian et al., 2003) after transfer into autoimmune-prone lymphopenic hosts. A complicating factor is that Th1 cells inhibit Th2 responses and vice versa (Parish, 1971; Parish and Liew, 1972), hence an antigen-specific Th2 cell may be viewed as a T_{reg} cell in Th1 responses against the same antigen. The same is true for Th1 cells if Th2 responses are assessed.

Natural T_{reg} development and the expression of an immunosuppressive phenotype by these cells is under the control of a specific transcription factor, forkhead box p3 (Foxp3), mutations in which lead to immune dysregulation in both mice and humans (Bennett et al., 2001) apparently as a direct consequence of T_{reg} deficiency (Fontenot et al., 2003; Khattri et al., 2003). Some T_{reg} suppressive effects, such as IL-10 production may also be accomplished by CD25–Foxp3– cells, highlighting the ability of other immune cells to also participate in "immune regulation" (Sundstedt et al., 2003).

T_{reg} cells function through the action of immunosuppressive cytokines, in particular TGF-β and IL-10. TGF-β appears to be particularly important in inducing a suppressive phenotype (Chen et al., 2003b; Fantini et al., 2004; Peng et al., 2004) and controlling T cell responses during autoimmunity (Green et al., 2003; Liu et al., 2003; Oida et al., 2003; Nakamura et al., 2004). In humans the reduced function of T_{regs} has been linked to certain autoimmune diseases (Ehrenstein et al., 2004; Kriegel et al., 2004; Viglietta et al., 2004), although it is not yet clear whether the lack of T_{reg} immunosuppression in these cases is a cause or effect of the autoimmune phenotype.

Adjuvants in the immunotherapy of allergy

Most allergies are immediate-type hypersensitivity reactions mediated by IgE and directed against normally innocuous antigens. Allergy is characterized by a sensitization phase that induces allergen-specific IgE, followed by allergic reactions upon reexposure to the allergen. Allergic diseases are driven by an aberrant immune response mediated through CD4+ T helper type 2 (Th2) cells and an associated cytokine pattern involving IL-4, IL-5, and IL-13. The Th2 cytokine pattern also promotes isotype switching in allergen-specific B cells to IgE, thereby sustaining the allergic phenotype.

Specific immunotherapy (SIT) against allergy was first attempted in 1911 (Noon, 1911) and remains a current treatment for allergy involving the administration of increasing doses of allergen in adjuvant. SIT is not ideal, however, as it requires extensive and long duration medical interventions for success, it is limited to certain antigens, and involves the risk of inducing anaphylaxis and even promoting allergies to other components of complex allergen mixtures (Valenta, 2002). Recent work has focused on improving safety by reducing the anaphylactogenic potential of allergens used in SIT (so called "hypoallergenics") and by using novel adjuvants, including, for example, TLR ligands, to decrease the time required for successful treatment. From a scientific point of view the mechanism of action for SIT remains unclear. A major hypothesis is that allergen-specific "blocking" antibody induced by SIT (usually IgG1 or IgG4) successfully competes with allergen-specific IgE (van Neerven et al., 1999). This may not, however, explain observations that the appearance of allergen-specific IgG4 often lags behind a successful therapeutic response in SIT; others have therefore proposed the mechanism of SIT involves a change in the cytokine milieu giving immune deviation towards Th1 (Jutel et al., 1995; McHugh et al., 1995) or the production of immunosuppressive cytokines such as IL-10 and TGF-β (Jutel et al., 2003). Successful SIT results in a reduction of immediate type I (IgE-mediated) hypersensitivity reactions, a response that occurs within minutes upon allergen exposure, suggesting that if a change in cytokine milieu is responsible for SIT, it must impact somehow in an antigen-specific manner on the production or function of allergen-specific IgE.

■ *Allergy as a Th2 bias*
Allergy is a rapidly growing disease area, with increasing incidence, severity, and mortality evident in industrialized countries. The well-publicized "hygiene hypothesis" grew out of a proposal to explain the inverse relationship between family size and hay fever incidence (Strachan, 1989). This epidemiological hypothesis has found ready support from the biological phenomena of Th1/Th2 immune deviation. Children indeed appear to have a

more "Th2-like" immune system in early childhood which becomes more balanced in non-atopic individuals (i.e., not genetically predisposed to allergy) as they age (Barrios et al., 1996; Prescott et al., 1998a, 1998b). Following this argument the treatment of allergic disease may best be accomplished by immune deviation towards a Th1 response.

The use of bacterial and viral products that act as adjuvants to induce Th1 immunity either as a general means to suppress Th2 responses or to generate allergen-specific Th1 cells are two active areas of investigation. Animal studies point to strong antiallergy effects both in prophylactic and therapeutic settings from treatment with bacteria such as live or heat-killed *Mycobacterium bovis* (BCG) (Erb et al., 1998; Hopfenspirger and Agrawal, 2002; Major et al., 2002), *M. vaccae* (Wang and Rook, 1998; Hopfenspirger and Agrawal, 2002; Zuany-Amorim et al., 2002), and listeria (Yeung et al., 1998; Hansen et al., 2000), or by treatment with bacterial products such as lipopolysaccharide (LPS) (Vannier et al., 1991; Tulic et al., 2000; Tulic et al., 2001) or MPL (Baldrick et al., 2001). The mechanism of protection provided by these bacterial compounds is thought to be due to the induction of a strong Th1 cytokine response, in particular IFN-γ (Erb et al., 1998); however, for *M. vaccae* treatment it may involve the induction of immunoregulatory T cells and depend on the production of IL-10 and TGF-β (Zuany-Amorim et al., 2002). When the principle of general Th1 stimulation by viral and bacterial products to protect from atopy is applied to humans from an epidemiological perspective, however, results have not been clear-cut (Strachan, 2000; Wills-Karp et al., 2001). Studies of children infected with measles (Shaheen et al., 1996; Paunio et al., 2000) or mycobacteria (Shirakawa et al., 1997; Gruber et al., 2001; Gruber et al., 2002) have given mixed evidence for protection against the subsequent development of allergic diseases. A more promising approach may be to combine the adjuvant effects of bacterial products with specific allergens by direct linkage, either in the same adjuvant formulation or by covalent linkage of the bacterial products to the allergens. The adjuvant effects of MPL (a ligand for TLR4) mixed with allergens have in fact been incorporated into SIT, with promising results in clinical trials in adults and children treated for pollen/grass allergies (Drachenberg et al., 2001; Drachenberg et al., 2003a, 2003b).

In a similar way to TLR4 stimuli, DNA containing unmethylated CpG motifs can act as an adjuvant, signaling through TLR9 (Hemmi et al., 2000) to induce a strong Th1 cytokine response, including the production of IL-12, IL-18, and IFN-γ (Akira et al., 2001; Klinman, 2004). Like the bacterial adjuvants described above, CpG DNA is able to protect experimental animals from allergic responses, including airway inflammation in both acute (Broide et al., 1998; Kline et al., 1998; Sur et al., 1999; Shirota et al., 2000) and chronic asthma disease models (Jain et al., 2002; Kline et al., 2002; Jain et al., 2003). Significantly, allergens can be coupled directly to CpG sequences, allowing a potentiation of the allergen-specific immune response (Tighe et al., 2000) and an enhanced effect of the CpG (Shirota et al., 2000). This is an important safety consideration for the use of CpG as an adjuvant, given that chronic exposure may have unwanted side effects (Heikenwalder et al., 2004; Storni et al., 2004) and that repeated treatments may be required to suppress allergic reactions (Broide et al., 2001). In humans a ragweed allergen linked to CpG has shown the ability to deviate the immune system towards Th1 (Simons et al., 2004). As for the mechanism of action of CpG DNA in modulating allergic disease, induction of Th1 cytokines such as IFN-γ and induction of IgG is thought to be important (Sur et al., 1999), although the appearance of IL-10 and TGF-β in some studies may also indicate a role for induced T_{regs} (Jain et al., 2002, 2003).

DNA vaccination using plasmid DNA encoding allergens has been effective at least in animal models in inducing strong Th1 immunity capable of protecting against allergy (Hsu et al., 1996; Hartl et al., 2004; Ludwig-Portugall et al., 2004). This adjuvant effect comes in part from the unmethylated CpG motifs in the plasmid backbone of the DNA vector (Sato et al., 1996; Klinman et al., 1997). Immunomodulatory proteins, such as cytokines, can be encoded either alone (Li et al., 1996; Kumar et al., 2001) or along with the allergen (Maecker et al., 2001) to enhance the antiallergy effects of immunization. Despite this, DNA vaccination has been very disappointing in humans and hopes to treat allergies by DNA vaccination remain limited.

The manipulation of the Th1/Th2 balance in allergy has also been attempted by the direct application of Th1 cytokines or the use of antagonists to block Th2 cytokines. The direct use of Th1 cytokines has had mixed results in animal models, with IFN-γ inhibiting allergen-induced symptoms of asthma in mice (Lack et al., 1994, 1996), but IL-12 showing contradictory results (Gavett et al., 1995; Hofstra et al., 1998) and IL-18 actually exacerbating asthma by increasing eosinophilia (Kumano et al., 1999; Wild et al., 2000). The use of antagonists to block Th2 cytokines as an allergy therapy also showed mixed success. sIL-4Ra was only limited in its effectiveness (Borish et al., 1999) and anti-IL-5 monoclonal antibody treatment did not change the airway hyperreactivity in asthmatic patients (Leckie et al., 2000; Kips et al., 2003) but nevertheless reduced eosinophilia. Since eosinophils appear to be the major cause for long-term damage in the asthmatic lung (fibrosis) (Humbles et al., 2004), blocking IL-5 remains an attractive strategy to treat asthma. As discussed above, an alternative to the use of expensive monoclonal antibodies against IL-5 may be active vaccination of the allergic host against IL-5, resulting in long-term depletion of the cytokine.

Other pathways may be used in the future to deviate the atopic immune system from Th2 towards Th1. For example, pulmonary plasmacytoid-like dendritic cells (pDCs) may play a role in inducing tolerance to inhaled substances as allergen-pulsed pulmonary pDCs can be used to protect mice from subsequent experimentally induced asthma (de Heer et al., 2004). A possible Th2 to Th1 deviation strategy may involve increasing IL-12 secretion by DCs, as retrovirally driven DC IL-12 overexpression can halt experimentally induced asthma, although, interestingly, cannot reverse disease in already sensitized animals (Kuipers et al., 2004).

Allergy as a deficiency of immune regulation

Recently there has been a renewed interest in the concept that allergy is not necessarily a Th1/Th2 imbalance, but that it reflects a defect in other "counter-regulatory" mechanisms such as inhibition by T_{regs} (Wills-Karp et al., 2001; Yazdanbakhsh et al., 2002). The hygiene hypothesis is not able to explain the paradox that there is an inverse correlation between exposure to Th2-inducing helminth infections and allergy, although helminths are known to be immunosuppressive and infected individuals may simply be immunosuppressed to a degree that they fail to mount an allergic reaction (King et al., 1993; Borkow et al., 2000).

Accumulating evidence points to the importance of immunosuppressive cytokines such as IL-10 and TGF-β in protection against allergy (Akdis et al., 1998; Akdis and Blaser, 2001; Jutel et al., 2003; Akdis et al., 2004). Current theories suggest that these immunosuppressive cytokines are produced by allergen-specific T_{reg} subsets induced in healthy individuals as a normal response to allergen exposure (Lewis, 2002; Kuipers and Lambrecht, 2004; Wahl et al., 2004). Some of the mechanistic details for the induction of these regulatory cells are now being worked out. For example, in the lung, allergen-specific T_{regs} are induced via pulmonary DCs, possibly of a plasmacytoid DC lineage (de Heer et al., 2004), involving an inducible costimulator (ICOS)-ICOSL pathway (Akbari et al., 2002). The induced T_{regs} are capable of transferring protection against airway hyperresponsiveness to previously sensitized mice. These observations are useful in understanding the interplay of allergen-specific cells and their phenotypes in the pathogenesis of allergic disease. The exploitation of the immunosuppressive power of allergen-specific T_{regs} will require more information about how these cells are formed and what vaccine formulations might increase their induction or improve their function.

Adjuvants in the immunotherapy of autoimmunity

Organ-specific autoimmunity is often considered to be driven by autoreactive inflammatory Th1 T cells producing cytokines such as IFN-γ and TNF-α (Ando et al., 1989; Campbell et al., 1991), although some autoimmune diseases (e.g., lupus) cannot be characterized in this way and many of the cytokines involved have a variety of immunosuppressive as well as inflammatory functions (O'Shea et al., 2002). Current treatments for autoimmunity involve the general suppression of inflammation as well as new biotherapeutics targeting specific cytokines, such as anti-TNF-α monoclonals. There are several difficulties to be overcome in developing new drugs for autoimmunity. Although target autoantigens recognized by autoimmune cells have been described for various autoimmune diseases, the broadening of the autoimmune response, a phenomenon termed "epitope spreading," means that autoreactivity may be induced to other antigens (Vanderlugt and Miller, 2002; Steinman, 2004). This implies that treatments targeting a single epitope might not be optimal, and rather the deviation of the immune system away from autoreactivity or the induction of antigen or organ-specific immunosuppression may be more feasible.

Immune deviation to treat autoimmunity

Several treatments for autoimmunity have emerged that may act by inducing immune deviation away from Th1 towards Th2 immunity. For example, a recent trial of IL-4 therapy for psoriasis reported immune deviation away from Th1, with decreased IFN-γ production and reduced Th1 phenotype CD4+ T cells (Ghoreschi et al., 2003). Similarly, immune deviation has been proposed as a mechanism to explain beneficial effects of statins (Youssef et al., 2002), PPAR-α agonists

(Lovett-Racke et al., 2004), and retinoids (Racke et al., 1995) in the treatment of EAE, an animal model for MS.

Immune deviation may also be induced by immunization with so-called "altered peptide ligands" (APLs). These are peptide analogs of autoantigens that are capable of engaging the TCR of autoreactive T cells but do not lead to full activation. The best-studied example of this is glatiramer acetate (GA, also known as copolymer-1 or by the trade name Copaxone®), a random copolymer of amino acids designed to mimic the composition of myelin basic protein (MBP). This is effective in preventing EAE (Teitelbaum et al., 1971) and is used to treat relapsing-remitting MS in humans (Johnson et al., 1995). It appears to act in several ways, including the induction of a Th2-dominated T cell response to myelin antigens (Aharoni et al., 2000; Duda et al., 2000). Despite the success of GA, other clinical trials of APLs have given mixed results. For example, two trials of APLs of MBP in MS patients had to be halted after an exacerbation of disease in some patients in one study (Bielekova et al., 2000) and the induction of allergic symptoms in the other (Kappos et al., 2000). In general the use of APLs may be a difficult strategy, because antagonists for one particular T cell clone may act as agonists for a related clone recognizing the same antigen.

Tolerance induction to prevent autoimmunity

In animal models of autoimmune disease, tolerance to autoantigens induced by oral antigen administration can be effective in reducing disease symptoms (Faria et al., 2003; Maiti et al., 2004; Min et al., 2004). While results in human trials have so far been less successful, a recent publication noted an improvement in the symptoms of juvenile arthritis patients after oral administration of type II collagen (Myers et al., 2001).

Antigen presentation by immature DCs is qualitatively different compared to activated, mature DCs (Lindquist et al., 2004) and may induce tolerance in peripheral antigen-specific T cells (Steinman et al., 2003). Recently the targeting of antigen to immature DCs by coupling the antigen to a DC-specific antibody led to antigen-specific tolerance (Bonifaz et al., 2002). A safety concern with this procedure is that bystander infections may allow activated DCs to present self antigens, thereby actually exacerbating disease.

T_{regs} and the prevention of autoimmunity

Autoimmunity and T_{reg} subsets have been closely linked since the finding that depletion of these cells can lead to autoimmunity (Sakaguchi et al., 1995). Conversely, autoimmunity in experimental animal models can be blocked by the transfer of T_{regs} (Asano et al., 1996; Tang et al., 2004). As a result, methods to boost this regulatory arm of the immune system, either through vaccination protocols that favor the development of induced T_{regs} or by the *ex vivo* expansion of T_{regs}, are being pursued for the treatment of autoimmunity (Bluestone and Tang, 2004; Tang et al., 2004). There are several developments that are of interest. A recent report showed that antigen-specific T_{regs} could be induced by low-level subcutaneous infusion of specific peptide (Apostolou and von Boehmer, 2004). The *in vivo* induction of T_{regs} has also been proposed as an explanation for the beneficial effects of anti-CD3 monoclonal antibody treatment in diabetes (Chatenoud et al., 1997; Herold et al., 2002; Belghith et al., 2003). Research to induce the production of T_{regs} is in its infancy and no reliable protocols have been established. In addition, as is true for other cell-based therapies, it will be difficult for such approaches to become clinically important, in part because such therapies are rarely commercially viable. They are simply too expensive.

Summary and conclusions

Therapeutic vaccines for the treatment of noninfectious diseases encompass a wide variety of possible formulations, antigens, and mechanisms of action. While some vaccines aim to stimulate a strong humoral or

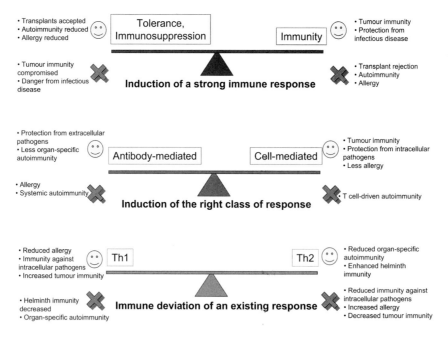

Figure 17.2 The balancing act of the immune system. Therapeutic vaccinations may conceivably alter the balance of immunosuppression and immunoreactivity, the class of immune response elicited, and the particular pathway of Th differentiation. All of these interventions could have positive and negative consequences that should be considered in vaccine and formulation design.

cell-mediated immune response, others are designed to induce the deviation or suppression of an existing reaction. Adjuvants, as a method of modifying the immune response, have an important part to play in fulfilling the potential of vaccination for noninfectious diseases.

Vaccination as a treatment for infectious disease has been hugely successful, but treatments for noninfectious diseases such as the induction of humoral responses against self antigens, T cell responses against tumors or immune deviation, and suppression of allergy and autoimmunity lead to their own special problems. The key will be balancing the competing requirements of treatment of these diseases vs. immunopathology by careful appreciation of the underlying disease mechanisms and the consequences of pushing the immune system too far in one direction (Figure 17.2). For example, humoral immunity sufficient to block the action of a self antigen may lead to increased susceptibility to certain diseases and special emphasis should be

placed on the reversibility of the effect. Also while strong cell-mediated immunity is almost certainly required for successful vaccination against cancer, care should be taken to choose antigens that will not lead to autoimmunity. Interference with the mechanisms of immunosuppression should also be made with care. Does overcoming immunosuppressive mechanisms in cancer therapy predispose to allergy or, more problematic, autoimmunity? Does enhancing immunosuppression to combat allergy and autoimmunity leave individuals at greater risk of cancer? The answers to these important questions will only become clear with the continued careful development of vaccines and their formulations.

■ References

Aharoni, R., Teitelbaum, D., Leitner, O., Meshorer, A., Sela, M., and Arnon, R. (2000). Specific Th2 cells accumulate in the central nervous system of mice protected against experimental autoimmune encephalomyelitis by copolymer 1. *Proc. Natl. Acad. Sci. USA* 97, 11472–11477.

Ahlers, J.D., Belyakov, I.M., Terabe, M., Koka, R., Donaldson, D.D., Thomas, E.K., and Berzofsky, J.A. (2002). A push-pull approach to maximize vaccine efficacy: abrogating suppression with an IL-13 inhibitor while augmenting help with granulocyte/macrophage colony-stimulating factor and CD40L. *Proc. Natl. Acad. Sci. USA* 99, 13020–13025.

Akbari, O., Freeman, G.J., Meyer, E.H., Greenfield, E.A., Chang, T.T., Sharpe, A.H., Berry, G., DeKruyff, R.H., and Umetsu, D.T. (2002). Antigen-specific regulatory T cells develop *via* the ICOS-ICOS-ligand pathway and inhibit allergen-induced airway hyperreactivity. *Nature Med.* 8, 1024–1032.

Akdis, C.A. and Blaser, K. (2001). Role of IL-10 in allergen-specific immunotherapy and normal response to allergens. *Microbes Infect.* 3, 891–898.

Akdis, C.A., Blesken, T., Akdis, M., Wuthrich, B., and Blaser, K. (1998). Role of interleukin 10 in specific immunotherapy. *J. Clin. Invest.* 102, 98–106.

Akdis, M., Verhagen, J., Taylor, A., Karamloo, F., Karagiannidis, C., Crameri, R., Thunberg, S., Deniz, G., Valenta, R., Fiebig, H., Kegel, C., Disch, R., Schmidt-Weber, C.B., Blaser, K., and Akdis, C.A. (2004). Immune responses in healthy and allergic individuals are characterized by a fine balance between allergen-specific T regulatory 1 and T helper 2 cells. *J. Exp. Med.* 199, 1567–1575.

Akira, S., Takeda, K., and Kaisho, T. (2001). Toll-like receptors: critical proteins linking innate and acquired immunity. *Nature Immunol.* 2, 675–680.

Akiyama, Y., Watanabe, M., Maruyama, K., Ruscetti, F.W., Wiltrout, R.H., and Yamaguchi, K. (2000). Enhancement of antitumor immunity against B16 melanoma tumor using genetically modified dendritic cells to produce cytokines. *Gene Ther.* 7, 2113–2121.

Alyanakian, M.A., You, S., Damotte, D., Gouarin, C., Esling, A., Garcia, C., Havouis, S., Chatenoud, L., and Bach, J.F. (2003). Diversity of regulatory CD4+ T cells controlling distinct organ-specific autoimmune diseases. *Proc. Natl. Acad. Sci. USA* 100, 15806–15811.

Ando, D.G., Clayton, J., Kono, D., Urban, J.L., and Sercarz, E.E. (1989). Encephalitogenic T cells in the B10.PL model of experimental allergic encephalomyelitis (EAE) are of the Th-1 lymphokine subtype. *Cell. Immunol.* 124, 132–143.

Apostolou, I. and von Boehmer, H. (2004). In vivo instruction of suppressor commitment in naive T cells. *J. Exp. Med.* 199, 1401–1408.

Asano, M., Toda, M., Sakaguchi, N., and Sakaguchi, S. (1996). Autoimmune disease as a consequence of developmental abnormality of a T cell subpopulation. *J. Exp. Med.* 184, 387–396.

Ashley, D.M., Faiola, B., Nair, S., Hale, L.P., Bigner, D.D., and Gilboa, E. (1997). Bone marrow-generated dendritic cells pulsed with tumor extracts or tumor RNA induce antitumor immunity against central nervous system tumors. *J. Exp. Med.* 186, 1177–1182.

Ault, K.A., Giuliano, A.R., Edwards, R.P., Tamms, G., Kim, L.L., Smith, J.F., Jansen, K.U., Allende, M.,

Taddeo, F.J., Skulsky, D., and Barr, E. (2004). A phase I study to evaluate a human papillomavirus (HPV) type 18 L1 VLP vaccine. *Vaccine* 22, 3004–3007.

Bachmann, M.F. and Dyer, M.R. (2004). Therapeutic vaccination for chronic diseases: a new class of drugs in sight. *Nature Rev. Drug Discov.* 3, 81–88.

Bachmann, M.F., Rohrer, U.H., Kundig, T.M., Burki, K., Hengartner, H., and Zinkernagel, R.M. (1993). The influence of antigen organization on B cell responsiveness. *Science* 262, 1448–1451.

Baldrick, P., Richardson, D., and Wheeler, A.W. (2001). Safety evaluation of a glutaraldehyde modified tyrosine adsorbed housedust mite extract containing monophosphoryl lipid A (MPL) adjuvant: a new allergy vaccine for dust mite allergy. *Vaccine* 20, 737–743.

Ball, J.M., Graham, D.Y., Opekun, A.R., Gilger, M.A., Guerrero, R.A., and Estes, M.K. (1999). Recombinant Norwalk virus-like particles given orally to volunteers: phase I study. *Gastroenterology* 117, 40–48.

Banchereau, J., Palucka, A.K., Dhodapkar, M., Burkeholder, S., Taquet, N., Rolland, A., Taquet, S., Coquery, S., Wittkowski, K.M., Bhardwaj, N., Pineiro, L., Steinman, R., and Fay, J. (2001). Immune and clinical responses in patients with metastatic melanoma to CD34+ progenitor-derived dendritic cell vaccine. *Cancer Res.* 61, 6451–6458.

Barrios, C., Brawand, P., Berney, M., Brandt, C., Lambert, P.H., and Siegrist, C.A. (1996). Neonatal and early life immune responses to various forms of vaccine antigens qualitatively differ from adult responses: predominance of a Th2-biased pattern which persists after adult boosting. *Eur. J. Immunol.* 26, 1489–1496.

Belghith, M., Bluestone, J.A., Barriot, S., Megret, J., Bach, J.F., and Chatenoud, L. (2003). TGF-β-dependent mechanisms mediate restoration of self-tolerance induced by antibodies to CD3 in overt autoimmune diabetes. *Nature Med.* 9, 1202–1208.

Bennett, C.L., Christie, J., Ramsdell, F., Brunkow, M.E., Ferguson, P.J., Whitesell, L., Kelly, T.E., Saulsbury, F.T., Chance, P.F., and Ochs, H.D. (2001). The immune dysregulation, polyendocrinopathy, enteropathy, X-linked syndrome (IPEX) is caused by mutations of Foxp3. *Nature Genet.* 27, 20–21.

Benson, E.M., Clarkson, J., Law, M., Marshall, P., Kelleher, A.D., Smith, D.E., Patou, G., Stewart, G.J., Cooper, D.A., and French, R.A. (1999). Therapeutic vaccination with p24-VLP and zidovudine augments HIV-specific cytotoxic T lymphocyte activity in asymptomatic HIV-infected individuals. *AIDS Res. Hum. Retroviruses* 15, 105–113.

Berzofsky, J.A., Terabe, M., Oh, S., Belyakov, I.M., Ahlers, J.D., Janik, J.E., and Morris, J.C. (2004). Progress on new vaccine strategies for the immunotherapy and prevention of cancer. *J. Clin. Invest.* 113, 1515–1525.

Bielekova, B., Goodwin, B., Richert, N., Cortese, I., Kondo, T., Afshar, G., Gran, B., Eaton, J., Antel, J., Frank, J.A., McFarland, H.F., and Martin, R. (2000). Encephalitogenic potential of the myelin basic protein peptide (amino acids

83–99) in multiple sclerosis: results of a phase II clinical trial with an altered peptide ligand. *Nature Med.* 6, 1167–1175.

Blattman, J.N. and Greenberg, P.D. (2004). Cancer immunotherapy: a treatment for the masses. *Science* 305, 200–205.

Bluestone, J.A. and Tang, Q. (2004). Therapeutic vaccination using CD4+CD25+ antigen-specific regulatory T cells. *Proc. Natl. Acad. Sci. USA* 101 (Suppl. 2), 14622–14626.

Bonifaz, L., Bonnyay, D., Mahnke, K., Rivera, M., Nussenzweig, M.C., and Steinman, R.M. (2002). Efficient targeting of protein antigen to the dendritic cell receptor DEC-205 in the steady state leads to antigen presentation on major histocompatibility complex class I products and peripheral CD8+ T cell tolerance. *J. Exp. Med.* 196, 1627–1638.

Borish, L.C., Nelson, H.S., Lanz, M.J., Claussen, L., Whitmore, J.B., Agosti, J.M., and Garrison, L. (1999). Interleukin-4 receptor in moderate atopic asthma. A phase I/II randomized, placebo-controlled trial. *Am. J. Respir. Crit. Care Med.* 160, 1816–1823.

Borkow, G., Leng, Q., Weisman, Z., Stein, M., Galai, N., Kalinkovich, A., and Bentwich, Z. (2000). Chronic immune activation associated with intestinal helminth infections results in impaired signal transduction and anergy. *J. Clin. Invest.* 106, 1053–1060.

Bretscher, P.A., Wei, G., Menon, J.N., and Bielefeldt-Ohmann, H. (1992). Establishment of stable, cell-mediated immunity that makes "susceptible" mice resistant to Leishmania major. *Science* 257, 539–542.

Brett, B.T., Smith, S.C., Bouvier, C.V., Michaeli, D., Hochhauser, D., Davidson, B.R., Kurzawinski, T.R., Watkinson, A.F., Van Someren, N., Pounder, R.E., and Caplin, M.E. (2002). Phase II study of anti-gastrin-17 antibodies, raised to G17DT, in advanced pancreatic cancer. *J. Clin. Oncol.* 20, 4225–4231.

Broide, D., Schwarze, J., Tighe, H., Gifford, T., Nguyen, M.-D., Malek, S., Van Uden, J., Martin-Orozco, E., Gelfand, E.W., and Raz, E. (1998). Immunostimulatory DNA sequences inhibit IL-5, eosinophilic inflammation, and airway hyperresponsiveness in mice. *J. Immunol.* 161, 7054–7062.

Broide, D.H., Stachnick, G., Castaneda, D., Nayar, J., Miller, M., Cho, J.Y., Roman, M., Zubeldia, J., Hayashi, T., and Raz, E. (2001). Systemic administration of immunostimulatory DNA sequences mediates reversible inhibition of Th2 responses in a mouse model of asthma. *J. Clin. Immunol.* 21, 175–182.

Brown, D.R., Fife, K.H., Wheeler, C.M., Koutsky, L.A., Lupinacci, L.M., Railkar, R., Suhr, G., Barr, E., Dicello, A., Li, W., Smith, J.F., Tadesse, A., and Jansen, K.U. (2004). Early assessment of the efficacy of a human papillomavirus type 16 L1 virus-like particle vaccine. *Vaccine* 22, 2936–2942.

Campbell, I.L., Kay, T.W., Oxbrow, L., and Harrison, L.C. (1991). Essential role for interferon-gamma and interleukin-6 in autoimmune insulin-dependent diabetes in NOD/WEHI mice. *J. Clin. Invest.* 87, 739–742.

Carroll, M.C. (2004). The complement system in regulation of adaptive immunity. *Nature Immunol.* 5, 981–986.

Chackerian, B., Lowy, D.R., and Schiller, J.T. (1999). Induction of autoantibodies to mouse CCR5 with recombinant papillomavirus particles. *Proc. Natl. Acad. Sci. USA* 96, 2373–2378.

Chackerian, B., Lowy, D.R., and Schiller, J.T. (2001). Conjugation of a self-antigen to papillomavirus-like particles allows for efficient induction of protective autoantibodies. *J. Clin. Invest.* 108, 415–423.

Chackerian, B., Lenz, P., Lowy, D.R., and Schiller, J.T. (2002). Determinants of autoantibody induction by conjugated papillomavirus virus-like particles. *J. Immunol.* 169, 6120–6126.

Chatenoud, L., Primo, J., and Bach, J.F. (1997). CD3 antibody-induced dominant self tolerance in overtly diabetic NOD mice. *J. Immunol.* 158, 2947–2954.

Chen, H.W., Lee, Y.P., Chung, Y.F., Shih, Y.C., Tsai, J.P., Tao, M.H., and Ting, C.C. (2003a). Inducing long-term survival with lasting anti-tumor immunity in treating B cell lymphoma by a combined dendritic cell-based and hydrodynamic plasmid-encoding IL-12 gene therapy. *Int. Immunol.* 15, 427–435.

Chen, W.J., Jin, W., Hardegen, N., Lei, K.-J., Li, L., Marinos, N., McGrady, G., and Wahl, S.M. (2003b). Conversion of peripheral CD4+CD25– naive T cells to CD4+CD25+ regulatory T cells by TGF-β induction of transcription factor Foxp3. *J. Exp. Med.* 198, 1875–1886.

Dalum, I., Jensen, M.R., Hindersson, P., Elsner, H.I., and Mouritsen, S. (1996). Breaking of B cell tolerance toward a highly conserved self protein. *J. Immunol.* 157, 4796–4804.

Dalum, I., Butler, D.M., Jensen, M.R., Hindersson, P., Steinaa, L., Waterston, A.M., Grell, S.N., Feldmann, M., Elsner, H.I., and Mouritsen, S. (1999). Therapeutic antibodies elicited by immunization against TNF-α. *Nature Biotechnol.* 17, 666–669.

De Heer, H.J., Hammad, H., Soullie, T., Hijdra, D., Vos, N., Willart, M.A.M., Hoogsteden, H.C., and Lambrecht, B.N. (2004). Essential role of lung plasmacytoid dendritic cells in preventing asthmatic reactions to harmless inhaled antigen. *J. Exp. Med.* 200, 89–98.

Drachenberg, K.J., Wheeler, A.W., Stuebner, P., and Horak, F. (2001). A well-tolerated grass pollen-specific allergy vaccine containing a novel adjuvant, monophosphoryl lipid A, reduces allergic symptoms after only four preseasonal injections. *Allergy* 56, 498–505.

Drachenberg, K.J., Heinzkill, M., Urban, E., and Woroniecki, S.R. (2003a). Efficacy and tolerability of short-term specific immunotherapy with pollen allergoids adjuvanted by monophosphoryl lipid A (MPL) for children and adolescents. *Allergol. Immunopathol.* (Madr.) 31, 270–277.

Drachenberg, K.J., Proll, S., Urban, E., and Woroniecki, S.R. (2003b). Single-course specific immunotherapy with mixed pollen allergoids: results of a multi-centre study. *Allergol. Immunopathol.* (Madr.) 31, 77–82.

Dranoff, G., Jaffee, E., Lazenby, A., Golumbek, P., Levitsky, H., Brose, K., Jackson, V., Hamada, H., Pardoll, D., and Mulligan, R.C. (1993). Vaccination with irradiated tumor cells engineered to secrete murine granulocyte-macrophage colony-stimulating factor stimulates potent, specific, and long-lasting anti-tumor immunity. *Proc. Natl. Acad. Sci. USA* 90, 3539–3543.

Duda, P.W., Schmied, M.C., Cook, S.L., Krieger, J.I., and Hafler, D.A. (2000). Glatiramer acetate (copaxone) induces degenerate, Th2-polarized immune responses in patients with multiple sclerosis. *J. Clin. Invest.* 105, 967–976.

Ehrenstein, M.R., Evans, J.G., Singh, A., Moore, S., Warnes, G., Isenberg, D.A., and Mauri, C. (2004). Compromised function of regulatory T cells in rheumatoid arthritis and reversal by anti-TNFα therapy. *J. Exp. Med.* 200, 277–285.

Erb, K.J., Holloway, J.W., Sobeck, A., Moll, H., and Le Gros, G. (1998). Infection of mice with Mycobacterium bovis-bacillus Calmette-Guerin (BCG) suppresses allergen-induced airway eosinophilia. *J. Exp. Med.* 187, 561–569.

Esslinger, C., Romero, P., and MacDonald, H.R. (2002). Efficient transduction of dendritic cells and induction of a T-cell response by third-generation lentivectors. *Hum. Gene Ther.* 13, 1091–1100.

Evans, T.G., Bonnez, W., Rose, R.C., Koenig, S., Demeter, L., Suzich, J.A., O'Brien, D., Campbell, M., White, W.I., Balsley, J., and Reichman, R.C. (2001). A Phase I study of a recombinant viruslike particle vaccine against human papillomavirus type 11 in healthy adult volunteers. *J. Infect. Dis.* 183, 1485–1493.

Fantini, M.C., Becker, C., Monteleone, G., Pallone, F., Galle, P.R., and Neurath, M.F. (2004). Cutting edge: TGF-β induces a regulatory phenotype in CD4+CD25– T cells through Foxp3 induction and down-regulation of Smad7. *J. Immunol.* 172, 5149–5153.

Faria, A.M., Maron, R., Ficker, S.M., Slavin, A.J., Spahn, T., and Weiner, H.L. (2003). Oral tolerance induced by continuous feeding: enhanced up-regulation of transforming growth factor-β/interleukin-10 and suppression of experimental autoimmune encephalomyelitis. *J. Autoimmun.* 20, 135–145.

Fife, K.H., Wheeler, C.M., Koutsky, L.A., Barr, E., Brown, D.R., Schiff, M.A., Kiviat, N.B., Jansen, K.U., Barber, H., Smith, J.F., Tadesse, A., Giacoletti, K., Smith, P.R., Suhr, G., and Johnson, D.A. (2004). Dose-ranging studies of the safety and immunogenicity of human papillomavirus type 11 and type 16 virus-like particle candidate vaccines in young healthy women. *Vaccine* 22, 2943–2952.

Finn, O.J. (2003). Cancer vaccines: between the idea and the reality. *Nature Rev. Immunol.* 3, 630–641.

Fontenot, J.D., Gavin, M.A., and Rudensky, A.Y. (2003). Foxp3 programs the development and function of CD4+CD25+ regulatory T cells. *Nature Immunol.* 4, 330–336.

Gabrilovich, D.I., Chen, H.L., Girgis, K.R., Cunningham, H.T., Meny, G.M., Nadaf, S., Kavanaugh, D., and Carbone, D.P. (1996a). Production of vascular endothelial growth factor by human tumors inhibits the functional maturation of dendritic cells. *Nature Med.* 2, 1096–1103.

Gabrilovich, D.I., Nadaf, S., Corak, J., Berzofsky, J.A., and Carbone, D.P. (1996b). Dendritic cells in antitumor immune responses: II. Dendritic cells grown from bone marrow precursors, but not mature DC from tumor-bearing mice, are effective antigen carriers in the therapy of established tumors. *Cell. Immunol.* 170, 111–119.

Gamvrellis, A., Leong, D., Hanley, J.C., Xiang, S.D., Mottram, P., and Plebanski, M. (2004). Vaccines that facilitate antigen entry into dendritic cells. *Immunol. Cell Biol.* 82, 506–516.

Gardiner, S.M., Auton, T.R., Downham, M.R., Sharp, H.L., Kemp, P.A., March, J.E., Martin, H., Morgan, P.J., Rushton, A., Bennett, T., and Glover, J.F. (2000). Active immunization with angiotensin I peptide analogue vaccines selectively reduces the pressor effects of exogenous angiotensin I in conscious rats. *Br. J. Pharmacol.* 129, 1178–1182.

Gavett, S.H., O'Hearn, D.J., Li, X., Huang, S.K., Finkelman, F.D., and Wills-Karp, M. (1995). Interleukin 12 inhibits antigen-induced airway hyperresponsiveness, inflammation, and Th2 cytokine expression in mice. *J. Exp. Med.* 182, 1527–1536.

Gelinas, D.S., DaSilva, K., Fenili, D., St. George-Hyslop, P., and McLaurin, J. (2004). Immunotherapy for Alzheimer's disease. *Proc. Natl. Acad. Sci. USA* 101, 14657–14662.

Ghoreschi, K., Thomas, P., Breit, S., Dugas, M., Mailhammer, R., van Eden, W., van der Zee, R., Biedermann, T., Prinz, J., Mack, M., Mrowietz, U., Christophers, E., Schlondorff, D., Plewig, G., Sander, C.A., and Rocken, M. (2003). Interleukin-4 therapy of psoriasis induces Th2 responses and improves human autoimmune disease. *Nature Med.* 9, 40–46.

Godfrey, D.I. and Kronenberg, M. (2004). Going both ways: immune regulation via CD1d-dependent NKT cells. *J. Clin. Invest.* 114, 1379–1388.

Golgher, D., Jones, E., Powrie, F., Elliott, T., and Gallimore, A. (2002). Depletion of CD25+ regulatory cells uncovers immune responses to shared murine tumor rejection antigens. *Eur. J. Immunol.* 32, 3267–3275.

Goodnow, C.C. (1992). Transgenic mice and analysis of B-cell tolerance. *Annu. Rev. Immunol.* 10, 489–518.

Goodnow, C.C. (1997). Balancing immunity, autoimmunity, and self-tolerance. *Ann. NY Acad. Sci.* 815, 55–66.

Green, E.A., Gorelik, L., McGregor, C.M., Tran, E.H., and Flavell, R.A. (2003). CD4+CD25+ T regulatory cells control anti-islet CD8+ T cells through TGF-β–TGF-β receptor interactions in type 1 diabetes. *Proc. Natl. Acad. Sci. USA* 100, 10878–10883.

Groh, V., Wu, J., Yee, C., and Spies, T. (2002). Tumour-derived soluble MIC ligands impair expression of NKG2D and T-cell activation. *Nature* 419, 734–738.

Gruber, C., Kulig, M., Bergmann, R., Guggenmoos-Holzmann, I., Wahn, U., and the MAS-90 Study Group (2001). Delayed hypersensitivity to tuberculin, total immunoglobulin E, specific sensitization, and atopic manifestation in longitudinally followed early bacille Calmette-Guerin-vaccinated and nonvaccinated children. *Pediatrics* 107, e36.

Gruber, C., Meinlschmidt, G., Bergmann, R., Wahn, U., and Stark, K. (2002). Is early BCG vaccination associated with less atopic disease? An epidemiological study in german preschool children with different ethnic backgrounds. *Pediatr. Allergy Immunol.* 13, 177–181.

Guermonprez, P., Valladeau, J., Zitvogel, L., Thery, C., and Amigorena, S. (2002). Antigen presentation and T cell stimulation by dendritic cells. *Annu. Rev. Immunol.* 20, 621–667.

Hansen, G., Yeung, V.P., Berry, G., Umetsu, D.T., and DeKruyff, R.H. (2000). Vaccination with heat-killed listeria as adjuvant reverses established allergen-induced airway hyperreactivity and inflammation: role of CD8+ T cells and IL-18. *J. Immunol.* 164, 223–230.

Harro, C.D., Pang, Y.Y., Roden, R.B., Hildesheim, A., Wang, Z., Reynolds, M.J., Mast, T.C., Robinson, R., Murphy, B.R., Karron, R.A., Dillner, J., Schiller, J.T., and Lowy, D.R. (2001). Safety and immunogenicity trial in adult volunteers of a human papillomavirus 16 L1 virus-like particle vaccine. *J. Natl. Cancer Inst.* 93, 284–292.

Hartl, A., Hochreiter, R., Stepanoska, T., Ferreira, F., and Thalhamer, J. (2004). Characterization of the protective and therapeutic efficiency of a DNA vaccine encoding the major birch pollen allergen Bet V 1a. *Allergy* 59, 65–73.

Heikenwalder, M., Polymenidou, M., Junt, T., Sigurdson, C., Wagner, H., Akira, S., Zinkernagel, R., and Aguzzi, A. (2004). Lymphoid follicle destruction and immunosuppression after repeated CpG oligodeoxynucleotide administration. *Nature Med.* 10, 187–192.

Heinzel, F., Sadick, M., Holaday, B., Coffman, R., and Locksley, R. (1989). Reciprocal expression of interferon γ or interleukin 4 during the resolution or progression of murine leishmaniasis. Evidence for expansion of distinct helper T cell subsets. *J. Exp. Med.* 169, 59–72.

Hemmi, H., Takeuchi, O., Kawai, T., Kaisho, T., Sato, S., Sanjo, H., Matsumoto, M., Hoshino, K., Wagner, H., Takeda, K., and Akira, S. (2000). A Toll-like receptor recognizes bacterial DNA. *Nature* 408, 740–745.

Herold, K.C., Hagopian, W., Auger, J.A., Poumian-Ruiz, E., Taylor, L., Donaldson, D., Gitelman, S.E., Harlan, D.M., Xu, D., Zivin, R.A., and Bluestone, J.A. (2002). Anti-CD3 monoclonal antibody in new-onset type 1 diabetes mellitus. *N. Engl. J. Med.* 346, 1692–1698.

Hertz, M., Mahalingam, S., Dalum, I., Klysner, S., Mattes, J., Neisig, A., Mouritsen, S., Foster, P.S., and Gautam, A. (2001). Active vaccination against IL-5 bypasses immunological tolerance and ameliorates experimental asthma. *J. Immunol.* 167, 3792–3799.

Hock, C., Konietzko, U., Streffer, J.R., Tracy, J., Signorell, A., Muller-Tillmanns, B., Lemke, U., Henke, K., Moritz, E., Garcia, E., Wollmer, M.A., Umbricht, D., de Quervain, D.J., Hofmann, M., Maddalena, A., Papassotiropoulos, A., and Nitsch, R.M. (2003). Antibodies against β-amyloid slow cognitive decline in Alzheimer's disease. *Neuron* 38, 547–554.

Hodi, F.S., Mihm, M.C., Soiffer, R.J., Haluska, F.G., Butler, M., Seiden, M.V., Davis, T., Henry-Spires, R., MacRae, S., Willman, A., Padera, R., Jaklitsch, M.T., Shankar, S., Chen, T.C., Korman, A., Allison, J.P., and Dranoff, G. (2003). Biologic activity of cytotoxic T lymphocyte-associated antigen 4 antibody blockade in previously vaccinated metastatic melanoma and ovarian carcinoma patients. *Proc. Natl. Acad. Sci. USA* 100, 4712–4717.

Hofstra, C.L., Van Ark, I., Hofman, G., Kool, M., Nijkamp, F.P., and Van Oosterhout, A.J. (1998). Prevention of Th2-like cell responses by coadministration of IL-12 and IL-18 is associated with inhibition of antigen-induced airway hyperresponsiveness, eosinophilia, and serum IgE levels. *J. Immunol.* 161, 5054–5060.

Hopfenspirger, M.T. and Agrawal, D.K. (2002). Airway hyperresponsiveness, late allergic response, and eosinophilia are reversed with mycobacterial antigens in ovalbumin-presensitized mice. *J. Immunol.* 168, 2516–2522.

Hosken, N.A., Shibuya, K., Heath, A.W., Murphy, K.M., and O'Garra, A. (1995). The effect of antigen dose on CD4+ T helper cell phenotype development in a T cell receptor-αβ -transgenic model. *J. Exp. Med.* 182, 1579–1584.

Houghton, A.N., Gold, J.S., and Blachere, N.E. (2001). Immunity against cancer: lessons learned from melanoma. *Curr. Opin. Immunol.* 13, 134–140.

Hsieh, C.S., Macatonia, S.E., Tripp, C.S., Wolf, S.F., O'Garra, A., and Murphy, K.M. (1993). Development of Th1 CD4+ T cells through IL-12 produced by listeria-induced macrophages. *Science* 260, 547–549.

Hsu, C.H., Chua, K.Y., Tao, M.H., Lai, Y.L., Wu, H.D., Huang, S.K., and Hsieh, K.H. (1996). Immunoprophylaxis of allergen-induced immunoglobulin E synthesis and airway hyperresponsiveness in vivo by genetic immunization. *Nature Med.* 2, 540–544.

Hudson, P.J. and Souriau, C. (2003). Engineered antibodies. *Nature Med.* 9, 129–134.

Humbles, A.A., Lloyd, C.M., McMillan, S.J., Friend, D.S., Xanthou, G., McKenna, E.E., Ghiran, S., Gerard, N.P., Yu, C., Orkin, S.H., and Gerard, C. (2004). A critical role for eosinophils in allergic airways remodeling. *Science* 305, 1776–1779.

Hurwitz, A.A., Yu, T.F., Leach, D.R., and Allison, J.P. (1998). CTLA-4 blockade synergizes with tumor-derived granulocyte-macrophage colony-stimulating factor for treatment of an experimental mammary carcinoma. *Proc. Natl. Acad. Sci. USA* 95, 10067–10071.

Iwasaki, A. and Medzhitov, R. (2004). Toll-like receptor control of the adaptive immune responses. *Nature Immunol.* 5, 987–995.

Jaffee, E.M., Hruban, R.H., Biedrzycki, B., Laheru, D., Schepers, K., Sauter, P.R., Goemann, M., Coleman, J., Grochow, L., Donehower, R.C., Lillemoe, K.D., O'Reilly, S., Abrams, R.A., Pardoll, D.M., Cameron, J.L., and Yeo, C.J. (2001). Novel allogeneic granulocyte-macrophage colony-stimulating factor-secreting tumor vaccine for pancreatic cancer: a phase I trial of safety and immune activation. *J. Clin. Oncol.* 19, 145–156.

Jain, V.V., Kitagaki, K., Businga, T., Hussain, I., George, C., O'Shaughnessy, P., and Kline, J.N. (2002). CpG-oligodeoxy-nucleotides inhibit airway remodeling in a murine model of chronic asthma. *J. Allergy Clin. Immunol.* 110, 867–872.

Jain, V.V., Businga, T.R., Kitagaki, K., George, C.L., O'Shaugh-nessy, P.T., and Kline, J.N. (2003). Mucosal immunotherapy with CpG oligodeoxynucleotides reverses a murine model of chronic asthma induced by repeated antigen exposure. *Am. J. Physiol. Lung Cell. Mol. Physiol.* 285, L1137–L1146.

Janssen, E.M., Lemmens, E.E., Wolfe, T., Christen, U., von Herrath, M.G., and Schoenberger, S.P. (2003). CD4+ T cells are required for secondary expansion and memory in CD8+ T lymphocytes. *Nature* 421, 852–856.

Jegerlehner, A., Storni, T., Lipowsky, G., Schmid, M., Pumpens, P., and Bachmann, M.F. (2002a). Regulation of IgG antibody responses by epitope density and CD21-mediated costimulation. *Eur. J. Immunol.* 32, 3305–3314.

Jegerlehner, A., Tissot, A., Lechner, F., Sebbel, P., Erdmann, I., Kundig, T., Bachi, T., Storni, T., Jennings, G., Pumpens, P., Renner, W.A., and Bachmann, M.F. (2002b). A molecular assembly system that renders antigens of choice highly repetitive for induction of protective B cell responses. *Vaccine* 20, 3104–3112.

Johnson, K.P., Brooks, B.R., Cohen, J.A., Ford, C.C., Goldstein, J., Lisak, R.P., Myers, L.W., Panitch, H.S., Rose, J.W., and Schiffer, R.B. (1995). Copolymer 1 reduces relapse rate and improves disability in relapsing-remitting multiple sclerosis: results of a phase III multicenter, double-blind placebo-controlled trial. Copolymer 1 Multiple Sclerosis Study Group. *Neurology* 45, 1268–1276.

Jutel, M., Pichler, W.J., Skrbic, D., Urwyler, A., Dahinden, C., and Muller, U.R. (1995). Bee venom immunotherapy results in decrease of IL-4 and IL-5 and increase of IFN-γ secretion in specific allergen-stimulated t cell cultures. *J. Immunol.* 154, 4187–4194.

Jutel, M., Akdis, M., Budak, F., Aebischer-Casaulta, C., Wrzyszcz, M., Blaser, K., and Akdis, C.A. (2003). IL-10 and TGF-β cooperate in the regulatory T cell response to mucosal allergens in normal immunity and specific immunotherapy. *Eur. J. Immunol.* 33, 1205–1214.

Kaplan, M. (2002). Eculizumab (Alexion). *Curr. Opin. Investig. Drugs* 3, 1017–1023.

Kappos, L., Comi, G., Panitch, H., Oger, J., Antel, J., Conlon, P., and Steinman, L. (2000). Induction of a non-encephalito-genic type 2 T helper-cell autoimmune response in multiple sclerosis after administration of an altered peptide ligand in a placebo-controlled, randomized phase II trial. Altered Peptide Ligand in Relapsing MS Study Group. *Nature Med.* 6, 1176–1182.

Kapsenberg, M.L. (2003). Dendritic-cell control of pathogen-driven T-cell polarization. *Nature Rev. Immunol.* 3, 984–993.

Kennedy, A.D., Beum, P.V., Solga, M.D., DiLillo, D.J., Lindorfer, M.A., Hess, C.E., Densmore, J.J., Williams, M.E., and Taylor, R.P. (2004). Rituximab infusion promotes rapid complement depletion and acute CD20 loss in chronic lymphocytic leukemia. *J. Immunol.* 172, 3280–3288.

Khattri, R., Cox, T., Yasayko, S.A., and Ramsdell, F. (2003). An essential role for scurfin in CD4+CD25+ T regulatory cells. *Nature Immunol.* 4, 337–342.

King, C.L., Mahanty, S., Kumaraswami, V., Abrams, J.S., Regunathan, J., Jayaraman, K., Ottesen, E.A., and Nutman, T.B. (1993). Cytokine control of parasite-specific anergy in human lymphatic filariasis. Preferential induction of a regulatory T helper type 2 lymphocyte subset. *J. Clin. Invest.* 92, 1667–1673.

Kips, J.C., O'Connor, B.J., Langley, S.J., Woodcock, A., Kerstjens, H.A., Postma, D.S., Danzig, M., Cuss, F., and Pauwels, R.A. (2003). Effect of SCH55700, a humanized anti-human interleukin-5 antibody, in severe persistent asthma: a pilot study. *Am. J. Respir. Crit. Care Med.* 167, 1655–1659.

Kline, J.N., Waldschmidt, T.J., Businga, T.R., Lemish, J.E., Weinstock, J.V., Thorne, P.S., and Krieg, A.M. (1998). Cutting edge: modulation of airway inflammation by CpG oligodeoxynucleotides in a murine model of asthma. *J. Immunol.* 160, 2555–2559.

Kline, J.N., Kitagaki, K., Businga, T.R., and Jain, V.V. (2002). Treatment of established asthma in a murine model using CpG oligodeoxynucleotides. *Am. J. Physiol. Lung Cell. Mol. Physiol.* 283, L170–L179.

Klinman, D.M. (2004). Immunotherapeutic uses of CpG oligodeoxynucleotides. *Nature Rev. Immunol.* 4, 249–258.

Klinman, D.M., Yi, A.-K., Beaucage, S.L., Conover, J., and Krieg, A.M. (1996). CpG motifs present in bacterial DNA rapidly induce lymphocytes to secrete interleukin 6, interleukin 12, and interferon γ. *Proc. Natl. Acad. Sci. USA* 93, 2879–2883.

Klinman, D.M., Yamshchikov, G., and Ishigatsubo, Y. (1997). Contribution of CpG motifs to the immunogenicity of DNA vaccines. *J. Immunol.* 158, 3635–3639.

Kopf, M., Le Gros, G., Bachmann, M., Lamers, M.C., Bluethmann, H., and Kohler, G. (1993). Disruption of the murine IL-4 gene blocks Th2 cytokine responses. *Nature* 362, 245–248.

Kriegel, M.A., Lohmann, T., Gabler, C., Blank, N., Kalden, J.R., and Lorenz, H.-M. (2004). Defective suppressor function of human CD4+ CD25+ regulatory T cells in autoimmune polyglandular syndrome type II. *J. Exp. Med.* 199, 1285–1291.

Kuipers, H. and Lambrecht, B.N. (2004). The interplay of dendritic cells, Th2 cells and regulatory T cells in asthma. *Curr. Opin. Immunol.* 16, 702–708.

Kuipers, H., Heirman, C., Hijdra, D., Muskens, F., Willart, M., van Meirvenne, S., Thielemans, K., Hoogsteden, H.C., and Lambrecht, B.N. (2004). Dendritic cells retrovirally overexpressing IL-12 induce strong Th1 responses to inhaled antigen in the lung but fail to revert established Th2 sensitization. *J. Leukoc. Biol.* 76, 1028–1038.

Kumano, K., Nakao, A., Nakajima, H., Hayashi, F., Kurimoto, M., Okamura, H., Saito, Y., and Iwamoto, I. (1999). Interleukin-18 enhances antigen-induced eosinophil recruitment into the mouse airways. *Am. J. Respir. Crit. Care Med.* 160, 873–878.

Kumar, M., Behera, A.K., Hu, J., Lockey, R.F., and Mohapatra, S.S. (2001). IFN-γ and IL-12 plasmid dnas as vaccine adjuvant in a murine model of grass allergy. *J. Allergy Clin. Immunol.* 108, 402–408.

Lack, G., Renz, H., Saloga, J., Bradley, K.L., Loader, J., Leung, D.Y., Larsen, G., and Gelfand, E.W. (1994). Nebulized but not parenteral IFN-γ decreases IgE production and normalizes airways function in a murine model of allergen sensitization. *J. Immunol.* 152, 2546–2554.

Lack, G., Bradley, K.L., Hamelmann, E., Renz, H., Loader, J., Leung, D.Y., Larsen, G., and Gelfand, E.W. (1996). Nebulized IFN-γ inhibits the development of secondary allergic responses in mice. *J. Immunol.* 157, 1432–1439.

Leach, D.R., Krummel, M.F., and Allison, J.P. (1996). Enhancement of antitumor immunity by CTLA-4 blockade. *Science* 271, 1734–1736.

Leckie, M.J., ten Brinke, A., Khan, J., Diamant, Z., O'Connor, B.J., Walls, C.M., Mathur, A.K., Cowley, H.C., Chung, K.F., Djukanovic, R., Hansel, T.T., Holgate, S.T., Sterk, P.J., and Barnes, P.J. (2000). Effects of an interleukin-5 blocking monoclonal antibody on eosinophils, airway hyper-responsiveness, and the late asthmatic response. *Lancet* 356, 2144–2148.

Lee, P., Wang, F., Kuniyoshi, J., Rubio, V., Stuges, T., Groshen, S., Gee, C., Lau, R., Jeffery, G., Margolin, K., Marty, V., and Weber, J. (2001). Effects of interleukin-12 on the immune response to a multipeptide vaccine for resected metastatic melanoma. *J. Clin. Oncol.* 19, 3836–3847.

Lewis, D.B. (2002). Allergy immunotherapy and inhibition of Th2 immune responses: a sufficient strategy? *Curr. Opin. Immunol.* 14, 644–651.

Lewis, J.J. (2004). Therapeutic cancer vaccines: using unique antigens. *Proc. Natl. Acad. Sci. USA* 101, 14653–14656.

Li, X.M., Chopra, R.K., Chou, T.Y., Schofield, B.H., Wills-Karp, M., and Huang, S.K. (1996). Mucosal IFN-γ gene transfer inhibits pulmonary allergic responses in mice. *J. Immunol.* 157, 3216–3219.

Lindquist, R.L., Shakhar, G., Dudziak, D., Wardemann, H., Eisenreich, T., Dustin, M.L., and Nussenzweig, M.C. (2004). Visualizing dendritic cell networks *in vivo*. *Nature Immunol.* 5, 1243–1250.

Liu, H., Hu, B., Xu, D., and Liew, F.Y. (2003). CD4+CD25+ regulatory T cells cure murine colitis: the role of IL-10, TGF-β, and CTLA4. *J. Immunol.* 171, 5012–5017.

Lovett-Racke, A.E., Hussain, R.Z., Northrop, S., Choy, J., Rocchini, A., Matthes, L., Chavis, J.A., Diab, A., Drew, P.D., and Racke, M.K. (2004). Peroxisome proliferator-activated receptor α agonists as therapy for autoimmune disease. *J. Immunol.* 172, 5790–5798.

Ludwig-Portugall, I., Montermann, E., Kremer, A., Reske-Kunz, A.B., and Sudowe, S. (2004). Prevention of long-term IgE antibody production by gene gun-mediated DNA vaccination. *J. Allergy Clin. Immunol.* 114, 951–957.

Macatonia, S., Hosken, N., Litton, M., Vieira, P., Hsieh, C., Culpepper, J., Wysocka, M., Trinchieri, G., Murphy, K., and O'Garra, A. (1995). Dendritic cells produce IL-12 and direct the development of Th1 cells from naive CD4+ T cells. *J. Immunol.* 154, 5071–5079.

Maecker, H.T., Hansen, G., Walter, D.M., DeKruyff, R.H., Levy, S., and Umetsu, D.T. (2001). Vaccination with allergen-IL-18 fusion DNA protects against, and reverses established, airway hyperreactivity in a murine asthma model. *J. Immunol.* 166, 959–965.

Maiti, P.K., Feferman, T., Im, S.H., Souroujon, M.C., and Fuchs, S. (2004). Immunosuppression of rat myasthenia gravis by oral administration of a syngeneic acetylcholine receptor fragment. *J Neuroimmunol.* 152, 112–120.

Major, T., Wohlleben, G., Reibetanz, B., and Erb, K.J. (2002). Application of heat killed Mycobacterium bovis-BCG into the lung inhibits the development of allergen-induced Th2 responses. *Vaccine* 20, 1532–1540.

Marshall, J.L., Hoyer, R.J., Toomey, M.A., Faraguna, K., Chang, P., Richmond, E., Pedicano, J.E., Gehan, E., Peck, R.A., Arlen, P., Tsang, K.Y., and Schlom, J. (2000). Phase I study in advanced cancer patients of a diversified prime-and-boost vaccination protocol using recombinant vaccinia virus and recombinant nonreplicating avipox virus to elicit anti-carcinoembryonic antigen immune responses. *J. Clin. Oncol.* 18, 3964–3973.

McHugh, S.M., Deighton, J., Stewart, A.G., Lachmann, P.J., and Ewan, P.W. (1995). Bee venom immunotherapy induces a shift in cytokine responses from a Th-2 to a Th-1 dominant pattern: comparison of rush and conventional immunotherapy. *Clin. Exp. Allergy* 25, 828–838.

Mettens, P. and Monteyne, P. (2002). Life-style vaccines. *Br. Med. Bull.* 62, 175–186.

Min, S.Y., Hwang, S.Y., Park, K.S., Lee, J.S., Lee, K.E., Kim, K.W., Jung, Y.O., Koh, H.J., Do, J.H., Kim, H., and Kim, H.Y. (2004). Induction of IL-10-producing CD4+CD25+ T cells in animal model of collagen-induced arthritis by oral administration of type II collagen. *Arthritis Res. Ther.* 6, R213–R219.

Morgan, D., Diamond, D.M., Gottschall, P.E., Ugen, K.E., Dickey, C., Hardy, J., Duff, K., Jantzen, P., DiCarlo, G., Wilcock, D., Connor, K., Hatcher, J., Hope, C., Gordon, M., and Arendash, G.W. (2000). A β-peptide vaccination prevents memory loss in an animal model of Alzheimer's disease. *Nature* 408, 982–985.

Moskophidis, D., Lechner, F., Pircher, H., and Zinkernagel, R.M. (1993). Virus persistence in acutely infected immuno-competent mice by exhaustion of antiviral cytotoxic effector T cells. *Nature* 362, 758–761.

Mosmann, T., Cherwinski, H., Bond, M., Giedlin, M., and Coffman, R. (1986). Two types of murine helper t cell clone: I. Definition according to profiles of lymphokine activities and secreted proteins. *J. Immunol.* 136, 2348–2357.

Moulton, H.M., Yoshihara, P.H., Mason, D.H., Iversen, P.L., and Triozzi, P.L. (2002). Active specific immunotherapy with a beta-human chorionic gonadotropin peptide vaccine in patients with metastatic colorectal cancer: antibody response is associated with improved survival. *Clin. Cancer Res.* 8, 2044–2051.

Murphy, K.M. and Reiner, S.L. (2002). The lineage decisions of helper T cells. *Nature Rev. Immunol.* 2, 933–944.

Myers, L.K., Higgins, G.C., Finkel, T.H., Reed, A.M., Thompson, J.W., Walton, R.C., Hendrickson, J., Kerr, N.C., Pandya-Lipman, R.K., Shlopov, B.V., Stastny, P., Postlethwaite, A.E., and Kang, A.H. (2001). Juvenile arthritis and autoimmunity to type II collagen. *Arthritis Rheum.* 44, 1775–1781.

Nair, S.K., Snyder, D., Rouse, B.T., and Gilboa, E. (1997). Regression of tumors in mice vaccinated with professional antigen-presenting cells pulsed with tumor extracts. *Int. J. Cancer* 70, 706–715.

Nakamura, K., Kitani, A., Fuss, I., Pedersen, A., Harada, N., Nawata, H., and Strober, W. (2004). TGF-β1 plays an important role in the mechanism of CD4+CD25+ regulatory T cell activity in both humans and mice. *J. Immunol.* 172, 834–842.

Nastala, C., Edington, H., McKinney, T., Tahara, H., Nalesnik, M., Brunda, M., Gately, M., Wolf, S., Schreiber, R., and Storkus, W. (1994). Recombinant IL-12 administration induces tumor regression in association with IFN-γ production. *J. Immunol.* 153, 1697–1706.

Nicoll, J.A., Wilkinson, D., Holmes, C., Steart, P., Markham, H., and Weller, R.O. (2003). Neuropathology of human Alzheimer disease after immunization with amyloid-beta peptide: a case report. *Nature Med.* 9, 448–452.

Nieda, M., Okai, M., Tazbirkova, A., Lin, H., Yamaura, A., Ide, K., Abraham, R., Juji, T., Macfarlane, D.J., and Nicol, A.J. (2004). Therapeutic Activation of Vα24+ Vβ11+NKT cells in human subjects results in highly coordinated secondary activation of acquired and innate immunity. *Blood* 103, 383–389.

Noon, L. (1911). Prophylactic inoculation against hay fever. *Lancet* 1, 1572–1573.

Oida, T., Zhang, X., Goto, M., Hachimura, S., Totsuka, M., Kaminogawa, S., and Weiner, H.L. (2003). CD4+CD25− T cells that express latency-associated peptide on the surface suppress CD4+CD45RBhigh-induced colitis by a TGF-β-dependent mechanism. *J. Immunol.* 170, 2516–2522.

Orgogozo, J.M., Gilman, S., Dartigues, J.F., Laurent, B., Puel, M., Kirby, L.C., Jouanny, P., Dubois, B., Eisner, L., Flitman, S., Michel, B.F., Boada, M., Frank, A., and Hock, C. (2003). Subacute meningoencephalitis in a subset of patients with AD after Aβ 42 immunization. *Neurology* 61, 46–54.

O'Shea, J.J., Ma, A., and Lipsky, P. (2002). Cytokines and autoimmunity. *Nature Rev. Immunol.* 2, 37–45.

Paglia, P., Chiodoni, C., Rodolfo, M., and Colombo, M.P. (1996). Murine dendritic cells loaded in vitro with soluble protein prime cytotoxic T lymphocytes against tumor antigen in vivo. *J. Exp. Med.* 183, 317–322.

Parish, C.R. (1971). Immune response to chemically modified flagellin: II. Evidence for a fundamental relationship between humoral and cell-mediated immunity. *J. Exp. Med.* 134, 21–47.

Parish, C.R. and Liew, F.Y. (1972). Immune response to chemically modified flagellin: 3. Enhanced cell-mediated immunity during high and low zone antibody tolerance to flagellin. *J. Exp. Med.* 135, 298–311.

Parronchi, P., Macchia, D., Piccinni, M.P., Biswas, P., Simonelli, C., Maggi, E., Ricci, M., Ansari, A.A., and Romagnani, S. (1991). Allergen- and bacterial antigen-specific T-cell clones established from atopic donors show a different profile of cytokine production. *Proc. Natl. Acad. Sci. USA* 88, 4538–4542.

Pastrana, D.V., Vass, W.C., Lowy, D.R., and Schiller, J.T. (2001). NHPV16 VLP vaccine induces human antibodies that neutralize divergent variants of HPV16. *Virology* 279, 361–369.

Paunio, M., Heinonen, O.P., Virtanen, M., Leinikki, P., Patja, A., and Peltola, H. (2000). Measles history and atopic diseases: a population-based cross-sectional study. *J. Am. Med. Assoc.* 283, 343–346.

Peng, Y., Laouar, Y., Li, M.O., Green, E.A., and Flavell, R.A. (2004). Tgf-{beta} regulates in vivo expansion of Foxp3-expressing CD4+CD25+ regulatory T cells responsible for protection against diabetes. *Proc. Natl. Acad. Sci. USA* 101, 4572–4577.

Petrovsky, N. and Aguilar, J.C. (2004). Vaccine adjuvants: current state and future trends. *Immunol. Cell Biol.* 82, 488–496.

Phan, G.Q., Yang, J.C., Sherry, R.M., Hwu, P., Topalian, S.L., Schwartzentruber, D.J., Restifo, N.P., Haworth, L.R., Seipp, C.A., Freezer, L.J., Morton, K.E., Mavroukakis, S.A., Duray, P.H., Steinberg, S.M., Allison, J.P., Davis, T.A., and Rosenberg, S.A. (2003). Cancer regression and autoimmunity induced by cytotoxic T lymphocyte-associated antigen 4 blockade in patients with metastatic melanoma. *Proc. Natl. Acad. Sci. USA* 100, 8372–8377.

Prasad, S.J., Farrand, K.J., Matthews, S.A., Chang, J.H., McHugh, R.S., and Ronchese, F. (2005). Dendritic cells loaded with stressed tumor cells elicit long-lasting protective tumor immunity in mice depleted of CD4+CD25+ regulatory T cells. *J. Immunol.* 174, 90–98.

Prescott, S.L., Macaubas, C., Holt, B.J., Smallacombe, T.B., Loh, R., Sly, P.D., and Holt, P.G. (1998a). Transplacental priming of the human immune system to environmental allergens: universal skewing of initial T cell responses toward the Th2 cytokine profile. *J. Immunol.* 160, 4730–4737.

Prescott, S.L., Macaubas, C., Smallacombe, T., Holt, B.J., Sly, P.D., Loh, R., and Holt, P.G. (1998b). Reciprocal age-related patterns of allergen-specific T-cell immunity in normal vs. atopic infants. *Clin. Exp. Allergy* 28 (Suppl. 5), 39–44; discussion 50–51.

Racke, M., Burnett, D., Pak, S., Albert, P., Cannella, B., Raine, C., McFarlin, D., and Scott, D. (1995). Retinoid treatment of experimental allergic encephalomyelitis. IL-4 production correlates with improved disease course. *J. Immunol.* 154, 450–458.

Reff, M., Carner, K., Chambers, K., Chinn, P., Leonard, J., Raab, R., Newman, R., Hanna, N., and Anderson, D. (1994). Depletion of B cells in vivo by a chimeric mouse human monoclonal antibody to CD20. *Blood* 83, 435–445.

Reichert, J.M. (2001). Monoclonal antibodies in the clinic. *Nature Biotechnol.* 19, 819–822.

Richard, M., Grencis, R.K., Humphreys, N.E., Renauld, J.-C., and Van Snick, J. (2000). Anti-IL-9 vaccination prevents worm expulsion and blood eosinophilia in Trichuris muris-infected mice. *Proc. Natl. Acad. Sci. USA* 97, 767–772.

Robinson, D.S., Hamid, Q., Ying, S., Tsicopoulos, A., Barkans, J., Bentley, A.M., Corrigan, C., Durham, S.R., and Kay, A.B. (1992). Predominant Th2-like bronchoalveolar T-lymphocyte population in atopic asthma. *N. Engl. J. Med.* 326, 298–304.

Robinson, S.R., Bishop, G.M., Lee, H.G., and Munch, G. (2004). Lessons from the AN 1792 Alzheimer vaccine: lest we forget. *Neurobiol. Aging* 25, 609–615.

Rosenberg, S.A., Yang, J.C., Schwartzentruber, D.J., Hwu, P., Marincola, F.M., Topalian, S.L., Restifo, N.P., Dudley, M.E., Schwarz, S.L., Spiess, P.J., Wunderlich, J.R., Parkhurst, M.R., Kawakami, Y., Seipp, C.A., Einhorn, J.H., and White, D.E. (1998). Immunologic and therapeutic evaluation of a synthetic peptide vaccine for the treatment of patients with metastatic melanoma. *Nature Med.* 4, 321–327.

Sad, S., Rao, K., Arora, R., Talwar, G.P., and Raghupathy, R. (1992). Bypass of carrier-induced epitope-specific suppression using a T-helper epitope. *Immunology* 76, 599–603.

Sakaguchi, S., Sakaguchi, N., Asano, M., Itoh, M., and Toda, M. (1995). Immunologic self-tolerance maintained by activated T cells expressing IL-2 receptor α-chains (CD25). Breakdown of a single mechanism of self-tolerance causes various autoimmune diseases. *J. Immunol.* 155, 1151–1164.

Salgia, R., Lynch, T., Skarin, A., Lucca, J., Lynch, C., Jung, K., Hodi, F.S., Jaklitsch, M., Mentzer, S., Swanson, S., Lukanich, J., Bueno, R., Wain, J., Mathisen, D., Wright, C., Fidias, P., Donahue, D., Clift, S., Hardy, S., Neuberg, D., Mulligan, R., Webb, I., Sugarbaker, D., Mihm, M., and Dranoff, G. (2003). Vaccination with irradiated autologous tumor cells engineered to secrete granulocyte-macrophage colony-stimulating factor augments antitumor immunity in some patients with metastatic non-small-cell lung carcinoma. *J. Clin. Oncol.* 21, 624–630.

Sato, Y., Roman, M., Tighe, H., Lee, D., Corr, M., Nguyen, M.D., Silverman, G.J., Lotz, M., Carson, D.A., and Raz, E. (1996). Immunostimulatory DNA sequences necessary for effective intradermal gene immunization. *Science* 273, 352–354.

Schenk, D., Barbour, R., Dunn, W., Gordon, G., Grajeda, H., Guido, T., Hu, K., Huang, J., Johnson-Wood, K., Khan, K., Kholodenko, D., Lee, M., Liao, Z., Lieberburg, I., Motter, R., Mutter, L., Soriano, F., Shopp, G., Vasquez, N., Vandevert, C., Walker, S., Wogulis, M., Yednock, T., Games, D., and Seubert, P. (1999). Immunization with amyloid-β attenuates Alzheimer-disease-like pathology in the PDAPP mouse. *Nature* 400, 173–177.

Schuler, G., Schuler-Thurner, B., and Steinman, R.M. (2003). The use of dendritic cells in cancer immunotherapy. *Curr. Opin. Immunol.* 15, 138–147.

Scott, P., Natovitz, P., Coffman, R., Pearce, E., and Sher, A. (1988). Immunoregulation of cutaneous leishmaniasis. T cell lines that transfer protective immunity or exacerbation belong to different t helper subsets and respond to distinct parasite antigens. *J. Exp. Med.* 168, 1675–1684.

Shaheen, S.O., Aaby, P., Hall, A.J., Barker, D.J., Heyes, C.B., Shiell, A.W., and Goudiaby, A. (1996). Measles and atopy in Guinea-Bissau. *Lancet* 347, 1792–1796.

Shankaran, V., Ikeda, H., Bruce, A.T., White, J.M., Swanson, P.E., Old, L.J., and Schreiber, R.D. (2001). IFNγ and lymphocytes prevent primary tumour development and shape tumour immunogenicity. *Nature* 410, 1107–1111.

Shedlock, D.J. and Shen, H. (2003). Requirement for CD4 T cell help in generating functional CD8 T cell memory. *Science* 300, 337–339.

Shirakawa, T., Enomoto, T., Shimazu, S., and Hopkin, J.M. (1997). The inverse association between tuberculin responses and atopic disorder. *Science* 275, 77–79.

Shirota, H., Sano, K., Kikuchi, T., Tamura, G., and Shirato, K. (2000). Regulation of murine airway eosinophilia and Th2 cells by antigen-conjugated CpG oligodeoxynucleotides as a novel antigen-specific immunomodulator. *J. Immunol.* 164, 5575–5582.

Siders, W.M., Vergilis, K.L., Johnson, C., Shields, J., and Kaplan, J.M. (2003). Induction of specific antitumor immunity in the mouse with the electrofusion product of tumor cells and dendritic cells. *Mol. Ther.* 7, 498–505.

Simms, M.S., Scholfield, D.P., Jacobs, E., Michaeli, D., Broome, P., Humphreys, J.E., and Bishop, M.C. (2000). Anti-GnRH antibodies can induce castrate levels of testosterone in patients with advanced prostate cancer. *Br. J. Cancer* 83, 443–446.

Simons, F.E., Shikishima, Y., Van Nest, G., Eiden, J.J., and HayGlass, K.T. (2004). Selective immune redirection in humans with ragweed allergy by injecting Amb a 1 linked to immunostimulatory DNA. *J. Allergy Clin. Immunol.* 113, 1144–1151.

Simons, J.W., Mikhak, B., Chang, J.F., DeMarzo, A.M., Carducci, M.A., Lim, M., Weber, C.E., Baccala, A.A., Goemann, M.A., Clift, S.M., Ando, D.G., Levitsky, H.I., Cohen, L.K., Sanda, M.G., Mulligan, R.C., Partin, A.W., Carter, H.B., Piantadosi, S., Marshall, F.F., and Nelson, W.G. (1999). Induction of immunity to prostate cancer antigens: results of a clinical trial of vaccination with irradiated autologous prostate tumor cells engineered to secrete granulocyte-macrophage colony-stimulating factor using ex vivo gene transfer. *Cancer Res.* 59, 5160–5168.

Smith, A.M., Morris, T., Justin, T., Michaeli, D., and Watson, S.A. (2001). Gastrimmune-induced antigastrin-17 antibodies inhibit acid secretion in a rat fistula model. *Aliment. Pharmacol. Ther.* 15, 1981–1988.

Snapper, C.M. and Paul, W.E. (1987). Interferon-γ and B cell stimulatory factor-1 reciprocally regulate Ig isotype production. *Science* 236, 944–947.

Soiffer, R., Lynch, T., Mihm, M., Jung, K., Rhuda, C., Schmollinger, J.C., Hodi, F.S., Liebster, L., Lam, P., Mentzer, S., Singer, S., Tanabe, K.K., Cosimi, A.B.,

Duda, R., Sober, A., Bhan, A., Daley, J., Neuberg, D., Parry, G., Rokovich, J., Richards, L., Drayer, J., Berns, A., Clift, S., and Dranoff, G. (1998). Vaccination with irradiated autologous melanoma cells engineered to secrete human granulocyte-macrophage colony-stimulating factor generates potent antitumor immunity in patients with metastatic melanoma. *Proc. Natl. Acad. Sci. USA* 95, 13141–13146.

Sondak, V.K., Liu, P.Y., Tuthill, R.J., Kempf, R.A., Unger, J.M., Sosman, J.A., Thompson, J.A., Weiss, G.R., Redman, B.G., Jakowatz, J.G., Noyes, R.D., and Flaherty, L.E. (2002). Adjuvant immunotherapy of resected, intermediate-thickness, node-negative melanoma with an allogeneic tumor vaccine: overall results of a randomized trial of the Southwest Oncology Group. *J. Clin. Oncol.* 20, 2058–2066.

Sosman, J.A., Unger, J.M., Liu, P.Y., Flaherty, L.E., Park, M.S., Kempf, R.A., Thompson, J.A., Terasaki, P.I., and Sondak, V.K. (2002). Adjuvant immunotherapy of resected, intermediate-thickness, node-negative melanoma with an allogeneic tumor vaccine: impact of HLA class I antigen expression on outcome. *J. Clin. Oncol.* 20, 2067–2075.

Spohn, G. and Bachmann, M.F. (2003). Therapeutic vaccination to block receptor–ligand interactions. *Expert Opin. Biol. Ther.* 3, 469–476.

Steinman, L. (2004). Immune therapy for autoimmune diseases. *Science* 305, 212–216.

Steinman, R.M., Hawiger, D., and Nussenzweig, M.C. (2003). Tolerogenic dendritic cells. *Annu. Rev. Immunol.* 21, 685–711.

Stevens, T.L., Bossie, A., Sanders, V.M., Fernandez-Botran, R., Coffman, R.L., Mosmann, T.R., and Vitetta, E.S. (1988). Regulation of antibody isotype secretion by subsets of antigen-specific helper T cells. *Nature* 334, 255–258.

Stift, A., Friedl, J., Dubsky, P., Bachleitner-Hofmann, T., Schueller, G., Zontsich, T., Benkoe, T., Radelbauer, K., Brostjan, C., Jakesz, R., and Gnant, M. (2003). Dendritic cell-based vaccination in solid cancer. *J. Clin. Oncol.* 21, 135–142.

Storni, T., Ruedl, C., Schwarz, K., Schwendener, R.A., Renner, W.A., and Bachmann, M.F. (2004). Nonmethylated Cg motifs packaged into virus-like particles induce protective cytotoxic T cell responses in the absence of systemic side effects. *J. Immunol.* 172, 1777–1785.

Strachan, D.P. (1989). Hay fever, hygiene, and household size. *Br. Med. J.* 299, 1259–1260.

Strachan, D.P. (2000). Family size, infection and atopy: the first decade of the "hygiene hypothesis". *Thorax* 55 (Suppl. 1), S2–S10.

Street, S.E.A., Hayakawa, Y., Zhan, Y., Lew, A.M., MacGregor, D., Jamieson, A.M., Diefenbach, A., Yagita, H., Godfrey, D.I., and Smyth, M.J. (2004). Innate immune surveillance of spontaneous B cell lymphomas by natural killer cells and $\gamma\delta$ T cells. *J. Exp. Med.* 199, 879–884.

Sundstedt, A., O'Neill, E.J., Nicolson, K.S., and Wraith, D.C. (2003). Role for IL-10 in suppression mediated by peptide-induced regulatory T cells in vivo. *J. Immunol.* 170, 1240–1248.

Sur, S., Wild, J.S., Choudhury, B.K., Sur, N., Alam, R., and Klinman, D.M. (1999). Long term prevention of allergic lung inflammation in a mouse model of asthma by CpG oligodeoxynucleotides. *J. Immunol.* 162, 6284–6293.

Sutmuller, R.P.M., van Duivenvoorde, L.M., van Elsas, A., Schumacher, T.N.M., Wildenberg, M.E., Allison, J.P., Toes, R.E.M., Offringa, R., and Melief, C.J.M. (2001). Synergism of cytotoxic T lymphocyte-associated antigen 4 blockade and depletion of CD25+ regulatory t cells in antitumor therapy reveals alternative pathways for suppression of autoreactive cytotoxic T lymphocyte responses. *J. Exp. Med.* 194, 823–832.

Talwar, G.P., Sharma, N.C., Dubey, S.K., Salahuddin, M., Das, C., Ramakrishnan, S., Kumar, S., and Hingorani, V. (1976). Isoimmunization against human chorionic gonadotropin with conjugates of processed beta-subunit of the hormone and tetanus toxoid. *Proc. Natl. Acad. Sci. USA* 73, 218–222.

Talwar, G.P., Singh, O., Pal, R., Chatterjee, N., Sahai, P., Dhall, K., Kaur, J., Das, S.K., Suri, S., Buckshee, K. et al. (1994). A vaccine that prevents pregnancy in women. *Proc. Natl. Acad. Sci. USA* 91, 8532–8536.

Tang, Q., Henriksen, K.J., Bi, M., Finger, E.B., Szot, G., Ye, J., Masteller, E.L., McDevitt, H., Bonyhadi, M., and Bluestone, J.A. (2004). In vitro-expanded antigen-specific regulatory T cells suppress autoimmune diabetes. *J. Exp. Med.* 199, 1455–1465.

Teitelbaum, D., Meshorer, A., Hirshfeld, T., Arnon, R., and Sela, M. (1971). Suppression of experimental allergic encephalomyelitis by a synthetic polypeptide. *Eur. J. Immunol.* 1, 242–248.

Terabe, M. and Berzofsky, J.A. (2004). Immunoregulatory T cells in tumor immunity. *Curr. Opin. Immunol.* 16, 157–162.

Terabe, M., Matsui, S., Noben-Trauth, N., Chen, H., Watson, C., Donaldson, D.D., Carbone, D.P., Paul, W.E., and Berzofsky, J.A. (2000). NKT cell-mediated repression of tumor immunosurveillance by IL-13 and the IL-4R-STAT6 pathway. *Nature Immunol.* 1, 515–520.

Terabe, M., Matsui, S., Park, J.-M., Mamura, M., Noben-Trauth, N., Donaldson, D.D., Chen, W., Wahl, S.M., Ledbetter, S., Pratt, B., Letterio, J.J., Paul, W.E., and Berzofsky, J.A. (2003). Transforming growth factor-β production and myeloid cells are an effector mechanism through which CD1d-restricted t cells block cytotoxic T lymphocyte-mediated tumor immunosurveillance: abrogation prevents tumor recurrence. *J. Exp. Med.* 198, 1741–1752.

Thomas, T.C., Rollins, S.A., Rother, R.P., Giannoni, M.A., Hartman, S.L., Elliott, E.A., Nye, S.H., Matis, L.A., Squinto, S.P., and Evans, M.J. (1996). Inhibition of complement activity by humanized anti-C5 antibody and single-chain Fv. *Mol. Immunol.* 33, 1389–1401.

Tighe, H., Takabayashi, K., Schwartz, D., Van Nest, G., Tuck, S., Eiden, J.J., Kagey-Sobotka, A., Creticos, P.S., Lichtenstein, L.M., Spiegelberg, H.L., and Raz, E. (2000). Conjugation of immunostimulatory DNA to the short ragweed allergen

Amb a 1 enhances its immunogenicity and reduces its allergenicity. *J. Allergy Clin. Immunol.* 106, 124–134.

Timmerman, J.M., Czerwinski, D.K., Davis, T.A., Hsu, F.J., Benike, C., Hao, Z.M., Taidi, B., Rajapaksa, R., Caspar, C.B., Okada, C.Y., van Beckhoven, A., Liles, T.M., Engleman, E.G., and Levy, R. (2002). Idiotype-pulsed dendritic cell vaccination for B-cell lymphoma: clinical and immune responses in 35 patients. *Blood* 99, 1517–1526.

Tulic, M.K., Wale, J.L., Holt, P.G., and Sly, P.D. (2000). Modification of the inflammatory response to allergen challenge after exposure to bacterial lipopolysaccharide. *Am. J. Respir. Cell. Mol. Biol.* 22, 604–612.

Tulic, M.K., Knight, D.A., Holt, P.G., and Sly, P.D. (2001). Lipopolysaccharide inhibits the late-phase response to allergen by altering nitric oxide synthase activity and interleukin-10. *Am. J. Respir. Cell. Mol. Biol.* 24, 640–646.

Turk, M.J., Guevara-Patino, J.A., Rizzuto, G.A., Engelhorn, M.E., and Houghton, A.N. (2004). Concomitant tumor immunity to a poorly immunogenic melanoma is prevented by regulatory T cells. *J. Exp. Med.* 200, 771–782.

Urban, J.F., Jr., Katona, I.M., Paul, W.E., and Finkelman, F.D. (1991). Interleukin 4 is important in protective immunity to a gastrointestinal nematode infection in mice. *Proc. Natl. Acad. Sci. USA* 88, 5513–5517.

Valenta, R. (2002). The future of antigen-specific immunotherapy of allergy. *Nature Rev. Immunol.* 2, 446–453.

Van Elsas, A., Sutmuller, R.P., Hurwitz, A.A., Ziskin, J., Villasenor, J., Medema, J.P., Overwijk, W.W., Restifo, N.P., Melief, C.J., Offringa, R., and Allison, J.P. (2001). Elucidating the autoimmune and antitumor effector mechanisms of a treatment based on cytotoxic T lymphocyte antigen-4 blockade in combination with a B16 melanoma vaccine: comparison of prophylaxis and therapy. *J. Exp. Med.* 194, 481–489.

Van Neerven, R.J., Wikborg, T., Lund, G., Jacobsen, B., Brinch-Nielsen, A., Arnved, J., and Ipsen, H. (1999). Blocking antibodies induced by specific allergy vaccination prevent the activation of CD4+ T cells by inhibiting serum-IgE-facilitated allergen presentation. *J. Immunol.* 163, 2944–2952.

Vanderlugt, C.L. and Miller, S.D. (2002). Epitope spreading in immune-mediated diseases: implications for immunotherapy. *Nature Rev. Immunol.* 2, 85–95.

Vannier, E., Lefort, J., Lellouch-Tubiana, A., Terlain, B., and Vargaftig, B.B. (1991). Lipopolysaccharide from Escherichia coli reduces antigen-induced bronchoconstriction in actively sensitized guinea pigs. *J. Clin. Invest.* 87, 1936–1944.

Viglietta, V., Baecher-Allan, C., Weiner, H.L., and Hafler, D.A. (2004). Loss of functional suppression by CD4+CD25+ regulatory T cells in patients with multiple sclerosis. *J. Exp. Med.* 199, 971–979.

Wahl, S.M., Vazquez, N., and Chen, W. (2004). Regulatory T cells and transcription factors: gatekeepers in allergic inflammation. *Curr. Opin. Immunol.* 16, 768–774.

Waldmann, T.A. (2003). Immunotherapy: past, present and future. *Nature Med.* 9, 269–277.

Wan, Y., Bramson, J., Carter, R., Graham, F., and Gauldie, J. (1997). Dendritic cells transduced with an adenoviral vector encoding a model tumor-associated antigen for tumor vaccination. *Hum. Gene Ther.* 8, 1355–1363.

Wang, C.C. and Rook, G.A. (1998). Inhibition of an established allergic response to ovalbumin in Balb/c mice by killed Mycobacterium vaccae. *Immunology* 93, 307–313.

Waterhouse, P., Penninger, J.M., Timms, E., Wakeham, A., Shahinian, A., Lee, K.P., Thompson, C.B., Griesser, H., and Mak, T.W. (1995). Lymphoproliferative disorders with early lethality in mice deficient in CTLA-4. *Science* 270, 985–988.

Watson, S.A., Morris, T.M., Varro, A., Michaeli, D., and Smith, A.M. (1999). A comparison of the therapeutic effectiveness of gastrin neutralisation in two human gastric cancer models: relation to endocrine and autocrine/paracrine gastrin mediated growth. *Gut* 45, 812–817.

Watson, S.A., Clarke, P.A., Morris, T.M., and Caplin, M.E. (2000). Antiserum raised against an epitope of the cholecystokinin B/gastrin receptor inhibits hepatic invasion of a human colon tumor. *Cancer Res.* 60, 5902–5907.

Weber, J., Cheinsong-Popov, R., Callow, D., Adams, S., Patou, G., Hodgkin, K., Martin, S., Gotch, F., and Kingsman, A. (1995). Immunogenicity of the yeast recombinant p17/p24:Ty virus-like particles (p24-VLP) in healthy volunteers. *Vaccine* 13, 831–834.

Wherry, E.J., Blattman, J.N., Murali-Krishna, K., van der Most, R., and Ahmed, R. (2003). Viral persistence alters CD8 T-cell immunodominance and tissue distribution and results in distinct stages of functional impairment. *J. Virol.* 77, 4911–4927.

Wierenga, E.A., Snoek, M., de Groot, C., Chretien, I., Bos, J.D., Jansen, H.M., and Kapsenberg, M.L. (1990). Evidence for compartmentalization of functional subsets of Cd2+T lymphocytes in atopic patients. *J. Immunol.* 144, 4651–4656.

Wild, J.S., Sigounas, A., Sur, N., Siddiqui, M.S., Alam, R., Kurimoto, M., and Sur, S. (2000). IFN-γ-inducing factor (IL-18) increases allergic sensitization, serum IgE, Th2 cytokines, and airway eosinophilia in a mouse model of allergic asthma. *J. Immunol.* 164, 2701–2710.

Wildbaum, G. and Karin, N. (1999). Augmentation of natural immunity to a pro-inflammatory cytokine (TNF-α) by targeted DNA vaccine confers long-lasting resistance to experimental autoimmune encephalomyelitis. *Gene Ther.* 6, 1128–1138.

Wildbaum, G., Westermann, J., Maor, G., and Karin, N. (2000). A targeted DNA vaccine encoding Fas ligand defines its dual role in the regulation of experimental autoimmune encephalomyelitis. *J. Clin. Invest.* 106, 671–679.

Wills-Karp, M., Santeliz, J., and Karp, C.L. (2001). The germless theory of allergic disease: revisiting the hygiene hypothesis. *Nature Rev. Immunol.* 1, 69–75.

Yamamura, M., Uyemura, K., Deans, R.J., Weinberg, K., Rea, T.H., Bloom, B.R., and Modlin, R.L. (1991). Defining protective responses to pathogens: cytokine profiles in leprosy lesions. *Science* 254, 277–279.

Yazdanbakhsh, M., Kremsner, P.G., and van Ree, R. (2002). Allergy, parasites, and the hygiene hypothesis. *Science* 296, 490–494.

Yeung, V.P., Gieni, R.S., Umetsu, D.T., and DeKruyff, R.H. (1998). Heat-killed Listeria monocytogenes as an adjuvant converts established murine Th2-dominated immune responses into Th1-dominated responses. *J. Immunol.* 161, 4146–4152.

Youssef, S., Wildbaum, G., Maor, G., Lanir, N., Gour-Lavie, A., Grabie, N., and Karin, N. (1998). Long-lasting protective immunity to experimental autoimmune encephalomyelitis following vaccination with naked DNA encoding C-C chemokines. *J. Immunol.* 161, 3870–3879.

Youssef, S., Wildbaum, G., and Karin, N. (1999). Prevention of experimental autoimmune encephalomyelitis by MIP-1α and MCP-1 naked DNA vaccines. *J. Autoimmun.* 13, 21–29.

Youssef, S., Maor, G., Wildbaum, G., Grabie, N., Gour-Lavie, A., and Karin, N. (2000). C-C chemokine-encoding DNA vaccines enhance breakdown of tolerance to their gene products and treat ongoing adjuvant arthritis. *J. Clin. Invest.* 106, 361–371.

Youssef, S., Stuve, O., Patarroyo, J.C., Ruiz, P.J., Radosevich, J.L., Hur, E.M., Bravo, M., Mitchell, D.J., Sobel, R.A., Steinman, L., and Zamvil, S.S. (2002). The HMG-CoA reductase inhibitor, atorvastatin, promotes a Th2 bias and reverses paralysis in central nervous system autoimmune disease. *Nature* 420, 78–84.

Zhou, S., Ou, R., Huang, L., Price, G.E., and Moskophidis, D. (2004). Differential tissue-specific regulation of antiviral CD8+ T-cell immune responses during chronic viral infection. *J. Virol.* 78, 3578–3600.

Zhu, M.Z., Marshall, J., Cole, D., Schlom, J., and Tsang, K.Y. (2000). Specific cytolytic T-cell responses to human CEA from patients immunized with recombinant avipox-CEA vaccine. *Clin. Cancer Res.* 6, 24–33.

Zinkernagel, R.M. (2003). On natural and artificial vaccinations. *Annu. Rev. Immunol.* 21, 515–546.

Zitvogel, L., Mayordomo, J.I., Tjandrawan, T., DeLeo, A.B., Clarke, M.R., Lotze, M.T., and Storkus, W.J. (1996). Therapy of murine tumors with tumor peptide-pulsed dendritic cells: dependence on T cells, B7 costimulation, and T helper cell 1-associated cytokines. *J. Exp. Med.* 183, 87–97.

Zuany-Amorim, C., Sawicka, E., Manlius, C., Le Moine, A., Brunet, L.R., Kemeny, D.M., Bowen, G., Rook, G., and Walker, C. (2002). Suppression of airway eosinophilia by killed Mycobacterium vaccae-induced allergen-specific regulatory T-cells. *Nature Med.* 8, 625–629.

Clinical evaluation of adjuvants

Jakub K. Simon and Robert Edelman
University of Maryland School of Medicine, Baltimore, Maryland

Introduction

The purpose of this chapter is to review the clinical evaluation of adjuvants in vaccine development. We review definitions, qualities of an ideal adjuvant, and components of adjuvant development, and discuss regulatory issues as well as examples of licensed and experimental adjuvants in human vaccines. The literature presented is published and peer-reviewed; because of proprietary issues relevant to adjuvants, much preclinical and clinical research has not been published and is not included in this chapter. Although relevant preclinical studies of adjuvants in clinical development are mentioned, adjuvants that have not been used in humans are not discussed. Also excluded are vehicles that do not have inherent immunopotentiating effect as well as alternative strategies at immunopotentiation such as nonspecific enhancers of the immune response, unique synthetic antigen constructs, and heterologous prime boost strategies. We hope that information presented herein will assist the reader in understanding issues surrounding the rational selection and clinical testing of adjuvants.

Definitions

The term "adjuvant" is used to describe a substance that in combination with a specific antigen produces more immunity than the antigen alone (Ramon, 1926). The enormous diversity of compounds that increase specific immune responses to an antigen and thus function as vaccine adjuvants makes any classification system arbitrary. The compounds in this review are grouped according to origin: (i) mineral salts, (ii) emulsions, (iii) particulate immunostimulators, (iv) microbial derivatives, (v) saponins, and (vi) endogenous human biologics (Table 18.1). A comprehensive list of adjuvants, beyond the scope of this chapter, is available and updated by the National Institute of Allergy and Infectious Diseases (NIAID; http://www.niaid.nih.gov/daids/vaccine/pdf/compendium.pdf).

A "carrier" is an immunogenic protein to which a "hapten," or a weakly immunogenic antigen, is bound (Edelman and Tacket, 1990). A carrier may also be a living organism (or vector) bearing genes for expression of the foreign hapten or antigen on its surface. Carriers increase the immune response by providing T cell help to the hapten or antigen.

A "vehicle" provides the substrate for the adjuvant, the antigen, or the antigen–carrier complex. Unlike carriers, vehicles are not themselves immunogenic. Like carriers, most vehicles can alone enhance antigens and so sometimes are considered to be another class of adjuvants, although their immunostimulatory effects are often augmented by the addition of conventional adjuvants to constitute "adjuvant formulations."

Characteristics of an ideal adjuvant

The characteristics of an ideal adjuvant include (i) safety of the adjuvant, including freedom from immediate and long-term side effects,

Table 18.1 Classes of modern vaccine adjuvants

Licensed	Antigens studied in humans	Antigens licensed	Comments
Aluminum salts	DPT[a], Hib[b], HBV[c], HIV[d], HAV[e], GBS[f], C. botulinum, malaria, pneumococcus, anthrax, cholera, rabies	DPT, Hib, HBV, HAV, pneumococcus, anthrax, cholera, rabies	Depot effect, APC[g] uptake, Th2[h] skew
Emulsion MF59	CMV[i], HBV, HSV[j], HIV, HCV, parvovirus, influenza	Influenza	APC uptake
Particulate virosome	HAV, HBV, influenza	HAV, influenza	APC uptake
Microbial product			
E. coli LT	Influenza	Influenza (withdrawn)	Binds gangliosides
MPL	HSV, HBV, HPV, malaria, melanoma	HBV, melanoma	TLR[k] 2 and 4
Ribi-529 (RC-529)	HBV, leishmania	HBV	TLR[k] 2 and 4
Cholera endotoxin B	Cholera, ETEC[l]	Cholera	

Experimental	Antigens studied in humans	Phase(s) of development	Comments
Microbial product			
Recombinant E. coli LT	ETEC, HBV, anthrax	Phase II ETEC	Transcutaneous
Detoxified E. coli LT	Influenza	Phase I influenza	Transcutaneous
CpG	HBV, cancer	Phase I/II HBV, cancer	TLR 9, Th1 skew
OM™ 174, 197, 294	Malaria, cancer	Phase I cancer	TLR 4
Endogenous human			
Cytokines	Leishmania, HIV, cancer	Phase II HIV, cancer	IL[m]-2, IL-6, IL-12, IL-18, GM-CSF[n], IFN[o]-γ
Hormones	HBV	Phase I (not successful)	DHEA[p]
Dendritic cells	HIV, cancer	Phase II cancer	
Saponins			
ISCOMS™	HPV[q], HCV, influenza, cancer	Phase I HPV, HCV	Th1 and Th2
QS-21	HIV, HSV, RSV[r], influenza, malaria, cancer	Phase II cancer	
Emulsions			
Montanides	HIV, malaria, cancer	Phase II HIV, cancer	
ASO2	HIV, HBV, HPV, malaria	Phase II malaria	Th1 and Th2
Particulate immunomodulators			
PLG	HIV	Phase I HIV	Cationic DNA[s], anionic protein
DC-Chol	HIV, H. pylori, cancer	Phase II cancer	

[a]DPT, diphtheria, pertussis, tetanus; [b]Hib, Haemophilus influenzae type b; [c]HBV, hepatitis B virus; [d]HIV, human immunodeficiency virus; [e]HAV, hepatitis A virus; [f]GBS, group B streptococcus; [g]APC, antigen-presenting cell; [h]Th, T helper (cell); [i]CMV, cytomegalovirus; [j]HSV, herpes simplex virus; [k]TLR, Toll-like receptor; [l]ETEC, enterotoxigenic E. coli; [m]IL, interleukin; [n]GM-CSF, granulocyte macrophage colony-stimulating factor; [o]IFN, interferon; [p]DHEA, dehydroepiandrosterone; [q]HPV, human papilloma virus; [r]RSV, respiratory syncitial virus; [s]DNA, deoxyribonucleic acid.

as discussed elsewhere (Edelman, 1980; Goldenthal et al., 1993) and summarized in Table 18.2; (ii) chemical and biological characterization so that lot-to-lot variations in the manufactured product are minimized, thereby ensuring consistent responses in vaccinees over time; (iii) enhancement of the protective immune response; (iv) improvement of efficacy with fewer doses of vaccine; (v) improvement in efficacy with a lower concentrations of antigen; (vi) stability on the shelf for at least two years; (vii) biodegradability and easy

Table 18.2 Real and theoretical risks of vaccine adjuvants

1	Local acute or chronic inflammation with formation of painful abscesses, persistent nodules, ulcers, or draining lymphadenopathy
2	Induction of influenza-like illness, with fever, malaise, myalgia, arthralgia, or headache
3	Anaphylactic reactions, angioedema, urticaria, and vasculitis
4	Systemic clinical toxicity to tissues or organs
5	Induction of hypersensitivity to host tissue, producing autoimmune arthritis, amyloidosis, anterior uveitis
6	Cross-reactions with human antigens, such as glomerular basement membranes or neurolemma, causing glomerulonephritis or meningoencephalitis
7	Sensitization to tuberculin or to other skin test antigens
8	Immune suppression
9	Predisposition to atopy, asthma, eczema, allergic rhinitis
10	Genetic events: carcinogenesis, teratogenesis, abortogenesis
11	Dissemination of live vector within the host to cause disease; spread of the vector to the environment and other persons

removal from the body after the adjuvant effect is exhausted; and (viii) low cost. To date, no adjuvant meets all of these goals.

Components of rational adjuvant development

Safety

The most important attribute of any adjuvanted vaccine is that it is more efficacious than the aqueous vaccine, and that this benefit outweighs its risk. During the past 75 years many adjuvants have been developed that were never accepted for routine vaccination because of their immediate toxicity and fear of delayed side effects. The current attitude regarding risks–benefits of vaccination favors safety over efficacy when a prophylactic vaccine is given to a healthy population of children and adults. In high-risk groups (including patients with cancer and acquired immune deficiency syndrome, AIDS) and for therapeutic vaccines, an additional level of toxicity may be acceptable if the benefit of the vaccine is substantial. The real or theoretical risks of administering vaccine adjuvants can be grouped as either local or systemic.

Local reactions

While the most frequent adverse side effects associated with parenteral adjuvanted vaccines are local tenderness and swelling, the most severe ones involve the formation of painful abscesses and nodules at the inoculum site. The mechanisms for such severe local reactions include: (i) contamination of the vaccine at the time of formulation with reactogenic chemicals and microbial products; (ii) instability of the vaccine on storage with breakdown into reactogenic side products; (iii) formation of inflammatory immune complexes at the inoculation site by combination of the adjuvanted vaccine with preexisting antibodies resulting in an arthus-type reaction; and (iv) poor biodegradability of the adjuvanted vaccine resulting in prolonged persistence in the tissues and reactive granuloma formation. Such local reactions are of special concern for depot-type adjuvants such as aluminum salts, oil emulsions, liposomes, biodegradable polymer microspheres, and living vectors such as BCG (Alving, 2002; Cano, 1999; Evans et al., 2001; Goldenthal et al., 1993; Hoffman et al., 1994; Keitel et al., 1993; Schultz et al., 1995). The route of injection (subcutaneous being more reactogenic than intramuscular), addition of excipients, change of the pH and buffer, or the addition of an anesthetic play a role in local reactions and may be optimized (Kenney et al., 2002). Fixed-drug recall reactions, characterized by immediate swelling, hives, and intense pruritis at the site of a prior antigen injection within 5–20 minutes after reexposure to that antigen at a remote site, have also been observed, particularly in association with peptide-based vaccines with alum or QS-21 (Edelman et al., 2002; Gordon et al., 1996; Kashala et al., 2002; Rinn et al., 1999). The reaction is likely to be IgE mediated, but the precise mechanism is unknown (Edelman et al., 2002).

■ *Systemic reactions*

Few studies have carefully evaluated systemic reactions to adjuvants. In a large systematic evaluation of the safety of preventive human immunodeficiency virus (HIV)-1 vaccines, 1398 HIV-negative healthy volunteers were followed for over 2000 person-years as part of 25 NIAID-sponsored AIDS Vaccine Evaluation Group phase I/II clinical trials (Keefer et al., 1997). The only adverse effects that were clearly related to vaccination were associated with adjuvants, including transient moderate to severe local pain and inflammation with alum plus deoxycholate, muramyl tripeptide dipalmitoyl phosphatidylethanolamine (MTP-PE), and QS21. MTP-PE was also associated with self-limited severe systemic febrile reactions that were similar to the fever and chills reported for MTP-PE with influenza vaccine (Keitel et al., 1993). There were no serious adverse laboratory toxicities and no evidence of significant immunosuppressive events after an average of 3.5 immunizations. To date, vaccine adjuvants have caused few severe, acute, systemic adverse effects. Interestingly, a theory of inadequate binding of low molecular weight peptides to adjuvant with subsequent crosslinking of IgE has been proposed (Edelman et al., 2002). It may be that the absence of adjuvant or adjuvant binding of antigen contributes to systemic hypersensitivity.

More theoretical risks of adjuvants include the induction of autoimmunity or cancer. Fortunately, in 10-, 18-, and 35-year follow-up studies, the incidence of cancer, autoimmune, and collagen disorders in 18,000 persons who received oil-emulsion influenza vaccine in the early 1950s was not different from that in persons given aqueous vaccines (Beebe et al., 1964, 1972; Davenport, 1968; Page et al., 1993). Adjuvant-associated arthritis (Kleinau et al., 1991; Murray et al., 1972; Pearson, 1963) has not been reported in humans, even after long-term follow-up (Beebe et al., 1972; Salk and Salk, 1977; Stuart-Harris 1969). Anaphylactic reactions, angioedema, urticaria, and vasculitis have been described following the administration of the majority of vaccines, although severe events are rare (Descotes et al., 2002). Finally, a syndrome known as macrophagic myofasciitis (MMF), characterized by diffuse arthromyalgias and fatigue in connection with muscle infiltration by macrophages and lymphocytes, has been attributed to alum-containing vaccinations in France (Gherardi et al., 2001), although a causal association has not been established. It requires decades of expensive and time-consuming follow-up for such low-incidence reactions to be identified, and at present a mechanism for the systematic, active follow-up of vaccinees given experimental adjuvants is not available (Jacobson et al., 2001). Active surveillance in preclinical and clinical studies has, however, resulted in the determination that certain adjuvants such as mineral oil emulsion incomplete Freund's adjuvant (IFA) and mycobacterial cell wall component muramyl dipeptide emulsion (MDP) may have an unfavorable risk–benefit ratio. Less toxic MDP derivatives including a butyl ester derivative (murabutide™) (Chedid et al., 1982; Telzak et al., 1986), threonyl-MDP (Byars et al., 1990; Ott et al., 1995), and MTP-PE (Ott et al., 1995; Sanchez-Pescador et al., 1988) have been developed.

While safety of new adjuvants is a major concern, particularly for those rare reactions that occur once in several thousand doses and that may not be detected until late in clinical development program, there are other factors that effect the orderly development of adjuvants, as summarized below (Gupta and Siber 1995).

■ Variable adjuvanticity

Adjuvants are often effective with some antigens and not others. For example, aluminum compounds typically provide strong adjuvanticity, yet they failed to augment vaccines against whooping cough (Butler et al., 1962), typhoid fever (Cvjetanovic and Uemura, 1965), trachoma (Woolridge et al., 1967), adenovirus hexon antigens (Kasel et al., 1971), influenza hemagglutinin (Davenport et al., 1968), and *Haemophilus influenzae* type b capsular polysaccharide conjugated to tetanus toxoid (Claesson et al., 1988). It is not always possible to predict compatible and incompatible adjuvant–vaccine combinations early in development (Alving, 2002). This situation is especially common when there are no reliable animal models. If possible, preclinical studies should be done with the antigen destined for clinical studies (Goldenthal et al., 1993; Gupta and Siber, 1995; Verdier 2002). Although ovalbumin is often used for preliminary screening, doses used are often too high to discriminate between small differences among adjuvant formulations (O'Hagan et al., 1993), and no functional antibody assays are available for this nonpathogenic antigen. Toxoids, such as diphtheria toxoid, which is a weak antigen, can be used at minimal threshold concentrations for preliminary evaluation of adjuvants instead of ovalbumin (Gupta and Siber, 1995).

■ Suboptimal use of aluminum adjuvants

Aluminum salts have become the reference preparations for evaluation of new adjuvants for human vaccines. Therefore, it is important that aluminum adjuvants be used optimally to allow correct evaluation of the experimental adjuvant (Baylor et al., 2002; Edelman, 1980; Gupta et al., 1995; Gupta and Siber, 1995). Aluminum adjuvants are difficult to manufacture in a physicochemically reproducible way, and this failure affects immunogenicity. Thus, during the adsorption of antigens on aluminum adjuvants, attention must be paid to the chemical and physical characteristics of the antigen, type of aluminum adjuvant, conditions of adsorption, and concentration of adjuvant (Baylor et al., 2002; Bumford, 1989; Gupta et al., 1995; Gupta and Siber, 1995; Jensen and Koch, 1988; World Health Organization, 1977). Although these adjuvants are commonly called "alum" in the literature, referring to all aluminum adjuvants as "alum" is misleading. Alum is $Al(SO_4)_2 \cdot 12H_2O$, and not all aluminum salts labeled "alum" are equally effective.

For instance, aluminum hydroxide is more potent than aluminum phosphate, which may be a result of its higher adsorption capacity at neutral pH (Gupta et al., 1995). To minimize the variations and to avoid nonreproducible results due to use of different preparations of aluminum compounds, it is advisable to state clearly the exact aluminum formulation used.

■ Animal models

Different animal species, and different strains within a species, may respond differently to the same adjuvant. Intraspecies variation in immune response to adjuvants and vaccines is particularly true among mouse strains (Alving, 2002; Gupta et al., 1993; Hardegree et al., 1972; Matsuhasi, 1991). For this reason, preclinical studies in one strain of a single animal species should be interpreted with caution. Biological differences between animal models and humans all too commonly lead to the clinical failure of formulations that are promising in preclinical studies.

Guinea pigs have been used widely for vaccine quality control, and may be the animal of choice for evaluating adjuvant formulations (Stewart-Tull, 1989). Guinea pigs respond consistently to adsorbed tetanus toxoid while mice show variable responses (Lyng and Nyerges, 1984). The guinea pig model was recently developed to test aluminum-adsorbed HiB conjugate vaccines (Siber et al., 1995). A useful rabbit model has been described by the US Food and Drug Administration (FDA) and National Institutes of Health (NIH) investigators to evaluate the toxicity and adjuvanticity of adjuvant formulations (Goldenthal et al., 1993). The rabbit model provides a much needed standard protocol for preclinical assessment of adjuvant formulations, and it should be utilized widely. However, the paucity of reagents to analyze guinea pig and rabbit cytokines and IgG subclasses may impede full utilization. The wide availability of murine cytokine and Ig subclass reagents, low husbandry costs, and ease of handling will ensure the continued use of mice despite their inconsistent responses to adjuvants. As per the International Conference on Harmonization (ICH) Guidance for Industry (S6 Preclinical Safety Evaluation of Biotechnology-Derived Pharmaceuticals available at http://www.fda.gov/cder/guidance/1859fnl.pdf), it is recommended that at least two strains of mice with different haplotypes be utilized, in addition to a nonrodent mammal that can receive a full dose. Vaccine alone, adjuvant, and vaccine–adjuvant combinations should be studied for toxicity and immunogenicity, and their concentrations should mimic or exceed human doses in quantity and number (Goldenthal et al., 1993; Gupta et al., 1993).

■ Immunoassays

In addition to measuring antibodies by enzyme-linked immunosorbent assay (ELISA) or other antigen–antibody binding assays, one should measure antibody function by neutralization, opsonophagocytic, or bactericidal assays if available. However, the most decisive test is protection against experimental challenge. For example, many adjuvant formulations induced high-titer antibody against malarial (Hunter and Lal, 1994) and simian immunodeficiency virus (SIV) antigens (Murphey-Corb et al., 1993), but antibody titers were not sufficient to predict protection even when the antigen contained protective epitopes and protection was mediated by antibody. The induction of protective immunity depended upon the quality rather than the quantity of antibody, that is, induction of antibody of the appropriate isotype and fine-epitope specificity. This induction was dependent upon unique, poorly understood interactions between the adjuvant, the antigen, and the host, in which the density of antigen/major histocompatability complex (MHC) binding may play a role (Celis, 2002). The conclusions from such experience suggests that the search for an effective vaccine must involve both antigens and adjuvants from the start of

preclinical development, and that no adjuvant can be considered a gold standard (Hunter, 2002; Hunter and Lal, 1994).

■ Regulatory issues

In concert with the ICH Technical Requirements for Registration of Pharmaceuticals for Human Use, worldwide regulatory guidance on the development and testing of vaccines has expanded significantly in the last few years. Documents covering nearly every aspect of drug and biologic development are being created and revised in an effort to enhance and standardize the quality, safety, and efficacy of pharmaceutical products. Developers of adjuvants and vaccines should familiarize themselves with the latest documents that are collected and published on several websites, including (i) the ICH website: http://www.ich.org; (ii) the FDA Center for Biologics Evaluation and Research (CBER) website: http://www.fda.gov/cber/guidelines.htm; and (iii) the European Agency for the Evaluation of Medicinal Products (EMEA) website: http://www.emea.eu.int. However, advice directed specifically at the development of adjuvants is relatively sparse. The EMEA has developed a Guideline on Adjuvants in Vaccines available at http://www.emea.eu.int/pdfs/human/veg/001703en.pdf in which nonclinical as well as clinical evaluation of adjuvants used in infectious disease vaccines is discussed. It is important to note that, as a rule, adjuvants are not licensed on their own. Because each combination of one or more antigens with an adjuvant has its own unique safety and efficacy profile, adjuvant formulations are licensed and regulated in combination. Regulatory requirements for adjuvant development in the US are similar to those in place for all biologics (see Code of Federal Regulations (CFR) Title 21 Parts 312 and 610 for specifics: http://www.accessdata.fda.gov/scripts/cdrh/cfdocs/cfcfr/cfrsearch.cfm).

■ Preclinical

Several guidance documents are available that provide advice regarding preclinical pharmacological and toxicological testing of vaccines, including ICH safety guidelines S5a and S6 as well as EMEA preclinical guidance CPMP/SWP/465/95. These documents discuss standard tests devised to ensure potency, safety, sterility, purity, and identity. Reactogenicity and toxicology tests of the adjuvant alone and the antigen–adjuvant combination are performed in a manner that is relevant to the intended clinical use, including route of administration, injection volume, and clinical formulation. When possible, preclinical immunogenicity and toxicity testing should be performed in species in which the adjuvant augments the immune response, and postvaccination challenge testing can be performed (Pink and Kieny, 2004). Special considerations apply to cholera toxin (CT) and *E. coli* heat-labile enterotoxin (LT) administered intranasally (IN), as inflammation in the olfactory nerves and bulb has been noted (Mutsch et al., 2004). For preclinical studies assessing IN administration of CT and LT more than one species and strain of the same species should be studied, the device intended for use in clinic should be used, and anatomy as well as physiology of the nasal cavity defined so as to assess proximity to olfactory bulb and brain (http://www.niaid.nih.gov/dmid/enteric/intranasal.htm).

■ Clinical

Clinical evaluation of vaccines with or without adjuvants includes phase I testing of safety and reactogenicity, phase II testing of safety and immunogenicity, and phase III testing of safety and efficacy. The good clinical practice (GCP) standard for design, conduct, analysis, and reporting of clinical trials must be followed as per ICH, FDA, and EMEA guidelines. Postlicensure phase IV studies continue to monitor safety of licensed vaccines to detect infrequent but potentially important effects of adjuvanted and nonadjuvanted vaccines. It is critical to note that preclinical testing in animals does not always predict toxicity, immunogenicity, or efficacy in humans. The effects of adjuvants when tested in humans for the first time in phase I trials may be completely different from the effects in animal models and cannot be accurately predicted; despite advances in the understanding of adjuvants and their function, the testing of new adjuvants in humans and determination of optimal dose, timing, and formulation is still empiric.

■ Adjuvants used in licensed vaccines for humans

Several adjuvants are licensed for human use in various countries, including aluminum compounds, MF-59, virosomes, monophosphoryl lipid A (MPL), and exotoxins.

■ Mineral salts

■ *Aluminum salts*

Aluminum salts are the only adjuvants used for licensed human vaccines in the USA. The following licensed, parenterally administered human vaccines are combined with aluminum: diphtheria pertussis, tetanus (DPT), acellular pertussis, DaPT *Haemophilus influenzae* type b (Hib) combinations, one of the Hib conjugates (PRP-OMPC), tetanus and diphtheria toxoid combinations, hepatitis B, hepatitis A, anthrax, pneumococcal, oral cholera, and a rabies vaccine.

The major advantage of using aluminum adjuvants is their record of safety after billions of doses, and the development of earlier, higher, and longer-lasting antibody after primary immunization compared to primary immunization with soluble vaccines (Edelman, 1980; Gupta et al., 1995). The mechanism of adjuvanticity includes formation of a depot at the injection site allowing slow release of antigen, stimulation of immunoreactive cells, activation of macrophages, and efficient uptake of aluminum-adsorbed antigen particles by antigen-presenting cells (because of their particulate nature and optimum particle size of <10 μg (Edelman, 1980; Gupta et al., 1995; Gupta, 1998; HogenEsch, 2002).

The limitations of aluminum adjuvants include the following. (i) The potential for induction of occasional painful nodules or swelling and erythema at the inoculation site and the induction of antigen-specific IgE antibody which correlates with such local reactions (Blennow et al., 1986; Mark et al., 1995). With perhaps one exception (Ratliff and Burns-Cox, 1984), there is no indication that aluminum induces clinically important, systemic immediate hypersensitivity when used according to current immunization schedules (Edelman, 1980; Gupta et al., 1995). (ii) Aluminum has been detected at the site of subcutaneous injections for up to one year in animals (Gupta et al., 1995), so it is not readily "biodegradable." In addition, the aluminum compounds have several immunological drawbacks, including (iii) the inability to enhance humoral immunity against certain vaccines in humans (Butler et al., 1962; Claesson et al., 1988; Cvjetanovic and Uemura, 1965; Davenport et al., 1968; et al., 1971; Woolridge et al.1967), (iv) lack of booster effect (Edelman, 1980; Gupta and Siber, 1995), and (v) near total inability to elicit cell-mediated immune (CMI) responses, particularly cytotoxic T cell responses to intracellular organisms (HogenEsch, 2002). The failure to induce CMI is a major limitation for vaccines against intracellular parasites such as malaria and HIV. Aluminum adjuvants may even selectively block development of CD8+ cytotoxic T lymphocytes (CTLs) by some antigens (Schirmbeck et al., 1994). (vi) Aluminum adjuvant preparations are not always reproducible, cannot be sterilized by filtration, and cannot be frozen or readily lyophilized (Gupta, 1998).

■ Emulsions

▪ *Microfluidized oil/water emulsion (MF59)*

A series of squalene emulsions were prepared using the Microfluidizer™ by Chiron Corporation investigators to generate small particle (200–300 nm), oil-in-water emulsions that had low viscosity and were biodegradable (Ott et al., 1995; Sanchez-Pescador et al., 1988). The most stable emulsion, termed MF59, consists of 4.3% (v/v) squalene, and 0.5% (v/v) each of the surfactants Tween 80 (polyoxyethylene sorbitan monooleate) and Span 85 (sorbitan trioleate). A small emulsion particle size of <400 nm was required for optimal antibody responses in large animals and in humans, but not in small animals (Ott et al., 1995). Overall, MF59 generates antibody titers consistently higher than those obtained with aluminum hydroxide, equal to or higher than IFA, and equal to or lower than complete Freund's adjuvant (CFA). Interestingly, injection of radiolabeled MF59 and herpes simplex virus (HSV) gD2 antigen suggests that the depot effect does not appear to be the mechanism of action of the oil/water emulsion MF59, and that detectable binding of the antigen to MF59 is also not necessary for adjuvant activity (Ott et al., 1995). Results of timed injection studies suggest that MF59 microdroplets activate the immune system in the absence of antigen. It is postulated that macrophage uptake of the emulsion droplets results in cytokine production, which leads to enhanced immune response in the presence of the antigen (Ott et al., 1995). MF59 has been tested in a variety of animal species showing a good safety profile and a significant increase of the immune response to several subunit antigens including cytomegalovirus (CMV), HSV, HIV, hepatitis C virus (HCV), hepatitis B virus (HBV), and influenza antigens.

Chiron Biocine (Sienna, Italy) has registered an influenza vaccine adjuvanted with MF59 as FLUAD in much of Europe, which has been given to more than a million people (De Donato et al., 1999). In all age groups, the clinical data have shown a potent adjuvant effect with an acceptable safety profile. The MF59 formulation has also been tested in combination with recombinant HSV glycoproteins, HBV PreS2/S antigens, and HIV envelope proteins. Study populations have included healthy adults (HSV, HBV, HIV, influenza) (Heineman et al., 1999), elderly populations (influenza) (Baldo et al., 2001), and infants and children (HIV) (Ott et al., 1995). Overall, MF59 has had acceptable reactogenicity profiles (Corey et al., 1999; Lambert et al., 1998; Langenberg et al., 1995) although efficacy of gD2gB2 MF59 HSV-2 vaccine was disappointing while efficacy of gD2 alum-MPL HSV-2 vaccine is promising (Corey et al., 1999; Stanberry et al., 2002). Ongoing clinical trials with HIV, influenza, and other antigens will continue to elucidate the reactogenicity and adjuvanticity profiles of MF59 formulations.

Particulate immunomodulators

Virosomes

Immunopotentiating reconstituted influenza virosomes (IRIV) are 150 nm proteoliposomes composed of influenza H1N1 surface glycoproteins intercalated in a mixture of natural and synthetic phospholipids. The influenza hemagglutinin (HA) antigen targets the virosomes to antigen-presenting cells (APCs) that take up the particles by receptor-mediated endocytosis. IRIV can act as antigen carriers to deliver many types of antigens bound or conjugated to the surface or internalized. Given the unique properties of the system, after proteolytic degradation the antigenic peptides can become complexed with both MHC class I and II molecules to be expressed on the surface of the APC.

The initial application of the virosome system was with hepatitis A vaccine Epaxal™. Berna Biologics Ltd (Bern, Switzerland) has registered Epaxal in several European, Asian, and South American countries after clinical testing, which showed a more rapid immune response and a significant reduction in local reactions compared to the conventional alum-adsorbed vaccine (Holzer et al., 1996).

An annually administered influenza vaccine was created by using the current HA and neuraminidase (NA) antigens jointly inserted in the vesicle membrane and given intranasally in combination with a low dose of LT for mucosal immunization (Baldo et al.; Gluck et al., 1999; Holzer et al., 1996). While this vaccine was initially registered in several countries in Europe, it has since been withdrawn due to concerns about a potential association with Bell's palsy (Mutsch et al., 2004). The mechanism for this appears to be the binding of the B subunit of LT and CT toxin to gangliosides, leading to toxin internalization (Couch, 2004). Future clinical testing of CT and LT mucosal administration will require special regulatory oversight (see above).

Microbial derivatives

Monophosphoryl lipid A (MPL®)

The adjuvant effect of lipopolysaccharide (LPS) was described in 1956 (Johnson et al., 1956). Most of the adjuvanticity and toxicity of LPS are associated with the lipid A region of the molecule (Luderitz et al., 1982). The LPS of *Salmonella minnesota* R595 has been detoxified without destroying its adjuvant activity by exposing the LPS to mild hydrolytic treatment (Myers et al., 1996; Qureshi et al., 1982; Ribi et al., 1982). The resultant monophosphoryl derivative of lipid A, called MPL® by Corixa Corporation (Seattle, WA), is a highly adaptable molecule that can be used effectively in many adjuvant formulations (Baldridge and Crane, 1999; Ulrich and Myers, 1995). Such formulations include antigen in saline (Schneerson et al., 1991), oil/water emulsions (Garg and Subbarao, 1992; Schneerson, et al., 1991), aluminum salts (Desombere et al., 2002; Leroux-Roels et al., 1993), and in liposomes (Fries et al., 1992; Zhou and Huang, 1993). The immunopotentiating nature of MPL® may be associated with its capacity to induce cytokines such as interleukin (IL)-12 (Ulrich and Myers, 1995), interferon (IFN)-γ, IL-1, and IL-2 in mouse and human macrophages

(Carozzi et al., 1989; Dijkstra et al., 1987; Ribi et al., 1986) via toll-like receptor (TLR) 2 and 4 (Martin et al., 2003). MPL® can exert adjuvant effects on both humoral and cellular responses by interfering with antigen-specific suppressor T cells (Baker et al., 1990; Domer et al., 1993). MPL® promotes antigen-specific delayed-type hypersensitivity (DTH) and a predominant murine IgG2a immunoglobulin response characteristic of Th1 help (Gustafson and Rhodes, 1992). Numerous animal and human studies testify to the utility MPL® as an adjuvant, used alone or combined effectively with other adjuvants and vehicles for capsular polysaccharide, protein, and peptide antigens for conventional (Baldridge and Crane, 1999; Ulrich and Myers, 1995; Vernacchio et al., 2002) and allergy vaccines (Wheeler and Woroniecki, 2004).

In the past decade, many clinical studies have utilized MPL® or DETOX™ (MPL® plus cell wall skeleton of *Mycobacterium phlei* in a squalane-in-water emulsion vehicle) as vaccine adjuvants in volunteers (Fries, et al., 1992; Hoffman, et al., 1994; McCormack et al., 2000; Schultz et al., 1995). The DETOX™ adjuvant formulation has been used in therapeutic vaccines for melanoma (Mitchell et al., 1988), ovarian cancer (MacLean et al., 1992), and breast cancer (MacLean et al., 1993) with modest clinical success. Melacine®, an allogenic melanoma tumor cell lysate with DETOX™, has been licensed in Canada for late-stage melanoma. Prophylactic HBV vaccine Fendrix® utilizing AS04 as an adjuvant has been licensed in Europe. Other prophylactic vaccines including vaccines against malaria (Hoffman et al., 1994), human papilloma virus (HPV) (Harper et al., 2004), and HSV (Stanberry et al., 2002) are in clinical trials. The malaria/DETOX™ vaccine was highly reactogenic; MPL® in liposomes + alum (Fries et al., 1992) and MPL® alone (Gordon et al., 1995) were better tolerated in two other malaria trials, and the vaccine formulations appeared more immunogenic than the same vaccines adsorbed to alum. The gD2 alum-MPL subunit HSV-2 vaccine shows promise

with 40% efficacy against infection and 74% efficacy against disease in double-seronegative women, but not men (Stanberry et al., 2002). The reason for this sex-specific efficacy is not known, but may be potentiated by sex-specific differences in TLR-4 polymorphism (Tiberio et al., 2004).

RC-529

Based on the adjuvanticity of MPL, a chemically distinct family of synthetic lipid A mimetics – the aminoalkyl glucosaminide 4-phosphates (AGP)s – have been developed by Corixa Corporation and tested in animals as well as humans (Baldridge et al., 2002; Evans et al., 2003). Ribi 529 (RC-529) is one of the library of Corixa's synthetic AGPs that has been combined with a recombinant hepatitis B antigen and licensed by Berna Biotech in Argentina. The addition of squalene to RC-529 (RC-529 SE) resulted in enhanced immunity of leishmania polyprotein Leish-111f and conferred protection from challenge in mice of up to 3 months (Coler et al., 2002).

Exotoxins (cholera toxin B subunit)

The bacterial ADP-ribosylating exotoxins (bAREs) represent a potent group of proteins that have been studied as enteric, nasal, and topical adjuvants for decades, and this category includes both licensed and experimental vaccines. Cholera toxin B subunit is used to enhance the mucosal immune response in a licensed whole cell cholera vaccine (Dukoral, PowderJect Pharmaceuticals, Oxford, UK) that contains 10^{11} killed *V. cholerae* O1 organisms including classic and El Tor Inaba and Ogawa strains (Ryan and Calderwood, 2000). The vaccine had a high level of protection (85%) against both classic and El Tor strains in the first six months (Clemens et al., 1986). However, the efficacy against El Tor waned by 36 months, particularly in young children (van Loon et al., 1996). The addition of the cholera toxin B subunit also provides short-lived efficacy (67% at 3 months) against traveler's diarrhea associated with LT producing enterotoxigenic *E. coli* (ETEC) (Clemens, et al., 1986; Ryan and Calderwood, 2000).

Experimental adjuvants in humans

The development of experimental adjuvants has been driven principally by the failure of aluminum compounds (i) to enhance many vaccines in humans (Edelman, 1980), (ii) to enhance subunit vaccine antigens in animals (Alving, 2002; Haigwood et al., 1992; Sanchez-Pescador et al. 1988), and (iii) to stimulate cytotoxic T cell responses (HogenEsch, 2002). The number of commercially feasible adjuvants tested in animals is too large to discuss in this short review. Instead, a smaller number of modern adjuvants or adjuvant formulations used to enhance a variety of experimental vaccines in humans are considered.

Microbial derivatives

Exotoxins (recombinant LT)

In addition to its use in a licensed intranasal virosomal influenza vaccine (see above), recombinant LT has been shown to be safe and immunogenic by transcutaneous immunization (TCI) in humans (Glenn et al., 2000). LT-specific IgG and IgA antibodies were present in both stool and urine, implying the induction of a strong mucosal immune response. The potent activation of epidermal Langerhans cells allows LT to adjuvant the response in humans to a coadministered antigen such as ETEC colonization factor CS6 (Guerena-Burgueno et al., 2002). Serological and antibody-secreting cell (ASC) responses to the LT and the *E. coli* surface antigen CS6 were comparable to those seen following a protective oral challenge. These results suggest that the use of TCI can potentially elicit effective immunity similar to natural infection with ETEC (Guerena-Burgueno et al., 2002). Other groups are using detoxified mutants of LT to explore the potential for oral or nasal vaccination (Barackman et al., 2001; Kotloff et al., 2001; Ryan et al., 1999) and generation of mutants LTK63 (serine to lysine substitution at position 63 in the A subunit) as well as LTR72 (alanine to arginine substitution at position 72 in the A subunit) reduce toxicity while maintaining adjuvanticity (Peppoloni et al., 2003). A phase I trial of intranasally delivered flu vaccine with LTK63 as an adjuvant is under way (Pink and Kieny, 2004).

Oligonucleotides

Just as bacterial deoxyribonucleic acid (DNA) can activate immune cells, synthetic oligodeoxynucleotides (ODN) containing unmethylated CpG dinucleotides in particular base contexts (CpG motifs) stimulate the innate immune system (signal 0) via TLR-9 (Takeshita et al., 2001) to induce protection in mice and primates (Davis et al., 2000; Krieg et al., 1995; Verthelyi et al., 2002). Either alone or in combination with a vaccine, they can activate human B cells, dendritic cells (DCs), and natural killer (NK) cells (Verthelyi et al., 2002), and trigger an immune cascade that includes the production of cytokines, chemokines, and IgM to protect against infection. CpG ODN are extremely efficient inducers of Th1 immunity and CTL, and can allow a 10- to 100-fold reduction in the dose of antigen, presumably because of the increased efficiency of antigen presentation by DCs (Krieg, 2001). Reports from animal and human studies indicate that ODN are safe when coadministered with allergen, cancer, and microbial antigens even at high doses (Agrawal and Kandimalla, 2002). Immunogenicity of hepatits B vaccination seems to be dramatically improved (Halperin et al., 2003; Siegrist et al., 2004b), along with the avidity of the antibodies formed (Siegrist et al., 2004a). Packaging synthetic CpGs into virus-like particles further enhances stability, presentation to APCs, and decreases toxicity (Storni et al., 2004). Of concern, subcutaneous immunization in mice with *H. pylori* lysate adjuvanted with CpG resulted in a strong local and systemic Th1 response, 10-fold reduction in bacterial density, yet significantly enhanced gastritis (Sommer et al., 2004). These findings highlight the difficulty of predicting *in vivo* biological effects of adjuvants from *in vitro* assays.

■ OM^TM 174, 197, and 294

Along with Corixa, a company named OM pharma has capitalized on the adjuvanticity of lipid A. OM^TM-174 is derived from *E. coli* lipid A with the retention of the diglucosamine diphosphate backbone and reduction of acyl chains, leaving the triacyl motif (Brandenburg et al., 2000). OM^TM-174 has been shown to induce humoral as well as cellular immune responses in animals and has been well tolerated at doses of 50 µg i.m. in humans (Engers et al., 2003). Antibody response and protection from *Plasmodium berghei* challenge in mice was similar between long-peptide PbCS242–310 with IFA and OM^TM-174 (Meraldi et al., 2003). Two new synthetic lipid A analogs OM^TM 197 and 294 have also been developed and induce DC maturation in mice, most likely via TLR-4 (Pink and Kieny, 2004).

■ Endogenous human agents

■ Cytokines

The use of cytokines as vaccine adjuvants has been encouraged by better understanding of cytokine mechanisms and by the commercial availability of recombinant IFN-γ and granulocyte macrophage colony-stimulating factor (GM-CSF). Cytokines offer several theoretical advantages compared to other adjuvants. First, cytokines are natural products of the human body, and so they may produce fewer long-term side effects after one injection compared to adjuvants derived from foreign plants, bacteria, and foreign chemicals. Second, if used with the correct dose and timing, specific cytokines may effectively direct the host response toward the appropriate Th1 cell and cell-mediated immune responses or toward the Th2 cell and humoral responses. For example, just as IL-12 enhanced the protective effect of leishmania-specific antigens and Th1 cells (Kenney et al., 1999), it may be possible to enhance antitoxin antibodies against a bacterial toxoid vaccine administered

with Th2 cytokines. Third, cytokines can be engineered in various ways to make them more potent. For example, cytokine molecules have been combined with liposomes or biodegradable polymers for slow release (Lachman et al., 1995) by conjugating them directly to vaccine haptens or antigens (Tao and Levy, 1993) as well as by cloning their genes into living vaccine vectors such as vaccinia virus or BCG for prolonged expression in the host (Murray et al., 1996).

Many cytokines (e.g., IL-3, IL-6, IL-11, GM-CSF) are capable of enhancing various immune responses when administered repeatedly, but the cytokines with the greatest potential are those administered in a single dose at or near the time of antigen injection; cytokines administered in this practical way include IFN-α, IFN-γ, IL-1, IL-2, IL-12, and GM-CSF. The adjuvant effects of these cytokines in animals or humans have been described and reviewed in detail (Stevenson et al., 2001; Chang et al., 2004; Heath and Playfair, 1992; Hughes and Babiuk, 1992; Lachman, et al., 1995; Lin et al., 1995; Patou et al., 1989; Scott, 1993). Although the immunopotentiating effects of cytokines appear to have great potential, the *in vivo* functions of cytokine networks are complex and incompletely understood. A cytokine can enhance, inhibit, or have no effect, depending on the dose, timing, and animal species, and which of these effects predominates is not always predictable (Heath and Playfair, 1992; Sturchler et al., 1989; Valensi et al., 1994).

■ Hormones

A promising immunomodulating steroid hormone, dehydroepiandrosterone (DHEA), enhanced hepatitis B vaccine (Araneo et al., 1993) and influenza vaccine (Danenberg et al., 1995) in aged mice, but clinical trials of DHEA have not been successful (Danenberg et al., 1997).

■ Dendritic cells

DCs are potent APCs and have been exploited as adjuvants by direct *in vitro* priming. Isolated DCs can be cultured and primed directly with soluble protein antigen, by use of viral vector systems, or by mRNA. Techniques such as hypertonic loading and electroporation have been used to stimulate MHC I vs. MHC II presentation; the cytokines mentioned above such as GM-CSF can also stimulate DCs (Arellano and Waller, 2004). Tumor-associated antigen (TAA) loading of DCs has been performed by injecting nonloaded DCs into tumor directly for subsequent cancer immuno-potentiation (Ragde et al., 2004). Early animal and human trials have revealed tumor protec-tion and pathogen clearance while others resulted in the induction of tolerance when antigen was delivered to DCs without a maturation signal. Antibodies such as antianti-gen uptake receptor CD205 have been utilized to target DCs while antidifferentiation substrate CD40 has been utilized to reverse tolerance (Moron et al., 2004). While low and short-lived CTL activity may be adequate to clear infection and small tumors, clinically established tumors may require sustained CTL activity that can be achieved with repeated DC vaccination. Sustained CTL activ-ity has, however, been associated with auto-immune disease in animal models and needs to be considered when tumor-specificity of antigen is determined. (Ludewig et al., 2000).

Saponins

Quil A and ISCOMS[TM]

Saponins are triterpene glycosides that can be isolated from the bark of the *Quillaja saponaria* Molina tree, a species native to South America (Kensil et al., 1991b). A partially purified saponin, Quil A, has been used widely as an adjuvant in veterinary vaccines (Campbell and Peerbaye, 1992). Quil A is a heterogeneous mixture of glycosides. Analysis by HPLC reveals at least 24 peaks that vary in their adjuvanticity and toxicity in mice (Kensil, 1991). Quil A has also been tested extensively as part of immune-stimulating complexes known as ISCOMs, which are cage-like 40 nm particles consisting of antigen, cholesterol, phospholipids, and Quil A (Morein et al.,

1984; Rimmelzwaan and Osterhaus, 1995). A highly protective ISCOM-based equine influenza vaccine is licensed in Sweden (Sundquist et al., 1988). ISCOMs have induced high titers of long-lasting functional antibodies and potent cytotoxic T cell responses in animals against viral antigens (Rimmelzwaan and Osterhaus, 1995). ISCOMS have induced mucosal immunity in mice after intranasal (Jones et al., 1988; Lovgren, 1988), parenteral, or intravaginal administration (Thapar et al., 1991), and thus may be particularly useful for protection against mucosal infections. The response to ISCOMs in which viral proteins have been incorporated closely resembles the antigen processing, presentation, and T cell stimulation elicited by replicating viruses. ISCOMs deliver antigen into the cytosolic compartment of APCs (Villacres et al., 1998), aided by their hydrophobic structure and saponins which can insert into cholesterol membranes (Ozel et al., 1989). Despite their potent adjuvanticity, ISCOM vaccines have only recently been administered to humans because of the local and systemic toxicity of Quil A in mice (Rimmelzwaan and Osterhaus, 1995; Ronnberg et al., 1995; Stieneker et al., 1995). An influenza ISCOM vaccine for humans containing a less toxic saponin frac-tion is under development and shows a strong cellular immune response (Ennis et al., 1999).

QS-21 (Stimulon[TM])

QS-21 is one of at least 24 structurally distinct triterpene glycosides isolated from Quil A. QS-21 was chosen for development by Antigenics, Inc. (Framingham, MA), because it demonstrated the proper balance of low mouse toxicity and maximum adjuvanticity, and eliminated the problem of lot-to-lot varia-tion characteristic of Quil A. It has many attractive features. QS-21 is lyophilized to produce a white powder effective in aqueous buffered vaccine solutions. It does not require emulsification. In the solid state, QS-21 is stable for many years at ambient temperatures, although stability is lower in aqueous solutions (Kensil et al., 1991b). It can be used alone or combined with other adjuvants including aluminum hydroxide and MPL. It has an acceptable toxicological profile in a variety of experimental animals including monkeys (Newman et al., 1992a). In rabbits, it is rapidly metabolized and eliminated in the urine and feces.

QS-21 is novel in that it can improve the immunogenicity of protein (Coughlin et al., 1995b; Kensil et al., 1991b; Marciani et al., 1991; Newman et al., 1992a), glycoprotein (Newman et al., 1992b, 1994; Powell et al., 1994), and polysaccharide antigens (Coughlin et al., 1995a) in a variety of small animals, dogs, or primates. It also uniquely stimulates both humoral and cell-mediated immunity, including potent class I-restricted CTL responses to subunit antigens (Newman et al., 1992b; Shirai et al., 1994; Wu et al., 1992). In mice immunized with *E. coli* polysaccharide, adding QS-21 not only increased IgG1 antibody titers, but it broadened the isotype response to include protective IgG2a antibodies and induced an anamnestic (memory) response on subsequent exposure to the polysaccharide (Coughlin et al., 1995a). QS-21 also enhanced the diphtheria toxoid-conjugated polysaccharide. QS-21 and a small number of other adjuvants (Baker et al., 1989; Fattom et al., 1995; Van Dam et al., 1989; Zigterman et al., 1989) may be able to improve the performance of polysaccharide-based vaccines. QS-21 is a component of a USDA-licensed, feline leukemia recombinant subunit antigen vaccine (Kensil et al., 1991a). In the first human clinical trial, QS-21 was mixed with the ganglioside melanoma antigen GM2, which was coupled to the protein carrier, keyhole limpet hemocyanin (KLH) (Livingston et al., 1994). Without QS-21 this antigen induced only low levels of IgM, and no IgG antibody in volunteers. The addition of $100\,\mu g$ of QS-21 to the vaccine resulted in six of six patients responding with IgG antibody to GM2, some as high as 1:1280 after four immunizations (Livingston et al., 1994).

Phase I clinical vaccine trials in progress with QS-21 include influenza, herpes simplex, HIV-1, hepatitis B, respiratory syncytial virus,

malaria, melanoma, colon cancer, and B-cell lymphoma (C.R. Kensil, personal communication, 2002). To date, more than 3000 healthy adult volunteers have received vaccines containing QS-21 without significant side effects other than occasional allergic reactions, depending upon the vaccine formulation (Edelman et al., 2002; Evans et al., 2001; Kashala et al., 2002; Kensil et al., 1995; Nardin et al., 2000; Newman et al., 1997). Toxicology studies are underway to determine if QS-21 is suitable for pediatric vaccines.

■ Emulsions

■ *Montanides*

Mineral oils in water/oil emulsions, such as IFA, stay at the injection site and are slowly eliminated by macrophages or metabolized to fatty acids, triglycerides, phospholipids, or sterols (Bollinger, 1970). Protein antigens are released very slowly from this matrix. Since IFA has not been accepted as a commercially viable adjuvant due to safety fears from animal studies (Alving, 2002), a proprietary, highly refined emulsifier from the mannide mono-oleate family in a natural metabolizable oil solution was developed by SEPPIC (Paris, France), named Montanide ISA 51. More than 1000 people have now been vaccinated with Montanide ISA 51 in malaria and cancer vaccine trials (Kenney et al., 2002; Slingluff et al., 2001; van Driel et al., 1999). The Montanide ISA 51 formulations are generally well tolerated systemically, although many subjects report mild to severe local reactions. Montanide ISA 720, which contains the same surfactant with a proprietary nonmineral oil that releases protein antigens more rapidly, has also been used in malaria and HIV vaccine trials (Cano, 1999; Genton et al., 2000; Lawrence et al., 1997; Lopez et al., 2001; Toledo et al., 2001). About half of the subjects developed mild to severe local pain and swelling that was sometimes delayed in onset by up to 10 days and required days to several weeks to resolve (Saul et al., 1999). Some volunteers developed painful local nodules and sterile abscesses, particularly those inoculated with higher doses of the vaccine formulations (Cano 1999; Genton et al., 2000; Lawrence et al., 2000). In summary, both Montanide adjuvants induce a strong immune response, but severe local reactions may limit their use.

■ *Other oil/water emulsion combinations (AS02)*

In addition to the inclusion of MF59 in various Chiron vaccines discussed above, several oil-in-water emulsions are under development by GlaxoSmithKline Biologicals in Rixensart, Belgium. AS02 (formerly known as SBAS2) is a proprietary oil-in-water emulsion containing MPL and QS-21 that causes strong antibody responses as well as Th1 and CTL cellular responses. Strong preclinical efficacy was found in a tuberculosis (TB) aerosol challenge model in guinea pigs where nearly as much protection was seen with AS02 (90%) as with BCG (100%). Phase I/II studies have been conducted in malaria, most recently with RTS,S, a circumsporozoite (CS) subunit antigen fused to the hepatitis S antigen (Stoute et al., 1997). RTS,S with AS02 demonstrated 34% efficacy in a phase IIb field trial in Gambia (Bojang et al., 2001) and an unprecedented 58% efficacy against severe malaria in Mozambique (Alonso et al., 2004). Similar emulsions are been studied with HPV-induced genital warts in a therapeutic setting (Gerard et al., 2001), with hepatitis BsAg (Desombere et al., 2002), and with multiple HIV vaccine formulations (McCormack et al., 2000).

■ Particulate immunomodulators

■ *Polylactide-co-glycolides (PLG)*

Biodegradable microspheres made of PLG provide strong adjuvanticity for subunit and DNA vaccines. Developed to provide a single-injection delivery system and replace the conventional need for boosting, antigen release occurs over weeks. Microspheres serve as depots for PLG which is phagocytozed by APCs and presented to CD4+ and CD8+ T cells. In mice and guinea pigs, both Th1 and Th2 responses to a single injection of tetanus toxoid were achieved with protection lasting up to one year. Multivalent formulations are feasible and preformed microspheres can be loaded to minimize antigen shearing (Diwan et al., 2001), but optimal formulations have yet to be determined. Cationic PLG is effective in presenting DNA vaccines, while anionic PLG may be better suited for protein vaccines. In HIV DNA vaccine development, anti-env antibody response induced by PLG/DNA in guinea pigs was equivalent to that of gp120 protein formulated with MF-59 while cationic PLG/DNA (HIV-1 gag) increased antibody priming over naked DNA in mice by 1,000- to 10,000-fold. A phase I trial of an HIV-*gag* DNA vaccine is currently in progress (Pink and Kieny, 2004).

■ *DC-Chol*

Cationic liposomes made of 3-N-(N',N'-dimethylaminoethane)-carbamoyl cholesterol (DC-Chol) have been developed as nonviral gene delivery systems (Gao and Huang, 1991) and subsequently exploited as immunostimulators with a balanced Th1/Th2 response (Brunel et al., 1999). Phase I studies of *H. pylori* and HIV *tat* candidate vaccines have revealed acceptable safety and reactogenicity as well as increased immunogenicity with DC-Chol. In the *H. pylori* study alum was also tested as an adjuvant and the cellular and humoral responses of DC-Chol were similar to those of alum (Pink and Kieny, 2004). Phase II studies of therapeutic antitumor vaccine tgDCC-E1A containing E1A plasmid and using DC-Chol as an adjuvant as well as delivery system have been performed. Although therapeutic response to the vaccine was limited and enrollment thereby curtailed to 24 patients, the safety and reactogenicity profile was judged acceptable (Villaret et al., 2002).

■ **Summary and conclusion**

Adjuvants typically have complex and multifactorial immunological mechanisms of action *in vivo*. As the signals induced and their interrelationships are being elucidated at the cellular and molecular level, a rational approach to adjuvant development is facilitated. Adjuvant safety, including the real and theoretical risks of administering vaccine adjuvants to humans, is a critical component that can enhance or retard the development process. In addition to the problem of safety, at least four other preclinical issues are critical to orderly clinical development of adjuvanted vaccines. These are (i) variable adjuvanticity, (ii) suboptimal use of aluminum adjuvants, (iii) inadequate animal models, and (iv) the inability to predict consistently protective or therapeutic efficacy by immunoassays.

An increasing array of adjuvants including aluminum compounds, MF59, virosomes, exotoxins, MPL, and RC-529 are becoming licensed around the world and set the stage for the development of novel adjuvants that will enhance prophylactic as well as therapeutic vaccine development. Experimental adjuvants in clinical trials include safer exotoxins, oligonucleotides, derivatives of lipid A other than MPL, cytokines, dendritic cells, saponins, montanides, nonionic block copolymers, PLG, and combination adjuvants such as AS04.

In addition to immunologic enhancement without toxicity and successful protection against challenge, choice of adjuvant for a clinical trial may depend upon cost and commercial availability. It is imperative that investigators in the private and public sectors alike work together to design and test novel adjuvants in an effort to improve existing and new vaccines.

■ References

Agrawal, S. and Kandimalla, E.R. (2002). Medicinal chemistry and therapeutic potential of CpG DNA. *Trends Mol. Med.* 8, 114–121.

Alonso, P.L., Sacarlal, J., Aponte, J.J., Leach, A., Macete, E., Milman, J., Mandomando, I., Spiessens, B., Guinovart, C., Espasa, M., Bassat, Q., Aide, P., Ofori-Anyinam, O., Navia, M.M., Corachan, S., Ceuppens, M., Dubois, M.C., Demoitie, M.A., Dubovsky, F., Menendez, C., Tornieporth, N., Ballou, W.R., Thompson, R., and Cohen, J. (2004).

Efficacy of the RTS,S/AS02A vaccine against Plasmodium falciparum infection and disease in young African children: randomised controlled trial. *Lancet* 364, 1411–1420.

Alving, C.R. (2002). Design and selection of vaccine adjuvants: animal models and human trials. *Vaccine* 20, S56–S64.

Araneo, B.A., Woods, M.L., and Daynes, R.A. (1993). Reversal of the immunosenescent phenotype by dehydroepiandrosterone: hormone treatment provides an adjuvant effect on the immunization of aged mice with recombinant hepatitis B surface antigen. *J. Infect. Dis.* 167, 830–840.

Arellano, M. and Waller, K. (2004). Granulocyte-macrophage-colony-stimulating factor and other cytokines: as adjuncts to cancer immunotherapy, stem cell transplantation, and vaccines. *Curr. Hematol. Rep.* 3, 424–431.

Baker, P.J., Fauntleroy, M.B., Stashak, P.W., Hiernaux, J.R., Cantrell, J.L., and Rudbach, J.A. (1989). Adjuvant effects of trehalose dimycolate on the antibody response to type III pneumococcal polysaccharide. *Infect. Immun.* 57, 912–917.

Baker, P.J., Haslov, K.R., Fauntleroy, M.B., Stashak, P.W., Myers, K., and Ulrich, J.T. (1990). Enrichment of suppressor T cells by means of binding to monophosphoryl lipid A. *Infect. Immun.* 58, 726–731.

Baldo, V., Menegon, T., Bonello, C., Floreani, A., and Trivello, R. (2001). Comparison of three different influenza vaccines in institutionalised elderly. *Vaccine* 19, 3472–3475.

Baldridge, J.R. and Crane, R.T. (1999). Monophosphoryl lipid A (MPL) formulations for the next generation of vaccines. *Methods* 19, 103–107.

Baldridge, J.R., Cluff, C.W., Evans, J.T., Lacy, M.J., Stephens, J.R., Brookshire, V.G., Wang, R., Ward, J.R., Yorgensen, Y.M., Persing, D.H., and Johnson, D.A. (2002). Immunostimulatory activity of aminoalkyl glucosaminide 4-phosphates (AGPs): induction of protective innate immune responses by RC-524 and RC-529. *J. Endotoxin Res.* 8, 453–458.

Barackman, J.D., Ott, G., Pine, S., and O'Hagan, D.T. (2001). Oral administration of influenza vaccine in combination with the adjuvants LT-K63 and LT-R72 induces potent immune responses comparable to or stronger than traditional intramuscular immunization. *Clin. Diagn. Lab. Immunol.* 8, 652–657.

Baylor, N.W., Egan, W., and Richman, P. (2002). Aluminum salts in vaccines: US perspective [correction appears in *Vaccine* (2002) 20, 3428]. *Vaccine* 20 (Suppl. 3), S18–S23.

Beebe, G.W., Simon, A.H., and Vivona, S. (1964). Follow-up study on army personnel who received adjuvant influenza virus vaccine 1951–1953. *Am. J. Med. Sci.* 247, 385–406.

Beebe, G.W., Simon, A.H., and Vivona, S. (1972). Long-term mortality follow-up of Army recruits who received adjuvant influenza virus vaccine in 1951–1953. *Am. J. Epidemiol.* 95, 337–346.

Blennow, M., Granstrom, M., Olin, P., Tiru, M., Jaatmaa, E., Askelof, P., and Sato, Y. (1986). Preliminary data from a clinical trial (phase 2) of an acellular pertussis vaccine, J-NIH-6. *Dev. Biol. Stand.* 65, 185–190.

Bojang, K.A., Milligan, P.J., Pinder, M., Vigneron, L., Alloueche, A., Kester, K.E., Ballou, W.R., Conway, D.J., Reece, W.H., Gothard, P., Yamuah, L., Delchambre, M., Voss, G., Greenwood, B.M., Hill, A., McAdam, K.P., Tornieporth, N., Cohen, J.D., and Doherty, T. (2001). Efficacy of RTS,S/AS02 malaria vaccine against Plasmodium falciparum infection in semi-immune adult men in The Gambia: a randomised trial. *Lancet* 358, 1927–1934.

Bollinger, J.N. (1970). Metabolic fate of mineral oil adjuvants using 14C-labeled tracers: I. Mineral oil. *J. Pharm. Sci.* 59, 1084–1088.

Brandenburg, K., Lindner, B., Schromm, A., Koch, M.H., Bauer, J., Merkli, A., Zbaeren, C., Davies, J.G., and Seydel, U. (2000). Physicochemical characteristics of triacyl lipid A partial structure OM-174 in relation to biological activity. *Eur. J. Biochem.* 267, 3370–3377.

Brunel, F., Darbouret, A., and Ronco, J. (1999). Cationic lipid DC-Chol induces an improved and balanced immunity able to overcome the unresponsiveness to the hepatitis B vaccine. *Vaccine* 17, 2192–2203.

Bumford, R. (1989). Aluminum salts: prospectives in their use as adjuvants. In Gregoriadis, G., Allison, A.C., and Poste, G. (Eds) *Immunological Adjuvants and Vaccines.* Plenum Press, New York, pp. 35–41.

Butler, N.R., Feng, S., Benson, P.F. et al. (1962). Response of infants to pertussis vaccine at one week and to poliomyelitis, diptheria, and tetanus vaccine at six months. *Lancet* 2, 112–114.

Byars, N.E., Allison, A.C., Harmon, M.W., and Kendal, A.P. (1990). Enhancement of antibody responses to influenza B virus haemagglutinin by use of a new adjuvant formulation. *Vaccine* 8, 49–56.

Campbell, J.B. and Peerbaye, Y.A. (1992). Saponin. *Res. Immunol.* 143, 526–530; discussion 577–578.

Cano, C.A.D. (1999). The multi-epitope polypeptide approach in HIV-1 vaccine development. *Genetic Anal. Biomolec. Eng.* 15, 149–153.

Carozzi, S., Salit, M., Cantaluppi, A., Nasini, M.G., Barocci, S., Cantarella, S., and Lamperi, S. (1989). Effect of monophosphoryl lipid A on the in vitro function of peritoneal leukocytes from uremic patients on continuous ambulatory peritoneal dialysis. *J. Clin. Microbiol.* 27, 1748–1753.

Celis, E. (2002). Getting peptide vaccines to work: just a matter of quality control? *J. Clin. Invest.* 110, 1765–1768.

Chang, D.Z., Lomazow, W., Joy, S.C., Stan, R., and Perales, M.A. (2004). Granulocyte-macrophage colony stimulating factor: an adjuvant for cancer vaccines. *Hematology* 9, 207–215.

Chedid, L.A., Parant, M.A., Audibert, F.M., Riveau, G.J., Parant, F.J., Lederer, E., Choay, J.P., and Lefrancier, P.L. (1982). Biological activity of a new synthetic muramyl peptide adjuvant devoid of pyrogenicity. *Infect. Immun.* 35, 417–424.

Claesson, B.A., Trollfors, B., Lagergard, T., Taranger, J., Bryla, D., Otterman, G., Cramton, T., Yang, Y., Reimer, C.B., and Robbins, J.B. (1988). Clinical and immunologic responses to the capsular polysaccharide of Haemophilus influenzae type b alone or conjugated to tetanus toxoid in 18- to 23-month-old children. *J. Pediatr.* 112, 695–702.

Clemens, J.D., Sack, D.A., Harris, J.R., Chakraborty, J., Khan, M.R., Stanton, B.F., Kay, B.A., Khan, M.U., Yunus, M., and Atkinson, W. (1986). Field trial of oral cholera vaccines in Bangladesh. *Lancet* 2, 124–127.

Coler, R.N., Skeiky, Y.A., Bernards, K., Greeson, K., Carter, D., Cornellison, C.D., Modabber, F., Campos-Neto, A., and Reed, S.G. (2002). Immunization with a polyprotein vaccine consisting of the T-cell antigens thiol-specific antioxidant, Leishmania major stress-inducible protein 1, and leishmania elongation initiation factor protects against leishmaniasis. *Infect. Immun.* 70, 4215–4225.

Corey, L., Langenberg, A.G., Ashley, R., Sekulovich, R.E., Izu, A.E., Douglas, J.M., Jr., Handsfield, H.H., Warren, T., Marr, L., Tyring, S., DiCarlo, R., Adimora, A.A., Leone, P., Dekker, C.L., Burke, R.L., Leong, W.P., and Straus, S.E. (1999). Recombinant glycoprotein vaccine for the prevention of genital HSV-2 infection: two randomized controlled trials. Chiron HSV Vaccine Study Group. *JAMA* 282, 331–340.

Couch, R.B. (2004). Nasal vaccination, Escherichia coli enterotoxin, and Bell's palsy. *N. Engl. J. Med.* 350, 860–861.

Coughlin, R.T., Fattom, A., Chu, C., White, A.C., and Winston, S. (1995a). Adjuvant activity of QS-21 for experimental E. coli 018 polysaccharide vaccines. *Vaccine* 13, 17–21.

Coughlin, R.T., Fish, D., Mather, T.N., Ma, J., Pavia, C., and Bulger, P. (1995b). Protection of dogs from Lyme disease with a vaccine containing outer surface protein (Osp) A, OspB, and the saponin adjuvant QS21. *J. Infect. Dis.* 171, 1049–1052.

Cvjetanovic, B. and Uemura, K. (1965). The present status of field and laboratory studies of typhoid and paratyphoid vaccines with special reference to studies sponsored by the World Health Organization. *Bull WHO* 32, 29–36.

Danenberg, H.D., Ben-Yehuda, A., Zakay-Rones, Z., and Friedman, G. (1995). Dehydroepiandrosterone (DHEA) treatment reverses the impaired immune response of old mice to influenza vaccination and protects from influenza infection. *Vaccine* 13, 1445–1448.

Danenberg, H.D., Ben Yehuda, A., Zakay-Rones, Z., Gross, D.J., and Friedman, G. (1997). Dehydroepiandrosterone treatment is not beneficial to the immune response to influenza in elderly subjects. *J. Clin. Endocrinol. Metab.* 82, 2911–2914.

Davenport, F.M. (1968). Seventeen years' experience with mineral oil adjuvant influenza virus vaccines. *Ann. Allergy* 26, 288–292.

Davenport, F.M., Hennessy, A.V., and Askin, F.B. (1968). Lack of adjuvant effect of AlPO$_4$ on purified influenza virus haemagglutinins in man. *J. Immunol.* 100, 1139–1140.

Davis, H.L., Suparto, I.I., Weeratna, R.R., Jumintarto, Iskandriati, D.D., Chamzah, S.S., Ma'ruf, A.A., Nente, C.C., Pawitri, D.D., Krieg, A.M., Heriyanto,

Smits, W., and Sajuthi, D.D. (2000). CpG DNA overcomes hyporesponsiveness to hepatitis B vaccine in orangutans. *Vaccine* 18, 1920–1924.

De Donato, S., Granoff, D., Minutello, M., Lecchi, G., Faccini, M., Agnello, M., Senatore, F., Verweij, P., Fritzell, B., and Podda, A. (1999). Safety and immunogenicity of MF59-adjuvanted influenza vaccine in the elderly. *Vaccine* 17, 3094–3101.

Descotes, J., Ravel, G., and Ruat, C. (2002). Vaccines: predicting the risk of allergy and autoimmunity. *Toxicology* 174, 45–51.

Desombere, I., Van der Wielen, M., Van Damme, P., Stoffel, M., De Clercq, N., Goilav, C., and Leroux-Roels, G. (2002). Immune response of HLA DQ2 positive subjects, vaccinated with HBsAg/AS04, a hepatitis B vaccine with a novel adjuvant. *Vaccine* 20, 2597–2602.

Dijkstra, J., Mellors, J.W., Ryan, J.L., and Szoka, F.C. (1987). Modulation of the biological activity of bacterial endotoxin by incorporation into liposomes. *J. Immunol.* 138, 2663–2670.

Diwan, M., Khar, R.K., and Talwar, G.P. (2001). Tetanus toxoid loaded "preformed microspheres" of cross-linked dextran. *Vaccine* 19, 3853–3859.

Domer, J.E., Human, L.G., Andersen, G.B., Rudbach, J.A., and Asherson, G.L. (1993). Abrogation of suppression of delayed hypersensitivity induced by Candida albicans-derived mannan by treatment with monophosphoryl lipid A. *Infect. Immun.* 61, 2122–2130.

Edelman, R. (1980). Vaccine adjuvants. *Rev. Infect. Dis.* 2, 370–383.

Edelman, R. and Tacket, C.O. (1990). Adjuvants. *Int. Rev. Immunol.* 7, 51–66.

Edelman, R., Wasserman, S.S., Kublin, J.G., Bodison, S.A., Nardin, E.H., Oliveira, G.A., Ansari, S., Diggs, C.L., Kashala, O.L., Schmeckpeper, B.J., and Hamilton, R.G. (2002). Immediate-type hypersensitivity and other clinical reactions in volunteers immunized with a synthetic multi-antigen peptide vaccine (PfCS-MAP1NYU) against Plasmodium falciparum sporozoites. *Vaccine* 21, 269–280.

Engers, H., Kieny, M.P., Malhotra, P., and Pink, J.R. (2003). Third meeting on novel adjuvants currently in or close to clinical testing, World Health Organization–Organization Mondiale de la Sante, Fondation Merieux, Annecy, France, 7–9 January 2002. *Vaccine* 21, 3503–3524.

Ennis, F.A., Cruz, J., Jameson, J., Klein, M., Burt, D., and Thipphawong, J. (1999). Augmentation of human influenza A virus-specific cytotoxic T lymphocyte memory by influenza vaccine and adjuvanted carriers (ISCOMS). *Virology* 259, 256–261.

Evans, J.T., Cluff, C.W., Johnson, D.A., Lacy, M.J., Persing, D.H., and Baldridge, J.R. (2003). Enhancement of antigen-specific immunity via the TLR4 ligands MPL adjuvant and Ribi.529. *Expert Rev. Vaccines* 2, 219–229.

Evans, T.G., McElrath, M.J., Matthews, T., Montefiori, D., Weinhold, K., Wolff, M., Keefer, M.C., Kallas, E.G., Corey, L., Gorse, G.J., Belshe, R., Graham, B.S., Spearman, P.W., Schwartz, D., Mulligan, M.J.,

Goepfert, P., Fast, P., Berman, P., Powell, M., and Francis, D. (2001). QS-21 promotes an adjuvant effect allowing for reduced antigen dose during HIV-1 envelope subunit immunization in humans. *Vaccine* 19, 2080–2091.

Fattom, A., Li, X., Cho, Y.H., Burns, A., Hawwari, A., Shepherd, S.E., Coughlin, R., Winston, S., and Naso, R. (1995). Effect of conjugation methodology, carrier protein, and adjuvants on the immune response to Staphylococcus aureus capsular polysaccharides. *Vaccine* 13, 1288–1293.

Fries, L.F., Gordon, D.M., Richards, R.L., Egan, J.E., Hollingdale, M.R., Gross, M., Silverman, C., and Alving, C.R. (1992). Liposomal malaria vaccine in humans: a safe and potent adjuvant strategy. *Proc. Natl. Acad. Sci. USA* 89, 358–362.

Gao, X. and Huang, L. (1991). A novel cationic liposome reagent for efficient transfection of mammalian cells. *Biochem. Biophys. Res. Commun.* 179, 280–285.

Garg, M. and Subbarao, B. (1992). Immune responses of systemic and mucosal lymphoid organs to Pnu: imune vaccine as a function of age and the efficacy of monophosphoryl lipid A as an adjuvant. *Infect. Immun.* 60, 2329–2336.

Genton, B., Al Yaman, F., Anders, R., Saul, A., Brown, G., Pye, D., Irving, D. O., Briggs, W.R., Mai, A., Ginny, M., Adiguma, T., Rare, L., Giddy, A., Reber-Liske, R., Stuerchler, D., and Alpers, M.P. (2000). Safety and immunogenicity of a three-component blood-stage malaria vaccine in adults living in an endemic area of Papua New Guinea. *Vaccine* 18, 2504–2511.

Gerard, C.M., Baudson, N., Kraemer, K., Bruck, C., Garcon, N., Paterson, Y., Pan, Z.K., and Pardoll, D. (2001). Therapeutic potential of protein and adjuvant vaccinations on tumour growth. *Vaccine* 19, 2583–2589.

Gherardi, R.K., Coquet, M., Cherin, P., Belec, L., Moretto, P., Dreyfus, P.A., Pellissier, J.F., Chariot, P., and Authier, F.J. (2001). Macrophagic myofasciitis lesions assess long-term persistence of vaccine-derived aluminium hydroxide in muscle. *Brain* 124, 1821–1831.

Glenn, G.M., Taylor, D.N., Li, X., Frankel, S., Montemarano, A., and Alving, C.R. (2000). Transcutaneous immunization: a human vaccine delivery strategy using a patch. *Nature Med* 6, 1403–1406.

Gluck, U., Gebbers, J.O., and Gluck, R. (1999). Phase 1 evaluation of intranasal virosomal influenza vaccine with and without Escherichia coli heat-labile toxin in adult volunteers. *J. Virol.* 73, 7780–7786.

Goldenthal, K.L., Cavagnaro, J.A., Alving, C.R., and Vogel, F.R. (1993). NCVDG working groups: safety evaluation of vaccine adjuvants: national cooperative vaccine development meeting working group. *AIDS Res. Hum. Retroviruses* 9, S47–S51.

Gordon, D.M., McGovern, T.W., Krzych, U. et al. (1995). Safety, immunogenicity, and efficacy of a recombinantly produced *Plasmodium falciparum* circumsporozoite protein-hepatitis B surface antigen subunit vaccine. *J. Infect. Dis.* 171, 1576–1585.

Gordon, D.M., Duffy, P.E., Heppner, D.G., Lyon, J.A., Williams, J.S., Scheumann, D., Farley, L., Stacey, D.,

Haynes, J.D., Sadoff, J.C., and Ballou, W.R. (1996). Phase I safety and immunogenicity testing of clinical lots of the synthetic Plasmodium falciparum vaccine SPf66 produced under good manufacturing procedure conditions in the United States. *Am. J. Trop. Med. Hyg.* 55, 63–68.

Guerena-Burgueno, F., Hall, E.R., Taylor, D.N., Cassels, F.J., Scott, D.A., Wolf, M.K., Roberts, Z.J., Nesterova, G.V., Alving, C.R., and Glenn, G.M. (2002). Safety and immunogenicity of a prototype enterotoxigenic Escherichia coli vaccine administered transcutaneously. *Infect. Immun.* 70, 1874–1880.

Gupta, R.K. (1998). Aluminum compounds as vaccine adjuvants. *Adv. Drug Deliv. Rev.* 32, 155–172.

Gupta, R.K. and Siber, G.R. (1995). Adjuvants for human vaccines: current status, problems and future prospects. *Vaccine* 13, 1263–1276.

Gupta, R.K., Relyveld, E.H., Lindblad, E.B., Bizzini, B., Ben-Efraim, S., and Gupta, C.K. (1993). Adjuvants: a balance between toxicity and adjuvanticity. *Vaccine* 11, 293–306.

Gupta, R.K., Rost, B.E., Relyveld, E., and Siber, G.R. (1995). Adjuvant properties of aluminum and calcium compounds. In Powell, M.F. and Newman, M.J. (Eds) *Vaccine Design: The Subunit and Adjuvant Approach.* Plenum Press, New York, pp. 229–248.

Gustafson, G.L. and Rhodes, M.J. (1992). Bacterial cell wall products as adjuvants: early interferon gamma as a marker for adjuvants that enhance protective immunity. *Res. Immunol.* 143, 483–488; discussion 573–574.

Haigwood, N.L., Nara, P.L., Brooks, E., Van Nest, G.A., Ott, G., Higgins, K.W., Dunlop, N., Scandella, C.J., Eichberg, J.W., and Steimer, K.S. (1992). Native but not denatured recombinant human immunodeficiency virus type 1 gp120 generates broad-spectrum neutralizing antibodies in baboons. *J. Virol.* 66, 172–182.

Halperin, S.A., Van Nest, G., Smith, B., Abtahi, S., Whiley, H., and Eiden, J.J. (2003). A phase I study of the safety and immunogenicity of recombinant hepatitis B surface antigen co-administered with an immunostimulatory phosphorothioate oligonucleotide adjuvant. *Vaccine* 21, 2461–2467.

Hardegree, M.C., Pittman, M., and Maloney, C.J. (1972). Influence of mouse strain on the assayed potency (unitage) of tetanus toxoid. *Appl. Microbiol.* 24, 120–126.

Harper, D.M., Franco, E.L., Wheeler, C., Ferris, D.G., Jenkins, D., Schuind, A., Zahaf, T., Innis, B., Naud, P., De Carvalho, N.S., Roteli-Martins, C.M., Teixeira, J., Blatter, M.M., Korn, A.P., Quint, W., and Dubin, G. (2004). Efficacy of a bivalent L1 virus-like particle vaccine in prevention of infection with human papillomavirus types 16 and 18 in young women: a randomised controlled trial. *Lancet* 364, 1757–1765.

Heath, A.W. and Playfair, J.H.L. (1992). Cytokines as immunological adjuvants. *Vaccine* 10, 427–434.

Heineman, T.C., Clements-Mann, M.L., Poland, G.A., Jacobson, R.M., Izu, A.E., Sakamoto, D., Eiden, J., Van Nest, G.A., and Hsu, H.H. (1999). A randomized, controlled study in adults of the immunogenicity of a novel hepatitis B vaccine containing MF59 adjuvant. *Vaccine* 17, 2769–2778.

Hoffman, S.L., Edelman, R., Bryan, J.P., Schneider, I., Davis, J., Sedegah, M., Gordon, D., Church, P., Gross, M., and Silverman, C. (1994). Safety, immunogenicity, and efficacy of a malaria sporozoite vaccine administered with monophosphoryl lipid A, cell wall skeleton of mycobacteria, and squalane as adjuvant. *Am. J. Trop. Med. Hyg.* 51, 603–612.

HogenEsch, H. (2002). Mechanisms of stimulation of the immune response by aluminum adjuvants. *Vaccine* 20 (Suppl. 3), S34–S39.

Holzer, B.R., Hatz, C., Schmidt-Sissolak, D., Gluck, R., Althaus, B., and Egger, M. (1996). Immunogenicity and adverse effects of inactivated virosome versus alumadsorbed hepatitis A vaccine: a randomized controlled trial. *Vaccine* 14, 982–986.

Hughes, H.P. and Babiuk, L.A. (1992). The adjuvant potential of cytokines. *Biotechnol. Ther.* 3, 101–117.

Hunter, R.L. (2002). Overview of vaccine adjuvants: present and future. *Vaccine* 20 (Suppl. 3), S7–S12.

Hunter, R.L. and Lal, A.A. (1994). Copolymer adjuvants in malaria vaccine development. *Am. J. Trop. Med. Hyg.* 50 (Suppl.), 52–58.

Jacobson, R.M., Adegbenro, A., Pankratz, V.S., and Poland, G.A. (2001). Adverse events and vaccination: the lack of power and predictability of infrequent events in pre-licensure study. *Vaccine* 19, 2428–2433.

Jensen, O.M. and Koch, C. (1988). On the effect of $Al(OH)_3$ as an immunological adjuvant. *Acta Pathol. Microbiol. Immun. Scand.* 96, 257–264.

Johnson, A.G., Gaines, S., and Landy, M. (1956). Studies on the O antigen of Salmonella typhosa: V. Enhancement of antibody response to protein antigens by the purified lipopolysaccharide. *J. Exp. Med.* 103, 225–246.

Jones, W.R., Bradley, J., Judd, S.J., Denholm, E.H., Ing, R.M., Mueller, U.W., Powell, J., Griffin, P.D., and Stevens, V.C. (1988). Phase I clinical trial of a World Health Organization birth control vaccine. *Lancet* 1, 1295–1298.

Kasel, J.A., Couch, R.B., and Douglas, R.G., Jr. (1971). Antigenicity of alum and aqueous adenovirus hexon antigen vaccines in man. *J. Immunol.* 107, 916–919.

Kashala, O., Amador, R., Valero, M.V., Moreno, A., Barbosa, A., Nickel, B., Daubenberger, C.A., Guzman, F., Pluschke, G., and Patarroyo, M.E. (2002). Safety, tolerability and immunogenicity of new formulations of the Plasmodium falciparum malaria peptide vaccine SPf66 combined with the immunological adjuvant QS-21. *Vaccine* 20, 2263–2277.

Keefer, M.C., Wolff, M., Gorse, G.J., Graham, B.S., Corey, L., Clements-Mann, M.L., Verani-Ketter, N., Erb, S., Smith, C.M., Belshe, R.B., Wagner, L.J., McElrath, M.J., Schwartz, D.H., and Fast, P. (1997). Safety profile of phase I and II preventive HIV type 1 envelope vaccination: experience of the NIAID AIDS Vaccine Evaluation Group. *AIDS Res. Hum. Retroviruses* 13, 1163–1177.

Keitel, W., Couch, R., Bond, N., Adair, S., Van Nest, G., and Dekker, C. (1993). Pilot evaluation of influenza virus vaccine (IVV) combined with adjuvant. *Vaccine* 11, 909–913.

Kenney, R.T., Sacks, D.L., Sypek, J.P., Vilela, L., Gam, A.A., and Evans-Davis, K. (1999). Protective immunity using recombinant human IL-12 and alum as adjuvants in a primate model of cutaneous leishmaniasis. *J. Immunol.* 163, 4481–4488.

Kenney, R.T., Regina, R.N., Pichyangkul, S., Price, V.L., and Engers, H.D. (2002). Second meeting on novel adjuvants currently in/close to human clinical testing. World Health Organization–Organization Mondiale de la Sante Fondation Merieux, Annecy, France, 5–7 June 2000. *Vaccine* 20, 2155–2163.

Kensil, C.R., Barrett, C., Kushner, N., Beltz, G., Storey, J., Patel, U., Recchia, J., Aubert, A., and Marciani, D. (1991a). Development of a genetically engineered vaccine against feline leukemia virus infection. *J. Am. Vet. Med. Assoc.* 199, 1423–1427.

Kensil, C.R., Patel, U., Lennick, M., and Marciani, D. (1991b). Separation and characterization of saponins with adjuvant activity from Quillaja saponaria Molina cortex. *J. Immunol.* 146, 431–437.

Kensil, C.R., Wu, J.Y., and Soltysik, S. (1995). Structural and immunological characterization of the vaccine adjuvant QS-21. *Pharm. Biotechnol.* 6, 525–541.

Kleinau, S., Erlandsson, H., Holmdahl, R., and Klareskog, L. (1991). Adjuvant oils induce arthritis in the DA rat: I. Characterization of the disease and evidence for an immunological involvement. *J. Autoimmun.* 4, 871–880.

Kotloff, K.L., Sztein, M.B., Wasserman, S.S., Losonsky, G.A., DiLorenzo, S.C., and Walker, R.I. (2001). Safety and immunogenicity of oral inactivated whole-cell Helicobacter pylori vaccine with adjuvant among volunteers with or without subclinical infection. *Infect. Immun.* 69, 3581–3590.

Krieg, A.M. (2001). From bugs to drugs: therapeutic immunomodulation with oligodeoxynucleotides containing CpG sequences from bacterial DNA. *Antisense Nucleic Acid Drug Dev.* 11, 181–188.

Krieg, A.M., Yi, A.K., Matson, S., Waldschmidt, T.J., Bishop, G.A., Teasdale, R., Koretzky, G.A., and Klinman, D.M. (1995). CpG motifs in bacterial DNA trigger direct B-cell activation. *Nature* 374, 546–549.

Lachman, L.B., Shih, L.C., Rao, X.M., Ullrich, S.E., and Cleland, J.L. (1995). Cytokine-containing liposomes as adjuvants for subunit vaccines. *Pharm. Biotechnol.* 6, 659–671.

Lambert, J.S., McNamara, J., Katz, S.L., Fenton, T., Kang, M., VanCott, T.C., Livingston, R., Hawkins, E., Moye, J., Jr., Borkowsky, W., Johnson, D., Yogev, R., Duliege, A.M., Francis, D., Gershon, A., Wara, D., Martin, N., Levin, M., McSherry, G., and Smith, G. (1998). Safety and immunogenicity of HIV recombinant envelope vaccines in HIV-infected infants and children. National Institutes of Health-sponsored Pediatric AIDS Clinical Trials Group (ACTG-218). *J. AIDS Hum. Retrovirol.* 19, 451–461.

Langenberg, A.G., Burke, R.L., Adair, S.F., Sekulovich, R., Tigges, M., Dekker, C.L., and Corey, L. (1995). A recombinant glycoprotein vaccine for herpes simplex virus type 2: safety and immunogenicity [corrected; published erratum appears in *Ann. Intern. Med.* (1995) 123, 395]. *Ann. Intern. Med.* 122, 889–898.

Lawrence, G., Cheng, Q.Q., Reed, C., Taylor, D., Stowers, A., Cloonan, N., Rzepczyk, C., Smillie, A., Anderson, K., Pombo, D., Allworth, A., Eisen, D., Anders, R., and Saul, A. (2000). Effect of vaccination with 3 recombinant asexual-stage malaria antigens on initial growth rates of Plasmodium falciparum in non-immune volunteers. *Vaccine* 18, 1925–1931.

Lawrence, G.W., Saul, A., Giddy, A.J., Kemp, R., and Pye, D. (1997). Phase I trial in humans of an oil-based adjuvant SEPPIC MONTANIDE ISA 720. *Vaccine* 15, 176–178.

Leroux-Roels, G., Moreux, E., Verhasselt, B. et al. (1993). Immunogenicity and reactogenicity of a recombinant HSV-2 glycoprotein D vaccine with or without monophosphoryl lipid A in HSV seronegative and seropositive subjects. 33rd Interscience Conference on Antimicrobial Agents and Chemotherapy, p. 341.

Lin, R., Tarr, P.E., and Jones, T.C. (1995). Present status of the use of cytokines as adjuvants with vaccines to protect against infectious diseases. *Clin. Infect. Dis.* 21, 1439–1449.

Livingston, P.O., Adluri, S., Helling, F., Yao, T.J., Kensil, C.R., Newman, M.J., and Marciani, D. (1994). Phase 1 trial of immunological adjuvant QS-21 with a GM2 ganglioside-keyhole limpet haemocyanin conjugate vaccine in patients with malignant melanoma. *Vaccine* 12, 1275–1280.

Lopez, J.A., Weilenman, C., Audran, R., Roggero, M.A., Bonelo, A., Tiercy, J.M., Spertini, F., and Corradin, G. (2001). A synthetic malaria vaccine elicits a potent CD8(+) and CD4(+) T lymphocyte immune response in humans. Implications for vaccination strategies. *Eur. J. Immunol.* 31, 1989–1998.

Lovgren, K. (1988). The serum antibody response distributed in subclasses and isotypes after intranasal and subcutaneous immunization with influenza virus immunostimulating complexes. *Scand. J. Immunol.* 27, 241–245.

Luderitz, O., Galanos, S., and Reitschel, E.T. (1982). Endotoxins of gram-negative bacteria. *Pharm. Ther.* 15, 383–402.

Ludewig, B., Ochsenbein, A.F., Odermatt, B., Paulin, D., Hengartner, H., and Zinkernagel, R.M. (2000). Immunotherapy with dendritic cells directed against tumor antigens shared with normal host cells results in severe autoimmune disease. *J. Exp. Med.* 191, 795–804.

Lyng, J. and Nyerges, G. (1984). The second international standard for tetanus toxoid (adsorbed). *J. Biol. Stand.* 12, 121–130.

MacLean, G.D., Bowen-Yacyshyn, M.B., Samuel, J., Meikle, A., Stuart, G., Nation, J., Poppema, S., Jerry, M., Koganty, R., and Wong, T. (1992). Active immunization of human ovarian cancer patients against a common carcinoma

(Thomsen-Friedenreich) determinant using a synthetic carbohydrate antigen. *J. Immunother.* 11, 292–305.

MacLean, G.D., Reddish, M., Koganty, R.R., Wong, T., Gandhi, S., Smolenski, M., Samuel, J., Nabholtz, J.M., and Longenecker, B.M. (1993). Immunization of breast cancer patients using a synthetic sialyl-Tn glycoconjugate plus Detox adjuvant. *Cancer Immunol. Immunother.* 36, 215–222.

Marciani, D.J., Kensil, C.R., Beltz, G.A., Hung, C.H., Cronier, J., and Aubert, A. (1991). Genetically engineered subunit vaccine against feline leukaemia virus: protective immune response in cats. *Vaccine* 9, 89–96.

Mark, A., Bjorksten, B., and Granstrom, M. (1995). Immunoglobulin E responses to diphtheria and tetanus toxoids after booster with aluminium-adsorbed and fluid DT-vaccines. *Vaccine* 13, 669–673.

Martin, M., Michalek, S.M., and Katz, J. (2003). Role of innate immune factors in the adjuvant activity of monophosphoryl lipid A. *Infect. Immun.* 71, 2498–2507.

Matsuhasi, T. (1991). Influence of mouse strain on the results of potency testing for diphtheria and tetanus toxoid components of D, T, DT and DTP vaccines. In Manclark, C.R. (Ed) *Proceedings of an Informal Consultation on the World Health Organization Requirements for Diphtheria, Tetanus, Pertussis and Combined Vaccines*. Publication No. (FDA) 91–1174. Department of Health and Human Services, US Public Health Service, Bethesda, MD, pp. 55–58.

McCormack, S., Tilzey, A., Carmichael, A., Gotch, F., Kepple, J., Newberry, A., Jones, G., Lister, S., Beddows, S., Cheingsong, R., Rees, A., Babiker, A., Banatvala, J., Bruck, C., Darbyshire, J., Tyrrell, D., Van Hoecke, C., and Weber, J. (2000). A phase I trial in HIV negative healthy volunteers evaluating the effect of potent adjuvants on immunogenicity of a recombinant gp120W61D derived from dual tropic R5X4 HIV-1ACH320. *Vaccine* 18, 1166–1177.

Meraldi, V., Audran, R., Romero, J.F., Brossard, V., Bauer, J., Lopez, J.A., and Corradin, G. (2003). OM-174, a new adjuvant with a potential for human use, induces a protective response when administered with the synthetic C-terminal fragment 242–310 from the circumsporozoite protein of Plasmodium berghei. *Vaccine* 21, 2485–2491.

Mitchell, M.S., Kan-Mitchell, J., Kempf, R.A., Harel, W., Shau, H.Y., and Lind, S. (1988). Active specific immunotherapy for melanoma: phase I trial of allogeneic lysates and a novel adjuvant. *Cancer Res.* 48, 5883–5893.

Morein, B., Sundquist, B., Hoglund, S., Dalsgaard, K., and Osterhaus, A. (1984). Iscom, a novel structure for antigenic presentation of membrane proteins from enveloped viruses. *Nature* 308, 457–460.

Moron, G., Dadaglio, G., and Leclerc, C. (2004). New tools for antigen delivery to the MHC class I pathway. *Trends Immunol.* 25, 92–97.

Murphey-Corb, M., Ohkawa, S., Martin, L. et al. (1993). Comparative efficacy of a whole killed SIV vaccine in combination with various adjuvants. Sixth Annual Meeting of the National Cooperative Vaccine Development Group for AIDS.

Murray, P.J., Aldovini, A., and Young, R.A. (1996). Manipulation and potentiation of antimycobacterial immunity using recombinant bacille Calmette-Guerin strains that secrete cytokines. *Proc. Natl. Acad. Sci. USA* 93, 934–939.

Murray, R., Cohen, P., and Hardegree, M.C. (1972). Mineral oil adjuvants: biological and chemical studies. *Ann. Allergy* 30, 146–151.

Mutsch, M., Zhou, W., Rhodes, P., Bopp, M., Chen, R.T., Linder, T., Spyr, C., and Steffen, R. (2004). Use of the inactivated intranasal influenza vaccine and the risk of Bell's palsy in Switzerland. *N. Engl. J. Med.* 350, 896–903.

Myers, K.R., Truchot, A.T., Ward, J. et al. (1996). A critical determinant of lipid A endotoxic activity. In Nowotny, A., Spitzer, J.J., and Ziegler, E.J. (Eds) *Cellular and Molecular Aspects of Endotoxin Reactions*. Elsevier, Amsterdam, pp. 145–156.

Nardin, E.H., Oliveira, G.A., Calvo-Calle, J.M., Castro, Z.R., Nussenzweig, R.S., Schmeckpeper, B., Hall, B.F., Diggs, C., Bodison, S., and Edelman, R. (2000). Synthetic malaria peptide vaccine elicits high levels of antibodies in vaccinees of defined HLA genotypes. *J. Infect. Dis.* 182, 1486–1496.

Newman, M.J., Wu, J.Y., Coughlin, R.T., Murphy, C.I., Seals, J.R., Wyand, M.S., and Kensil, C.R. (1992a). Immunogenicity and toxicity testing of an experimental HIV-1 vaccine in nonhuman primates. *AIDS Res. Hum. Retroviruses* 8, 1413–1418.

Newman, M.J., Wu, J.Y., Gardner, B.H., Munroe, K.J., Leombruno, D., Recchia, J., Kensil, C.R., and Coughlin, R.T. (1992b). Saponin adjuvant induction of ovalbumin-specific CD8+ cytotoxic T lymphocyte responses. *J. Immunol.* 148, 2357–2362.

Newman, M.J., Munroe, K.J., Anderson, C.A., Murphy, C.I., Panicali, D.L., Seals, J.R., Wu, J.Y., Wyand, M.S., and Kensil, C.R. (1994). Induction of antigen-specific killer T lymphocyte responses using subunit SIVmac251 gag and env vaccines containing QS-21 saponin adjuvant. *AIDS Res. Hum. Retroviruses* 10, 853–861.

Newman, M.J., Wu, J.Y., Gardner, B.H., Anderson, C.A., Kensil, C.R., Recchia, J., Coughlin, R.T., and Powell, M.F. (1997). Induction of cross-reactive cytotoxic T-lymphocyte responses specific for HIV-1 gp120 using saponin adjuvant (QS-21) supplemented subunit vaccine formulations. *Vaccine* 15, 1001–1007.

O'Hagan, D.T., Jeffery, H., and Davis, S.S. (1993). Long-term antibody responses in mice following subcutaneous immunization with ovalbumin entrapped in biodegradable microparticles. *Vaccine* 11, 965–969.

Ott, G., Barchfeld, G.L. et al. (1995). MF59: design and evaluation of a safe and potent adjuvant for human vaccines. In Powell, M.F. and Newman, M.J. (Eds) *Vaccine Design: The Subunit and Adjuvant Approach*. Plenum Press, New York, pp. 277–296.

Ozel, M., Hoglund, S., Gelderblom, H.R., and Morein, B. (1989). Quaternary structure of the immunostimulating complex (iscom). *J. Ultrastruct. Mol. Struct. Res.* 102, 240–248.

Page, W.F., Norman, J.E., and Benenson, A.S. (1993). Long-term follow-up of army recruits immunized with Freund's incomplete adjuvanted vaccine. *Vaccine Res.* 2, 141–149.

Patou, G., Scott, G.M., Kelsey, M.C., and Playfair, J.H.L. (1989). Gamma interferon as an adjuvant to hepatitis B vaccine. *J. Interferon Res.* 9, S261.

Pearson, C.M. (1963). Experimental joint disease: observations on adjuvant-induced arthritis. *J. Chronic Dis.* 16, 863–874.

Peppoloni, S., Ruggiero, P., Contorni, M., Morandi, M., Pizza, M., Rappuoli, R., Podda, A., and Del Giudice, G. (2003). Mutants of the Escherichia coli heat-labile enterotoxin as safe and strong adjuvants for intranasal delivery of vaccines. *Expert Rev. Vaccines.* 2, 285–293.

Pink, J.R. and Kieny, M.P. (2004). Fourth meeting on novel adjuvants currently in/close to human clinical testing. World Health Organization–Organization Mondiale de la Sante Fondation Merieux, Annecy, France, 23–25 June 2003. *Vaccine* 22, 2097–2102.

Powell, M.F., Cleland, J.L., Eastman, D.J., Lim, A., Murthy, K., Newman, M.J., Nunberg, J.H., Weissburg, R.P., Vennari, J.C., and Wrin, T. (1994). Immunogenicity and HIV-1 virus neutralization of MN recombinant glycoprotein 120/HIV-1 QS21 vaccine in baboons [published erratum appears in *AIDS Res. Hum. Retroviruses* (1995) 11, 661]. *AIDS Res. Hum. Retroviruses* 10 (Suppl. 2), S105–S108.

Qureshi, N., Takayama, K., and Ribi, E. (1982). Purification and structural determination of nontoxic lipid A obtained from the lipopolysaccharide of *Salmonella typhimurium*. *J. Biol. Chem.* 257, 11808–11815.

Ragde, H., Cavanagh, W.A., and Tjoa, B.A. (2004). Dendritic cell based vaccines: progress in immunotherapy studies for prostate cancer. *J. Urol.* 172, 2532–2538.

Ramon, G. (1926). Procedes pour accroitre la production des antitoxines. *Ann. Inst. Pasteur* 40, 1–10.

Ratliff, D.A. and Burns-Cox, C.J. (1984). Anaphylasix to tetanus toxoid. *Br. Med. J.* 288, 114.

Ribi, E., Amano, K., Cantrell, J., Schwartzman, S. et al. (1982). Preparation and antitumor activity of nontoxic lipid A. *Cancer Immunol. Immunother.* 12, 91–96.

Ribi, E., Cantrell, J., Takayama, K. et al. (1986). Modulation of humoral and cell-mediated immune responses by a structurally established nontoxic lipid A. In Szentivanyi, A. and Friedman, H. (Eds) *Immunobiology and Immunopharmacology of Bacterial Endotoxins*. Plenum Press, New York, pp. 407–420.

Rimmelzwaan, G.F. and Osterhaus, A.D.M.E. (1995). A novel generation of viral vaccines based on the ISCOM matrix. In Powell, M.F. and Newman, M.J. (Eds) *The Subunit and Adjuvant Approach*. Plenum Press, New York, pp. 543–558.

Rinn, K., Schiffman, K., Otero, H.O., and Disis, M.L. (1999). Antigen-specific recall urticaria to a peptide-based vaccine. *J. Allergy Clin. Immunol.* 104, 240–242.

Ronnberg, B., Fekadu, M., and Morein, B. (1995). Adjuvant activity of non-toxic Quillaja saponaria Molina components for use in ISCOM matrix. *Vaccine* 13, 1375–1382.

Ryan, E.J., McNeela, E., Murphy, G.A., Stewart, H., O'Hagan, D., Pizza, M., Rappuoli, R., and Mills, K.H. (1999). Mutants of Escherichia coli heat-labile toxin act as effective mucosal adjuvants for nasal delivery of an acellular pertussis vaccine: differential effects of the nontoxic AB complex and enzyme activity on Th1 and Th2 cells. *Infect. Immun.* 67, 6270–6280.

Ryan, E.T. and Calderwood, S.B. (2000). Cholera vaccines. *Clin. Infect. Dis.* 31, 561–565.

Salk, J. and Salk, D. (1977). Control of influenza and poliomyelitis with killed virus vaccines. *Science* 195, 834–847.

Sanchez-Pescador, L., Burke, R.L., Ott, G., and Van Nest, G. (1988). The effect of adjuvants on the efficacy of a recombinant herpes simplex virus glycoprotein vaccine. *J. Immunol.* 141, 1720–1727.

Saul, A., Lawrence, G., Smillie, A., Rzepczyk, C.M., Reed, C., Taylor, D., Anderson, K., Stowers, A., Kemp, R., Allworth, A., Anders, R.F., Brown, G.V., Pye, D., Schoofs, P., Irving, D.O., Dyer, S.L., Woodrow, G.C., Briggs, W.R., Reber, R., and Sturchler, D. (1999). Human phase I vaccine trials of 3 recombinant asexual stage malaria antigens with Montanide ISA720 adjuvant. *Vaccine* 17, 3145–3159.

Schirmbeck, R., Kuhrober, A., Janowicz, Z.A., and Reimann, J. (1994). Immunization with soluble hepatitis B virus surface protein elicits murine H-2 class I-restricted CD8+ cytotoxic T lymphocyte responses in vivo. *J. Immunol.* 152, 1110–1119.

Schneerson, R., Fattom, A., Szu, S.C., Bryla, D., Ulrich, J.T., Rudbach, J.A., Schiffman, G., and Robbins, J.B. (1991). Evaluation of monophosphoryl lipid A (MPL) as an adjuvant. Enhancement of the serum antibody response in mice to polysaccharide-protein conjugates by concurrent injection with MPL. *J. Immunol.* 147, 2136–2140.

Schultz, N., Oratz, R., Chen, D., Zeleniuch-Jacquotte, A., Abeles, G., and Bystryn, J.C. (1995). Effect of DETOX as an adjuvant for melanoma vaccine. *Vaccine* 13, 503–508.

Scott, P. (1993). IL-12: initiation cytokine for cell-mediated immunity [comment]. *Science* 260, 496–497.

Shirai, M., Pendleton, C.D., Ahlers, J., Takeshita, T., Newman, M., and Berzofsky, J.A. (1994). Helper-cytotoxic T lymphocyte (CTL) determinant linkage required for priming of anti-HIV CD8+ CTL in vivo with peptide vaccine constructs. *J. Immunol.* 152, 549–556.

Siber, G.R., Anderson, R., Habafy, M., and Gupta, R.K. (1995). Development of a guinea pig model to assess immunogenicity of Haemophilus influenzae type b capsular polysaccharide conjugate vaccines. *Vaccine* 13, 525–531.

Siegrist, C.A., Pihlgren, M., Tougne, C., Efler, S.M., Morris, M.L., AlAdhami, M.J., Cameron, D.W., Cooper, C.L., Heathcote, J., Davis, H.L., and Lambert, P.H. (2004a). Co-administration of CpG oligonucleotides enhances the late affinity maturation process of human anti-hepatitis B vaccine response. *Vaccine* 23, 615–622.

Slingluff, C.L., Jr., Yamshchikov, G., Neese, P., Galavotti, H., Eastham, S., Engelhard, V.H., Kittlesen, D., Deacon, D., Hibbitts, S., Grosh, W.W., Petroni, G., Cohen, R., Wiernasz, C., Patterson, J.W., Conway, B.P., and Ross, W.G. (2001). Phase I trial of a melanoma vaccine with gp100(280–288) peptide and tetanus helper peptide in adjuvant: immunologic and clinical outcomes. *Clin. Cancer Res.* 7, 3012–3024.

Sommer, F., Wilken, H., Faller, G., and Lohoff, M. (2004). Systemic Th1 immunization of mice against Helicobacter pylori infection with CpG oligodeoxynucleotides as adjuvants does not protect from infection but enhances gastritis. *Infect. Immun.* 72, 1029–1035.

Stanberry, L.R., Spruance, S.L., Cunningham, A.L., Bernstein, D.I., Mindel, A., Sacks, S., Tyring, S., Aoki, F.Y., Slaoui, M., Denis, M., Vandepapeliere, P., and Dubin, G. (2002). Glycoprotein-D-adjuvant vaccine to prevent genital herpes. *N. Engl. J. Med.* 347, 1652–1661.

Stevenson, M.M., Su, Z., Sam, H., and Mohan, K. (2001). Modulation of host responses to blood-stage malaria by interleukin-12: from therapy to adjuvant activity. *Microbes. Infect.* 3, 49–59.

Stewart-Tull, D.E.S. (1989). Recommendations for the assessment of adjuvants (immunopotentiators). In Gregoriadis, G., Allison, A.C., and Poste, G. (Eds) *Immunological Adjuvants and Vaccines.* Plenum Press, New York, pp. 213–226.

Stieneker, F., Kersten, G., van Bloois, L., Crommelin, D.J., Hem, S.L., Lower, J., and Kreuter, J. (1995). Comparison of 24 different adjuvants for inactivated HIV-2 split whole virus as antigen in mice. Induction of titres of binding antibodies and toxicity of the formulations. *Vaccine* 13, 45–53.

Storni, T., Ruedl, C., Schwarz, K., Schwendener, R.A., Renner, W.A., and Bachmann, M.F. (2004). Nonmethylated CG motifs packaged into virus-like particles induce protective cytotoxic T cell responses in the absence of systemic side effects. *J. Immunol.* 172, 1777–1785.

Stoute, J.A., Slaoui, M., Heppner, D.G., Momin, P., Kester, K.E., Desmons, P., Wellde, B.T., Garcon, N., Krzych, U., and Marchand, M. (1997). A preliminary evaluation of a recombinant circumsporozoite protein vaccine against Plasmodium falciparum malaria. RTS,S Malaria Vaccine Evaluation Group [see comments]. *N. Engl. J. Med.* 336, 86–91.

Stuart-Harris, C.H. (1969). Adjuvant influenza vaccines. *Bull. WHO* 41, 617–621.

Sturchler, D., Berger, R., Etlinger, H., Fernex, M., Matile, H., Pink, R., Schlumbom, V., and Just, M. (1989). Effects of interferons on immune response to a synthetic peptide malaria sporozoite vaccine in non-immune adults. *Vaccine* 7, 457–461.

Sundquist, B., Lovgren, K., and Morein, B. (1988). Influenza virus ISCOMs: antibody response in animals. *Vaccine* 6, 49–53.

Takeshita, F., Leifer, C.A., Gursel, I., Ishii, K.J., Takeshita, S., Gursel, M., and Klinman, D.M. (2001). Cutting edge: role of Toll-like receptor 9 in CpG DNA-induced activation of human cells. *J. Immunol.* 167, 3555–3558.

Tao, M.H. and Levy, R. (1993). Idiotype/granulocyte-macrophage colony-stimulating factor fusion protein as a vaccine for B-cell lymphoma [see comments]. *Nature* 362, 755–758.

Telzak, E., Wolff, S.M., Dinarello, C.A., Conlon, T., el Kholy, A., Bahr, G.M., Choay, J.P., Morin, A., and Chedid, L. (1986). Clinical evaluation of the immunoadjuvant murabutide, a derivative of MDP, administered with a tetanus toxoid vaccine. *J. Infect. Dis.* 153, 628–633.

Thapar, M.A., Parr, E.L., Bozzola, J.J., and Parr, M.B. (1991). Secretory immune responses in the mouse vagina after parenteral or intravaginal immunization with an immunostimulating complex (ISCOM). *Vaccine* 9, 129–133.

Tiberio, L., Fletcher, L., Eldridge, J.H., and Duncan, D.D. (2004). Host factors impacting the innate response in humans to the candidate adjuvants RC529 and monophosphoryl lipid A. *Vaccine* 22, 1515–1523.

Toledo, H., Baly, A., Castro, O., Resik, S., Laferte, J., Rolo, F., Navea, L., Lobaina, L., Cruz, O., Miguez, J., Serrano, T., Sierra, B., Perez, L., Ricardo, M. E., Dubed, M., Lubian, A. L., Blanco, M., Millan, J.C., Ortega, A., Iglesias, E., Penton, E., Martin, Z., Perez, J., Diaz, M., and Duarte, C.A. (2001). A phase I clinical trial of a multi-epitope polypeptide TAB9 combined with Montanide ISA 720 adjuvant in non-HIV-1 infected human volunteers. *Vaccine* 19, 4328–4336.

Ulrich, J.T. and Myers, K.R. (1995). Monophosphoryl lipid A as an adjuvant: past experiences and new directions. In Powell, M.F. and Newman, M.J. (Eds) *The Subunit and Adjuvant Approach.* Plenum Press, New York, pp. 495–524.

Valensi, J.P., Carlson, J.R., and Van Nest, G.A. (1994). Systemic cytokine profiles in BALB/c mice immunized with trivalent influenza vaccine containing MF59 oil emulsion and other advanced adjuvants. *J. Immunol.* 153, 4029–4039.

Van Dam, G.J., Verheul, A.F., Zigterman, G.J., De Reuver, M.J., and Snippe, H. (1989). Nonionic block polymer surfactants enhance the avidity of antibodies in polyclonal antisera against Streptococcus pneumoniae type 3 in normal and Xid mice. *J. Immunol.* 143, 3049–3053.

Van Driel, W.J., Ressing, M.E., Kenter, G.G., Brandt, R.M., Krul, E.J., van Rossum, A.B., Schuuring, E., Offringa, R., Bauknecht, T., Tamm-Hermelink, A., van Dam, P.A., Fleuren, G.J., Kast, W.M., Melief, C.J., and Trimbos, J.B. (1999). Vaccination with HPV16 peptides of patients with advanced cervical carcinoma: clinical evaluation of a phase I–II trial. *Eur. J. Cancer* 35, 946–952.

Van Loon, F.P., Clemens, J.D., Chakraborty, J., Rao, M.R., Kay, B.A., Sack, D.A., Yunus, M., Ali, M., Svennerholm, A.M., and Holmgren, J. (1996). Field trial of inactivated oral cholera vaccines in Bangladesh: results from 5 years of follow-up. *Vaccine* 14, 162–166.

Verdier, F. (2002). Non-clinical vaccine safety assessment. *Toxicology* 174, no37–43.

Vernacchio, L., Bernstein, H., Pelton, S., Allen, C., MacDonald, K., Dunn, J., Duncan, D.D., Tsao, G., LaPosta, V., Eldridge, J., Laussucq, S., Ambrosino, D.M., and Molrine, D.C. (2002). Effect of monophosphoryl lipid A (MPL) on T-helper cells when administered as an adjuvant with pneumocococcal-CRM197 conjugate vaccine in healthy toddlers. *Vaccine* 20, 3658–3667.

Verthelyi, D., Kenney, R.T., Seder, R.A., Gam, A.A., Friedag, B., and Klinman, D.M. (2002). CpG oligodeoxynucleotides as vaccine adjuvants in primates. *J. Immunol.* 168, 1659–1663.

Villacres, M.C., Behboudi, S., Nikkila, T., Lovgren-Bengtsson, K., and Morein, B. (1998). Internalization of iscom-borne antigens and presentation under MHC class I or class II restriction. *Cell Immunol.* 185, 30–38.

Villaret, D., Glisson, B., Kenady, D., Hanna, E., Carey, M., Gleich, L., Yoo, G.H., Futran, N., Hung, M.C., Anklesaria, P., and Heald, A.E. (2002). A multicenter phase II study of tgDCC-E1A for the intratumoral treatment of patients with recurrent head and neck squamous cell carcinoma. *Head Neck* 24, 661–669.

Wheeler, A.W. and Woroniecki, S.R. (2004). Allergy vaccines: new approaches to an old concept. *Expert Opin. Biol. Ther.* 4, 1473–1481.

Woolridge, R.L., Grayston, J.T., Chang, I.A. et al. (1967). Long-term follow-up of the initial (1959–1960) trachoma vaccine field on Taiwan. *Am. J. Ophthalmol.* 63, 1650–1653.

World Health Organization (1977). *Manual for the Production and Control of Vaccines: Tetanus Toxoid.* World Health Organization.

Wu, J.Y., Gardner, B.H., Murphy, C.I., Seals, J.R., Kensil, C.R., Recchia, J., Beltz, G.A., Newman, G.W., and Newman, M.J. (1992). Saponin adjuvant enhancement of antigen-specific immune responses to an experimental HIV-1 vaccine. *J. Immunol.* 148, 1519–1525.

Zhou, F. and Huang, L. (1993). Monophosphoryl lipid A enhances specific CTL induction by a soluble protein antigen entrapped in liposomes. *Vaccine* 11, 1139–1144.

Zigterman, G.J., Schotanus, K., Ernste, E.B., Van Dam, G.J., Jansze, M., Snippe, H., and Willers, J.M. (1989). Nonionic block polymer surfactants modulate the humoral immune response against Streptococcus pneumoniae-derived hexasaccharide- protein conjugates. *Infect. Immun.* 57, 2712–2718.

Regulatory considerations in the nonclinical safety assessment of adjuvanted preventive vaccines

Elizabeth M. Sutkowski and Marion F. Gruber
US Food and Drug Administration, Rockville, Maryland

Introduction

The regulatory considerations for vaccines are, for the most part, also applicable to vaccines formulated with adjuvant(s). However, for the latter products, additional issues may be considered that are unique to novel adjuvants. Preventive and therapeutic vaccines for infectious disease indications are regulated by the Office of Vaccines Research and Review in the Center for Biologics Evaluation and Research (CBER) within the US Food and Drug Administration (FDA). This is in contrast to vaccines for other indications such as cancer vaccines, which have different risk–benefit considerations and are regulated by a different office within CBER, the Office of Cell, Tissue, and Gene Therapies (OCTGT). Topics covered in this chapter include a brief overview of the Investigational New Drug Application (IND) regulations as they apply to preventive vaccines, an overview of the information to be included in the IND submission, and a discussion of the utility of the pre-IND meeting.

Furthermore, this chapter includes recommendations regarding the nonclinical safety program for preventive adjuvanted vaccines, with emphasis on approaches to the design of preclinical toxicity studies to support initiation of phase I clinical trials.

Safety assessment of preventive vaccines is a continuous process that begins with the development of a vaccine candidate at the pre-IND stage and continues through the various stages of clinical development to postlicensure surveillance. Such assessment includes characterization of the product by physical, chemical and biological testing, adequate control of the manufacturing process, and the development and establishment of adequate lot release tests to assure the safety, purity, and potency of the product. In the past, nonclinical safety assessments of preventive vaccines had not routinely included good laboratory practices (GLP)-compliant toxicity studies in animal models. Vaccines have been enormously successful in eradication of preventable infectious diseases and the continued successful implementation of vaccination programs requires the assurance of vaccine safety. Additionally, a broad range of novel vaccines are currently in development and the composition of these products has evolved from attenuated or inactivated whole cell organisms to protein–polysaccharide conjugates, peptides, recombinant proteins, plasmid DNA vaccines, and gene transfer products. These vaccines are frequently combined with novel adjuvants, administered using new delivery systems, and may be administered by new routes of administration. As biotechnology has advanced to produce antigens that are expressed using recombinant DNA technology and/or are more highly purified (but may be less immunogenic), and our knowledge of the mechanism of adjuvant action has developed, it follows that the number of novel adjuvants being evaluated in clinical studies has increased (Kenney et al., 2002; Engers et al., 2003; Kenney and Edelman, 2003).

Adjuvants work in many ways and at many stages in the dendritic cell migration and maturation process (Degen et al., 2003; Hunter, 2002; Lien and Golenbock, 2003; Lima et al., 2004; and as described in Chapter 1). Adjuvants are often divided into two main types: those that enhance the delivery of antigens and those that act directly on the immune system to augment the immune response (Petrovsky and Aguilar, 2004; Vogel and Hem, 2004). Multiple reports from preclinical and clinical studies of various types of adjuvants have been published (Alving, 2002; Baylor et al., 2002; Kenney and Edelman, 2003; Vogel and Hem, 2004; Vogel and Powell, 1995; Vogel et al., http://www.niaid.nih.gov/daids/vaccine/pdf/compendium.pdf), including mineral salts/gel-type adjuvants, e.g., aluminum hydroxide and aluminum or calcium phosphate gels; microbial (natural and synthetic) adjuvants, e.g., 3-O-deacylated monophosphoryl lipid A (MPL), CpG motifs, and mutants of *E. coli* heat-labile enterotoxin (LT) and cholera toxin (CT); oil emulsions and surfactant-based adjuvants, e.g., MF59, Montanide ISA 51; particulate adjuvants, e.g.,

virosomes, immunostimulating complexes (ISCOMS), poly(lactide-co-glycolides) (PLG); endogenous human immunomodulators, e.g., cytokines; and combinations thereof. The development of new adjuvants presents challenges to manufacturers as well as regulatory authorities, as criteria to evaluate their safety profile may not exist and toxicity study designs established for conventional small drug molecules may not be sufficiently relevant.

In addition, in contrast to other biological products that are predominantly developed to treat ill patients, preventive vaccines are primarily indicated and administered to large numbers of healthy individuals, predominantly healthy infants and children, and this places significant emphasis on their safety (Verdier, 2002). Also, the incidence of the infectious disease that a vaccine candidate is intended to prevent may be quite low in a particular population. Therefore, depending on the situation, a high percentage of vaccinated subjects may never benefit from the vaccine. Thus, the benefit of the vaccine in preventing the infectious disease may be difficult to appreciate on an individual level. These types of considerations have led to a low tolerance for adverse events from vaccines in general. Given these findings, in the context of novel vaccine development, there is an increased focus on vaccine safety assessment in animal models prior to the initiation of clinical trials. However, toxicity assessment of vaccines is an evolving field and it should be recognized that approaches to toxicity assessments may change as the field evolves.

■ Definitions

Preclinical assessment: Product characterization and animal safety testing conducted prior to human use of the product (a subset of nonclinical assessment).

Nonclinical assessment: Preclinical assessment plus continued testing conducted throughout product/clinical development. Examples include (i) testing deemed necessary when significant changes have been made to the manufacture or formulation of a product in development and (ii) additional testing required for evaluation of potential safety concerns identified in phase I or II clinical trials.

Vaccine: As defined in CBER's guidance document entitled, "Content and Format of Chemistry, Manufacturing and Controls Information and Establishment Description Information for a Vaccine or Related Product," a vaccine is an immunogen, the administration of which is intended to stimulate the immune system to result in the prevention, amelioration, or therapy of any disease or infection. A vaccine may be a live attenuated preparation of bacteria, viruses, or parasites; inactivated (killed) whole organisms; living irradiated cells; crude fractions or purified immunogens, including those derived from recombinant DNA in a host cell; conjugates formed by covalent linkage of components; synthetic antigens; polynucleotides (such as plasmid DNA vaccines); living vectored cells expressing specific heterologous immunogens; or cells pulsed with immunogen. It may also be a combination of vaccines listed above. Therapeutic vaccines (e.g., viral vector-based gene therapy, tumor vaccines, and certain antiidiotypic vaccines) and therapeutic vaccine-related products are not considered here.

Phase I clinical trial: Initial study of the product's safety in humans.

New products: New products may include products that have undergone significant changes in the production process (e.g., a previous version was already tested in humans), previously licensed products administered by a novel route of administration and/or for a new indication, and previously licensed products formulated with novel adjuvants or excipients.

Novel products: Novel products include antigens and adjuvants that belong to a new product class for which there is little or no prior clinical experience.

Route of administration: The means by which the candidate vaccine product is introduced to the host. Routes of administration may include the intravenous, intramuscular, subcutaneous, transcutaneous, intradermal, oral, intranasal, intranodal, intravaginal, and intrarectal routes.

Adjuvant: An agent that is added to a vaccine antigen to augment (and possibly target) the specific immune response to the antigen.

Constituent materials: As listed in Title 21 of the Code of Federal Regulations, Part 610.15 (21 CFR 610.15) includes (a) ingredients, preservatives, diluents, and adjuvants, (b) extraneous protein; cell culture produced vaccines, and (c) antibiotics.

Preclinical toxicity study: A study designed with the primary purpose of demonstrating the safety and tolerability of a candidate vaccine product. The preclinical toxicity study design should meet the general criteria outlined in a later section (Toxicity studies for preventive vaccines) to be considered supportive for the intended phase I clinical trial. Preclinical toxicity studies should be designed to mimic the way in which the vaccine is to be administered in the clinic and either evaluate responses in animals after a single dose administration or after episodic, repeat dose administrations.

GLP: Good laboratory practices as defined in 21 CFR 58 consist of regulations that govern the procedures, practices, and conditions under which nonclinical laboratory studies (*in vitro* and *in vivo* experiments) are conducted to determine the safety of a test article.

GMP: Good manufacturing practices as defined in 21 CFR 210 and 211 consist of regulations that govern the procedures and practices under which manufacturing is controlled and the quality of manufacturing is assured.

■ Current status of relevant, global regulatory guidance and initiatives

In recent years, several initiatives have been put in place to develop guidelines for the evaluation of adjuvants and adjuvanted vaccines. In 1993 a summary article from a workshop convened at the Fifth Annual Meeting of the National Cooperative Vaccine Development Groups for AIDS entitled "Safety Evaluation of Vaccine Adjuvants" was published by Dr. Karen Goldenthal of CBER and others (Goldenthal et al., 1993), which summarized approaches to the preclinical evaluation of adjuvants combined with preventive vaccines. Afterward, the World Health Organization (WHO) began sponsoring regular meetings on novel adjuvants currently in or close to clinical testing (Kenney et al., 2002; Engers et al., 2003). Also, the Committee for Proprietary Medicinal Products (CPMP) of the European Medicines Evaluation Agency (EMEA) published regulatory guidances that are also applicable, at least in part, to the evaluation of new adjuvants, such as the CPMP document entitled "Note for Guidance on Preclinical, Pharmacological, and Toxicological Testing of Vaccines," published in 1997.

The FDA's CBER and Office of Women's Health, together with the Society of Toxicology (Contemporary Concepts in Toxicology Section) co-sponsored a workshop in December 2002 entitled "Nonclinical Safety Evaluation of Preventive Vaccines: Recent Advances and Regulatory Considerations." The objectives of this workshop were to reach a consensus on the most appropriate currently available approaches that can be applied to toxicity assessments of preventive vaccines and to discuss the type of information that can be derived from such studies to assure that it will be relevant and useful for assessment of human risk. In addition, the meeting offered a venue to discuss issues concerning specific methodologies that can be used to screen for potential adverse effects of new investigational vaccines and vaccine adjuvants, and it also addressed the subject of reproductive/developmental toxicity studies for these products. Discussions focused on relevant animal models, toxicity study design for vaccines and vaccine adjuvants, parameters to be evaluated, and alternative methods for nonclinical safety

assessment of vaccines. For a transcript of the meeting, the reader is referred to CBER's website on meetings and workshops accessible at http://www.fda.gov/cber/minutes/workshop-min.htm and/or the Society of Toxicology's website at http://www.toxicology.org/ai/meet/cct-vaccines.asp, where the speakers' slides are also available.

With respect to preventive vaccines, the WHO has issued a guideline entitled "WHO Guidelines on Nonclinical Evaluation of Vaccines," which was accepted by the 54th meeting of the WHO Expert Committee on Biological Standardization held on November 17–21, 2003. In addition to discussing general toxicity assessments, the WHO guideline addresses special considerations, such as adjuvanted vaccines and vaccines given by novel routes of administration. This document was generated with significant contributions by CBER and the EU regulatory authorities as well as other experts in the field of vaccine safety. The WHO Guidelines on Nonclinical Evaluation of Vaccines is available at http://www.who.int/biologicals/publications/nonclinical_evaluation_vaccines_nov_2003.pdf. Representatives of CBER have also contributed along with others to a very useful article entitled "Vaccine Preclinical Toxicology Testing," which is available on the website of the National Institute of Allergy and Infectious Diseases (NIAID) (Chang et al., http://www.niaid.nih.gov/daids/vaccine/Science/VRTT/00_Main.htm). This website also addresses immunologic adjuvants and has a link to "A Compendium of Vaccine Adjuvants and Excipients" (Vogel et al., http://www.niaid.nih.gov/daids/vaccine/pdf/compendium.pdf).

In June 2004 the Global Advisory Committee on Vaccine Safety (GACVS), an expert clinical and scientific advisory body to WHO, met in Geneva to consider the safety of adjuvants. The committee received an update on preclinical and clinical studies of various adjuvants by industry representatives and heard presentations regarding regulatory guidelines and draft guidelines on vaccines and vaccine adjuvants (presented by representatives of industry as well as the CPMP of the EMEA, the US FDA, and the WHO). The committee recommended a new clinical, scientific, and regulatory approach to this complex area, with attention to the short- and long-term safety of adjuvants. A summary of this meeting appeared in the July 2004 issue of the *Weekly Epidemiological Record*. Lastly, in January 2005 the CPMP published a guidance entitled "Guideline on Adjuvants in Vaccines for Human Use," which addresses quality, nonclinical, and clinical issues arising from the use of new or established adjuvants in vaccines (http://www.emea.eu.int/pdfs/human/vwp/13471604en.pdf; see also Sesardic and Dobbelaer, 2004).

It is hoped that the regulatory guidelines and documents mentioned above will promote consistent and harmonized approaches to nonclinical safety testing of vaccines and vaccine adjuvants. The approaches to nonclinical safety evaluation of vaccines and adjuvanted vaccines discussed in this chapter are a result of numerous working group efforts, such as the internal CBER Preclinical Safety of Preventive Vaccines Working Group, the FDA/Society of Toxicology Workshop of 2002, the drafting group of the WHO Guidelines on Nonclinical Evaluation of Vaccines, the WHO-sponsored meetings on novel adjuvants currently in or close to clinical testing, and discussions on the safety of adjuvants which took place at the meeting convened by the WHO GACVS in 2004.

■ Relevant US (FDA) regulatory requirements and considerations

Assuring the safety of biological products is at the forefront of CBER's mission. Safety is defined in 21 CFR 600.3 as "the relative freedom from harmful effect to persons affected, directly or indirectly, by a product when prudently administered, taking into consideration the character of the product in relation to the condition of the recipient at the time." The key components of safety assessment of a biologic product include control of the manufacture process, nonclinical safety evaluation, prelicensure clinical evaluation, postlicensure surveillance, and postlicensure studies. The extent of control of the manufacture process depends on the phase of the investigation and develops from having control over the raw materials to developing in-process controls for intermediates and validated process procedures, and finally to developing lot release specifications (to ensure consistency in manufacture) and demonstrating stability.

In addition, nonclinical safety assessments may include (i) immunogenicity studies (with and without adjuvant), which may be a measure of potency; (ii) pyrogenicity studies (as part of the evaluation of vaccine purity); (iii) demonstration of adequate attenuation for live organisms; (iv) demonstration of adequate inactivation (and control for reversion to toxicity, where applicable) for inactivated organisms or toxoids; (v) adventitious agent testing; (vi) biodistribution and persistence/integration studies for nucleic acid vaccines and nonreplicating recombinant viral vectors; (vii) lack of replication-competent viruses (RCV) in preparations of nonreplicating viral vectors; and (viii) neurovirulence testing. For guidance in these areas, reference is made to applicable guidance documents including CBER's guidance document entitled "Content and Format of Chemistry, Manufacturing and Controls Information and Establishment Description Information for a Vaccine or Related Product"; the International Conference on Harmonization (ICH) guidance entitled "Quality of Biotechnological/Biological Products: Derivation and Characterization of Cell Substrates Used for Production of Biotechnological/Biological Products, Q5D, 7/16/1997"; the ICH guidance on "Viral Safety Evaluation of Biotechnology Products Derived From Cell Lines of Human or Animal Origin, Q5A 3/5/1997"; CBER's guidance document entitled "Points to Consider in the Characterization of Cell Lines Used to Produce

Biologicals (1993), May 17, 1993"; CBER's guidance for industry document entitled "Considerations for Plasmid DNA Vaccines for Infectious Disease Indications, February, 2005"; CBER's guidance document entitled "Points to Consider in the Production and Testing of New Drugs and Biologicals Produced by Recombinant DNA Technology, Draft April 10, 1985"; CBER's guidance document entitled "Supplement to the Points to Consider in the Production and Testing of New Drugs and Biologicals Produced by Recombinant DNA Technology: Nucleic Acid Characterization and Genetic Stability, April 6, 1992"; and CBER's guidance for industry document entitled "Evaluation of Combination Vaccines for Preventable Diseases: Production, Testing and Clinical Studies, 1997" (http://www.fda.gov/cber/gdlns/combvacc.txt).

This chapter discusses general approaches to preclinical toxicity study design(s) including considerations for nonclinical safety assessments of adjuvants. However, the discussion of specific toxicity protocol designs (e.g., carcinogenicity, tumorigenicity, and developmental toxicity studies) and considerations for specific product categories (e.g., DNA vaccines, live, attenuated vaccines, etc.) is beyond the scope of this chapter. For additional guidance, reference is made to applicable guidance documents including the ICH document entitled "Preclinical Safety Evaluation of Biotechnology-Derived Pharmaceuticals, S6, 1997"; the ICH document entitled "Non-Clinical Safety Studies for the Conduct of Human Clinical Trials for Pharmaceuticals", M3, published in 1997, M3(M), amended on November 9, 2000; the ICH document entitled "Safety Pharmacology Studies for Human Pharmaceuticals", S7A, 2001; CBER's "Guidance for Industry: Nonclinical Studies for Development of Pharmaceutical Excipients, 2002"; the WHO Guidelines on Nonclinical Evaluation of Vaccines; the CPMP 2005 Guideline on Adjuvants in Vaccines for Human Use; and CBER's guidance for industry document entitled "Considerations for

Reproductive Toxicity Studies for Preventive Vaccines for Infectious Disease Indications," August 2000.

■ Investigational new drug applications (INDs)
   (21 CFR 312)

Under current regulations, any use in the USA of a drug product not previously authorized for marketing in the USA first requires submission of an IND to the FDA. The IND regulations, found in 21 CFR 312, describe the circumstances for which an IND is required; these regulations apply to both drugs and biologics, including vaccines. Information on the submission of INDs can be found in the guidance for industry document entitled "Content and Format of Investigational New Drug Applications (INDs) for Phase 1 Studies of Drugs, Including Well-characterized, Therapeutic, Biotechnology-derived Products, 1995."

When a new IND application is submitted to the FDA, an acknowledgement letter providing the IND number and listing the date of receipt of the original submission is issued to the sponsor within several weeks of receipt. A statutory review period of 30 days begins from the date of receipt of the IND; the clinical study may not proceed before the end of this period unless the sponsor is notified (21 CFR 312.40(b)). When the review is completed, the sponsor is informed whether the study proposed under the IND may proceed or has been placed on clinical hold. If the sponsor has not been contacted by the end of the 30-day review period, the study may proceed. The regulations relating to the grounds for imposition of clinical hold (e.g., the IND does not contain sufficient information to assess the risks to subjects of the proposed studies, etc.) are located in 21 CFR 312.42(b). Phase I clinical studies are usually conducted in a small number of subjects to evaluate the initial safety of the product, and these studies are placed on clinical hold if there is concern regarding the safety of the subjects. If a study is placed on clinical hold, the sponsor can expect to receive a letter within 30 days of being notified of the hold by telephone; this letter will define the reasons for the clinical hold. The study will remain on clinical hold until complete responses to these issues are submitted for CBER review, FDA determines the responses to be satisfactory, and FDA notifies the sponsor, either by telephone or in writing, that the study may proceed.

Regulations covering investigational products to be used under an IND are located in Part 312 of the CFR and regulations relating to the manufacture and standards for lot release of licensed biological products are found in Part 610 of the CFR. Part 610 describes tests for potency, general safety, sterility, purity, and identity of the product. Part 610.15 covers constituent materials, which includes (a) ingredients, preservatives, diluents, and adjuvants, (b) extraneous protein; cell culture produced vaccines, and (c) antibiotics. Part 610.15(a) states, "All ingredients...shall meet generally accepted standards of purity and quality." In addition, Part 610.15(a) states, "An adjuvant shall not be introduced into a product unless there is satisfactory evidence that it does not affect adversely the safety or potency of the product." This implies that adequate nonclinical safety information regarding the adjuvant (chemistry, manufacturing, and control information, and pharmacologic and toxicologic information) needs to be provided to the IND (or to a cross-referenced master file as discussed below). Part 610.15(a) also lists limits for the amount of aluminum allowed in a recommended individual dose of a biologic product. Aluminum-derived adjuvants are the only types of adjuvants included in US licensed vaccines to date (Baylor et al., 2002; Finn and Egan, 2004); however, there is no prohibition against other types of adjuvants. It is stressed that adjuvants alone are not licensed; each specific antigen/adjuvant combination is licensed.

The various sections of the IND application as prescribed in the IND regulations (21 CFR 312.23(a)) are discussed in detail elsewhere (Chandler et al., 1999). The CFR (21 CFR 312.23(a)(7)) states that an IND should include chemistry, manufacturing, and control (CMC) information as appropriate for the particular investigations covered by the IND. In each phase of the investigation, however, sufficient information is required to ensure the proper identification, quality, purity, and strength of the biologic. In addition, the CFR (21 CFR 312.23(a)(8)) states that an IND should include data from pharmacologic and toxicologic studies (in laboratory animals or *in vitro*) that allow the sponsor to conclude that it is reasonably safe to conduct the proposed clinical investigations. Also, the type, duration, and scope of animal and other tests required varies with the duration and nature of the proposed clinical investigations.

For an adjuvanted preventive vaccine, sufficient CMC information regarding the antigen(s), adjuvant(s), and combined antigen/adjuvant formulation intended for clinical use should be provided in the original submission to an IND (or in a referenced master file, see below). This would include information on raw materials, purification/inactivation procedures, characterization data, stability data, and lot release testing to include sterility or bioburden testing. For example, data might be provided on antigen load, degree of adsorption or association of the vaccine antigen to the adjuvant, particle size and size distribution of the adjuvant and the final adjuvanted vaccine formulation, and stability of adsorption or emulsion, etc.

In addition, "proof of concept" information regarding the antigen(s), adjuvant(s), and combined antigen/adjuvant formulation intended for clinical use should be provided in the IND. This would include the rationale for the choice of particular adjuvant(s) (e.g., to enhance delivery, to enhance or target a particular type of immune response, or a combination of these) as well as the choice of antigen(s). Also, data supporting the clinically proposed ratio of adjuvant to antigen (from pilot optimization studies) should be included. This may include data from exploratory (non-GLP) "proof of concept"/safety studies.

The pharmacologic and toxicologic information submitted to the IND should be adequate to identify/characterize potential toxic effects. Documentation should include, but not be limited to, data demonstrating the safety of the clinically intended dose (i.e., the full human dose, which has not been adjusted based on weight), frequency of administration, and route of administration. The general approach to designing toxicity studies for adjuvanted preventive vaccines and novel adjuvants is described in detail later in this chapter.

■ Pre-IND meetings

A sponsor should consult with CBER for guidance early and throughout product development. Communication with FDA representatives before submission of an IND may be especially important if a manufacturer or sponsor has not previously interacted with FDA/CBER and has no experience with IND submissions or if a new product, technology, or assay is under development. If an IND is being prepared for a new vaccine, the initial contact should be with the branch chiefs in the Division of Vaccines and Related Products Applications (DVRPA) in the Office of Vaccines Research and Review, CBER. The branch chief can provide specific guidance and recommendations. Even if a sponsor believes that a pre-IND meeting is not necessary, it is recommended to consult with the branch chief to see if CBER agrees. An IND packet is available, which contains copies of selected sections of the regulations pertaining to vaccine INDs, Form 1571, Form 1572 for the clinical investigator, and relevant articles and reprints, including a copy of the guidance for industry document entitled "Content and Format of Investigational New Drug Applications (INDs) for Phase 1 Studies of Drugs, Including Well-Characterized, Therapeutic, Biotechnology-derived Products." The IND packet can be requested from the Division of Vaccines and Related Products Applications, OVRR, CBER at 301-827-3070.

When the branch chief is contacted, the sponsor may be advised to submit a request for a formal pre-IND meeting. The purpose of this meeting is to discuss manufacturing, product characterization, lot release testing, animal safety and immunogenicity, and the proposed phase I clinical protocol. CBER should be consulted to determine whether toxicity studies are necessary for a particular vaccine. A guidance for industry document on formal meetings with sponsors and applicants for PDUFA products describes procedures for requesting, scheduling, conducting, and documenting such formal meetings. The meeting request should include information such as a list of the specific objectives/outcomes expected from the meeting, a preliminary proposed agenda, and a draft list of specific questions, grouped by discipline. At the time the meeting is scheduled by CBER, the sponsor is notified of the date by which CBER will need to receive the background package. For a pre-IND (Type B) meeting, the sponsor should submit a background package to FDA so that it is received at least 4 weeks prior to the formal meeting.

The background package should include chemistry, manufacturing, and control information such as a description of the manufacturing facility, if available, a description of the product, a summary of the manufacturing process (e.g., a flow chart), a description of in-process testing, biochemical characterization, and, if available, tentative lot-release specifications for the product. Also, the package should include a summary of preclinical safety studies that have been conducted to support a clinical study (e.g., immunogenicity studies, neutralization assays, investigations in animal protection models, and any toxicity studies) as well as a clinical data summary (e.g., previous human data for the vaccine or a related vaccine, if available, a proposed phase I clinical protocol, and the clinical development plan). Sponsors may include proposed toxicity protocols in the pre-IND background package for CBER to comment on/concur with the study design prior to study initiation. In this regard, if necessary, it may be possible to obtain informal advice prior to the pre-IND meeting regarding the need for a toxicity study and/or toxicity study design.

■ Master files

A master file (MF) is a submission of information to the FDA that may be used to provide confidential information about the methods used in the manufacturing, processing, packaging, and storing of biological products. Biologic MFs are generally used by MF holders to allow sponsors of an IND to cross-reference the material in the MF in support of an IND without disclosure of the contents of the MF to the IND sponsor. FDA reviews information in a MF only when a sponsor or applicant incorporates material in the MF by reference. The MF holder must authorize the FDA to incorporate the material by reference for a specific IND in writing. Copies of the written authorization should be sent to the IND and the MF. MFs should be submitted in duplicate and should contain a complete list of IND sponsors currently authorized to incorporate by reference any information in the MF. Original submissions to Biologic MFs and updates should be sent to CBER rather than to CDER, and MF holders should update their MFs annually as discussed in the "Guideline for Drug Master Files."

When information about the adjuvant is not submitted as part of the IND, it needs to be submitted as a MF, and more often adjuvant manufacturers submit a Type II MF (for drug substance, drug substance intermediate, and material used in their preparation, or drug product), rather than a Type IV MF (for excipient, colorant, flavor, essence, or material used in their preparation). Since adjuvants are not licensed on their own, if an adjuvant is to be used as part of a vaccine for which licensure is being sought, full details on adjuvant manufacture, characterization, toxicology and preclinical characterization, and quality control should be provided, preferably as part of the vaccine BLA, alternatively as part of a detailed MF held by the adjuvant manufacturer. Inspection of the adjuvant manufacturing facility may be performed as part of the license review process.

■ Toxicity studies for preventive vaccines

■ Objectives

The objective of a toxicity study prior to initiation of clinical trials should be to screen adequately for toxic effects. Furthermore, the study should characterize the identified toxic effects of the vaccine in order to conclude that it is reasonably safe to conduct the proposed clinical investigation. Potential toxic effects of the product should be evaluated with regard to target organs, dose, route(s) of exposure, duration and frequency of exposure, and potential reversibility of observed toxic effects. In general, for preventive vaccines, healthy individuals are enrolled in phase I clinical trials and the animal model chosen for the toxicity assessments are healthy animals. Thus, rare toxicities, or potential effects in subpopulations, might only be addressed in humans. Therefore, it is important to recognize the limitations of an animal model with regard to its ability to predict safety and effectiveness in humans.

Despite these limitations, safety assessments in animal models are valuable tools to determine a safe dose, schedule, and route of administration, and to identify potential or unknown toxicities. When designing a toxicity study, it is important to evaluate very broad measures because most toxicities are not predictable. In certain instances, i.e., due to the specific nature of the product, there may be specific theoretical concerns regarding product safety. In these cases, specific assays may be included for addressing those key theoretical concerns.

The determination of whether a preclinical toxicity study is needed for a particular investigational vaccine will depend on numerous parameters, including, but not limited to, the intended target population, the proposed clinical route of administration, available preclinical and clinical data from the use of related products, availability of animal models, available information on the mechanism of action of the product, features of the product, such as novelty, homology with a human protein, and risk/benefit considerations. Examples follow for situations when preclinical toxicity studies may be needed or not needed. However, because preventive vaccines present a diverse class of biological products and because new approaches develop over time, this list is not meant to be all-inclusive.

If the product is formulated with a novel adjuvant, and insufficient clinical or preclinical data are available to support the safety of the novel adjuvant, preclinical toxicity studies will need to be conducted with adjuvanted product prior to initiating phase I clinical trials. Similarly, if the vaccine antigen(s) belongs to a novel product class for which there is inadequate prior clinical experience, preclinical toxicity studies likely will be needed. If the vaccine is administered via a novel route of administration (e.g., intranasal route or inhaled route), preclinical toxicity studies are needed, regardless of whether the product is investigational or licensed, to support the safety of the product being administered via the novel route. Simultaneous administration of two or more vaccines may raise concerns about adverse safety outcomes, e.g., adverse effects/interactions of preservatives or adjuvants with vaccine antigens. The need for toxicity studies in these situations would be decided on a case-by-case basis.

For some products, e.g., certain live viral vaccines, animal toxicity studies may not be feasible due to the lack of an animal model. In these cases, specific vaccine potency and attenuation testing *in vivo* and *in vitro* may be accepted in lieu of preclinical toxicity studies. Also, data demonstrating the absence of adventitious agents are critical for initiating phase I clinical trials in these instances.

For vaccines belonging to a category for which extensive clinical experience exists with similar products, it may be sufficient to cite clinical data from related products to support initiation of phase I clinical trials. Similarly, if the vaccine consists of a combination of either licensed and/or investigational vaccine antigens, data from preclinical toxicity studies and/or clinical data using the individual vaccine antigens may be sufficient to support initiation of phase I clinical trials.

■ Timing

CBER will determine, per 21 CFR 312.23(a)(8), whether or not a preclinical toxicity study is needed to support initiation of phase I clinical trials and provide the scientific rationale for the decision. As discussed earlier, the decision would usually be communicated to the sponsor during the pre-IND meeting if one occurs and if not, through other means, e.g., telephone discussions between the sponsor and CBER. If it is determined that a toxicity study is necessary to evaluate the safety of an investigational vaccine, the toxicity study will be conducted *prior* to initiating the phase I clinical trial. If a sponsor thinks a preclinical toxicity study is not needed or is not feasible, the branch chiefs in DVRPA in the Office of Vaccines Research and Review (CBER) should be contacted for their advice. A sponsor may be advised to provide supportive safety data or the scientific rationale for not performing a toxicity study (including supportive data) in the pre-IND meeting background package. In this case, CBER will advise the sponsor of their decision at the pre-IND meeting, or in some cases earlier.

In addition to toxicity assessments necessary to establish product safety prior to the initiation of clinical trials, it may be necessary to conduct additional nonclinical safety assessments in parallel with clinical product development (Figure 19.1). Examples where additional safety assessment may be necessary include changes in the manufacturing process or product formulation for a product already undergoing clinical investigation, changes in the route of administration, addition of novel

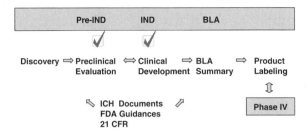

Figure 19.1 Vaccine development. When to perform toxicology studies.

or different adjuvants, evaluation of potential safety concerns that may have arisen from phase I and II clinical studies or that have been described in the literature for similar products, or to establish the no observed adverse effect level (NOAEL) and maximum tolerated doses (MTD). Special nonclinical safety studies may be needed to evaluate the product safety in specific target populations. For example, if the target population for a preventive vaccine product includes pregnant women, reproductive toxicity studies will be required prior to conducting phase I studies in pregnant women. If the target population for a preventive vaccine product includes females of child-bearing potential, reproductive toxicity studies to assess potential adverse effects on fetal developmental will be needed prior to submitting the BLA or these data will need to be included in the BLA.

■ Approaches to study design

Safety concerns for drug products in general include potential inherent toxicities of the product, potential toxicities of impurities and contaminants, and potential toxicities due to interactions of the components present in the final formulation. Vaccines act through a complex mechanism by which elements of the immune system are the effectors; thus, for vaccines, the immune response induced by the vaccine product may lead to undesired

toxic side effects in addition to the safety concerns listed above. Also, in contrast to most conventional drug products, vaccines are administered using episodic dosing over months or even years. Thus, given the complexity of these issues, toxicity testing programs applicable to conventional chemical drug products (i.e., small molecules) may not always be applicable to preventive vaccines, necessitating modifications of traditional toxicity study designs and/or the development of new approaches to toxicity testing for these products.

It is emphasized that no one study design fits all product categories, and thus, the nonclinical study design will need to be tailored to the particular vaccine product and will depend on the product features, specific safety concerns, and available test systems. Parameters to be considered in general in designing animal toxicology studies include choice of a relevant animal species/strain, product formulation, clinically intended dose and route of administration, timing and techniques of vaccine administration, timing of evaluation of endpoints, etc. When evaluating the safety profile of the antigen/adjuvant combination or the adjuvant alone, the exact formulation proposed for use in the clinic should be used. The toxicity study should be conducted with clinical lots of GMP material.

Some nonclinical laboratory studies, including pilot experiments such as dose-finding and "proof-of-concept" challenge studies, may not need to be in compliance with GLP regulations (21 CFR Part 58). However, pivotal toxicity studies should be conducted in compliance with GLP regulations. For each nonclinical laboratory study subject to GLP regulations under part 58, a statement documenting that the study was conducted in compliance with the GLP regulations under part 58 is necessary. If the study was not conducted in compliance with the GLP regulations under part 58, a brief statement of the reason for the non-compliance should be included (21 CFR 312.23(a)(8)(iii)).

■ Animal species

When deciding which animal model is appropriate for nonclinical safety assessment of the investigational vaccine product, it is helpful to choose an animal model for which good historical data exist. To the extent possible, the safety profile of the product should be characterized in an animal model able to develop an immune response to the vaccine. Thus, prior to conducting the definitive toxicity study, data regarding the immune response induced by the vaccine in animal model(s) are important. In some situations, it may be possible to minimize animal use by combining toxicity studies and certain immunogenicity evaluations. If the vaccine is formulated with adjuvant, it should be demonstrated that the proposed adjuvant enhances the immune response in the animal model chosen. Consideration should also be given to whether to use naive versus partially immune or immune animals for optimal safety assessment. In addition, it may be important to consider which animal model is most appropriate for the planned route of administration (e.g., intranasal administration).

There may be situations where, due to the species-specific nature of the vaccine or adjuvant (e.g., bacterial vectored vaccines, use of cytokines as adjuvants), a relevant animal model does not exist. In these situations, the use of homologous proteins, e.g., murine counterparts of a protein or agent, may need to be considered. In such situations, it may still be useful to perform a safety study in an animal model to assess the intrinsic toxicity of the antigen/adjuvant formulation and/or other components in the vaccine formulation (e.g., preservatives, stabilizers, etc.). In some instances, *in vitro* studies (with human cells) may be performed to fully characterize products. The rationale/need for preclinical toxicity studies in these situations should be discussed between the sponsor and CBER.

Currently, CBER proposes that the toxicity study conducted to support initiation of phase I clinical trials for a preventive vaccine can be performed in one rather than two relevant animal species. Rodents and rabbits are usually adequate; nonhuman primates usually are not necessary. However, there may be situations where two or more species may be necessary to characterize adequately the toxicity of a product, in particular when the biological activity of the product is not well understood. Examples would include the use of immuno-modulating adjuvants, such as cytokines, chemokines, or costimulatory signaling molecules and/or their ligands. For the chosen species, the number of animals studied per sex, group, and time interval should be sufficient to allow meaningful scientific interpretation of the data generated. The size of the treatment group will depend on the animal model chosen, i.e., the number of animals included in studies using nonhuman primates would be expected to be less than the number included in studies using rodents. For small animal models, e.g., mice and rats, it is recommended that approximately ten animals/sex/group/ time interval be used.

■ Route of administration, dose, and controls

The route of administration should correspond to that intended for use in the clinic. If toxic effects are observed in safety studies using a particular route of administration (e.g., intranasal), separate toxicity studies using a different route of administration (e.g., intravenous) may be helpful in understanding the full spectrum of toxicity of the product. When the vaccine is to be administered in the clinic using a particular device, the same device should be used in the animal study, where feasible. Ideally, the effects of low, intermediate, and high doses of the vaccine formulation should be evaluated in the animal model to identify potential dose–response relationships with respect to adverse effects. At a minimum, the highest human dose to be used in the proposed clinical trial (not scaled for body weight/ surface area) should be evaluated in the animal model, if feasible. If the volume of the highest human dose exceeds the maximum volume that can be administered (by a single injection) to a particular animal model, a dose that has been scaled for body weight (but exceeds the human dose on a mg/kg basis) may be used. Alternatively, it may be possible to administer the full human dose by dividing it among multiple sites using the same route of administration.

When a vaccine is to be administered more than one time in a clinical trial, the number of doses administered in the animal model should exceed by at least one the number of doses proposed in humans (i.e., for n doses to be given in the clinic, the toxicity study should include at least $n + 1$ doses). To better simulate the proposed clinical usage, repeat vaccine doses should be given as episodic doses, rather than daily doses. The dosing schedule may be compressed, but sufficient time (usually more than two weeks) should be allowed between repeat doses for the host immune response to develop.

The study design should include appropriate control groups to evaluate a baseline level of treatment with vehicle alone and adjuvant alone, for comparison to treatment with an active formulation. In addition, the study should include an additional treatment group to be sacrificed and evaluated as described below at later time points after treatment to evaluate reversibility of potential adverse effects.

■ Parameters monitored

Toxicity studies should address the potential for local inflammatory reactions, systemic toxicities, and immune-mediated toxicities. A broad spectrum of information should be obtained from the toxicity studies. The immune response in a group of treated animals should be evaluated to confirm that the anticipated immune response occurred in the toxicity study, and the quality of the immune response should be evaluated, if possible. In-life parameters to be monitored include daily clinical observations, weekly body weights, weekly feed consumption, weekly

physical examinations, ophthalmologic examinations, injection site observations, and limb use impairment. Serum chemistries including liver and renal function tests (e.g., ALT, AST, creatine kinase, and BUN) and hematologic analyses (CBC and differentials) should be evaluated. Data should be collected at specified intervals during treatment, at scheduled necropsies, and following recovery periods (e.g., one to three days and two weeks or more following the last dose administration) to evaluate the reversibility of any potential adverse effects. At study termination, final body weights (fasted), terminal blood collection and analysis, and a complete gross necropsy (including gross lesions and organ weights) and full tissue collection and preservation should be conducted. Injection site histopathology and histopathology on select tissues, including target organs, organs local to the route of administration, and immune organs, e.g., see tissues listed in the WHO guidelines on nonclinical evaluation of vaccines, should be conducted and data should be reported in full. Full toxicity study reports with well-organized tables should be provided. These should include narrative and tabular summary data, statistics, and data suitable for detailed review, consisting of line listings of individual animal data points for each animal organized by study group (including local reaction site scores, histopathology reports, ophthalmology reports, etc.).

Special considerations for adjuvanted vaccines

■ Additional safety assessment of the adjuvant alone

If an adjuvant is to be used in a vaccine, the benefit of adding the adjuvant should be demonstrated, e.g., by conducting preclinical immunogenicity studies in which the immune response obtained with the antigen/adjuvant combination is compared to that obtained with the antigen alone. If no preclinical toxicity data or clinical safety data exist for the adjuvant, the safety profile of the adjuvant will need to be characterized. In this case, toxicity studies of the type discussed above should be conducted with the adjuvant alone as well as with the antigen/adjuvant formulation. In addition, it may be helpful to evaluate whether the antigen/adjuvant combination exerts a synergistic adverse effect in the animal model compared to the individual components. Data from preclinical toxicity studies, in which the adjuvant was formulated with a vaccine antigen that differed from that proposed for the clinical study, provide supportive information, but may not be sufficient.

For certain adjuvants, additional safety studies as described in toxicity guidelines for chemical entities, biotechnology-derived pharmaceuticals, or pharmaceutical excipients may be applicable. For example, the safety of an adjuvant may need to be further assessed in additional repeat dose studies, safety pharmacology studies, pharmacokinetic or "depot" studies, genotoxicity studies, and/or carcinogenicity studies. Additional safety assessments may need to be considered when an IND for a particular adjuvanted vaccine progresses to phase III studies, or if the adjuvant will be a "platform" for multiple products.

■ Considerations for bacterial toxin adjuvants delivered intranasally

Results from preclinical and clinical studies, which raised certain concerns about the safety of bacterial toxin adjuvants delivered intranasally, were presented at a meeting entitled "Safety Evaluation of Toxin Adjuvants Delivered Intranasally," convened by NIAID on July 9, 2001 (www.niaid.nih.gov/dmid/enteric/intranasal.htm). Data derived from studies conducted in Balb/c mice indicated that toxins (cholera toxin (CT), *E. coli* heat-labile enterotoxin (LT), and attenuated point mutants derived from each) administered intranasally could transit the cribiform plate via olfactory nerve fibers to reach the olfactory bulb and nerves and cause inflammation in the olfactory region of the brain. However, data from other studies conducted in rabbits

or CD-1 mice did not replicate the finding described above, i.e., no inflammatory reactions in the olfactory bulbs were reported. It was proposed that the observed outcomes may have differed due to the animal strains and/or species used. However, in this context, it is of interest to note that clinical data regarding an inactivated intranasal influenza vaccine used in Switzerland, which contained LT as an adjuvant, indicated a higher than background rate of Bell's palsy cases in vaccine recipients. Additional analyses of the data indicated a strong association between the influenza vaccine used in Switzerland and risk of Bell's palsy in Switzerland (Mutsch et al., 2004; Couch, 2004). Of note is that this particular vaccine is no longer in clinical use.

In addition to the considerations for toxicity study designs outlined above for adjuvanted vaccines, meeting attendees recommended that safety studies for toxin adjuvants administered via the intranasal route may need to be conducted in two different mice strains, i.e., Balb/c and CD-1, and possibly one other species, such as the guinea pig or a species that is receptive to administration via nasal spray rather than droplets. It was noted that the anatomy and physiology of the nasal cavity determines the accessibility of the olfactory region and brain, e.g., differences among species in the nasal surface area as well as the complexity of the nasal cavities may require a dose adjustment based on weight or surface area of the nasal mucosa. Parameters to be monitored should include the potential passage of the toxin into the brain (histology), impact of the presence of the toxin in brain tissue (inflammation, etc.), and potential impact on neurological function.

■ Clinical assessment of adjuvanted preventive vaccines

The safety and immunogenicity of bacterial toxin adjuvants and toxin mutants in human subjects are frequently evaluated in the absence of vaccine antigen prior to evaluating the antigen/toxin adjuvant combination.

Although a placebo group is not required in a phase I study, inclusion of a placebo group may enhance interpretation of the initial safety data. The use of a saline placebo is favored over an adjuvant alone arm, if there is only to be one control group. However, to evaluate the safety of the adjuvant in the phase I study, the inclusion of a second control group with adjuvant alone may be useful. In advanced development (e.g., for a phase III efficacy trial, which will often provide the definitive safety data for the new vaccine), however, a saline placebo would be preferred. The immunologic benefit of the inclusion of an adjuvant in a vaccine should also be demonstrated clinically. Ideally, the comparison between the antigen alone and the antigen/adjuvant combination will be made early in clinical development where appropriate.

Conclusions

Strategies and approaches for the development and delivery of vaccine antigens have expanded over the last decade leading to a broad range of novel products. Moreover, the ability of adjuvants to increase the immunogenicity of these vaccine antigens holds great promise for improved preventive vaccines in the future. Nonclinical safety assessment of preventive vaccines is a critical component in vaccine development and has necessitated the development of national and international guidelines to address study designs and parameters relevant for the toxicity assessment of these products. However, better models and technologies are needed to optimize the safety evaluation of vaccines. For novel adjuvants in particular, a better understanding of their mechanism of action is critical. Methods and/or animal models need to be developed to address immunological aspects of adjuvant safety, including potential side effects such as hypersensitivity reactions, the generation of autoimmunity, and tolerance induction.

Global harmonization efforts are critical to developing improved and consistent standards for the nonclinical and clinical evaluation of vaccines formulated with adjuvants. Even though progress has been made in formulating regulatory policy and guidelines, approaches to safety assessment of preventive vaccines is still evolving. As increased scientific knowledge is gained, regulatory approaches may need to be optimized and refined to better assess the safety of preventive vaccines and to predict their toxicity.

Additional information

The recommendations provided in this chapter do not reflect official US FDA policy. As FDA guidance in this area is under development, the reader is encouraged to contact the Office of Vaccines Research and Review (OVRR) in the CBER at the FDA regarding preclinical safety testing requirements for particular vaccine candidates to support INDs. In addition, specific guidance on regulatory requirements for a particular product should be sought from the FDA.

Acknowledgments

The authors thank Richard McFarland, Karen Goldenthal, and Norman Baylor for their critical review of this work.

References

Alving, C.R. (2002). Design and selection of vaccine adjuvants: animal models and human trials, *Vaccine* 20, S6–S4.

Baylor, N.W., Egan, W., and Richman, P. (2002). Aluminum salts in vaccines: US perspective. *Vaccine* 20, S18–S23.

Chandler, D.K.F., McVittie, L.D., and Novak, J.M. (1999). In Paoletti, L.C. and McInnes, P.M. (Eds) *Vaccines from Concept to Clinic: A Guide to the Development and Clinical Testing of Vaccines for Human Use*, IND Submissions for Vaccines: Perspectives of IND Reviewers. CRC Press, Washington, DC, pp. 107–126.

Chang, P.Y., Sheets, R., Shapiro, S., Hargus, S., and Gruber, M. Vaccine pre-clinical toxicology testing (http://www.niaid.nih.gov/daids/vaccine/Science/VRTT/00_Main.htm).

Code of Federal Regulations (2004). Title 21. US Government Printing Office, Washington, DC (http://www.access.gpo.gov/cgi-bin/cfrassemble.cgi?title=200121).

Couch, R.B. (2004). Nasal vaccination, *Escherichia coli* enterotoxin, and Bell's palsy. *N. Engl. J. Med.* 350, 860–861.

CPMP document (1997). Note for Guidance on Preclinical Pharmacological and Toxicological Testing of Vaccines (http://www.emea.eu.int/pdfs/human/swp/046595en.pdf).

CPMP document (2005). Guideline on Adjuvants in Vaccines for Human Use (http://www.emea.eu.int/pdfs/human/vwp/13471604en.pdf).

Degen, W.G.J., Jansen, T., and Schijns, V.E.J.C. (2003). Vaccine adjuvant technology: from mechanistic concepts to practical applications. *Expert Rev. Vaccines* 2, 327–335.

Engers, H., Kieny, M.P., Malhotra, P., and Pink, R.J. (2003). Meeting report: third meeting on novel adjuvants currently in/close to human clinical testing, WHO, Foundation Merieux, Annecy, France, 7–9 January 2002. *Vaccine* 21, 3503–3524.

Finn, T.M. and Egan, W. (2004). In Plotkin, S.A. and Orenstein, W.A. (Eds) *Vaccines*, 4th edn. Elsevier New York, pp. 81–90.

Global Advisory Committee on Vaccine Safety, 10–11 June 2004. *Weekly Epidemiological Record* 29, 269–270.

Goldenthal, K.L., Cavagnaro, S.A., Alving, C.R., and Vogel, F.R. (1993). Safety evaluation of vaccine adjuvants: National Cooperative Vaccine Development Meeting Working Group. *AIDS Res. Hum. Retroviruses* 9 (Suppl. 1), S47–S51.

Guidance for Industry (1995). Content and format of investigational new drug applications (INDs) for phase 1 studies of drugs, including well-characterized, therapeutic, biotechnology-derived products (http://www.fda.gov/cber/gdlns/ind1.pdf).

Guidance for Industry (1997). Evaluation of combination vaccines for preventable diseases: production, testing and clinical studies (http://www.fda.gov/cber/gdlns/combvacc.txt).

Guidance for Industry (1999). Content and format of chemistry, manufacturing and controls information and establishment description information for a vaccine or related product (http://www.fda.gov/cber/gdlns/cmcvacc.pdf).

Guidance for Industry (2000). Considerations for reproductive toxicity studies for preventive vaccines for infectious disease indications, August (http://www.fda.gov/cber/gdlns/reprotox.pdf).

Guidance for Industry (2000). Formal meetings with sponsors and applicants for PDUFA products (http://www.fda.gov/cber/gdlns/mtpdufa.pdf).

Guidance for Industry (2005). Nonclinical studies for the safety evaluation of pharmaceutical excipients (http://www.fda.gov/cber/gdlns/dvpexcp.pdf).

Guidance for Industry (2005). Considerations for plasmid DNA vaccines for infectious disease indications (http://www.fda.gov/cber/gdlns/plasdnavac.pdf).

Guideline for Drug Master Files (1989). http://www.fda.gov/cder/guidance/dmf.htm.

Hunter, R.L. (2002). Overview of vaccine adjuvants: present and future. *Vaccine* 20, S7–S12.

ICH Guidance on Preclinical Safety Evaluation of Biotechnology-Derived Pharmaceuticals, S6 (1997) (http://www.ich.org).

ICH Guidance on Quality of Biotechnological/Biological Products: Derivation and Characterization of Cell Substrates Used for Production of Biotechnological/Biological Products, Q5D, 7/16/1997 (http://www.ich.org).

ICH Guidance on Viral Safety Evaluation of Biotechnology Products Derived From Cell Lines of Human or Animal Origin, Q5A 3/5/1997 (http://www.ich.org).

ICH Guidance on Non-Clinical Safety Studies for the Conduct of Human Clinical Trials for Pharmaceuticals, M3 (1997), M3(M), amended on November 9, 2000 (http://www.ich.org).

ICH Guidance on Safety Pharmacology Studies for Human Pharmaceuticals, S7A, July 13, 2001 (http://www.fda.gov/cber/gdlns/ichs7a071201.pdf).

Kenney, R.T. and Edelman, R. (2003). Survey of human-use adjuvants. *Expert Rev. Vaccines* 2, 167–188.

Kenney, R.T., Rabinovich, N.R., Pichyangkul, S., Price, V.L., and Engers, H.D. (2002). Meeting report: second meeting on novel adjuvants currently in/close to human clinical testing, WHO, Foundation Merieux, Annecy, France, 5–7 June 2000. *Vaccine* 20, 2155–2163.

Lien, E. and Golenbock, D.T. (2003). Adjuvants and their signaling pathways: beyond TLRs. *Nature Immunol.* 4, 1162–1164.

Lima, K.M., Aparecida dos Santos, S., Rodrigues, Jr., J.M., and Silva, C.L. (2004). Vaccine adjuvant: it makes the difference. *Vaccine* 22, 2374–2379.

Mutsch, M., Zhou, W., Rhodes, P., Matthias, B., Chen, R., Linder, T., Spyr, C., and Steffen, R. (2004). Use of the inactivated intranasal influenza vaccine and the risk of Bell's palsy in Switzerland. *N. Engl. J. Med.* 350, 896–903.

Petrovsky, N. and Aguilar, J.C. (2004). Vaccine adjuvants: current state and future trends. *Immunol. Cell Biol.* 82, 488–496.

Points to Consider in the Production and Testing of New Drugs and Biologicals Produced by Recombinant DNA Technology, draft April 10, 1985 (http://www.fda.gov/cber/gdlns/ptcdna.pdf).

Points to Consider in the Characterization of Cell Lines Used to Produce Biologicals, May 17, 1993 (http://www.fda.gov/cber/gdlns/ptccell.pdf).

Sesardic, D. and Dobbelaer, R. (2004). European Union regulatory developments for new vaccine adjuvants and delivery systems. *Vaccine* 22, 2452–2456.

Supplement to the Points to Consider in the Production and Testing of New Drugs and Biologicals Produced by Recombinant DNA Technology: Nucleic Acid Characterization and Genetic Stability, April 6, 1992 (http://www.fda.gov/cber/gdlns/ptcsupdna.pdf).

Verdier, F. (2002). Non-clinical vaccine safety assessment. *Toxicology* 174, 37–43.

Vogel, F.R. and Hem, S.L. (2004). In Plotkin, S.A. and Orenstein, W.A. (Eds) *Vaccines*, 4th edn. Elsevier New York, pp. 69–79.

Vogel, F.R. and Powell, M.F. (1995). In Powell, M.F. and Newman, M.J. (Eds) *A Compendium of Vaccine Adjuvants and Excipients*. Plenum Press, New York, pp. 141–228.

Vogel, F.R., Powell, M.F., and Alving, C.R. *A Compendium of Vaccine Adjuvants and Excipients*, 2nd edn. (http://www.niaid.nih.gov/daids/vaccine/pdf/compendium.pdf).

Weekly Epidemiological Record (July 2004). Global Advisory Committee on Vaccine Safety, 10–11 June 2004 (http://www.who.int/wer).

WHO (2003). Guidelines on Nonclinical Evaluation of Vaccines (http://www.who.int/biologicals/Nonclinical_evaluation_vaccines_Nov_2003.pdf).

Index